Blood and Marrow
Stem Cell Transplantation

The Jones and Bartlett Series in Oncology

Basic Steps in Planning Nursing Research, Third Edition, Brink/Wood

Biotherapy: A Comprehensive Overview, Rieger

Bone Marrow Transplantation: Administrative and Clinical Strategies, Buchsel/Whedon

Budgeting and Financial Management for Nurse Managers, Swansburg

Cancer Chemotherapy: A Nursing Process Approach, Second Edition, Barton Burke

Cancer and HIV Clinical Nutrition Pocket Guide, Wilkes

Cancer Nursing: Principles and Practice, Fourth Edition, Groenwald et al.

Cancer Pain Management, Second Edition, McGuire/Yarbro/Ferrell

A Cancer Source Book for Nurses, Seventh Edition, American Cancer Society

Cancer Symptom Management, Groenwald et al.

Cancer Symptom Management Patient Self-Care Guides, Groenwald et al.

Chemotherapy Care Plans: Designs for Nursing Care, Barton Burke et al.

Chemo Girl: Saving the World One Treatment at a Time, Richmond

Chronic Illness: Impact and Intervention, Third Edition, Lubkin

A Clinical Guide to Stem Cell and Bone Marrow Transplantation, Shapiro et al.

Comprehensive Cancer Nursing Review, Groenwald et al.

Comprehensive Perioperative Nursing Review, Fairchild et al.

Contemporary Issues in Breast Cancer, Hassey Dow

Desk Reference for Critical Care Nursing, Wright/Shelton

Fundamentals of Nursing Research, Brockopp/Hastings-Tolsma

Gynecologic Nurse Oncologists Women and Cancer: A Gynecologic Oncology Nursing Perspective, Moore

Handbook of Oncology Nursing, Second Edition, Gross/Johnson

Health Policy and Nursing: Crisis and Reform in the U.S. Health Care Delivery System, Second Edition, Harrington/Estes

Hospice and Palliative Care: Concepts and Practice, Sheehan/Forman

Intravenous Therapy, Nentwich

Introductory Management and Leadership for Clinical Nurses: A Text Workbook, Swansburg

Management and Leadership for Nurse Managers, Second Edition, Swansburg

Medical Instrumentation for Nurses and Allied Health-Care Professionals, Aston/Brown

Memory Bank for Chemotherapy, Third Edition, Preston/Wilfinger

Nursing Staff Development, Swansburg

Oncology Nursing in the Ambulatory Setting: Issues and Models of Care, Buchsel/Yarbro

Oncology Nursing Drug Reference, Second Edition, Wilkes et al.

Oncology Nursing Homecare Handbook, Barton Burke

Oncology Nursing Society's *Instruments for Clinical Health-Care Research, Second Edition,* Frank-Stromborg/Olsen

Oncology Nursing Society's *Suffering: A Communication Manual for Nurses,* Ferrell

Ready Reference for Critical Care, Second Edition, Strawn/Stewart

Risk Management in Health Care Institutions, Kavaler/Speigel

Blood and Marrow Stem Cell Transplantation

Principles, Practice, and Nursing Insights

SECOND EDITION

Edited by

Marie Bakitas Whedon, RN, MS, AOCN, FAAN

Oncology/Hematology Clinical Nurse Specialist
Norris Cotton Cancer Center
Dartmouth-Hitchcock Medical Center
Lebanon, New Hampshire

Debra Wujcik, RN, MSN, AOCN

Clinical Director
Vanderbilt Cancer Center
Nashville, Tennessee

Jones and Bartlett Publishers
Sudbury, Massachusetts
Boston   London   Singapore

Editorial, Sales, and Customer Service Offices

Jones and Bartlett Publishers
40 Tall Pine Drive
Sudbury, MA 01776
(508) 443-5000
(800) 832-0034
info@jbpub.com
http://www.jbpub.com

Jones and Bartlett Publishers International
Barb House, Barb Mews
London W6 7PA
UK

Library of Congress Cataloging-in-Publication Data

Blood and marrow stem cell transplantation : principles, practice, and
  nursing insights / [edited by] Marie Bakitas Whedon, Debra Wujcik — 2nd ed.
      p.   cm.
    Rev. ed. of: Bone marrow transplantation. c1991.
    Includes bibliographical references and index.
    ISBN 0-7637-0356-7
    1. Bone marrow—Transplantation. 2. Hematopoietic stem cells—
Transplantation. 3. Bone marrow—Transplantation—Nursing.
4. Hematopoietic stem cells—Transplantation—Nursing. I. Whedon,
Marie Bakitas. II. Wujcik, Debra. III. Blood marrow transplantation.
    [DNLM: 1. Bone Marrow Transplantation—nursing. 2. Bone Marrow
Transplantation—adverse effects. 3. Stem Cells—transplantation.
WH 380 B6545 1997]
RD123.5.B56 1997
617.4´4—dc21
DNLM/DLC
for Library of Congress   97-2860
                                                                        CIP

Production Editor: Marilyn E. Rash
Editorial Production Service: Joan M. Flaherty
Illustrations/Design: Katherine Harvey
Typesetting: Bookwrights
Cover Concept: Brian Russo
Cover Design: Hannus Design Associates
Printing and Binding: Courier Companies

Printed in the United States of America
01 00 99 98 97   10 9 8 7 6 5 4 3 2 1

To my husband, Jim, sons, Jimmy and Ryan, and in memory of my parents, Thomas and Helen Bakitas—my never-ending sources of love and support.

M.B.W.

To my husband, Dan, and daughters, Kristy and Kari, who support me in all of my professional activities and encourage me to pursue all of my dreams. I dedicate this book to my mother, Corabel Shiley, the nurse who inspired me the most.

D.W.

Contents

Foreword *xi*
Preface *xiii*
Contributors *xvii*

Part I **Basics of Transplantation** **1**

1 **Bone Marrow to Blood Stem Cells: Past, Present, Future** 3
   J. R. Wingard

2 **Hematopoiesis** 25
   D. Wujcik

3 **Transplant Immunology: HLA and Issues of Stem Cell Donation** 43
   J. Hegland

4 **Blood and Marrow Stem Cell Transplantation: Indications, Procedure, Process** 66
   S. A. O'Connell, K. Schmit-Pokorny

5 **Pharmacologic and Biologic Agents** 100
   S. P. Dix, G. C. Yee

6 **Radiation Therapy in Transplantation** 151
   R. A. Strohl

7 **Genetics and Gene Therapy** 162
   J. Jenkins

Part II **Acute Effects** **175**

8 **Graft-versus-Host Disease** 177
   K. A. Caudell

9   Hematologic Effects of Transplantation   205
     F. Walker, S. Burcat

10   Gastrointestinal Effects   220
     C. Engelking, D. M. Rust

11   Pulmonary and Cardiac Effects   266
     T. Wikle Shapiro

12   Renal and Hepatic Effects   298
     B. Ballard, K. J. Mitchell

13   Neurological Effects   326
     D. K. Meriney, P. Grimm

14   Psychosocial Effects: Pretransplant and
     Acute Treatment Phase   355
     S. Walch, T. A. Ahles

Part III   Issues of Recovery   375

15   Fertility and Sexuality Issues   377
     A. B. Moadel, J. S. Ostroff, L. M. Lesko

16   Quality of Life after Transplantation   400
     E. DeMeyer, M. B. Whedon, B. R. Ferrell

17   Patients' Perspectives   429
     S. Stewart

18   Family Issues and Perspectives of Transplantation   442
     J. G. Eilers

Part IV   The Care Environment   457

19   The Bone Marrow and Blood Stem Cell Marketplace   459
     M. K. Bedell, W. T. Mroz

20   Transplant Networks and Standards of Care:
     International Perspectives   474
     S. A. Ezzone, M. Fliedner

21   Nursing Research in Blood Cell and
     Marrow Transplantation   497
     M. Haberman

22   Ethical Issues of Transplantation   506
     P. Plunkett

23   Models of Ambulatory Care for Blood Cell and
     Bone Marrow Transplantation   525
     P. C. Buchsel, P. M. Kapustay

     Index   563

Foreword

The few short years since the first edition of this book have been marked by an almost exponential increase in the number of patients receiving marrow transplants, in the number of institutions doing marrow transplants, and in the number of scientific publications about marrow transplantation and related fields. Clearly, it is time for the second edition.

A major change in the field has been the development of techniques for stem cell separation. The recognition that stem cells express the CD34 antigen and the development of appropriate monoclonal antibodies have made it possible to separate stem cells from the marrow and to achieve marrow grafts with small numbers of these cells. The technique is used to separate marrow cells from unwanted cells, T cells, and malignant cells.

Perhaps the most significant change has been in the development of sources of stem cells other than marrow. The number of stem cells in the circulating blood can be increased by chemotherapy and/or by the administration of hematopoietic growth factors (GM-CSF or G-CSF), and these cells can be collected by advanced centrifuge technology. The advantages of peripheral blood stem cells are that the donor does not have to receive a general anesthetic and collections can be repeated. Peripheral blood cells are now replacing the use of marrow in most transplants. The discovery that cord blood is rich in stem cells has led to their use for selected marrow transplants.

The third major change has been in the increasing use of marrow grafts from unrelated donors. Only about one fourth of transplant recipients have a matched sibling donor. The National Marrow Donor Program has recruited 1.8 million volunteers who have agreed to be marrow donors. Collaboration with other national centers for marrow donors has established a pool of approximately 3 million potential donors. At present, an unrelated donor can be found for about one half of the Caucasian candidates for transplants. Recruitment of donors from other ethnic populations is under way.

The final major change has been in the use of autologous marrow grafts or autologous peripheral blood stem cell grafts. The patient's own stem cells can be collected from marrow or peripheral blood, processed to remove malignant cells if present, and given back to the patient after intensive chemo-irradiation therapy. Autologous grafts are being used increasingly to treat hematological diseases and solid tumors. Most notable is the use of autologous grafts in patients with breast cancer. Increased numbers of complete remissions are being described in patients with metastatic disease. An increased number of long-term freedom from recurrence and possible cure is being seen in patients with nodes positive for tumor at the time of surgery. Several different antitumor preparative regimens are being studied. Long-term follow-up will be needed for definitive evaluation.

There are many other developments in the field of stem cell transplantation. One thing that has not changed, however, is the need for skilled care of the patient. Skilled care implies the best of medical and nursing care before, during, and after the transplant. It also includes emotional and psychological support for the patient and family. The nurse plays the central role in skilled care. The challenge for the nurse is to play that role while keeping up with and participating in the rapid developments in the field.

E. Donnall Thomas, MD
Professor of Medicine Emeritus
University of Washington School of Medicine
Member, Fred Hutchinson Cancer Research Center
1990 Nobel Laureate, Medicine/Physiology

Preface

Although it seems like only yesterday, six years have passed since the first edition of this book was written. The pace of change in the field of transplantation since that time has been unimaginable. This has resulted in a complete overhaul of the organization and content of this second edition, a new title, and the addition of an editor. I am pleased to have Debra Wujcik join me in developing this edition of *Blood and Marrow Stem Cell Transplantation: Principles, Practice, and Nursing Insights.* The expanded new title reflects the most current developments in transplantation including incredible changes in even the foundational concepts of transplant nursing—a shift from the traditional use of bone marrow to the growing use of blood stem cells for transplantation.

When faced with so much change it is stabilizing to take a moment to reflect: When we entered the field of oncology nursing more than twenty years ago, bone marrow transplantation was an investigational therapy being performed in a few select centers. Patients had to leave even academic university hospitals and travel long distances for a treatment that was the last hope to control a deadly disease. Most of the patients we knew personally did not survive the process. Central venous catheters were not available, HLA typing was in its infancy, the supportive care armamentarium was minimal, and the literature describing these procedures was limited to what was happening in the laboratory or single patient reports. Years later, we entered the world of bone marrow transplantation to find how far this subspecialty had developed.

Bone marrow transplantation is now a standard treatment for certain leukemias and lymphomas and has shown promise for treating other cancers like multiple myeloma and breast cancer. Its application to the cure of previously incurable diseases with solid tumors now surpasses its original application to childhood immunodeficiencies and leukemias. International registries and umbilical cord blood have increased the pool of available donors and increased the number of allogeneic bone marrow transplants performed. Technologic developments now allow successful engraftment using either stem cells harvested from the bone marrow or progenitor cells from the peripheral circulation. Triple lumen venous access devices are commonplace to administer multiple infusions of antibiotics, blood components, total parenteral nutrition, and growth factors. They have reduced treatment-related mortality to an insignificant percentage.

Research in bone marrow transplantation extends beyond technologic advancements. Nurses have taken a leading role in important areas of transplant research including testing the efficacy of care procedures (e.g., oral care, catheter care), quality of life, and survivorship issues. The special needs of patients and families are well documented. Clinicians continue to develop strategies to prevent and treat the long-term sequelae of transplant such as graft-versus-host disease.

The challenge of the 1990s has been to reduce costs of transplant while pushing forward the development of new drugs and processes, and their applications to new diseases. The care of patients has again shifted, this time from specialized academic inpatient units to community outpatient clinics and to the home. Now many family members must not only provide the emotional support through this difficult treatment, but also function as surrogate nurses in the home or outpatient residences. The traditional team has been extended to include family members in more active roles as outpatient and home care providers.

This second edition reflects the many changes in transplantation. Part I, Basics of Transplantation, contains updated chapters on history, processes of transplantation, and immunology, in addition to new chapters on hematologic concepts, pharmacologic and biologic agents, radiation therapy, and gene therapy. Major advances in HLA technology and our understanding of immunology at the molecular level have caused a major reorganization of the material in this chapter. Material on the procedural aspects of transplantation has been added to reflect the fact that the use of peripherally derived stem cells has caused clinicians to shift their practices in carrying out the procedure. The chapters addressing the procedural aspects of autologous and allogeneic transplantation are now combined with material on the use of peripherally derived blood stem cells.

Part II still focuses on acute effects after transplantation, however each chapter has been totally revised to reflect recent changes and developments in the occurrence and management of these symptoms. Part III addresses issues of recovery, including a totally revised and updated compilation of material on the important issues of fertility and sexuality. Survivorship issues have been expanded and are now viewed from a quality-of-life perspective. Additionally, the important aspect of the role of family during and following transplant has resulted in a new chapter in this part. New patients' stories have been compiled by former BMT patient Susan Stewart.

Finally, Part IV addresses important issues in the transplant care environment. The chapter on economic issues has been expanded to include information on the ever-changing environment of health-care financing and focus on "marketplace." Clinicians who are new to transplant will appreciate a one-stop primer in the new chapter on transplant networks and standards. This chapter gives a comprehensive overview of how the field is organized in terms of resources, professional networks, and standards of care. A chapter detailing where nurses have been and where we are going in furthering science through research adds to the total view of transplant science. A revised chapter on ethical issues matches the new challenges patients face with changes in transplant technology. The final chapter provides an overview of caring for patients who are now treated primarily in the outpatient arena. Care plans have been replaced with clinical paths; therefore, the Nursing Care Plans appendix no longer appears. A list of centers is no longer included because the economic environment, and competition, makes the identification of centers a moving target.

Nurses new to the specialty can use *Blood and Marrow Stem Cell Transplantation: Principles, Practice, and Nursing Insights* as a core curriculum for developing clinical expertise in transplantation. Experienced transplant nurses will find this a valuable volume to help them incorporate current research findings into their practice. Transplant specialty clinicians from other disciplines also will find many useful chapters to enhance their clinical knowledge. In addition, this book will serve as a useful reference to nurses in all care settings as the care of bone marrow and blood cell transplant moves into the next century.

Acknowledgments

With any major work there are ups and downs, but the projects that get completed successfully are those that have a strong team. We are grateful to many people who assisted us through the development and production of this book. In the interest of time and space we can only recognize and thank a few of them: Joan Flaherty, our production editor, for always having a sense of humor, even under the tightest of deadlines; Marilyn Rash from Jones and Bartlett for guidance and answers to impossible questions; Carolyn Vardell (Vanderbilt) for her help in manuscript editing; Beverly Cavanaugh (DHMC) for secretarial support and encouragement; the staff of the Matthews-Fuller Health Sciences Library (DHMC) for immediate responses to every reference question; and, of course, our many contributors, a very professional team, who were always timely when we needed action. This was a blessing.

We also wish to thank people who have contributed indirectly and in unique ways: Margaret Barton Burke who is always available for personal and professional advice and support; Brian Russo for his creative cover design idea under deadline; Colleen Haley for her freshness and inspiration as a new pediatric nurse, which energized me (M.B.W.) when I grew weary; and Tom and Cindy Bakitas whose pride about this book was a source of motivation when motivation was hard to find.

Contributors

Tim A. Ahles, PhD
Program Director
Center for Psychooncology Research
Department of Psychiatry
Dartmouth-Hitchcock Medical Center
Lebanon, New Hampshire

Bruce Ballard, RN, BSN
Center Coordinator
IMPACT Center of St. Paul
Response Oncology, Inc.
St. Paul, Minnesota

Marilyn K. Bedell, RN, MSN, OCN
Director
Medical and Oncology Services
Norris Cotton Cancer Center
Dartmouth-Hitchcock Medical Center
Lebanon, New Hampshire

Patricia Corcoran Buchsel, RN, MSN
Senior Research Associate
University of Washington
School of Nursing
Seattle, Washington

Shelley Burcat, RN, MSN
Clinical Nurse Specialist
Bone Marrow Transplant Unit
Thomas Jefferson University Hospital
Philadelphia, Pennsylvania

Kathryn Ann Caudell, PhD, RN
Assistant Professor
University of New Mexico
College of Nursing
Albuquerque, New Mexico

Elaine DeMeyer, RN, MSN, OCN
*Bone Marrow Transplant Clinical Nurse
  Specialist*
Baylor University Medical Center
Dallas, Texas

Suzanne P. Dix, PharmD
BMT Clinical Specialist
Oncology and Hematology Associates of
  Kansas City
Kansas City, Missouri

June G. Eilers, PhD, RN, CS
*Oncology/Hematology Clinical Nurse
  Specialist*
Clinical Nurse Researcher
University of Nebraska Medical Center
Omaha, Nebraska

Constance Engelking, RN, MS, OCN
Executive Director
Zalmen A. Arlin Cancer Institute
Westchester County Medical Center
Valhalla, New York

Susan A. Ezzone, RN, MS, ANP
BMT Clinical Nurse Specialist
Ohio State University Medical Center
Arthur G. James Cancer Hospital
 and Research Institute
Columbus, Ohio

Betty R. Ferrell, PhD, FAAN
Associate Research Scientist
City of Hope National Medical Center
Duarte, California

Monica C. Fliedner, RN, MSN
Hematology/BMT Clinical Nurse Specialist
University Hospital Utrecht
Utrecht, The Netherlands

Patricia Grimm, PhD, RN, CS
American Cancer Society Professor of
 Oncology Nursing
Assistant Professor
Johns Hopkins University School of Nursing
Psychiatric Consultation Liaison Nurse–BMT
Johns Hopkins Oncology Center
Baltimore, Maryland

Mel Haberman, PhD, RN, FAAN
Director of Research
Oncology Nursing Society
Pittsburgh, Pennsylvania
Assistant Staff Scientist
Fred Hutchinson Cancer Research Center
Seattle, Washington

Janet Hegland, BS, MT
Director of Research and Scientific Services
National Marrow Donor Program
Minneapolis, Minnesota

Jean Jenkins, MSN, RN
Clinical Nurse Specialist/Consultant
National Institutes of Health
National Center for Human Genome Research
Bethesda, Maryland

Pamela M. Kapustay, RN, MN
Nursing Director
The Westlake Comprehensive Cancer
 Center
 A Salick Health Care Affiliate
Westlake Village, California

Lynna M. Lesko, MD, PhD
Associate Director
Clinical Research
General Medicine Division
Boehringer Ingelheim Corporation
Ridgefield, Connecticut

Deborah K. Meriney, RN, MN, OCN
Instructor
University of Pittsburgh School of Nursing
Pittsburgh, Pennsylvania

Karin Mitchell, RN, BSN, CCRN
Critical Care Education Specialist
Fred Hutchinson Cancer Research
 Center
Seattle, Washington

Alyson B. Moadel, PhD
Post Doctoral Psychooncology Fellow
Psychiatry Service
Memorial Sloan-Kettering Cancer
 Center
New York, New York

William Mroz, BSN, MBA
Administrator
Transplant Programs
Dartmouth-Hitchcock Medical Center
Lebanon, New Hampshire

Susan A. O'Connell, MSN, RN, OCN
Clinical Nurse Specialist/BMT
The University of Michigan Medical
 Center
Ann Arbor, Michigan

Jamie S. Ostroff, PhD
Assistant Attending Psychologist
Psychiatry Service
Memorial Sloan-Kettering Cancer Center
New York, New York

Deborah M. Rust, RN, MSN, CRNP, OCN
Program Manager
Oncology Nurse Practitioner Program
University of Pittsburgh School of Nursing

Nurse Practitioner
BMT Program
University of Pittsburgh Cancer Institute
Pittsburgh, Pennsylvania

Kim Schmit-Pokorny, RN, MSN, OCN
Manager/Coordinator
Bone Marrow/Peripheral Stem Cell
 Transplantation Program
Department of Internal Medicine
University of Nebraska Medical Center
Omaha, Nebraska

Terry Wikle Shapiro, RN, MSN, CFNP
Adult and Pediatric Nurse Practitioner
Bone Marrow Transplant Program
University of Arizona Health Sciences
 Center
Tucson, Arizona

Peggy Plunkett, MSN, ARNP, CS
*Psychiatric Liaison Clinical Nurse
 Specialist*
Norris Cotton Cancer Center
Dartmouth-Hitchcock Medical Center
Lebanon, New Hampshire

Susan Stewart
Editor
BMT Newsletter
Highland Park, Illinois

Roberta Strohl, RN, MN, OCN
Clinical Nurse Specialist
Department of Radiation Oncology
University of Maryland
Baltimore, Maryland

Susan E. Walch, PhD
Research Associate
Center for Psychooncology Research
Department of Psychiatry
Dartmouth-Hitchcock Medical Center
Lebanon, New Hampshire

Frances Walker, RN, MSN, AOCN
Nursing Care Coordinator, BMT
Thomas Jefferson University Hospital
Philadelphia, Pennsylvania

John R. Wingard, MD
Professor of Medicine
Director
Bone Marrow Transplant Program
University of Florida Health Science Center
Gainesville, Florida

Gary C. Yee, PharmD, FCCP
Associate Professor
Department of Pharmacy Practice
College of Pharmacy
University of Florida Health Science Center
Gainesville, Florida

PART I
Basics of Transplantation

1

Bone Marrow to Blood Stem Cells
Past, Present, Future

John R. Wingard

The mythical figure of the chimera has often been used to symbolize the field of bone marrow transplantation (BMT). The chimera was a fire-spouting monster with a lion's head, a goat's body, and a serpent's tail. This creature was feared because it killed many animals and people. The monster was eventually killed with the consent of the gods, with the hope that the earth would be freed of this scourge.

In the field of BMT, the term *chimera* was first used by Ford and colleagues in 1956 to describe animals lethally irradiated and then given bone marrow from another animal: this maneuver resulted in the recipient's carrying a foreign hematopoietic system derived from the other animal. It is somewhat ironic that this creature, which originally evoked fear and revulsion and represented a cruel perversion of nature, now symbolizes a medical therapy offered with hope and concern and represents one of modern medicine's successful attempts to correct a number of nature's ailments afflicting human beings.

EVOLUTION OF BMT AS A TREATMENT OF HUMAN DISEASE

Human bone marrow administration as a treatment for disease has been attempted sporadi-

cally since the late 19th century. Many of the early applications involved feeding or injecting bone marrow or spleen extracts into patients who had a variety of ailments, such as several kinds of anemia, including the "anemia of rapid growth, overwork and underfeeding," leukemia, and chlorosis (Quine, 1896). Sometimes, arsenic and iron were given adjunctively. While some benefits were ascribed to the bone marrow treatments, the reason for improvement was unclear, and these efforts now seem quaint and unscientific.

In the modern era, human bone marrow transplantation began in 1957 when French and Yugoslav physicians treated several laboratory workers who had been exposed to radiation during the Vinca nuclear reactor accident (Mathe et al., 1959). One patient received fetal spleen and liver cells but died from hemorrhage. Four patients were given allogeneic bone marrow cells and all recovered marrow function. However, although there was some evidence of temporary engraftment, whether the bone marrow transplant conveyed any lasting benefit was uncertain (van Bekkum and de Vries, 1967).

Almost three decades later, in 1986, at Chernobyl a nuclear reactor accident of significantly larger proportions in Russia hospitalized hundreds of individuals and led to the employment of marrow transplants once again to attempt to reverse the hematologic toxicity from accidental exposure to radiation (Baranov et al., 1989). Of the 33 persons estimated to have received more than 600 cGy, half had severe nonhematologic toxicity (mainly burns), which made survival unlikely. Thirteen received marrow transplants and one was given fetal liver because no histocompatible donor was available. Of the marrow transplants, ten were from siblings (five HLA-identical, the remainder one-haplotype identical). Although transient hematologic recovery occurred in most patients, there were only two long-term survivors. Most of the deaths were due to burns and other nonhematologic radiation injury. Thus, even three decades later, despite a wealth of new knowledge and advances in supportive care, we are reminded of the limitations of BMT and other treatment modalities used to deal with radiation accidents—the mortality related to the nonhematologic toxic effects of radiation, such as burns, gastrointestinal, pulmonary, or central nervous system injuries, are not affected. However, although BMT has not proved a useful tool for treating the devastating effects of accidental irradiation, enormous utility has been found in a variety of medical applications.

During the early years of human BMT, attention was directed to determining the optimal source of bone marrow cells and methods of preserving the cells, achieving safe techniques for administering marrow intravenously to avoid pulmonary emboli, estimating the number of cells needed, and defining the types of illnesses to which BMT could be applied (Thomas et al., 1957; Thomas and Storb, 1970).

In 1970 a review of the reported human bone marrow transplant experience indicated that approximately 200 transplants had been performed during the preceding decade (see Table 1.1) (Bortin, 1970). The early results did not auger well. More than half of the patients had failed to engraft; three fourths had died before being reported in the literature. There was evidence of chimerism in only a few of the cases in which there were markers of donor cells and only three chimeric patients were alive at the time of reporting. Of the patients with aplastic anemia treated by allogeneic marrow none engrafted, but five of seven patients given syngeneic marrow transplants recovered.

Because of this very disappointing early experience, the number of marrow transplants performed during the early 1960s declined (see

TABLE 1.1   Results of 203 reported human bone marrow transplants

Disease	Number of patients	Number with no engraftment	Number with secondary disease	Number of allogeneic diseases
Aplastic anemia	73	66	5	0
Leukemia	84	33	32	3
Malignant disease	31	23	1	1
Immune deficiency	15	3	11	7
Total	203	125	49	11*

*Three alive at the time of this report.

SOURCE: M.M. Bortin, A compendium of reported human bone marrow transplants, *Transplantation* 9(6):571–587, © Williams & Wilkins, 1970. Reprinted with permission.

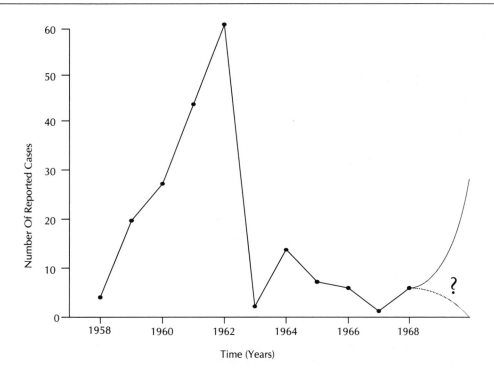

Figure 1.1 Reported human bone marrow transplants

SOURCE: M.M. Bortin, A compendium of reported human bone marrow transplants, *Transplantation* 9(6):571-587, © Williams & Wilkins, 1970. Used with permission.

Figure 1.1). Improvements in the results of BMT awaited developments in several ancillary fields: supportive care (especially transfusion support and antibiotics), histocompatibility testing, conditioning regimens, and control of graft-versus-host disease (GVHD).

As a result of the advances in these related fields, a resurgence of interest in bone marrow transplantation took place in the late 1960s. At this time human tissue typing permitted intentionally matched marrow transplants, which were applied to the treatment of genetic immunodeficiency syndromes. These disorders are rare but have provided important biologic insights.

The wider application of BMT in the 1970s occurred initially in the therapy of severe aplastic anemia or acute leukemia, for which other treatment had failed. Improved results were reported in 1975 (Thomas et al., 1975) (see Figure 1.2). As supportive care of patients improved and more effective conditioning regimens were applied, 6-month survival rates increased from less than 20% to greater than 70%.

Since then, steady increases in interest have paralleled improved long-term outcomes and

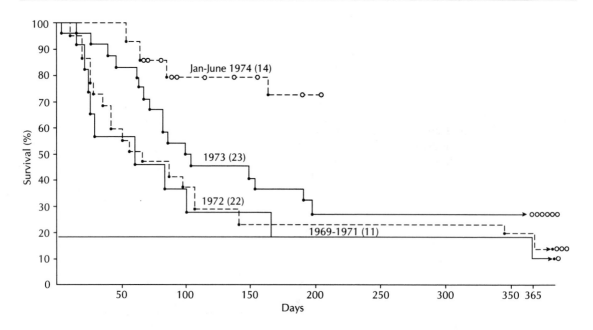

Figure 1.2 Survival curves in 70 patients with acute leukemia given a marrow graft from a major-histocompatibility-complex-matched sibling

NOTE: Open circles indicate living patients.
SOURCE: Reprinted by permission of the *New England Journal of Medicine* 292:841, 1975.

wider applications. By 1986 more than 200 bone marrow transplant centers (60% established since 1980) were performing almost 5000 transplants annually (Bortin et al., 1988) (see Figure 1.3). Expansion of transplant activity has continued unabated (Sobocinski et al., 1994).

An important advance that has evolved slowly is the refinement of criteria for performing BMT. It has become recognized that certain factors (both related and unrelated to the disease to be treated by BMT) must be considered in selecting patients. Examples of factors unrelated to the disease to be treated that increase

the risk of performing a BMT include advanced age of the patient, significantly impaired ventilatory function, abnormal hepatic function, and the presence of an active infection.

The status of the disease to be treated by BMT is an important determinant of the outcome for the patient. When BMT was performed in patients with acute leukemia in full relapse, long-term disease-free survival rates of approximately 15% were seen. In contrast, when BMT was done in patients in chemotherapy-induced remission, the mortality rate fell dramatically, due to both a lower relapse rate and a decreased rate of transplant-associated mortality. Similarly, the earlier in the course of the disease the transplant is performed the better: the risk of relapse is lower and the likelihood of toxicity from the conditioning regimen is less than if the transplant is performed after multiple relapses or multiple courses of therapy.

By adopting patient selection criteria one can minimize the risk of failure from toxicity. By performing the transplant at the appropriate time in the course of an individual's disease one can optimize the likelihood of control of the underlying disease.

During the 1980s, the capability to cryopreserve hematopoietic progenitor cells was developed, initially using glycerol as a cryopreservative, but subsequently dimethylsulfoxide (DMSO) (Barnes and Loutit, 1955). Numerous animal models demonstrated that cryopreserved marrow could reconstitute hematopoiesis following lethal irradiation. The first attempts in humans in the late 1950s to exploit this in autologous BMT (ABMT) were disappointing (Kurnick et al., 1958). However, a number of clinical trials conducted since 1975 have been more promising. Because of potential contamination by tumor cells, especially for lymphohematopoietic malignancies, attempts to define effective purging methods have been made. The role for ex vivo purging using either pharmacologic or antibody-mediated means remains uncertain because of the absence of controlled trials.

During the last decade, the frequency of autologous transplantation has increased tremendously (Applebaum, 1996). The use of autologous peripheral blood progenitor cells during the early 1980s demonstrated the capacity for hematologic reconstitution (Goldman et al., 1980; Juttner et al., 1985). Hematopoietic growth factors or the combination of cytotoxic agents plus growth factors can increase the number of hematopoietic progenitor cells in the circulating blood and permit collection by apheresis of "enriched" progenitor cells capable

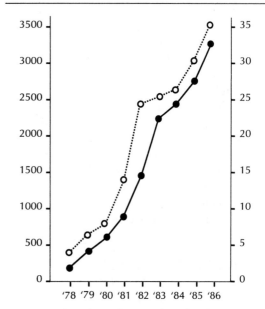

● ● Number of patients transplanted per year
○····○ Number of new transplant teams formed per year

Figure 1.3   Annual number of patients receiving allogeneic bone marrow transplants and annual number of new transplant teams formed

SOURCE: M.M. Bortin, Current status of BMT in humans: report from the International Bone Marrow Transplant Registry. *Nat Immun Cell Growth Regul* 7:339, © S. Karger A.G., Basel. Used with permission.

of speedy engraftment. Not only has autologous BMT become more common than allogeneic BMT but peripheral blood is now more commonly used than marrow as a source of progenitor cells to effect engraftment following marrow-lethal cytoreductive therapies.

Autologous BMT was initially a treatment modality mostly for lymphopoietic malignancies as salvage treatment. During the last 5 years, however, the use of autologous BMT has expanded to new applications in the therapy of solid tumors such as neuroblastoma, breast cancer, testicular cancer, and ovarian cancer. In recent years, the use of ABMT for breast cancer has surpassed the use of ABMT for lymphoma (Antman et al., 1994).

The majority of patients who could benefit from an allogeneic BMT do not have suitably matched family members to serve as donors. The development of the National Bone Marrow Transplant Donor Registry in the United States in 1986 and similar donor registries in other countries throughout the world have made it possible for patients without family donors who would otherwise not be candidates for BMT, to undergo this treatment.

CONDITIONING REGIMENS

Some form of conditioning is necessary for BMT candidates, except in certain rare situations in which a monozygotic twin is the donor or in which the recipient has a certain form of immunodeficiency and the donor is HLA identical. From animal experiments, it was learned early on that there are several prerequisites for a conditioning regimen (Santos, 1974). The conditioning regimen must first suppress the recipient's immunity to prevent graft rejection. Second, it must create "space" for the donor marrow: not physical space, but rather an effect (still poorly understood) on the marrow microenvironment that permits the establishment and growth of hematopoietic progenitors. A third requirement for patients to receive transplants for malignant disease is an antitumor effect, to eradicate residual tumor cells.

Total body irradiation (TBI), cyclophosphamide, or a combination of the two, were the first conditioning regimens. Both agents possess all three properties desirable in conditioning agents.

Experiments in mammals (reviewed by van Bekkum and de Vries, 1967) had demonstrated three types of syndromes after exposure to irradiation. Animals exposed to lethal TBI up to 1200 cGy die 8 to 14 days later from the effects of marrow aplasia (the so-called hematopoietic syndrome). Mice given 1200 cGy to 12,000 cGy die 4 to 5 days later due to the sequelae from gut damage (the gastrointestinal syndrome). Animals subjected to more than 12,000 cGy die within hours or 1 to 2 days after exposure due to toxicity to the central nervous system (the cerebral syndrome). Infusions of syngeneic bone marrow will reverse the hematopoietic syndrome, but have no effect on the other two syndromes. In animals subjected to less than lethal irradiation, the frequency and persistence of engraftment after marrow transplant was found to be related to the TBI dose. In general, supralethal TBI doses were necessary for long-lasting chimerism.

Aside from the extensive experience with TBI in animals, there were several other reasons TBI was a good choice as a preparative regimen. Irradiation was known to be effective in killing leukemic cells. It was able to bypass supposed sanctuary sites, such as the testes and central nervous system, to eliminate any occult contaminating tumor cells. One of its major organ toxicities, bone marrow, is not a concern when it is to be replaced by donor marrow. Initially, TBI doses of 800 cGy to 1000 cGy were given at a rate of 3 cGy to 6 cGy/min as a single dose. This was successful in achieving engraftment, but was not very effective in eradicating leukemia.

Experience with cyclophosphamide in animals (Santos et al., 1970) similarly led to its use in humans. The combination of cyclophosphamide and total body irradiation (CyTBI) was introduced very early, and since has become the most common conditioning regimen in the treatment of malignant disease (Thomas et al., 1977). During the 1970s it was recognized that the risk for another major nonhematologic toxicity, interstitial pneumonitis, could be reduced by fractionation of the TBI, rather than administration in a single dose (Meyers et al., 1983). Another regimen, busulfan plus cyclophosphamide (BuCy), was developed as an alternative preparative regimen to CyTBI. Busulfan has very little immunosuppressive potency, but has excellent antitumor and space-making properties. The combination regimen of BuCy has been shown to be at least as effective as CyTBI in the treatment of acute nonlympho-cytic leukemia (ANLL) (Santos et al., 1983). In recent years it has also been found to be effective as a conditioning regimen for chronic myelogenous leukemia (CML), Hodgkin's disease, non-Hodgkin's lymphoma, and beta-thalassemia.

Other agents have also been introduced into preparative regimens to try to improve the antitumor efficacy. One agent used increasingly is etoposide (VP 16), which has excellent antitumor activity, as well as some immuno-suppressive activity although not as much as cyclophosphamide (Gassman et al., 1988). Caution must be exercised in allogeneic transplantation to avoid agents with little or no immunosuppressive properties, especially in situations where there is an increased risk of graft rejection such as with a nonsibling donor, a mismatched donor, or a marrow graft manipulated ex vivo to remove T lymphocytes. In recent years, the addition of antithymocyte globulin or thiotepa to the preparative regimen has been explored to reduce the risk of graft rejection in high-risk transplants.

With autologous BMT, there is no such concern for graft rejection or the need for immunosuppression, and thus a panoply of preparative regimens have been and continue to be explored. The major objective is to develop combinations of drugs and/or radiotherapy with additive or synergistic antitumor activity and toxicities that do not overlap or are minimal nonhematologic toxicities.

With respect to severe aplastic anemia there is no necessity for antitumor activity, but the risk of graft rejection is substantive, and immunosuppression of the host is the paramount consideration in choosing a conditioning regimen. Of the first 66 patients transplanted with allogeneic marrow for aplastic anemia, none benefitted, and none demonstrated chimerism (Bortin, 1970). This was due in large measure to the fact that none received vigorous immunosuppressive pretreatment. Santos developed the use of high-dose cyclophosphamide alone as a conditioning regimen for patients with aplastic anemia (Santos, 1974). This continues to be the most common preparative regimen for allogeneic BMT for aplastic anemia. For patients who have been sensitized to the donor through blood transfusions or prior pregnancy (by exposure to fetal alloantigens), one of the major difficulties to overcome was graft rejection. It was learned that by increasing the immunosuppression in the conditioning regimen rejection could be reduced. Initially this was done by adding TBI to cyclophosphamide; the rejection rate decreased, however, there was no increase in survival due to the sequelae of the irradiation toxicity. Subsequently, the use of cyclosporin or total lymphoid irradiation has provided better immunosuppression without the added mortality from toxicity.

DEVELOPMENTS IN TISSUE TYPING

Dausset (1954, 1958) first presented evidence of leukoantigens in patients receiving multiple transfusions. Initially thought to be autoantibodies, they were later shown to be alloantibodies to antigens expressed on the leukocytes. Family studies showed the leukocyte antigens to be genetically determined. These antigens are the gene products of the HLA (or major histocompatibility) complex, which is a series of genes located on human chromosome 6. Although initially thought to be leukocyte specific, the HLA antigens subsequently were found to be broadly distributed tissue antigens. The HLA system plays a critical role in the cellular interactions that occur as part of immune reactions to viruses and other foreign antigens in that T lymphocytes only recognize foreign antigens when they are physically associated with HLA gene products. HLA gene products have been recognized as important determinants of allograft rejection.

In 1964 Terasaki and McClelland introduced the microlymphocytotoxicity assay, which continues to be the major procedure to perform HLA typing. During the 1960s two serologically defined loci (the A and B loci) were identified, and in 1970 the C locus was defined. These now are grouped as class I loci. The D region was initially assessed by the mixed lymphocyte reaction. It has subsequently been learned that there are several loci within the region, some of which can be defined serologically (such as DR and DQ). The D loci are grouped as class II loci.

The dismal results of the initial human bone marrow transplantation experience were in large measure due to the lack of tissue typing in the selection of donors. In the compilation of early human BMT experience by Bortin (1970), matched donors (using the mixed leukocyte culture test) were used in only three cases, and all three lived; only two of the 200 patients who received transplants without histocompatibility matching survived.

Beatty and colleagues (1985) have shown the importance of HLA identity between the host and the donor in determining the outcome of the allogeneic BMT. As the number of HLA antigens not shared by both donor and recipient increases, the rate and severity of GVHD increase, the risk for delayed engraftment or nonengraftment increases, and the rate of survival decreases. Attempts to improve the potential success for transplantation using donors who are unrelated or who are only partially matched is in the developmental stages in the field of BMT, and the issues involved are discussed in subsequent chapters. The development of new DNA techniques to more precisely define the class II alleles permits the selection of more closely matched unrelated donors (Schreuder et al., 1991).

DEVELOPMENTS IN SUPPORTIVE CARE

Blood Banking

The presence of different blood groups has been known since the early part of the 20th century. Initially, the major ABO groups were defined in the first decade of this century, and in 1940 the Rh system was described. Subsequently, more than 200 blood group systems have been discovered. Blood preservation and anticoagulation were also developed in the first half of the 20th century. The first blood banks were organized in the 1930s, and during the 1940s blood transfusion was available in many U.S. hospitals. The introduction of plastic equipment in the late 1940s facilitated wider applications of transfusion. Refrigeration, improved preservative solutions, automated equipment for separating and processing blood, and serologic testing for viruses all have led to improved utilization and safety of blood components.

The introduction in the 1960s of component therapy, in which whole blood could be divided into red cells, plasma, platelets, and other components, enabled the targeted use of blood products to replace specific needed elements and avoid unnecessary components. This led to improved safety and efficacy, and has allowed better utilization of donor supplies because a larger number of therapeutic units are derived from each donation.

The advances of BMT have depended heavily on the availability of blood component support. In the early 1960s platelet transfusions were available only at some large hospitals with cancer treatment programs. The use of platelets has subsequently grown meteorically. For example, the American Red Cross Blood Services distributed 196,000 units in 1972, but more than 3 million units in 1986. This increase is attributable to the development of standardized criteria for the use of these products, the increasing use of aplasia-producing cytotoxic therapy in the treatment of malignant diseases, and improved technology with the advent of differential centrifugation increasing the availability of these products. In 1963, the relationship between the number of circulating platelets and the risk for hemorrhage was described (Gaydos et al., 1962). The incidence of spontaneous hemorrhage was found to not significantly increase until the count fell below 20,000/μl. The risk of hemorrhage also was shown to be reduced by transfusion (Freireich et al., 1963). Using these data, in many centers, the general practice has evolved to prophylactically transfuse patients at counts less than 15,000/μl to 20,000/μl in chemotherapy-treated patients. Platelets can be obtained either by concentration of pooled multiple donor components or by single-donor platelets obtained by plateletpheresis. Both techniques are used widely, but the latter is preferred because it exposes the patient to fewer different HLA antigens, reduces the chance for alloimmunization, and lessens the risk of exposure to infectious agents in the product.

Neutropenic patients were found to be at greater risk for infection, especially with neutrophil counts less than 500/μl. The initial attempts to correct neutropenia used transfusions from patients with chronic myelogenous leukemia (CML) with high circulating neutrophil counts. During the early 1970s the source of neutrophils shifted from CML patients to normal donors with a yield of only 10% of that used in early studies. One early technique to obtain neutrophils was removal of cells from donors by leukopheresis and passage of the cells over nylon wool columns to which neutrophils selectively adhered. This provided an excellent yield, but some damage to the neutrophils impaired their functional capacity; most important, donors occasionally suffered potentially serious toxicities such as activation of complement, and signs and symptoms of leukostasis. Accordingly, this technique was abandoned and the technique of flow centrifugation has become prominent with the use of an erythrocyte sedimenting agent, such as hydroxymethyl starch, to facilitate the separation. Sometimes, corticosteroids are also used to elevate the donor's neutrophil count and improve the yield. Generally, 1×10^9 to 1.5×10^9 cells are obtained. Neutrophil transfusions have been shown to be efficacious in the treatment of bacterial sepsis. Trials in which neutrophil transfusions are given prophylactically during neutropenia have generally shown a reduction in infections but no reduction in deaths.

During the late 1970s, several BMT studies (Winston et al., 1980) demonstrated that the risk of death from infection by cytomegalovirus (CMV), which is transmitted via blood products, was significantly increased in BMT patients given neutrophil transfusions. Subsequently, the routine use of neutrophil transfusions has largely been abandoned in the management of aplasia soon after BMT, due to the concern of exposure to CMV. In recent years, the use of hematopoietic growth factors has permitted the collection of even larger numbers of granulocytes. These "enriched" granulocytes are being evaluated as adjunctive therapy in life-threatening fungal and antibiotic-resistant bacterial infections.

There are several unique challenges in the area of transfusion support in BMT. In the setting of profound immunosuppression present shortly after BMT, donor lymphocytes in blood transfusions can transiently engraft and produce GVHD. Transfusions of all types of cellular blood products have been shown to cause GVHD. Therefore, all cellular blood products should be irradiated with 1500 cGy to 3000 cGy to eliminate the proliferative potential of lymphocytes.

As mentioned, infection with CMV is a major cause of morbidity and death after BMT (Meyers et al., 1983). Seropositive patients can reactivate latent endogenous virus, and to date, there is no effective preventive strategy. However, seronegative patients can acquire the virus through the marrow graft (if the donor is seropositive) or through blood transfusions since the majority of adult Americans who constitute the donor pool are seropositive. One possible way to avoid acquisition of CMV is through the use of blood products screened to eliminate CMV-positive donors; this approach has been found to eliminate CMV primary infection (Bowden et al., 1986). It is applicable to only the situation in which both donor and recipient are seronegative, however. Fortunately, the risk of CMV disease in such patients is low even without CMV screening (Wingard et al., 1990). Also, the use of CMV-screened blood products in syngeneic and autologous BMT patients does not appear necessary since studies have shown the risk of CMV disease to be low (Wingard et al., 1988), although some advocate its use in this setting (Rowe et al., 1994).

Filtration of blood products is an area of interest in recent years, offering the potential for reducing transmission of viral pathogens such as CMV that reside mostly within leukocytes, reduction of alloimmunization, and reduction of febrile and other transfusion reactions. High-efficiency leukocyte filters are currently available for erythrocyte and platelet products and several studies suggest a benefit (De Witte et al., 1990). An alternative strategy is to filter the products as they are collected, which may reduce the level of cytokines in the product during storage, which may mediate some of the reactions.

The genes controlling the major blood groups are located on chromosome 9, not chromosome 6 where the HLA complex resides. Thus, it is possible for a patient and donor to be HLA identical yet ABO mismatched. Because red cells make up a substantial part of the marrow product, techniques had to be developed to avoid major hemolytic transfusion reactions when the patients were infused. One early technique was intensive plasma exchange of the recipient to remove anti-A and/or anti-B isohemagglutinins. With the advent of cell separators, the most common technique now is to differentially centrifuge the marrow product using hydroxymethyl starch to remove the donor erythrocytes, and resuspend the marrow in recipient-type erythrocytes (Braine et al., 1982). The recipient is also given copious fluids and monitored closely to minimize the hazard for an ABO-incompatible transfusion reaction.

Antimicrobial Therapy

As previously mentioned, life-threatening infection has been a major obstacle to advances in BMT (Winston et al., 1979). Infection was the most common cause of death in the early history not only of BMT, but also in the chemotherapy of leukemia (Hersh et al., 1965; Levine et al., 1974).

One of the first advances in this area was the recognition of the association between neutropenia and the risk for infection (Bodey et al., 1966). The incidence of any type of infection has been found to increase as the number of circulating neutrophils falls below 500/μl; the incidence of serious infection was noted to be particularly high at neutrophil counts below 100/μl. The duration of neutropenia also was found to be significantly correlated with the risk of infection. The major type of infection in neutropenia was due to enteric gram-negative bacteria. During the second or third week of neutropenia, fungi, especially *Candida* and *Aspergillus*, emerged as important pathogens. In recent years, with the routine use of indwelling venous catheters, gram-positive bacteria have become increasingly important pathogens during neutropenia.

An equally important advance in the control of infection was the recognition that fever during neutropenia was usually caused by infection, and that the use of empiric broad-spectrum antibiotics was much more effective in treating the infection than waiting until the infection was documented by blood culture or some other diagnostic test. Initially, various combinations of a semisynthetic penicillin plus an aminoglycoside were used, but more recently, single-agent therapy with ceftazidime and several other agents has been found to be effective (Pizzo et al., 1986).

A variety of antimicrobial agents have been used over the years to prevent infections. Combinations of nonabsorbable agents (such as orally administered vancomycin, gentamycin, and nystatin) and absorbable agents (such as trimethoprim-sulfamethoxazole) have been studied in multiple centers but have not been found to be consistently useful. In recent years the advent of the quinolone family of antibiotics has provided a group of agents that can be administered orally and have a wide antibacterial spectrum, including *Pseudomonas*. Norfloxacin, one member of this family, has been found to be an effective prophylaxis against gram-negative bacterial infection in neutropenic patients treated for leukemia. Ciprofloxacin is also effective in BMT patients (Lew et al., 1995). With the emergence of gram-positive bacterial pathogens, many of which are resistant to methicillin, some clinicians advocate the use of intravenous vancomycin prophylactically (Karp et al., 1986). Because of the emergence

of vancomycin-resistant enterococci, caution needs to be exercised by limiting the use of vancomycin to situations in which the need is great and alternatives are not possible.

The most elaborate strategy to prevent infections is isolation of the patient in a laminar air flow (LAF) room along with the use of topical and oral antibiotics and sterile food. This has been shown to be effective but is very expensive. It also exacts an emotional toll on the patient because of the isolation from human contact. In addition, several studies showed no increase in survival (Bodey, 1984; Armstrong, 1984). One study showed a reduced rate of GVHD in patients with aplastic anemia who received transplants in LAF (Storb et al., 1983). However, in the absence of a substantial benefit of LAF, and with its high cost, most BMT units do not use LAF. Moreover, with the introduction of a panoply of safe and effective antibiotics with a wide spectrum of activity, death from bacterial infections has diminished. Many BMT units use simple reverse isolation, with patients placed in single rooms or rooms equipped with high-efficiency particulate air (HEPA) filters.

As the control of bacterial infections has been refined, attention has turned to the more problematic fungal infections, which continue to be the most common cause of death from infection before engraftment. Because of the difficulty in early diagnosis and the poor success rate when therapy is delayed, efforts to prevent *Candida* infection have been numerous. Orally administered agents have not been consistently effective, in part, because of poor tolerance of oral medications after chemotherapy. Two strategies (empiric therapy and prophylaxis) have been found to be effective. Amphotericin B given intravenously, started empirically 3 to 7 days after the start of the antibacterial empiric regimen in persistently febrile patients reduces fungal infections (Pizzo et al., 1982; EORTC, 1989). Fluconazole, another azole, has been shown to be highly efficacious given prophylactically (Goodman et al., 1992) and is widely used, and may offer a survival advantage (Slavin et al., 1995). Unfortunately, fluconazole, which is less toxic than amphotericin B, is not effective against *Aspergillus*. In the past, *Aspergillus* infections were uniformly fatal, despite the use of amphotericin B. In recent years, however, use of the CT scan to detect early distinctive pulmonary lesions, coupled with the use of early, high-dose amphotericin B has improved control rates (Kuhlman et al., 1987; Burch et al., 1987). Although itraconazole offers a less toxic alternative to amphotericin B with good activity against *Aspergillus*, its bioavailability is variable soon after BMT.

Over the years the major postengraftment infectious complication has been CMV pneumonitis; indeed, this has represented one of the most common causes of death after BMT. Until recently, there was no effective therapy. Thus, over the past decade, efforts have focused on prevention through the use of CMV-negative blood products, anti-CMV immunoglobulin, and high-dose acyclovir. However, even in the absence of such measures, the incidence of CMV pneumonia in some centers has decreased in recent years, without any change in the rates of CMV infection. This may be due to the adoption of cyclosporin as anti-GVHD prophylaxis and to improved control of GVHD. More recently, several studies have shown the combination of ganciclovir plus intravenous immunoglobulin to be an effective therapy for CMV pneumonitis, with 50% to 70% survival rates (Reed et al., 1988). Ganciclovir prophylaxis or "preemptive" therapy initiated at the first detection of active infection have been shown to prevent illness from CMV infection (Goodrich et al., 1991; Goodrich et al., 1993; Winston et al., 1993). Acyclovir prophylaxis has similarly

been shown to reduce the risk for CMV disease (Prentice et al., 1994).

Hematopoietic Growth Factors

A variety of glycoprotein cytokines have been identified which have important roles in the regulation of the proliferation and maturation of bone marrow progenitor cells of all lineages. With the recombinant DNA technology, erythropoietin and several myeloid growth factors have become commercially available. Erythropoietin has been shown to be beneficial in the anemia associated with chronic renal failure and in some cases of anemia associated with cancer. Studies have suggested promise in some BMT situations (Link et al., 1994), but the definition of its precise role after BMT has yet to be elucidated.

Both G-CSF and GM-CSF have been shown in controlled randomized trials to have significant shortening of time to neutrophil recovery after both autologous and allogeneic BMT. In addition, these myeloid growth factors have been found to be extremely effective in mobilizing primitive hematopoietic progenitor cells from the bone marrow compartment to the peripheral blood. Collection of large numbers of "stem cells" are now possible by pheresis and a number of uncontrolled trials have suggested more rapid recovery of neutrophil and platelet function through the use of these "enriched" stem cell products. Although durable engraftment was an initial concern, it is now clear that stable engraftment after myeloablative regimens occurs. Thus, an enriched peripheral blood stem cell product collected after mobilization of hematopoietic growth factors (HGF) or chemotherapy represents a viable alternative to bone marrow and its use in autologous transplantation is well established; it is being explored for allogeneic transplantation as well (Lane et al., 1995). HGF have had less substantial benefit in the reduction of infectious morbidity but shortening of duration of antibiotics, duration of hospitalization, and the interval of fever have frequently been noted. A reduction in the use of health-care resources and costs also have been a welcome accompaniment.

Several multilineage cytokines including IL-3, IL-6, IL-11 are being investigated as to whether not only neutrophil engraftment can be shortened, but platelet function can be restored more quickly as well. The discovery and synthesis of thrombopoietin and recognition of its role in megakaryocyte growth and differentiation have led to the recent entry of this molecule into clinical trials. They offer the potential for reducing the reliance on blood product transfusions and reduce accompanying morbidity and cost associated with transfusion support.

Nutritional Considerations

The gastrointestinal side effects of the chemoradiotherapy in the conditioning regimen include anorexia, nausea, vomiting, and diarrhea. Additionally, graft-versus-host disease and enteric viruses can cause severe, prolonged diarrhea. Up to half of BMT patients have enteritis severe enough to cause a protein losing enteropathy (Weisdorf et al., 1983). Mucositis often makes oral intake of fluid and nutrients difficult. In summary, loss of nitrogen results from reduced intake of nutrients, enteral loss in diarrhea, and the direct catabolic effect of the cytotoxic therapy, infection, graft-versus-host disease and corticosteroids, and immobilization.

Early in the history of BMT, when patients referred for BMT often had residual leukemia, malnutrition was frequently present. Animal studies demonstrated that hematopoietic recovery without adequate nutrition was compromised (Stuart and Sensenbrenner, 1979). Thus,

many BMT centers routinely used total parenteral nutritional (TPN) support to replete nutrition and ensure marrow engraftment. In recent years, the character of transplant patients has changed. Patients are frequently in remission at time of transplant and are well nourished. Thus, the goal has changed from nutritional repletion to maintenance. Many studies of well-nourished patients undergoing chemotherapy and radiotherapy have shown no benefits from total parenteral nutrition (Koretz, 1984), although some have noted more rapid hematologic recovery (Hays et al., 1983). One randomized trial in BMT patients compared patients given TPN to those given maintenance IV fluids plus enteral feedings as tolerated (Weisdorf et al., 1987). Patients who received TPN had improved overall survival and disease-free survival rates. In contrast, another study of BMT patients compared TPN and an enteral feeding program in a randomized trial (Szeluga et al., 1987). The Weisdorf study began the trial during cytoreductive therapy, the Szeluga study started the nutritional program just before marrow infusion (after completion of the conditioning regimen). Both studies found that patients were unable to achieve maintenance nutritional status with an enteral feeding program. The Szeluga study, in contrast, found no long-term benefit in survival or disease-free survival. Szeluga and colleagues (1987) speculate that TPN may have potentiated the effects of the antineoplastic therapy rather than supported marrow recovery; thus, an effect might be seen when given during chemotherapy, but in the absence of a gross nutritional deficiency, TPN would not offer a benefit.

A survey of BMT centers in 1987 indicated that various methods were being used to provide oral nutritional support (Dezenhall et al., 1987). Sterile food was rarely used due to cost and poor acceptance by patients. Most commonly used were either a reduced-bacterial diet or a house diet without fresh vegetables or fruit. Frequently, patients have prolonged poor oral intake after marrow engraftment. In the past, this necessitated delays in hospital discharge. Now, with the availability of home IV therapy, many patients can be discharged and continue to receive TPN without compromising their nutrition (Lenssen et al., 1983).

BMT in the Outpatient Setting

Several developments have occurred that have led to the performance of transplant care in the outpatient setting that was traditionally done in the hospital setting. The availability of home health services has permitted the delivery of infusional therapies in an outpatient residential setting. This has been facilitated by the availability of programmable portable infusion pumps, computerized informational services, and skilled nursing professionals with both infusional expertise and knowledge of oncologic principles. The creation of "day" hospitals has permitted timely skilled clinical and laboratory assessments, the administration of fluids, electrolytes, antibiotic infusions, and blood products, and the delivery of a variety of supportive care measures (Peters et al., 1994). The introduction of oral antibiotics with broad-spectrum activity and the demonstration that antibiotic prophylaxis and once-daily infusional antibiotic for neutropenic fever to be effective has made feasible the therapy of neutropenic fever in the outpatient setting (Gilbert et al., 1994). Careful analyses of neutropenic fever have led to the recognition of low-risk and high-risk cases so patients can be grouped according to which treatment in the outpatient setting is likely to be successful and which may be too risky.

These advances in medical technology have arrived at a time when the public is demanding lower-cost health care. These initiatives are likely to lower the cost of transplantation at a time when the application of transplantation is accelerating in volume. Finally, many patients want greater autonomy and a larger role in their own care.

For these activities to be successfully performed in the outpatient setting, communication between the patient and the health-care team is vital to ensure that important clinical events are recognized by the patient and brought to the attention of the health-care team. Moreover, in the event of a complication requiring immediate care by health professionals, prompt access to a full range of inpatient services is needed. Generally, it is desirable that a partner be available to the patient to assist in the provision of care. The initial efforts of outpatient transplants have been performed in solid tumor autotransplants. Regimens causing little gastrointestinal toxicity have been particularly appropriate for the outpatient setting. Moreover, the preparative regimens have been less intensive than some of the regimens for allogeneic transplantation or those for leukemia. Exploration of this in other patients is now being evaluated in several centers.

DEVELOPMENTS IN THE CONTROL OF GVHD

Once techniques to ensure engraftment by adequate conditioning were developed, it became clear that GVHD was a major obstacle for allogeneic BMT. From animal studies it was recognized that GVHD was caused by donor T lymphocytes. It was learned that the frequency and severity of GVHD depended on the degree of HLA compatibility and the dose of lymphocytes. Although GVHD had harmful effects, being one of the major causes of death, it was found to also have beneficial effects, associated with an antileukemic effect (Weiden et al., 1979). Thus, the goal of prevention and treatment of GVHD was moderation of its severity without complete elimination.

Based on studies in dogs, methotrexate was employed as a prophylaxis against GVHD in some centers, and based on studies in rodents, cyclophosphamide was used in other centers. In recent years cyclosporin has been found to be an effective preventive measure and has been substituted as the preferred GVHD prophylaxis by many centers (Santos et al., 1987). Some centers employ a combination of methotrexate and cyclosporin.

High doses of corticosteroids have been the mainstay of treatment of GVHD over the years. In cases of refractory GVHD, antithymocyte globulin (ATG) has sometimes been useful.

Another strategy investigated in the past decade is the removal of the T lymphocytes from the donor marrow. A variety of techniques have been used: anti-T cell monoclonal antibodies, corticosteroids, lectins, counterflow centrifugal elutriation. These have been shown to reduce GVHD in a variety of studies. Unfortunately, these techniques have also been associated with increased rates of relapse (Goldman et al., 1988), apparently eliminating the graft-versus-leukemia (GVL) effect seen with allogeneic BMT (reviewed in Wingard et al., 1992a). Techniques to deplete selected cell subpopulations to preserve the GVL effect while diminishing GVHD are being explored (Champlin et al., 1996).

For chronic GVHD, combination therapy with steroids plus azathioprine was the preferred treatment for many years (Sullivan, 1983). A study comparing prednisone plus azathioprine versus prednisone showed prednisone alone to be as effective and to be associated with fewer infectious complications (Sullivan et al., 1988). For high-risk patients, the combination of steroids plus cyclosporin is more effective (Sullivan et al., 1988a, b). Thalidomide has been shown to be active in the treatment of chronic GVHD and currently trials are investigating its role in the treatment of GVHD (Vogelsang et al., 1987).

NURSING CARE

As the field of bone marrow transplantation has evolved, so too has BMT nursing, which has become one of the most challenging nursing specialties. Its roles have become more complex and have expanded enormously in recent years.

The traditional major concern of attending to the acute care needs of patients has become increasingly difficult. BMT patients are generally young, but span the age range from infancy to the middle years of life: thus, skill in managing pediatric, adolescent, and adult concerns are prerequisites. BMT nurses are frequently called upon to provide the highly technical critical care services needed to manage the problems of nutritional support, electrolyte and fluid management, aplasia, sepsis, severe graft-versus-host disease, transfusion management, and vital organ failure (O'Quin and Moravec, 1988). Knowledge of general oncologic principles and a detailed understanding of an array of chemotherapeutic agents is fundamental. The introduction of computerized information systems to the clinical setting have required mastery of automated data systems. Within the Oncology Nursing Society (ONS) a special interest group (SIG) has developed, focusing solely on the concerns of BMT nurses. These concerns include efforts to develop national standards of BMT nursing care, especially with respect to management of mucositis, skin care, indwelling venous catheter care, and isolation procedures.

The role of nursing in patient and family education has also expanded. Patients and their families require orientation to the treatment modalities and to the specific objectives in the plan of care. Although many patients have been under the care of an oncology treatment team before referral, few have a good understanding of what is to be undertaken. Specific issues that require emphasis in patient orientation include a prolonged hospitalization with some type of isolation, the attendant loss of control associated with the restrictions of a hospital environment, the unique problems of graft-versus-host disease, and the need for avoidance of crowds for several months after recovery of marrow function to avoid contagious illness until the slower recovery of cellular immunity occurs. Teaching self-care tasks, especially with respect to exercise, nutrition, and indwelling catheters, and to encourage the patient to exercise as much control over his or her care, is very important. For patients newly referred to the transplant center, orientation to the inpatient and outpatient units enables them to best use the center's resources.

A greater emphasis on the psychosocial needs of patients and families has also emerged (Haberman, 1988). Nurses play a pivotal role in the recognition of patients' psychosocial needs and are called on to ensure that appropriate resources are directed to dealing with them. Patients who do not reside in the same community as the transplant center are especially in need of psychosocial resources since their network of family and friends is unable to be physically present during much of the BMT experience. Changes in family roles are universal concerns for patients and significant others. The primary nurse or case manager must be adept at engaging the services of social workers, psychiatric liaison nurses, child life specialists, occupational therapists, and so forth. Passage between inpatient and outpatient units must be accomplished seamlessly because more care is being delivered in the outpatient setting; communication, assessment of patient and family resources, and support to both the patient and his or her nonprofessional caregivers are crucial to assess continuity of care, to allay stress, and to encourage confidence in success.

Follow-up care is becoming increasingly important because there are more and more long-term survivors (Nims and Strom, 1988). During the first year after transplant the patient and primary care team must be vigilant for the possible occurrence of chronic graft-versus-host disease, infections, obstructive airway disease, and recurrence (if transplanted for malignancy). Ovarian failure, which requires hormonal replacement, is a concern for adult women. Issues regarding sexuality are frequent concerns for both men and women (Wingard et al., 1992b). For children, growth and development must be monitored to detect pituitary, thyroid, or adrenal insufficiency (Sanders et al., 1988). Resumption of employment and former family social roles emerges as a task for patients as the acute illness recedes into the background. Recognition of these "late" concerns, and assisting patients and families in dealing with these issues of survivorship, have become important roles for nursing.

CONSIDERATIONS FOR THE FUTURE

In the nearly four decades of human bone marrow transplantation, enormous strides have occurred in the treatment of human disease. Currently, success rates in severe aplastic anemia exceed 70%, in acute nonlymphoblastic leukemia in first remission 55%, in relapsed Hodgkin's or non-Hodgkin's lymphoma 50%, and chronic myelogenous leukemia 40% to 50%. There are a variety of other less common diseases for which success rates exceed 50%. In recognition of the importance of this medical discipline and the singular contributions of E. Donnall Thomas, the Nobel prize in Medicine in 1990 was awarded to Dr. Thomas for bone marrow transplantation.

There remain a variety of limitations to the greater application of BMT, which require further improvements. The major causes of failure are graft-versus-host disease, immunodeficiency and infection, toxicities from the preparative regimen, and relapse. Further, only one third of patients have an HLA-identical sibling as a potential donor.

One strategy to address the lack of a compatible donor is the further development of the National Bone Marrow Donor Registry. This is addressed in a subsequent chapter. The use of related donors who are haplo-identical is another alternative, but remains limited as an option at present until better techniques are developed to control graft-versus-host disease.

With ex vivo purging of T cells from the donor graft, serious GVHD can be prevented. Unfortunately, this and other measures successful in preventing GVHD have generally resulted in an increased relapse rate, by abrogation of the graft-versus-leukemia effect. There is some experimental evidence that the cell populations that mediate the GVL effect differ from the lymphocytes that mediate GVHD, although other data do not support this (reviewed in Wingard, 1992a). In the future there will certainly be attempts to identify, characterize, and grow cells that mediate GVL and not GVHD. If successful, the marrow graft can be engineered to contain enriched populations of GVL cells and depleted of cells that mediate GVHD. Attempts to enrich the marrow with natural killer (NK) cells or lymphokine-activated killer (LAK) cells to enhance the antileukemic potential are also likely in the near future.

Recent studies suggest that the graft-versus-leukemia effect is much more potent than previously appreciated. Infusions of donor buffy coat cells in relatively small numbers in patients with early relapse after allogeneic transplant have been shown to re-establish durable remissions (Kolb et al., 1990; Drobyski et al., 1992). One current shortcoming of this approach is a substantial risk of graft-versus-host disease or aplasia. With improved understanding of the

effector cells responsible for this antitumor activity, infusions of selected populations may provide the beneficial antitumor effect without the deleterious complications. Using cell culture techniques now available, large numbers of cloned cytotoxic T lymphocytes with desired specificity can be administered to the transplant recipient. Already clinical trials are underway to explore the use of donor cytotoxic T cells to treat CMV and EBV disease in the transplant setting (Riddell et al., 1994; Papadopopoulos et al., 1994). Patients at high risk for relapse may benefit from staged infusions of these effector cells at intervals after the transplant to prevent relapse.

An alternative way to avoid the limitations of GVHD and unavailability of a donor is with the use of autologous BMT. Results with autologous BMT have been improving in recent years, especially with lymphomas and acute nonlymphocytic leukemia (Santos et al., 1989). With the absence of GVHD, the early posttransplant mortality is lower than after allogeneic BMT. However, the relapse rate is generally substantially higher, due to the frequent contamination of the marrow graft with occult tumor cells and also to the absence of any GVL effect. Efforts to improve elimination of contaminating tumor cells are under development. Use of pharmacologic methods, such as 4-hydroperoxycyclophosphamide, monoclonal antibodies directed against tumor-associated antigens, immunoabsorption columns, and cell separation techniques are being studied. The role of various biologic response modifiers to reduce the risk for relapse after autologous BMT will be more fully explored. Interferon is being studied for a possible antileukemic effect (Meyers et al., 1987). Alternatively, administration of an antibody (by itself or linked with a cellular toxin or radioisotope) specific for tumor antigens, or the administration of immuno-modulatory cytokines such as IL-2, IL-4 or IL-12 can be performed after transplant. Such immunoadjuvant therapeutics would be expected to be most effective at a time of minimal residual disease, shortly after transplant.

Additionally, the deliberate creation of autologous GVHD is being investigated as a potential adjunctive to exert an immunotherapeutic effect. In humans (as shown earlier in animals) autologous or syngeneic GVHD can be produced routinely after autologous BMT when low-dose cyclosporin is administered (Jones et al., 1989). Cells that mediate this autologous GVHD are very similar to the cells that mediate chronic GVHD after allogeneic BMT; they are autoreactive against target cells that express Ia antigens (Hess and Fisher, 1989). Ia antigens are expressed on lymphoma and nonlymphocytic leukemia cells. Thus, these effector cells may be capable of mediating an antileukemic effect, similar to that seen with chronic GVHD after allogeneic BMT (Weiden et al., 1981). Fortunately, autologous GVHD, unlike acute GVHD after allogeneic BMT, is generally mild, and is easily controlled with either no therapy or a short course of corticosteroids. Studies are under way to purposely create autologous GVHD, with a goal of demonstrating an antitumor effect. If successful, the results of autologous BMT will exploit the benefits of the antileukemic effect of chronic GVHD without the harmful effects of acute GVHD with attendant immunodeficiency and risk of life-threatening infection.

With the delivery of transplant care in the outpatient setting the utility of multiple tandem transplants with dose-intensive therapy is possible. Each course is followed by an infusion of stem cells to provide a tolerable, multicourse dose-intensive treatment regimen. This might be particularly attractive for epithelial tumors for which multiple treatments may be more efficacious than a single-dose treatment.

Techniques to select hematopoietic stem cells by immunophenotypic differences from tumor cells and other cells not necessary for engraftment permit the exploration of transplantation of small numbers of pluripotent HSC to effect engraftment and to provide a product free of contaminating tumor cells. This is being explored in transplantation for lymphoma, multiple myeloma, and breast cancer. Highly purified stem cell populations also permit the exploration of techniques to expand the numbers of cells ex vivo through incubation of small numbers of cells with cocktails of growth factors. Thus, one might be able to effect BMT through the use of very few donor cells that will enhance the acceptability of volunteer HSC donations (Brugger et al., 1995). Similarly the use of peripheral blood after HGF mobilization is being explored in allogeneic transplantation. Again, the hope is to make HSC donation more palatable. An area of active investigation is the insertion of genes into hematopoietic stem cells to correct a genetic deficiency, to provide resistance to chemotherapeutic drugs, or to convey resistance to certain viral pathogens such as HIV. The use of gene insertion techniques might broaden the applicability of BMT to other disease processes.

One concern increasing in emphasis in recent years is the quality of life of survivors of various cancer treatments. Several small studies suggest that outcomes are similar to other types of cancer (Andrykowski et al., 1989a, b).

Survivors have reported both positive and negative changes in plans and activities, relationships, physical status, and existential concerns, but positive changes often exceeded the negative changes, except in physical status (Wingard et al., 1991; Baker et al., 1991; Curbow et al., 1993a, 1993b). Life satisfaction has been rated favorably by most (Baker et al., 1994). High levels of function and excellent health has been reported by many patients. Most survivors have returned to work or school. Twenty to thirty percent reported improved family relations, greater compassion, redirected life goals, and existential recovery, and

36% reported psychological gains after recovery from the transplant. While most appear to have been successful in reintegrating their lives, some reported significant losses: 16% reported their health to be ill or bad, 9% said social function was limited "a good bit," and 13% reported moderate to severe pain (Baker et al., 1994). The role of the family has been recognized as an important predictor of posttransplant emotional distress (Syrjala et al., 1993). A variety of challenges need to be addressed and studied in further psychosocial research of BMT survivors (Wingard, 1994).

In summary, the historical developments of BMT have occurred because of the dedication and perseverance of specialists in many fields. Advances in the biological sciences, supportive care, and nursing care have resulted in improved outcomes for patients undergoing BMT and other types of cancer therapy as well. These developments bode well for the future of BMT as an important treatment modality with expanding applications.

REFERENCES

Andrykowski, M.D., Henslee, P.J., Farrall, M.G. 1989a. Physical and psychosocial functioning of adult survivors of allogeneic bone marrow transplantation. *BMT* 4:75-81.

Andrykowski, M.A., Henslee, P.J., and Barnett, R.L. 1989b. Longitudinal assessment of psychosocial functioning of adult survivors of allogeneic bone marrow transplantation. *BMT* 4:505-509.

Antman, K.O., Armitage, J.O., Horowitz, M.M., Rowlings, P.A. For the North America Autologous Bone Marrow Transplant Registry (NAABMTR). 1994. Autotransplants for breast cancer in north America. *Proc ASCO* 13:67 (abstr 69).

Applebaum, F.R. 1996. The use of bone marrow and peripheral blood stem cell transplantation in the treatment of cancer. *CA—Canc J Clinicians* 46(3):42-164.

Armstrong, D. 1984. Protected environments are discomforting and expensive and do not offer meaningful protection. *Am J Med* 76: 685-689.

Baker, F., Curbow, B., Wingard, J.R. 1991. Role retention and quality of life of bone marrow transplant survivors. *Soc Sci Med* 32:697-704.

Baker, F., et al. 1994. Quality of life of bone marrow transplant long-term survivors. *BMT* 13:589-596.

Baranov, A., et al. 1989. Bone marrow transplantation after the Chernobyl nuclear accident. *N Engl J Med* 321:205-212.

Barnes, D.W.H., Loutit, J.F. 1955. The radiation recovery factor: preservation by the Polge-Smith-Parkes technique. *J Natl Cancer Inst* 15:901.

Beatty, P.G., et al. 1985. Marrow transplantation from related donor other than HLA-identical siblings. *N Engl J Med* 313:765-771

Bodey, G.P. 1984. Current status of prophylaxis of infection with protected environments. *Am J Med* 76:678-684.

Bodey, G.P., et al. 1966. Quantitative relationships between circulating leukocytes and infection in patients with acute leukemia. *Ann Intern Med* 64:328-340.

Bortin, M.M. 1970. A compendium of reported human bone marrow transplants. *Transplantation* 9:571-587.

Bortin, M.M., Horowitz, M.M., Gale, R.P. 1988. Current status of bone marrow transplantation in humans: report from the International Bone Marrow Transplant Registry. *Nat Immun Cell Growth Regul* 7:334-350.

Bowden, R.A., et al. 1986. Cytomegalovirus immune globulin and seronegative blood products to prevent primary cytomegalovirus infection after marrow transplantation. *N Engl J Med* 314:1006 -1010.

Braine, H.G., et al. 1982. Bone marrow transplantation with major ABO blood group incompatibility using erythrocyte depletion of marrow prior to infusion. *Blood* 60:420-425.

Brugger, W., Heimfeld, S., Berenson, et al. 1995. Reconstitution of hematopoiesis after high-dose chemotherapy by autologous progenitor cells generated ex vivo. *N Engl J Med* 333:283-7.

Burch, P.A., et al. 1987. Favorable outcome of invasive aspergillosis in patients with acute leukemia. *J Clin Oncol* 5:1985-1993.

Champlin, R., Giralt, S., Gajewski, J. 1996. T cells, graft-versus-host disease and graft-versus-leukemia: innovative approaches for blood and marrow transplantation. *Acta Hematol* 95(3-4):157-163.

Curbow, B., Baker, F., Somerfield, et al. 1993a. Personal changes, dispositional optimism and psychological adjustment to bone marrow transplantation. *J Behav Med* 16:423-443.

Curbow, B., Legro, M.W., Baker, et al. 1993b. Loss and recovery themes of long-term survivors of bone marrow transplants. *J Psychosoc Oncol* 10:1-20.

Dausset, J. 1954. Leukoagglutinins. IV. Leukoagglutinins and blood transfusions. *Vox Sang* 4:190.

Dausset, J. 1958. Iso-leuco-anticorps. *Acta Haematol (Basel)* 20:156:166.

De Witte, T., et al. 1990. Prevention of primary cytomegalovirus infection after allogeneic bone marrow transplantation by using leukocyte-poor random blood products from cytomegalovirus-unscreened blood-bank donors. *Transplantation* 50:964.

Dezenhall, A., et al. 1987. Food and nutrition services in bone marrow transplant centers. *J Am Dietetic Assoc* 87:1351-1353.

Drobyski, W.R., Roth, R.S., Thibodeau, S.N., et al. 1992. Molecular remission occurring after donor leukocyte infusions for the treatment of relapsed chronic myelogenous leukemia after allogeneic bone marrow transplantation. *BMT* 10:301-304.

EORTC International Antimicrobial Therapy Cooperative Group. 1989. Empiric antifungal therapy in febrile granulocytopenic patients. *Am J Med* 86:668-672.

Ford, C.E., Hamerton, J.L., Barnes, D.W.H., Loutit, J.F. 1956. Cytological identification of radiation-chimaeras. *Nature* 177:452-454.

Freireich, E.J., et al. 1963. Response to repeated platelet transfusions from the same donor. *Annu Intern Med* 59:277-287.

Gassmann, W., et al. 1988. Comparison of cyclophosphamide, cytarabine, and etoposide as immunosuppressive agents before allogeneic bone marrow transplantation. *Blood* 72:1574-1579.

Gaydos, L.A., Freireich, E.J., Mantel, N. 1962. The quantitative relation between platelet count and hemorrhage in patients with acute leukemia. *N Engl J Med* 266:905-909.

Gilbert, C., et al. 1994. Sequential prophylactic oral and empiric once-daily parenteral antibiotics for neutropenia and fever after high-dose chemotherapy and autologous bone marrow support. *J Clin Oncol* 12:1005-11.

Goldman, J.M., et al. 1980. Haematological reconstitution after autografting for chronic granulocytic leukaemia in transformation: the influence of previous splenomegaly. *Br J Haematol* 45:223.

Goldman, J.M., et al. 1988. Bone marrow transplantation for chronic myelogenous leukemia in chronic phase: increased risk of relapse associated with T cell depletion. *Ann Intern Med* 108:806-814.

Goodman, J.L., et al. 1992. A controlled trial of fluconazole to prevent fungal infections in patients undergoing bone marrow transplantation. *N Engl J Med* 326:845-51.

Goodrich, J.M., Bowden, R.A., Fisher, L., et al. 1993. Ganciclovir prophylaxis to prevent cytomegalovirus disease after allogeneic marrow transplant. *Ann Intern Med* 118:173-178.

Goodrich, J.M., Mori, M., Gleaves, C.A., et al. 1991. Early treatment with ganciclovir to prevent cytomegalovirus disease after allogeneic bone marrow transplant. *N Engl J Med* 325:1601-1607.

Haberman, M.R. 1988. Psychosocial aspects of bone marrow transplantation. *Sem Oncol Nurs* 4:55-59.

Hays, D.M., et al. 1983. Effect of total parenteral nutrition on marrow recovery during induction therapy for acute nonlymphocytic leukemia in childhood. *Med Pediatr Oncol* 11:134-140.

Hersh, E.M., et al. 1965. Causes of death in acute leukemia. *JAMA* 193:99-103.

Hess, A.D., Fischer, A.D. 1989. Immune mechanisms in cyclosporin-induced syngeneic graft-versus-host disease. *Transplantation* 48:895-900.

Jones, R.J., et al. 1989. Preliminary communication: induction of graft-versus-host disease after autologous bone marrow transplantation. *Lancet* 1:754-757.

Juttner, C.A., et al. 1985. Circulating autologous stem cells collected in very early remission from acute nonlymphoblastic leukemia produce prompt but incomplete haemapoietic reconstitution after high dose melphalan or supralethal chemoradiotherapy. *Br J Haematol* 61:739.

Karp, J.E., et al. 1986. Empiric use of vancomycin during prolonged treatment-induced granulocytopenia: randomized, double-blind, placebo-controlled clinical trial in patients with acute leukemia. *Am J Med* 106:1-7.

Kolb H.J., et al. 1990. Donor leukocyte transfusions for treatment of recurrent chronic myelogenous leukemia in marrow transplant patients. *Blood* 76:2462-2465.

Koretz, R.L. 1984. Parenteral nutrition. Is it oncologically logical? *J Clin Oncol* 2:534-538.

Kuhlman, J.E., et al. 1987. Invasive pulmonary aspergillosis in acute leukemia. *Chest* 92:95-99.

Kurnick, N.B., et al. 1958. Preliminary observations and treatment of post irradiation haematolopoietic depression in man by the infusion of stored autogenous bone marrow. *Ann Intern Med* 49:969.

Lane, T.A., et al. 1995. Harvesting and enrichment of hematopoietic progenitor cells mobilized into the peripheral blood of normal donors by granulocyte-macrophage colony-stimulating factor (GM-CSF) or G-CSF: potential role in allogeneic marrow transplantation. *Blood 85*: 275-282.

Lenssen, P., et al. 1983. Parenteral nutrition in marrow transplant recipients after discharge from the hospital. *Exp Hematol 11*:974-981.

Levine, A.S., et al. 1974. Hematologic malignancies and other marrow failure states: progress in the management of complicating infections. *Semin Hematol 11*:141-202.

Lew, M.A., et al. 1995. Ciprofloxacin versus trimethoprim/sulfamethoxazole for prophylaxis of bacterial infections in bone marrow transplant recipients: a randomized, controlled trial. *J Clin Oncol 13*:239-250.

Link, H., et al. 1994. A controlled trial of recombinant human erythropoietin after bone marrow transplant. *Blood 84*:3327-3335.

Mathe, G., et al. 1959. Transfusions et greffes de moeille osseuse homologue chez les humains irradiés à hautes doses accidentellement. *Rev Fr Etudes Clin Biol 4*:238.

Meyers, J.D., et al. 1983. Biology of interstitial pneumonia after marrow transplantation. In Gale, R.P. (Ed.) *Recent Advances in Bone Marrow Transplantation*. New York: A.R. Liss, 405-423.

Meyers, J.D., et al. 1987. Prophylactic use of human leukocyte interferon after allogeneic marrow transplantation. *Ann Intern Med 107*:809-816.

Nims, J.W., Strom, S. 1988. Late complications of bone marrow transplant recipients: nursing care issues. *Semin Oncol Nurs 4*:47-54.

O'Quin, T., Moravec, C. 1988. The critically ill bone marrow transplant patient. *Sem Oncol Nurs 4*:25-30.

Papadopopoulos, E.B., et al. 1994. Infusions of donor leukocytes to treat Epstein-Barr virus-associated lymphoproliferative disorders after allogeneic bone marrow transplantation. *N Engl J Med 330*:1185-91.

Peters, W.P., et al. 1994. The use of intensive clinic support to permit outpatient autologous bone marrow transplantation for breast cancer. *Semin Oncol 21*: 25-31.

Pizzo, P.A., et al. 1982. Empiric antibiotic and antifungal therapy for cancer patients with prolonged fever and granulocytopenia. *Am J Med 72*:101-111.

Pizzo, P.A., et al. 1986. A randomized trial comparing ceftazidime along with combination antibiotic therapy in cancer patients with fever and neutropenia. *N Engl J Med 315*:552-558.

Prentice, H.G., et al. 1994. Impact of long-term acyclovir on cytomegalovirus infection and survival after allogeneic bone marrow transplantation. *Lancet 343*:749.

Quine, W.E. 1896. The remedial application of bone marrow. *JAMA 26*:1012-1013.

Reed, E.C., et al. 1988. Treatment of cytomegalovirus pneumonia with ganciclovir and intravenous cytomegalovirus immunoglobulin in patients with bone marrow transplant. *Ann Intern Med 109*:783-788.

Riddell, S.R., Walter, B.A., Gilbert, M.J., Greenberg, P.D. 1994. Selective reconstitution of CD8+ cytotoxic T lymphocyte responses in immunodeficient bone marrow transplant recipients by the adoptive transfer of T cell clones. *BMT 14*:S78-S84.

Rowe, J.M., et al. 1994. Recommended guidelines for the management of autologous and allogeneic bone marrow transplanation: a report from the Eastern Cooperative Oncology Group (ECOG). *Ann Intern Med 120*:143-158.

Sanders, J.E., et al. 1988. Growth and development of children after bone marrow transplantation. *Horm Res 30*:92-97.

Santos, G.W., et al. 1970. Rationale for the use of cyclophosphamide as immunosuppression for marrow transplants in man. In Bertelli, A., Monoco, A.P. (Eds.) *International Symposium on Pharmacological Treatment in Organ and Tissue Transplantation*. Amsterdam: Experta Medical Found., 24.

Santos, G.W. 1974. Immunosuppression for clinical marrow transplantation. *Semin Hematol 11*:341-351.

Santos, G.W., et al. 1983. Marrow transplantation for acute nonlymphocytic leukemia after treatment with busulfan and cyclophosphamide. *N Engl J Med 309*: 1347-1353.

Santos, G.W., et al. 1987. Cyclosporin plus methylprednisolone versus cyclophosphamide plus methylprednisolone as prophylaxis for graft-versus-host disease: a randomized, double-blind study in patients undergoing allogeneic marrow transplantation. *Clin Transpl 1*:21-28.

Santos, G.W., Yeager, A.M., Jones, R.J. 1989. Autologous bone marrow transplantation. *Ann Rev Med 40*:99-112.

Schreuder, G.M.T.H., et al. 1991. Increasing complexity of HLA-DR2 as detected by serology and oligonucleotide typing. *Hum Immunol 32*:141-149.

Slavin, M.A., et al. 1995. Efficacy and safety of fluconazole prophylaxis for fungal infections after marrow transplantation: a prospective, randomized, double-blind study. *J Infect Dis 171*:1545-52.

Sobocinski, K.A., et al. 1994. Bone marrow transplantation–1994: a report from the International Bone Marrow Transplant Registry and the North American Autologous Bone Marrow Transplant Registry. *J Hematother 3*:95-102.

Storb, R., et al. 1983. Graft-versus-host disease and survival in patients with aplastic anemia treated by marrow grafts from HLA-identical siblings: beneficial effect of a protective environment. *N Engl J Med 308*:302-307.

Stuart, R.K., Sensenbrenner, L.L. 1979. Adverse nutritional deprivation of transplanted hematopoietic cells. *Exp Hematol 7*:435-442.

Sullivan, K.M. 1983. Graft-versus-host disease. In Blume, K.G., Petz, L.D. (Eds.) *Clinical Bone Marrow Transplantation.* New York: Churchill Livingston, 91-130.

Sullivan, K.M., et al. 1988a. Prednisone and azathioprine compared with prednisone and placebo for treatment of chronic graft-versus-host disease: prognostic influence of prolonged thrombocytopenia after allogeneic marrow transplantation. *Blood 72*:546-554.

Sullivan, K.M., et al. 1988b. Alternating-day cyclosporin and prednisone for treatment of high-risk chronic graft-v-host disease. *Blood 72*:555-561.

Syrjala, K.L., Chapko, M.K., Vitaliano, et al. 1993. Recovery after allogeneic marrow transplantation: prospective study of predictors of long-term physical and psychosocial functioning. *BMT 11*:319-327.

Szeluga, D.J., et al. 1987. Nutritional support of bone marrow transplant recipients: a prospective, randomized clinical trial comparing total parenteral nutrition to an enteral feeding program. *Cancer Res 47*:3309-3316.

Terasaki, P.I., McClelland, J.D. 1964. Microdroplet assay of human serum cytotoxins. *Nature 204*:998-1000.

Thomas, E.D., et al. 1957. Intravenous infusion of bone marrow in patients receiving radiation and chemotherapy. *N Engl J Med 257*:491-496.

Thomas, E.D., et al. 1975. Bone marrow transplantation. *N Engl J Med 292*:832-843, 895-902.

Thomas, E.D., et al. 1977. One hundred patients with acute leukemia treated by chemotherapy, total body irradiation and allogeneic marrow transplantation. *Blood 49*:511-533.

Thomas, E.D., Storb, R. 1970. Techniques for human marrow grafting. *Blood 36*:507-515.

van Bekkum, D.W., de Vries, J.J. 1967. *Radiation Chimeras.* London: Logos.

Vogelsang, G.B., et al. 1987. Thalidomide therapy of chronic graft-versus-host disease. *Blood 70*:1116.

Weiden, P.L., Flournoy, N., Thomas, E.D. 1979. Antileukemic effect of graft-versus-host disease in human recipients of allogeneic marrow grafts. *N Engl J Med 300*:1068-1073.

Weiden, P.L., et al. 1981. Antileukemic effect of chronic graft-verus-host disease. *Med Intelligence 304*:1529-1533.

Weisdorf, S.A., et al. 1983. Graft-versus-host disease of the intestine: a protein losing enteropathy characterized by fecal alpha-1-antitrypsin. *Gastroenterology 85*:1076-1081.

Weisdorf, S.A., et al. 1987. Positive effect of prophylactic total parenteral nutrition on long-term outcome of bone marrow transplantation. *Transplantation 43*:833-838.

Wingard, J.R. 1994. Functional ability and quality of life of patients after allogeneic marrow transplantation: factors affecting social and occupational functions: strategies to improve social and job reintegration. *BMT 14*:S29-S33.

Wingard, J.R., et al. 1988. Cytomegalovirus infection after autologous bone marrow transplantation with comparison to infection after allogeneic bone marrow transplantation. *Blood 71*:1432-1437.

Wingard, J.R., et al. 1990. Cytomegalovirus infections in patients treated by intensive cytoreductive therapy with marrow transplant. *Rev Infect Dis 12*(suppl 7): 805-810.

Wingard, J.R., et al. 1991. Health, functional status, and employment of long-term survivors after bone marrow transplantation. *Ann Intern Med 114*:113-118.

Wingard, J.R., et al. 1992a. Bone marrow transplantation: a form of adoptive immunotherapy. In Mitchell, M.D. (Ed.) *Biological Approaches to Cancer Treatment: Biomodulation.* New York: McGraw-Hill, 554-573.

Wingard, J.R., Curbow, B., Baker, F., et al. 1992b. Sexual satisfaction in survivors of bone marrow transplantation. *BMT 9*:185-190.

Winston, D.J., et al. 1979. Infectious complications of human bone marrow transplantation. *Medicine 58*:1-31.

Winston, D.J., et al. 1980. Cytomegalovirus infections associated with leukocyte transfusions. *Ann Intern Med 93*:671-675.

Winston, D.J., et al. 1993. Ganciclovir prophylaxis of cytomegalovirus infection and disease in allogeneic bone marrow transplant recipients. *Ann Intern Med 118*:179-184.

2

Hematopoiesis

Debra Wujcik

Hematopoiesis, or blood cell production, is a complex, multistep process. The formation of blood cells begins in fetal life. By the 20th week of fetal development, the bone marrow is producing the cellular components of the blood in the liver, marrow, and spleen. By the 7th month, the bone marrow is the primary site of blood formation and remains so throughout life. The products of hematopoiesis, red blood cells, leukocytes, and platelets, are essential for life.

Bone marrow transplantation (BMT) is a treatment for malignant and nonmalignant conditions that replaces diseased or treatment-damaged marrow. The patient receives high doses of chemotherapy and/or total body irradiation followed by a rescue with pluripotent stem cells. The chemoradiotherapy produces severe and prolonged pancytopenia and the effects are lethal without stem cell reconstitution. Engraftment of the new stem cells, evidenced by peripherally circulating neutrophils, can take from a few days after a peripheral blood cell transplant to many weeks after a transplant from a human-leukocyte-antigen–matched but unrelated donor. Antibiotics, growth factors, and transfusion support are all critical during this time.

To understand the complications and outcomes of transplantation, the nurse must first understand normal hematopoiesis. Upon that

base, the implications of obtaining stem cells from a variety of sources can be understood. The issue of stem cells obtained from the bone marrow versus blood continues to be investigated.

HEMATOPOIESIS: STRUCTURE AND PROCESS

Hematopoiesis is the formation and development of the various blood cells from the pluripotent stem cell. This process includes proliferation, differentiation, and maturation of cells (Wujcik, 1992). *Proliferation* is simply the division of the cells to form two daughter cells. *Differentiation* consists of acquiring specialized functions and characteristics different from the immature cell. *Maturation* refers to the cell developing into a functionally active cell.

The classic depiction of blood cell growth is a treelike cascade with orderly progression from immature to fully mature cells (see Figure 2.1). As more has been understood about hematopoiesis, additional cells and the proteins that direct this growth have been identified.

Blood-Forming Organs

Bone Marrow
The blood-forming organs include the bone marrow, spleen, and liver (Caudell and

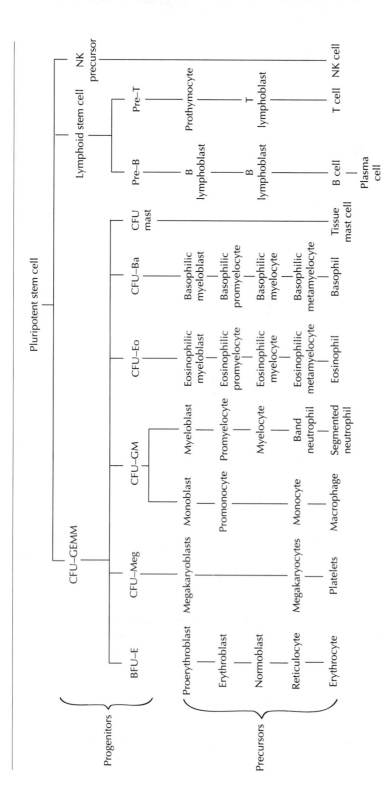

Figure 2.1 Growth of blood cells

SOURCE: Wujcik, D., 1997.

Whedon, 1991). The bone marrow milieu is a delicate balance of cells in various stages of development and sinusoidal spaces surrounded by the bone marrow stroma, a framework of supportive tissue. The bone marrow contains endothelial cells, fibroblasts, adipocytes, and macrophages and produces collagen and adhesive proteins. The immature cells adhere to the collagen and proteins while maturation and development occur. The growth and proliferation of the bone marrow cells are influenced by hematopoietic growth factors (HGF).

Hematopoiesis occurs in the flat bones including the sternum, ribs, skull, pelvis, shoulder, vertebrae, and inominates. The marrow capable of producing cells, or "red marrow," is found in the distal ends. With aging, inactive marrow is replaced by fatty tissue and is referred to as "yellow marrow." In times of increased demand for blood cells, the yellow marrow can again become active red marrow.

The bone marrow microenvironment can be damaged by chemotherapy and radiation. Successful engraftment of transplanted stem cells depends on the quality and quantity of stem cells and the integrity of the marrow's microenvironment (Charbord, 1994).

Spleen

The spleen contains both lymphoid and reticuloendothelial cells. The spleen has many functions which support hematopoiesis (Griffin, 1986). These include removing old and dead red blood cells (RBCs) and platelets, culling activity (removing particles from RBCs without injuring the cell), platelet storage, antigen filtration, and preparation of antigens for phagocytosis.

Liver

The liver contributes to hematopoiesis through production of fibrinogen, prothrombin, and other procoagulant and anticoagulant factors.

If needed, the liver can contribute to production of red blood cells (RBCs).

Blood Cells

Stem Cells

All production of blood cells begins with the pluripotent stem cell. The stem cells have the capacity for (1) self-renewal, (2) multilineage (both myeloid and lymphoid) differentiation, and (3) proliferation (Wujcik, 1995; Coiffier et al., 1994). The stem cell must be capable of reconstituting or repopulating the empty bone marrow with both myeloid and lymphoid cells (Spangrude, 1994). It is also characterized by renewal capability, producing two daughter cells, one capable of self-renewal and one committed to differentiating (Charbord, 1994). It is estimated that adult humans possess only 1×10^6 or 1×10^7 stem cells and about 5% of normal cells are needed to repopulate the marrow after transplant.

From the noncommitted, pluripotent state, the committed cells must differentiate, proliferate, and mature to fully functional "adult" cells. The earliest identifiable stem cell is the colony-forming unit blast cell (CFU-blast). This cell can differentiate to form mature cells in both the myeloid and lymphoid cell lines. This cell can also renew itself.

Progenitor

The first level of commitment to a cell line is the progenitor cell. The progenitors have limited proliferative capacity and are irreversibly committed to one of several lineages of differentiation.

Precursors

Precursors, or postprogenitors, are a heterogenous population and are committed to a single lineage. Some have proliferative capacity, some are becoming morphologically recognizable, and some are mature, fully functional end cells.

Mature Cells

Fully mature cells can carry out specific functions (see Table 2.1). Leukocytes, or white blood cells (WBC), fight infection, red blood cells carry oxygen, and platelets assist with hemostasis. Some cells complete maturation in the bone marrow (neutrophils), some in circulating blood (erythrocytes), and others in the tissue (macrophages). Granulocytes comprise 50% to 70% of the WBC count. The body's main defense against bacterial infection is provided by granulocytes, which include neutrophils, eosinophils, and basophils.

Neutrophils

Neutrophils are the most numerous of the granulocytes, constituting 50% to 70% of the circulating WBCs. The maturation of the neutrophil in the bone marrow occurs over 10 to 11 days (Wujcik, 1992). During the first 4 to 5 days, cellular division takes place as the myeloblast matures into a promyelocyte, then a myelocyte. At the metamyelocyte level, the cells lose their ability to divide but continue to mature. Once matured, the neutrophil is released into the peripheral blood. About one half of the released neutrophils circulate freely for 6 to 8 hours (circulating pool), then migrate into tissue. The rest of the neutrophils adhere to vessel walls (marginating pool). Three times as many neutrophils are stored in the bone marrow as are circulating peripherally. This keeps a neu-

TABLE 2.1 Normal blood cells

Blood cell	Normal cells/mm³	Percentage of WBC	Function
Neutrophil	3000–6000	50–70	Phagocytizes bacteria
Eosinophil	150–300	1–4	Phagocytizes parasites and fungus
Basophil	0–100	0.05	Elevated in asthma, allergies
Monocytes/Macrophages	300–600	6–8	Fights fungal, protozoan, parasitic infections
B Lymphocytes	200–1200	9	Provides humoral immunity
T Lymphocytes	800–3600	26	Provides cellular immunity
Helper/inducer			Assists B-cell production of antibodies
Cytotoxic			Recognizes and binds to antigens
Suppressor			Inhibits B and T lymphocyte functions
T memory			Produces memory effect
Erythrocytes			Transport oxygen for tissue oxygenation
Male	4.6–6.2 million		
Female	4.1–5.4 million		
Thrombocytes	150,000–350,000		Assists with hemostasis

trophil pool in reserve for immediate release in an event of injury.

Neutrophils are also referred to as *segs* (segmented neutrophils) and *polys* or *PMNs* (polymorphonuclear granulocytes). These mature cells contain neutrophilic granules, which attack and destroy bacteria. They are the first and most numerous cells to arrive at an area of disease or tissue injury. The neutrophils are attracted to microorganisms through a process of chemotaxis.

Eosinophil

Eosinophils are a second type of granulocyte that comprise 2% to 4% of the circulating WBCs. The colony-forming unit-eosinophil (CFU-EO) is the committed progenitor and the precursors are the eosinophilic myeloblast, promyelocyte, and myelocyte. Eosinophils also circulate freely for a short time (about 8 hours) before migrating into tissue to ingest bacteria and modulate the inflammatory response. Eosinophils generally increase in response to parasitic infections. In addition, eosinophils inactivate mediators released from mast cells during allergic reactions (Caudell and Whedon, 1991).

Basophil

Basophils divide and mature in the same pattern as the other granulocytes. The progenitor is the colony-forming unit-basophil (CFU-B) and the precursors are basophilic myeloblast, promyelocyte, myelocyte, metamyelocyte, and mature basophil. Basophils contribute to hypersensitivity reactions by releasing heparin, histamine, and other substances contained in their granules when stimulated. Basophils comprise only 0.05% of circulating WBCs and levels are increased in patients with asthma, allergies, and some types of cancers. Activated basophils release histamine, bradykinin, and serotonin.

Monocyte/Macrophages

The progenitor colony-forming unit-granulocyte-macrophage (CFU-GM) produces both neutrophils and macrophages. The earliest precursor is the monoblast, then promonocytes and monocytes. The mature monocyte circulates longer than the granulocyte (1 to 3 days) before migrating into the tissue. The monocyte transforms to a macrophage in the tissue and contributes to nonspecific immunity against fungal, protozoan, and parasitic infections. Monocytes comprise 6% to 8% of circulating WBCs.

Erythrocytes

The progenitor for the erythrocyte is the burst-forming unit-erythrocyte (BFU-E). The precursor proerythroblast and erythroblast continue to divide. Proliferative ability is lost at the next level, the normoblast. The slightly immature erythrocyte, the reticulocyte, is released to the bloodstream for final maturation over 1 to 2 days. The mature erythrocyte carries oxygen to tissue and removes carbon dioxide via the hemoglobin molecule. The normal range of RBCs in men is 4.6 to 6.2 cells/mm^3 and in women is 4.2 to 5.4 cells/mm^3 (DiJulio, 1991).

Thrombocytes

Thrombocytes protect from uncontrolled bleeding by releasing platelets that form plugs at the site of bleeding. In addition, thrombocytes facilitate conversion of fibrinogen to fibrin to initiate clotting. The progenitor is the colony-forming unit-megakaryocyte (CFU-MEG) and the precursors are megakaryoblasts and megakaryocytes. Mature thrombocytes circulate for 7 to 8 days in the bloodstream. The normal platelet count is 150,000 to 350,000 cells/mm^3.

Lymphocytes

Lymphocytes arise from the lymphoid stem cell. The T- and B-cell lineages develop differently. Pre-T lymphocytes migrate to the thymus for maturation from prothymocytes, to lymphoblasts, and then T lymphocytes. T lymphocytes provide cellular immunity that cannot be transferred in plasma. The major functions of T lymphocytes are protection against viruses and fungi, mediation of cutaneous delayed hypersensitivity, rejection of transplanted organs, immunological surveillance against cancer cells, and modulation of the overall immune response with helper or suppressor cells.

There are four subsets of T cells that participate in many phases of the immune response. Helper/inducer cells secrete lymphokines to assist B-lymphocytic production of an antibody (Ab). Cytotoxic cells, stimulated by helper T lymphocytes, recognize and bind to cells with altered self antigens (Ag) or various antigen and release mediators that cause altered cells to lyse or kill target cells. Suppressor cells inhibit or down regulate immune functions of both T and B lymphocytes. They are responsible for tolerance to a self antigen as well. The other subset, T memory cells, is responsible for the memory effect for future responses.

Pre-B lymphocytes migrate to various lymphatic tissue such as the spleen and lymph nodes to mature. B lymphocytes provide humoral immunity or immunity transferrable by serum. When the B lymphoblast is stimulated by an antigen, the antigen-antibody binding produces mature B lymphocytes. Final maturation of the B lymphocyte results in a plasma cell that secretes a specific antibody called *immunoglobulin*. Humoral immunity involves two systems: antibody and complement.

Homeostasis

Homeostasis is maintained when cellular death is equivalent to cellular production. Under normal conditions, the bone marrow produces 2.5 billion RBCs, 2.5 billion platelets, and 1.0 billion granulocytes per kilogram per day (Erslev et al., 1983). The rates can increase five- to tenfold when altered by stress, infection, hem-orrhage, and bone marrow injury or depletion. This balance is maintained by an interaction between the hematopoietic stem cells, the supportive structure of the bone marrow (stroma), and cells that regulate growth.

HEMATOPOIETIC GROWTH FACTORS

A complex feedback system controls the entire process of hematopoiesis. This system consists of proteins produced by T lymphocytes, monocytes, and stromal cells called hematopoietic growth factors (HGF). The HGFs regulate blood cell production by stimulating cells to divide and mature in a systematic manner. These same proteins are released during inflammatory and specific immune responses. A number of HGFs have been identified and their actions continue to be described (Table 2.2).

The original molecules described were named colony-stimulating factors (CSFs) due to the mature colonies formed in response to the growth factor (Wujcik, 1995). The first CSFs identified were granulocyte CSF (G-CSF), granulocyte-macrophage CSF (GM-CSF), and monocyte CSF (M-CSF). Interleukin-3 (IL-3) was identified as a multipotential CSF. These cells are now referred to as HGFs. Some HGFs are available commercially and are administered to overcome the effects of chemotherapy. A growing list of molecules that influence hematopoietic cells are called *interleukins* (ILs). The ILs stimulate both multipotent progenitors and lineage-restricted precursors and communicate among white cells (Sharp, 1995) (Table 2.3).

Classification of Hematopoietic Growth Factors

Lineage Specific

The classification of HGFs is based on the type of mature cells that grow in the colonies in

TABLE 2.2 Hematopoietic growth factors

FDA status	HGF	Generic name (trade name)	Effect on hematopoiesis	FDA indication
Approved	Erythropoietin	epoetin-alfa (Epogen®, Procrit®)	Stimulates maturation of red blood cells	Treatment of anemia due to cancer chemotherapy
	Granulocyte-colony-stimulating factor	filgrastim (Neupogen®)	Stimulates proliferation and differentiation of neutrophils and affects functional activity of mature cells	Decrease infections in patients with non-myeloid malignancies
	Granulocyte macrophage-colony-stimulating factor	sargramostim (Leukine®, Prokine®)	Stimulates proliferation and differentiation of multilineage colonies (neutrophils, eosino-phils, macrophages)	Accelerate myeloid recovery in selected patients undergoing autologous BMT
Investigational	Monocyte-colony-stimulating factor	molgrastim (Leucomax®, Macstim®, Macrolin®)	Proliferates and activates monocytes	
	Interleukin-3		Acts at level of CFU-GEMM	
	Stem cell factor		Acts at level of pluri-potent stem cell	
	Thrombopoietin		Matures megakaryocytes	

TABLE 2.3 Role of interleukins in hematopoiesis

Interleukin (IL)	Biological function related to hematopoiesis
IL-1	Activates resting T cells and macrophages, enhances NK cells and inflammatory response
IL-2	Proliferates all subpopulations of T cells; enhances NK cells
IL-3	Stimulates proliferation at level of CFU-GEMM
IL-4	Stimulates activated B cells, resting T cells; stimulates activated macrophages
IL-5	Induces B-cell differentiation; induces eosinophil differentiation
IL-6	Differentiates myeloid cells; differentiates B cells and plasma cells
IL-7	Supports the growth of B-cell precursors
IL-8	Aids neutrophil function in phagocytosis
IL-9	Stimulates helper T cell growth
IL-10	Suppresses helper T cells
IL-11	Affects early progenitor cells
IL-12	Stimulates cytotoxic T cells

SOURCE: Data from Sharp, E., 1995.

response to the HGF (Wujcik, 1995). HGFs that influence production and growth of one cell line are called lineage specific. For example, erythropoietin only stimulates production and maturation of erythrocytes. G-CSF influences only neutrophils.

Multilineage

Other HGFs are multilineage, affecting several cell lines. GM-CSF stimulates production of granulocytes and macrophages. IL-3 may stimulate RBCs, granulocytes, and platelets. Multilineage HGFs affect pluripotent and progenitor cells and lineage-specific HGFs act on more mature precursors.

Biologic Activity of HGFs

Mechanism of Action

Each blood cell has receptors on the cellular surface that receive one or more specific HGF. Direct and indirect actions occur when the HGF binds to the cell's surface receptors (Crosier and Clark, 1992). The HGF may signal the cell to divide or mature. An indirect effect occurs when the binding of the HGF with the cell causes the release of another protein product. For example, GM-CSF causes maturation and division of granulocytes and macrophages. In addition, there is release of macrophages, tumor necrosis factor, and gamma interferon. These secondary cytokines are responsible for the fever and chills experienced when endogenous GM-CSF is administered. The HGFs act as signals between cells. They are called *pleiotropic* because they have different actions in different cells. In addition, the action of HGF may inhibit or precipitate the action of another cytokine or HGF in a cascade effect.

These three HGFs have FDA approval for clinical use to treat symptoms related to chemotherapy. Both G and GM-CSF have specific indications for patients undergoing transplantation. There is shorter time to neutrophil recovery, fewer infections, and fewer hospital days in patients receiving G or GM-CSF after BMT. In addition, both are used to mobilize peripheral progenitor cells for blood cell transplantation (BCT) (Singer, 1992).

Granulocyte Colony-Stimulating Factor

Granulocyte colony-stimulating factor is produced by monocyte-macrophages, endothelial cells, and fibroblasts. G-CSF stimulates the proliferation and differentiation of neutrophils. In addition, G-CSF affects the functional activity of mature cells in response to bacteria. There is enhancement of several infection-fighting processes: phagocytosis, cellular metabolism, antibody-dependent killing, and antigen processing.

Administration of G-CSF is indicated for patients receiving myelosuppressive chemotherapy. G-CSF, administered 24 hours after chemotherapy, stimulates more rapid recovery of neutrophils. There may be an early rise in the neutrophil count as the reserve neutrophils are released from the marrow. The stimulation by the G-CSF causes increased cellular division and more rapid maturation of cells. Studies have shown tendencies toward shorter hospital stays and fewer days of fever in patients receiving autologous BMT and G-CSF (Sheridan et al., 1990). G-CSF is also used to increase levels of circulating committed progenitor cells. Exogenous administration of growth factors provides a fairly predictable response both in timing and numbers of cells (Sheridan et al., 1989).

Granulocyte-Macrophage Colony-Stimulating Factor

Granulocyte-macrophage colony-stimulating factor stimulates the division and maturation of multilineage colonies, specifically neutrophils, eosinophils, and macrophage progenitor cells. In vitro, there is evidence of stimulation of megakaryocyte and erythroid precursor cells.

GM-CSF also affects the functional activity of mature neutrophils, macrophages, and eosinophils. GM-CSF is secreted by many cellular sources, including T lymphocytes, monocytes, fibroblasts, and endothelial cells.

The first approved HGF for patients undergoing autologous BMT was GM-CSF, specifically for patients with non-Hodgkin's lymphoma, Hodgkin's lymphoma, or acute lymphocytic leukemia. The nadir phase is decreased from 18 to 12 days when GM-CSF is administered after BMT (Nemunaitis et al., 1990; Nemunaitis et al., 1988). In addition, patients receiving GM-CSF after BMT have fewer days of fever, decreased numbers of platelet transfusions, and fewer days of hospitalization (Aurer et al., 1990). Another application for GM-CSF is in patients who are experiencing graft failure after BMT and elderly patients with acute myeloid leukemia (AML) (Nemunaitis et al., 1990).

Erythropoietin

Erythropoietin (EPO) selectively acts upon the erythroid progenitor cells to stimulate maturation of the RBCs. Endogenous EPO is produced in response to decreased oxygenation in the kidneys. As the anemic blood circulates through the kidneys, EPO is released by renal tubules. The protein travels to the BM and stimulates the BFU-E to proliferate and differentiate. The role of exogenous EPO in patients undergoing transplantation continues to be investigated since the response to EPO is seen 2 to 6 weeks after beginning therapy (Metcalf and Morstyn, 1991).

Other Hematopoietic Growth Factors

Many other HGFs have been identified and described. Their role in patients undergoing transplantation is yet to be defined. IL-3 is a multilineage HGF that acts on the earliest progenitors. IL-3 acts on the CFU-GEMM and ap-

pears to be a more potent stimulator of megakaryopoiesis (platelet production) than any other HGF (Lindemann and Martelsmann, 1993). Stem cell factor (SCF) interacts with the most primitive cells and when used in combination with other HGFs, supports growth of all colonies of cells (Henon, 1993a). Macrophage CSF (M-CSF) is another lineage-specific HGF that supports proliferation and activation of monocytes and their committed progenitors. M-CSF is being evaluated in BMT patients for effectiveness in treating fungal infections refractory to amphotericin B therapy (Nemunaitis et al., 1993). Finally, thrombopoietin is another promising HGF. This factor has demonstrated activity in megakaryocyte maturation and platelet production and holds promise as an effective agent to improve platelet recovery after transplantation (Banu et al., 1994).

IMMUNITY

Immunity is characterized as a series of events that protect the body against foreign substances (Griffin, 1986; Gallucci and McCarthy, 1995; Claman, 1992). To be effective, the immune system must recognize proteins, viruses, bacteria, and parasites that are not part of the body's normal environment, and it must subsequently destroy the invaders. A great deal of immunity is acquired in childhood. By the time a child enters school, he or she has a mature immune system responding to infection, preserving the internal environment through removal of dead and damaged cells, and providing surveillance against malignant cells.

The immune system consists of both natural (nonspecific) and acquired (specific) immunity. White blood cells are the cells that provide immunity. Granulocytes (neutrophils, eosinophils, and basophils), monocytes, and their tissue complements provide nonspecific immunity while lymphocytes are responsible for specific immunity. Both nonspecific and specific immunity are altered by the effects of conditioning chemotherapy and total body irradiation. These treatments alter all normal defenses against infection for months to several years.

Natural Nonspecific Defenses

Natural, nonspecific immunity matures over a lifetime of exposure to antigens. These natural defenses include intact barriers (skin and mucosa), inflammatory response, acidic environment of the stomach, preformed antibodies from the biological mother, and the cleansing effect of tears and saliva. In addition, WBCs provide the ability for phagocytosis.

Inflammatory Response

Inflammation is a series of sequential changes in the tissues in response to injury. The injury causes release of chemical mediators such as histamine, bradykinin, and serotonin. There is "walling off" of tissue spaces as lymphatics are blocked due to fibrinogen clots. This delays spread of bacteria or toxins.

Next, the neutrophils leave the bloodstream and flow along the vessel to the site of inflammation. The cells then begin to adhere to the surface of endothelial cells (margination). The neutrophils, which are very loose and flexible, begin to penetrate between the cells into tissue (diapedesis). By following the chemical signals, the cells migrate to the site of infection (chemotaxis). Neutrophils begin invading organisms, killing them with intracellular peroxide and superoxide. The neutrophils continue to ingest and digest the organisms until toxic substances from the digestive process kill the neutrophils or depletes them of essential enzymes. This is usually after each neutrophil has engulfed from 5 to 25 bacteria.

Neutrophils accumulate at the site of injury or infection. They are quickly replaced by monocytes residing in the tissue called *macro-*

phages. These macrophages are found as histiocytes in subcutaneous tissue, alveolar tissue in lungs, Kupffer cells in the liver, and glial cells in the brain. They are the cells able to respond during the first hour of injury.

The monocytic response to infection is a slower but longer, continuing process. Monocytes migrate to the site and in 8 to 12 hours swell and mature into macrophages. The macrophages then phagocytose and digest the dead neutrophils. After several days, a cavity is formed in the inflamed tissue. The cavity contains necrotic tissue, dead neutrophils, and macrophages, and causes pus to form. The monocytes process the antigen they phagocytose and present it to the other WBCs such as lymphocytes. This processed antigen can stimulate specific immunity. Monocytes bridge the gap between a nonspecific and specific immunity. If the nonspecific immunity fails, the acquired specific defense, also called adaptive immunity, is enlisted.

Acquired Specific Host Defenses

Acquired immunity requires recognition of foreign substances and a memory response. To be effective, this system must also identify and tolerate its own cells and their products. Lymphocytes are responsible for recognizing antigens and inducing specific host defenses. Lymphocytes have surface molecules called *cluster of differentiation (CD) antigens*. These CD markers allow identification of subtypes of lymphocytes.

Cell-Mediated Immunity

B lymphocytes are precursors of the antibody-secreting T lymphocyte, the plasma cell. Antibodies are released from the plasma cell. The function of the plasma cells is to secrete immunoglobulin (Ig) or antibodies. Plasma cells are formed when groups of antigen-specific B lymphocytes or clones respond to the presence of antigens. Antigen specificity is determined by a receptor site on the B lymphocyte's membrane. Each plasma cell produces only one type of antibody. Other activated B lymphocytes remain quiescent and turn into memory cells.

The primary response to the antigen takes 4 to 10 days. The first antibody formed is immunoglobulin M (IgM). As the response continues, IgM matures and ultimately produces IgG. The secondary response is also called the *memory response* and is much faster with antibodies produced within 1 to 2 days and the antibody titre increased up to 50 times that of the primary response.

Humoral Immunity

Humoral immunity is provided through antigen-antibody (Ag-Ab) reactions and the complement system. The antigen-antibody response causes death of the antigens through one or more processes. The first is precipitation. The insoluble antibodies, in combination with the soluble antigens, lead to precipitation of the complex. A clump is formed that is quickly destroyed through phagocytosis. *Agglutination* is the process whereby an antigen attaches itself to particulate matter and the antigen-antibody complexes form clumps. This is the process during a transfusion reaction when the antigen-antibody reaction causes RBCs to clump. Neutralization occurs where the antibody neutralizes bacterial toxins. Finally, *opsonization* is the reaction between antigen and antibody that causes the antigen to become sticky, which makes it easier for phagocytes to engulf them.

The *complement system* is a series of enzymatic reactions resulting in antigen destruction of antigens by lysis. *Complement* is an encompassing term for 11 serum proteins circulating in inactive forms. The complement protein recognizes and binds with a specific antibody. The antigen is coated with immunoglobulin, which complement recognizes as a red flag. The antibody destroys any cell marked with the immunoglobulin. The complement response hinges on the ability to recognize self. Once the body identifies self as foreign, the complement system mechanism can be catastrophic. For example, in graft-versus-host disease (GVHD), this process can be life threatening. The complement system serves to bridge the two interdependent processes, cellular and humoral immunity.

IMPACT OF TRANSPLANTATION ON HEMATOPOIESIS

Transplantation is performed for malignant and nonmalignant conditions to replace a defective marrow or a marrow that has been damaged by treatment. The patient receives high-dose chemotherapy and/or total body irradiation which destroys (ablates) myeloid and lymphoid cells. All protection against infection and immunity is removed. The patient is "rescued" with bone marrow or blood stem cells. These stem cells are able to repopulate the marrow quickly, allowing immediate recovery from the severe myelosuppression. The stem cells also provide for long-term engraftment evidenced by the onset of hematopoietic recovery within 21 days after marrow infusion (Orlic and Bodine, 1994). Repopulation should be established between 21 and 35 days.

IDENTIFICATION OF CELLS FOR TRANSPLANTATION

Physical properties distinguish stem cells needed for transplantation from others contained in the marrow and blood. A number of quantitative assays are used to identify and isolate these primitive hematopoietic cells based on their physical characteristics (Sacher, 1993; Eaves and Eaves, 1994; Di Nicola et al., 1993).

Colony-Forming Units-Spleen

The first method to measure the number of pluripotent cells in the marrow was the spleen colony assay. In the early 1960s, McCulloch and Till (1960) described the ability of injected bone marrow cells to form colonies in the spleens of mice that had received lethal doses of irradiation. For the next 30 years, this colony-forming unit-spleen (CFU-S) assay was used as an indicator of stem cell frequency in infused cell suspensions. These cells are useful for preventing postengraftment infections and bleeding. However, these cells do not have long-term repopulating ability and are not the cells responsible for long-term engraftment. Thus the CFU-S does not identify the "true" stem cell (McNiece and Briddell, 1994).

From this beginning, a number of other systems have been developed to identify the various subpopulations of hematopoietic cells. Cell culture assays were developed in animal models, then adapted for human cells (Messner and McCullough, 1994). Semisolid culture mediums are used to identify clones of progenitor cells at levels of differentiation (McNiece and Briddell, 1994). The most immature population of cells that can be identified by this method is denoted CFU-BLAST. These colonies give rise to cells with blast morphology (shapes). The CFU-BLAST cells, if left to grow in culture, develop into megakaryocytes, erythrocytes, and granulocytes in 6 to 8 weeks. These cells can be cloned to form exact colonies, but do not have the same indefinite self-renewal ability (McNiece and Briddell, 1994).

Competitive Repopulating Unit

The competitive repopulating unit (CRU) is an in vivo assay to identify cells that are each able to regenerate at least 5% of the entire hematopoietic system. In addition, these cells must sustain cell production for at least 6 months (Eaves and Eaves, 1994).

Long-Term Culture-Initiating Cells

Cells in colonies that give rise to mature cells after an interval of as many as 5 to 8 weeks in marrow culture systems are called long-term culture-initiating cells (LTC-IC) (Orlic and Bodine, 1994). The LTC-ICs can be used with both marrow and blood stem cells and are also called long-term marrow culture (LTMC) (Kessinger, 1993a; Eaves and Eaves, 1994; Charbord, 1994).

High-Proliferative Potential Cultures

High-proliferative potential cultures measure cells between LTC-IC and assays for CFU-GM, CFU-E, CFU-GEMM. They are considered to be very primitive cells (Charbord, 1994). Stem cell factor was described using HPPC assays.

CD34-Positive Cells

Another method to distinguish cell populations relies on staining cell surface molecules with a monoclonal antibody linked to fluorescent dyes. These cluster differentiation (CD) antigens and the monoclonal antibodies that attach to them are assigned CD numbers. For example, CD5 marks both T and B lymphocytes; CD1, CD3, and CD7 are markers only for T lymphocytes; CD21, CD22, CD37, and CD40 are associated only with B lymphocytes.

The CD34 assay is the most common way to identify cells for engraftment (Bensinger, 1994; Hogge et al., 1993; Shpall et al., 1993). The stem cells are found in the mononuclear fraction of the marrow suspension and their morphology resembles "blast" cells. The CD34 marker was identified when a monoclonal antibody was developed against a leukemia cell line, separating cells that could give rise to all hematopoietic colonies.

Within the CD34-positive cells there is a subpopulation that has the property of self-renewal (Berenstein et al., 1991). It is estimated that the actual number of "true stem cells" ranges from 1×10^4 to 2×10^5 cells. Efforts continue to separate the rich subpopulations such as lineage-negative (lin– cells), cells in G_o phase, and others. CD34-positive cells are present in fetal cord blood and in low concentrations in normal peripheral blood (Bender et al., 1994). In addition to using CD34 assays to identify cells for a transplant, these cells are being manipulated ex vivo to increase their numbers. Expansion of small populations of cells could decrease the number of phereses required or could make specific cells available for therapeutic gene transfer (Brugger et al., 1993).

CD34 antigens are not found on breast tumors, neuroblastoma, lymphoma, and multiple myeloma cells (Shpall et al., 1994). In theory, stem cell isolates from these patients should be free of tumor contamination. In other words CD34-positive selection should deplete cancer cells from the marrow or peripheral blood (Berenson, 1993). However, the purity of the cells is not complete. For example, one third of the cells collected using a common system, the Avidin-biotin system, are neither stem cell nor progenitors (Bensinger, 1994). In addition, the CD34 antigen is also expressed in certain types of leukemia cells. Efforts continue to identify ways to purify marrow and blood cells from patients with leukemia (Berenson, 1993). The measurement of CD34-positive cells is used mostly when obtaining stem cells from peripheral blood.

Number of Stem Cells

There are a number of devices for stem cell separation (Bensinger, 1994). The fluorescence-activated cell sorter (FACS) sorts out cells labeled with an anti-CD34 antibody. Cell loss with this machine exceeds 50%. Immunorosetting methodology with red cells, floating beads, or magnetic beads is used to manipulate marrow cells. The manipulation can be purging stem cells of T lymphocytes or tumor cells, or indirectly removing nonprogenitor cells.

Immunoabsorption uses a protein (Avidin) and vitamin (biotin) for stem cell isolation. This process typically recovers only 30% to 60% of the CD34-positive cells originally present (Bensinger, 1994). All methods currently being used have problems with variability and reproducibility (Valbonesi, 1993).

There are several potential benefits of obtaining pure or enriched stem cells either from blood or marrow:

1. increased numbers of the stem cells needed for successful allografts,
2. decreased contamination with cancer cells,
3. decreased number of leukophereses needed to obtain the desired quantity of cells, and
4. use of the cells as a vehicle to introduce new or modified genes for genetic engineering (Gale et al., 1994).

SOURCE OF CELLS FOR TRANSPLANTATION

Bone marrow transplantation has been used as a treatment for some diseases for more than 30 years. Stem cells for transplantation can be obtained from an HLA-matched related or unrelated donor (allogeneic) or from self (autologous). The stem cells can be harvested from the marrow for a bone marrow transplant or from the blood for a blood cell transplant.

Bone Marrow

Allogeneic BMT

Marrow for an allogeneic BMT can be obtained from an identical twin, an HLA-matched related donor (usually a sibling), or an HLA-matched unrelated donor (Beatty and Anasetti,

1990; Bortin et al., 1992). The marrow stem cells are harvested in the operating room usually while the patient is under general anesthesia (Buckner et al., 1984). The mixture obtained contains marrow stem cells and some peripheral blood. Between 50 and 100 aspirations are needed from both iliac crests to obtain sufficient cells for a transplant. The required dose is usually equal to 10 ml/kg of the recipient's body weight or between 400 and 600 ml and accounts for about 5% of the body's marrow pool (Meagher and Herzig, 1993). The marrow is placed in a heparinized tissue culture medium, filtered to remove bone and fat particles, then processed for administration.

Autologous BMT

Autologous BM is obtained when the patient is in remission. The procedure is the same as for allogeneic BMT but the donor is also the recipient. If there is a possibility of malignant cells remaining in the marrow, it can be purged using chemotherapeutic drugs or immune modulation. The marrow is processed in the laboratory, then frozen in a preservative, dimethyl sulfoxide (DMSO). Viability of stem cells can be maintained even after years in storage in liquid nitrogen (Kessinger, 1993a). The preservative prevents cell lysis when the marrow is later thawed at the bedside.

Blood Cells

Since the mid 1980s, peripheral blood has been used as a source of cells for transplantation in humans. The terminology for transplants using cells obtained from peripheral blood is evolving. *Peripheral blood stem cell transplant (PBST)* is a general term that refers to a transplant of an unspecified number of true pluripotent cells, with or without committed progenitor cells and precursor cells (Craig et al., 1995; Coiffier et al., 1994). The term *blood cell*

transplant (BCT) is considered more precise and preferred to PBSC transplant. *BCT* is analogous to *BMT*.

Autologous BCT

Peripheral blood stem cells represent from 1% to 10% of marrow progenitors. The number of cells can be increased rapidly, up to 500 fold through use of HGFs (Sacher, 1993). BCT is replacing autologous BMT due to lower morbidity and more rapid hematologic recovery (Coiffier et al., 1994). Neutrophil recovery is more rapid with BCT than BMT although platelet recovery is not consistent (Gale et al., 1994). It is not clear whether stem cells collected from the blood have the same characteristics as those found in the marrow (Lowry and Tabbara, 1992; Hogge et al., 1993). Immediate hematologic recovery after BCT is influenced by prior damage to bone marrow, cryopreservation of the cells, and the method used to mobilize the blood cells (Coiffier et al., 1994).

To increase the number of CD34-positive cells collected for BCT, a process of mobilization is used. Chemotherapy, HGFs, or a combination of both are used to produce a temporary increase in the number of peripheral progenitor cells (To, 1994; Berenstein et al., 1991). The cells are harvested through one or more leukophereses sessions, processed, and frozen. The cells are reinfused after cytotoxic chemotherapy has been administered.

Blood cell transplant is a useful option when the possibility of marrow involvement precludes autologous BMT. In addition, harvesting blood cells does not require general anesthesia so may have fewer complications than harvesting marrow. Also, studies have now documented the more rapid recovery of neutrophils and platelets when progenitor cells are used (Sheridan et al., 1990; Sacher, 1993). Currently, autologous BCT is indicated for some patients with acute myelogenous leukemia, low-grade non-Hodgkin's lymphoma, multiple myeloma, some solid tumors, and even chronic myelogenous leukemia (Henon, 1993b).

A number of issues concerning BCT remain unresolved. One is whether these blood-derived cells can restore long-term hematopoiesis. Clinicians question whether the cells needed for rapid engraftment after BCT have been identified. Current data suggests engraftment endures at least 5 years after BCT (Gale et al., 1994). Although the type and number of these cells remain controversial, the apparent success of BCT indicates the cells needed for long-term engraftment are present (Kessinger, 1993b; Bender et al., 1992). Investigators continue to strive to predict accurately the number of CD34-positive cells needed for engraftment (Urashima et al., 1993).

Allogeneic BCT

Harvesting blood stem cells from allogeneic donors is undergoing active investigation. At times they are used to enhance effectiveness of the allogeneic BMT. BCT has also been used when the matched related donor is unable to have the bone marrow harvested due to medical conditions. In the future, donors may prefer leukopheresis to surgery for harvest of cells (Gale et al., 1994).

Umbilical Cord Blood

Another source of stem cells for transplantation is human umbilical cord blood. The majority of these transplants to date have been from HLA-matched siblings. Because the fetal immune system is not developed, there is little allorecognition and GVHD expected. This means cord blood may be a very desirable option for unrelated and mismatched transplants (Miniero et al., 1993). Another source of fetal stem cells being investigated is the liver of fetuses aborted

during the first trimester (Westgren et al., 1994). It has been demonstrated that if the cord is clamped within 20 seconds of delivery, the number of CFU-GM harvested is adequate for transplant in adults weighing 50 to 70 kilograms (Bertolini et al., 1993).

The results of these transplants is being closely documented and monitored by a registry of international cord blood transplantation (Gluckman et al., 1993). There are immense ethical considerations related to the use of fetal tissue and umbilical stem cells for transplantation (Lind, 1994).

PATIENT EDUCATION RELATED TO HEMATOPOIESIS

Education of patients undergoing BMT and BCT is individualized, progressive, and continuous (Buchsel, 1993). The first step in obtaining informed consent for transplantation is to provide information about the process, the expected complications, and the outcomes. The nurse must be knowledgeable about the various types of transplants, the sources of stem cells, and the indications for a transplant specific to the type and stage of disease.

The patient with a hematologic disorder such as acute leukemia will have had chemotherapy prior to being considered for BMT or BCT. Teaching will build on prior education related to myelosuppression after chemotherapy (Wujcik, 1993). The added component will be the impact of immune suppression in addition to myelosuppression (Lum, 1990). This means the patient will be more susceptible to viral and fungal infections for an extended period of time (6 months to several years). Some patients undergoing BMT may not have had such intensive therapy, such for patients with chronic-phase CML. These patients need more extensive teaching that includes normal hematopoiesis, the defect due to the disease, and the effects of both immunosuppression and myelosuppression.

The transplant nurse progressively builds on a base of knowledge. This begins with normal blood cell production and the function of WBCs, RBCs, and platelets. Then the expected impact of transplant is described. The nurse uses clinical expertise to prepare the patient for the expected length and severity of myelosuppression related to the type of transplant. The patient must learn strategies for self-care along with the interventions the transplant team will use to minimize the complications of neutropenia, thrombocytopenia, and anemia. Finally, the nurse reviews the procedure for obtaining and infusing the cells for transplant.

REFERENCES

Aurer, I., Ribas, A., Gale, R., et al. 1990. What is the role of recombinant colony-stimulating factors in bone marrow transplantation? *BMT* 6:79-87.

Banu, N., Deng, B., Wang, J., et al. 1994. Modulation of megakaryocytopoiesis by human c-Mpl ligand. *Blood* 84:390 (abstr).

Beatty, P.G., Anasetti, C. 1990. Marrow transplantation from donors other than HLA-identical siblings. *Hematol Oncol Clin North Am* 4:677-688.

Bender, J.G., To, L.B., Williams, S., Schwartzberg, L.S. 1992. Defining a therapeutic dose of peripheral blood stem cells. *J Hematother* 1(4):329-341 (review).

Bender, J.G., Unverzagt, K., Walker, D.E., Lee, W., Smith, S., Williams, S., Van Epps, D.E. 1994. Phenotypic analysis and characterization of CD34-positive cells from normal human bone marrow, cord blood, peripheral blood, and mobilized peripheral blood from patients undergoing autologous stem cell transplantation. *Clin Immunol Immunopathol* 70(1):10-18.

Bensinger, W. 1994. Isolating stem and progenitor cells. *Blood Stem Cell Transplants*. New York: Cambridge University Press, 32-42.

Berenson, R. 1993. Human stem cell transplantation (review). *Leuk & Lymphoma* 11(suppl 2):137-139.

Berenstein, I.D., Andrews, R.G., Zsebo, K.M. 1991. Recombinant human stem cell factor enhances the formation of colonies by CD34-positive and CD34-positive lin– cells, and the generation of colony-forming progeny from CD34-positive lin– cells cultured with interleukin-3 (IL-3), granulocyte-macrophage colony-stimulating factor (GM-CSF), or granulocyte-colony stimulating factor (G-CSF). *Blood* 77:2316-2321.

Bertolini, F., Lazzari, L., Corsini, C., Lauri, E., Gorini, F., Sirchia, G. 1993. Cord blood banking for stem cell transplant. *Int J Artif Organs* 16(suppl 5):111-112.

Bortin, M.M., Horowitz, M.M., Rimm, A.A. 1992. Increasing utilization of allogeneic bone marrow transplantation. *Ann Intern Med* 116:505-512.

Brugger, W., Mocklin, W., Heimfeld, S., Berenson, R.J., Mertelsmann, R., Kanz, L. 1993. Ex vivo expansion of enriched peripheral blood CD34-positive progenitor cells by stem cell factor, interleukin-1 beta (IL-1beta), IL-6, IL-3, interferon-gamma, and erythropoietin. *Blood* 81(10):2579-2584.

Buchsel, P.C. 1993. Bone marrow transplantation. In Groenwald, S. L. Frogge, M.H. Goodman, M. Yarbro C.H. (Eds.) *Cancer Nursing: Principles and Practice.* Boston: Jones & Bartlett, 393-434.

Buckner, C.D., Clift, R.A., Sanders, J.E., et al. 1984. Marrow harvesting from normal donors. *Blood* 64:630-634.

Caudell, K.A., Whedon, M.B. 1991. Hematopoietic complications. In Whedon, M.B. (Ed.) *Bone Marrow Transplantation: Principles, Practice, and Nursing Insights.* Boston: Jones & Bartlett, 135-159.

Charbord, P. 1994. Hemopoietic stem cells: analysis of some parameters critical for engraftment. *Stem Cells* 12:545-562.

Claman, H. 1992. The biology of the immune response. *JAMA* 268(20):2790-2796.

Coiffier, B., Philip, T., Burnett, A.K., et al. 1994. Consensus conference on intensive chemotherapy plus hematopoietic stem cell transplantation in malignancies, Lyon, June 4–6, 1993. *Ann Oncol* 5(1):19-23.

Craig, J.I.O., Turner, M.L., Parker, A.C. 1995. Peripheral blood stem cell transplantation. *Blood Rev* 6(2):59-67.

Crosier, P., Clark, S. 1992. Basic biology of the hematopoietic growth factors. *Semin Oncol* 19(4):349-361.

DiJulio, J. 1991. Hematopoiesis: an overview. *Oncol Nurs Forum* 15:325-330.

Di Nicola, M., Siena, S., Bregni, M., et al. 1993. Quantization of CD34-positive peripheral blood hematopoietic progenitors for autografting in cancer patients. *Int J Artif Organs* 16(suppl 5):80-82.

Eaves, C.J., Eaves, A.C. 1994. Stem and progenitor cells in the blood. *Blood Stem Cell Transplants*. New York: Cambridge University Press, 20-31.

Erslev, A.J., Weiss, L. 1983. Structure and function of marrow. In Williams, W. Beutler, E, Erslev, A.J. (Eds.) *Hematology.* New York: McGraw-Hill, 75-81.

Gale, R.P., Henon, P., Juttner, C.A. 1994. Overview of blood stem cell transplants. *Blood Stem Cell Transplants.* New York: Cambridge University Press, 1-5.

Gallucci, B.B., McCarthy, D. 1995. The Immune System. In Rieger, P.T. (Ed.) *Biotherapy: A Comprehensive Overview.* Boston: Jones & Bartlett, 15-42.

Gluckman, E., Wagner, J., Hows, J., et al. 1993. Cord blood banking for hematopoietic stem cell transplantation: an international cord blood transplant registry. *BMT 11*(3):199-200.

Griffin, J.P. 1986. Immunity. In Griffin, J.P. (Ed.) *Hematology and Immunology for Nurses.* Norwalk, CT: Appleton-Century-Crofts, 41-54.

Henon, P.R. 1993a. Peripheral blood stem cell transplantation: critical review. *The Int J Artif Organs 16*: 64-70.

Henon, P.R. 1993b. Peripheral blood stem cell transplantations: past, present and future (review). *Stem Cells 11*(3):154-172.

Hogge, D.E., Sutherland, H.J., Lansdrop, P.M., et al. 1993. The elusive peripheral blood hemopoietic stem cell. *Semin Hematol 30*(4, suppl 4):82-91.

Kessinger, A. 1993a. Utilization of peripheral blood stem cells in autotransplantation. *Hematol Oncol Clin North Am 7*(3):535-545.

Kessinger, A. 1993b. Is blood or bone marrow better? (review). *Stem Cells 11*(4):290-295.

Lind, S.E. 1994. Ethical considerations related to the collection and distribution of cord blood stem cells for transplantation to reconstitute hematopoietic function (review). *Transfusion 34*(9):828-834.

Lindemann, A., Martelsmann, R. 1993. Interleukin-3: structure and function. *Cancer Invest 11*(5):609-623.

Lowry, P., Tabbara, A. 1992. Peripheral hematopoietic stem cell transplantation: current concepts. *Exp Hematol 20*:937-942.

Lum, L.G. 1990. Immune recovery after bone marrow transplantation. *Hematol Oncol Clin North Am 4*(3): 659-675.

McCulloch, E.A., Till, J.E. 1960. The radiation sensitivity of normal mouse bone marrow cells, determined by quantitative marrow tranplantation into irradiated mice. *Radiat Res 13*:115-125.

McNiece, I.K., Briddell, R.A. 1994. Primitive hematopoietic colony-forming cells with high proliferative potential. In Freshney, R.I., Pragnell, I.B., Freshney,

M.G. (Eds.) *Culture of Hematopoietic Cells.* New York: Wiley, 23-39.

Meagher, R.C., Herzig, R.H. 1993. Techniques of harvesting and cryopreservation of stem cells. *Hematol Oncol Clin North Am 7*(3):501-533.

Messner, H.A., McCullough, E.A. 1994. Mechanisms of human hematopoiesis. In Forman, S.J., Blume, K.G., Thomas, E.D. (Eds.) *Bone Marrow Transplantation.* Boston: Blackwell Scientific, 41-54.

Metcalf, D., Morstyn, G. 1991. Colony-stimulating factors: general biology. In DeVita, V., Hellman, S., Rosenberg, S. (Eds.) *Biologic Therapy of Cancer.* Philadelphia: Lippincott, 417-444.

Miniero, R., Ramenghi, U., Crescenzio, N., et al. 1993. Umbilical cord blood stem cell transplantation. *Int J Artif Organs 16*(suppl 5):113-115.

Nemunaitis, J., Singer, J., Buckner, C. 1988. Use of recombinant human granulocyte-macrophage colony-stimulating factor in autologous marrow transplantation for lymphoid malignancies. *Blood 72*(2):834-836.

Nemunaitis, J., Singer, J., Buckner, C., et al. 1990. Use of recombinant human granulocyte-macrophage colony-stimulating factor in graft failure after bone marrow transplantation. *Blood 76*(1):245-253.

Nemunaitis, J., Meyers, J., Buckner, C., et al. 1993. Phase I/II trial of recombinant human macrophage colony-stimulating factor (M-CSF) in patients with invasive fungal infection. *Proc Am Soc Clin Oncol 12*:159.

Orlic, D., Bodine, D.M. 1994. What defines a pluripotent hematopoietic stem cell (PHSC): will the real PHSC please stand up! *J Am Soc Hematol 84*(12):3991-3994.

Sacher, R.A. 1993. Bone marrow and stem cell transplantation—where are we going? *Semin Hematol 30*(4, suppl 4):130-133.

Sharp, E. 1995. The Interleukins. In Rieger, P.T. (Ed.) *Biotherapy: A Comprehensive Overview.* Boston: Jones & Bartlett, 93-111.

Sheridan, W., Morstyn, G., Wolf, M., et al. 1989. Granulocyte-colony-stimulating factor and neturophil recovery after high-dose chemotherapy and bone marrow transplantation. *Lancet 2*(8668):891-895.

Sheridan, W., Juttner, C., Szer, J., et al. 1990. Granulocyte-colony-stimulating factor (G-CSF) in peripheral blood stem cell (PBSC) and bone marrow (BM) transplantation. *Blood 76*(5):565.

Shpall, E.J., Jones, R.B., Bearman, S.I., et al. 1993. Positive selection of CD34-positive hematopoietic progenitor cells for transplantation. *Stem Cells 11*(suppl 3):48-49.

Shpall, E.J., Jones, R.B., Bearman, S.I., et al. 1994. Transplantation of enriched CD34-positive autologous marrow into breast cancer patients following high-dose chemotherapy: influence of CD34-positive peripheral-blood progenitors and growth factors on engraftment. *J Clin Oncol* 12(1):28-36.

Singer, J. 1992. Role of colony-stimulating factors in bone marrow transplantation. *Semin Oncol* 19(3): 27-31.

Spangrude, G.J. 1994. Biological and clinical aspects of hematopoietic stem cells (review). *Ann Rev Med 45*: 93-104.

To, L.B. 1994. Mobilizing and collecting blood stem cells. *Blood Stem Cell Transplants*. New York: Cambridge University Press, 56-74.

Urashima, M., Uchiyama, H., Hoshi, Y., et al. 1993. Prediction of engraftment after peripheral blood stem cell transplantation by CD34-positive cells in grafts. *Acta Paediatr Jpn 35*(4):325-331.

Valbonesi, M. 1993. Hemopoietic stem cells: technical and methodological considerations (review). *Stem Cells 11*(suppl 3):58-63.

Westgren, M., Ek, S., Bui, T.H., et al. 1994. Establishment of a tissue bank for fetal stem cell transplantation. *Acta Obstet Gynecol Scand 73*(5):385-388.

Wujcik, D. 1992. Overview of colony-stimulating factors: focus on the neutrophil. *A Case Management Approach to Patients Receiving G-CSF 1*(1):8-13.

Wujcik, D. 1997. Leukemia. In Groenwald, S.L., Frogge, M.H., Goodman, M., Yarbro, C.H. (Eds.) *Cancer Nursing: Principles and Practice,* 2d ed. Boston: Jones & Bartlett.

Wujcik, D. 1995. Hematopoietic growth factors. In Rieger, P.T. (Ed.) *Biotherapy: A Comprehensive Overview*. Boston: Jones & Bartlett, 113-133.

3

Transplant Immunology
HLA and Issues of Stem Cell Donation

Janet Hegland

Sixty-five to seventy percent of patients with diseases potentially curable by bone marrow transplantation are deprived of use of this modality because of lack of a human leukocyte antigen (HLA)-compatible marrow donor in their family. (Perkins and Hansen, 1994)

The human leukocyte antigen (HLA) system in humans distinguishes, from an immunological standpoint, foreign pathogens and tissue from self. In this capacity, the system plays a major role in the immunologic regulation of allogeneic (between two members of the same species) bone marrow transplantation. A key factor to the success of an allogeneic bone marrow transplant is the ability to closely match the patient and the donor for a group of proteins found on the surface of most of the cells of the body. These proteins are called human leukocyte antigens or HLAs. HLA typing (or tissue typing, as it is commonly called) includes a number of tests to determine the histocompatibility, or "sameness," of the tissue of two individuals.

THE HUMAN LEUKOCYTE ANTIGEN SYSTEM

The discovery of the HLA system began in the late 1930s when English pathologist, Peter Gorer, discovered that each individual expresses a variety of markers on the surface of most of his or her cells, which differentiate individuals of the same species from one another. Because these markers determined tissue compatibility, they were termed *histocompatibility molecules*. Later, in the mid 1950s, antibodies known to clump white blood cells (leukoagglutinating antibodies) were found in the sera of both multiply transfused patients and in 20% to 30% of multiparous women. The importance of matching these antigens for success in organ transplantation was soon realized and provided an impetus for studying the genes that determine human leukocyte antigens.

Nomenclature

In 1968 the HLA Nomenclature Committee, formed under the auspices of the World Health Organization (WHO), recommended a universal HLA nomenclature system to replace the various local terminologies used to name HLA antigens. Modifications of this original system have evolved to the two HLA nomenclature systems in use today (Figure 3.1). The serologic nomenclature system was established in 1984 to describe serologically characterized HLA antigens. The molecular nomenclature system was established in 1987 to describe HLA alleles

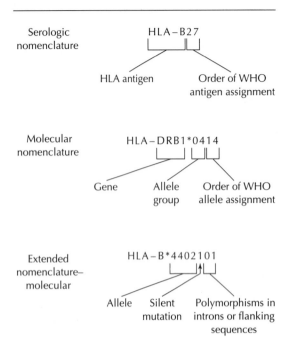

Serologic nomenclature — HLA–B27
- HLA antigen
- Order of WHO antigen assignment

Molecular nomenclature — HLA–DRB1*0414
- Gene
- Allele group
- Order of WHO allele assignment

Extended nomenclature– molecular — HLA–B*4402101
- Allele
- Silent mutation
- Polymorphisms in introns or flanking sequences

Figure 3.1 WHO nomenclature for HLA

*This names areas of defined noncoding sequences.

(alternative forms of an HLA gene) defined by nucleotide sequencing. Both systems are used internationally by scientists, laboratories, and clinicians when referring to components of the HLA system.

Human leukocyte antigens following the serologic nomenclature system are described by listing the HLA molecule or gene product (HLA-A, -B, -C, -DR, -DQ, -DP) first, followed by a number, assigned sequentially according to the order of discovery. Historically, HLA-A and -B were considered one group of antigens and were combined in the assignment of sequential numbers. For example, HLA-A1 was the first HLA-A antigen recognized by the WHO Nomenclature Committee and HLA-A28 was the 28th antigen recognized. More recently, since the advent of DNA-based HLA

typing procedures, new serologic HLA specificities are named according to their associated HLA allele rather than being numbered sequentially. For example, HLA-A*210 is the antigen expressed by the HLA allele, HLA-A*0210. Table 3.1 presents antigens officially recognized by WHO.

HLA antigens found on a single HLA molecule (and no others) are called *private antigens.* In contrast, HLA *public antigens* are antigenic determinants or epitopes common to several HLA molecules, each of which also bears a distinct HLA private antigen. HLA-Bw4 and -Bw6 are the best known examples of HLA public antigens. We all type positive for one or both of these HLA public antigens in addition to typing positive for our respective HLA-B private antigens. The distribution of HLA-Bw4 and -Bw6 is shown in Table 3.2. When we match a donor and a patient for HLA-B private antigens, we are, by default, matching the public antigens. Consequently, the public antigens HLA-Bw4 and -Bw6 are not usually considered independently in matching patients and donors.

In several instances, an HLA that was initially thought to be a single private antigen was later found to be a group of two or more closely related antigens, each of a narrower specificity. These closely related antigens are called *splits* of the original broad-specificity antigen. Relationships of split antigens to older, broadly defined serologic specificities are shown in parentheses in Table 3.1. For example, HLA-A68(28) and HLA-A69(28) antigens are splits of the broad antigen, HLA-A28. When we match a donor and patient for split antigens, we are, by default, matching the broad specificity. However, if we only match the broad specificity, then the donor and recipient may express different splits, possibly resulting in a mismatch for that gene product. It is therefore important to have the HLA typing laboratory type for the split rather than the broad specificities.

TABLE 3.1 Serologic HLA specificities recognized by WHO

A	B	B *(cont.)*	C	DR	DQ
A1	B5	B51(5)	Cw1	DR1	DQ1
A2	B7	B5102	Cw2	DR103	DQ2
A203	B703	B5103	Cw3	DR2	DQ3
A210	B8	B52(5)	Cw4	DR3	DQ4
A3	B12	B53	Cw5	DR4	DQ5(1)
A9	B13	B54(22)	Cw6	DR5	DQ6(1)
A10	B14	B55(22)	Cw7	DR6	DQ7(3)
A11	B15	B56(22)	Cw8	DR7	DQ8(3)
A19	B16	B57(17)	Cw9(w3)	DR8	DQ9(3)
A23(9)	B17	B58(17)	Cw10(w3)	DR9	
A24(9)	B18	B59		DR10	
A2403	B21	B60(40)		DR11(5)	
A25(10)	B22	B61(40)		DR12(5)	
A26(10)	B27	B62(15)		DR13(6)	
A28	B35	B63(15)		DR14(6)	
A29(19)	B37	B64(15)		DR1403	
A30(19)	B38(16)	B65(14)		DR1404	
A31(19)	B39(16)	B67		DR15(2)	
A32(19)	B3901	B70		DR16(2)	
A33(19)	B3902	B71(70)		DR17(3)	
A34(10)	B40	B72(70)		DR18(3)	
A36	B4005	B73			
A43	B41	B75(15)		DR51	
A66(10)	B42	B76(15)		DR52	
A68(28)	B44(12)	B77(15)		DR53	
A69(28)	B45(12)	B77(15)			
A74(19)	B46	B7801			
	B47				
	B48	Bw4			
	B49(21)	Bw6			
	B50(21)				

SOURCE: Data from Bodmer, J.G., et al. 1992. Nomenclature for factors of the HLA system, 1991. In Tsuji, T., Aizawa, M., Sasazuki, T. (Eds.) *HLA 1991*. Oxford: Oxford University Press, 17-31.

HLA private antigens can be organized into groups based on apparent serologic cross-reactivity among members of the same group. These groups are called *cross-reactive groups (CREGS)*. Table 3.3 lists the common cross-reactive groups. It is believed that the basis for the cross-reactivity is a public HLA antigen common to all members of the CREG. In the area of allogeneic marrow transplantation, it has been generally assumed that if a mismatch must occur between a donor and a recipient because of lack of a perfectly matched donor,

TABLE 3.2 Distribution of HLA-B public antigens

Public antigen	Associated private antigens
Bw4	B5, B5102, B5103, B13, B17, B27, B37, B38(16), B44(12), B47, B49(21), B51(15), B52(5), B53, B57(17), B58(17), B59, B63(15), B77(15), A9, A23(9), A24(9), A2403, A25(10), A32(19)
Bw6	B7, B703, B8, B14, B18, B22, B35, B39(16), B3901, B3902, B40, B4005, B41, B42, B45(12), B46, B48, B50(21), B54(22), B55(22), B56(22), B60(40), B61(40), B62(15), B64(14), B67, B70, B71(70), B72(70), B73, B75(15), B76(15), B7801

SOURCE: Adapted from Dupont, B., Yang, S.Y. 1994. *Histocompatibility*. In Forman, S.J., Blume, K.G., Thomas, E.D. (Eds.) *Bone Marrow Transplantation*. Cambridge, MA: Blackwell Scientific Publications, 37. Used with permission.

TABLE 3.3 Cross-reactive antigen groups

A LOCUS

1.	A1	A3	A11	A36		
2.	A9	A23	A24			
3.	A10	A25	A26	A34	A66	A43
4.	A19	A29	A30	A31	A32	A33	A74
5.	A2	A28	A68	A69		

B LOCUS

1.	B5	B18	B35	B51	B52	B53	B70	B71	B72			
2.	B12	B21	B44	B45	B49	B50						
3.	B14	B64	B65									
4.	B8	B59										
5.	B15	B17	B46	B57	B58	B62	B63	B70	B71	B72	B75	B76	B77
6.	B16	B38	B39	B67								
7.	B37											
8.	B7	B27	B42	B73								
9.	B7	B22	B54	B55	B56	B67						
10.	B7	B40	B41	B48	B60	B61						
11.	B13	B47										

that matching within the same cross-reactive group (i.e., a minor mismatch) would be preferred to a mismatch outside the CREG (i.e., a major mismatch). This assumption is now being challenged based on the availability of DNA-based HLA typing methods. These methods can discern actual structural differences between two mismatched HLA molecules based on the differences between the nucleotide sequence of the two defined alleles.

The molecular HLA Nomenclature System describes the HLA allele that encodes the expressed HLA molecule. The HLA gene (HLA-A, -B, -C, -DRB1, -DRB3, -DRB4, -DRB5, -DQB1, -DQA1, -DPB1, -DPA1) is followed by an asterisk, then the allele. The first two digits of the allele generally correspond to the serologically characterized antigen or group of antigens encoded by the allele with which it shares structural similarities. The third and fourth digits are assigned sequentially, in order of discovery. For example, the allele

DRB1*0414 is the fourteenth allele described of the DRB1*04 allele group. Tables 3.4 and 3.5 list the HLA alleles currently recognized by WHO. The large number of alleles in this table is evidence of the extreme polymorphism (or many forms) of the HLA system. In fact, this list is constantly being updated as new alleles are discovered.

The molecular HLA Nomenclature System has recently been extended to include fifth,

TABLE 3.4 HLA DNA-based nomenclature for class I alleles

A*0101	A*2601	B*0702	B*1520	B*3802	B*4801	Cw*0101	Cw*1504
A*0102	A*2602	B*0703	B*1521	B*39011	B*4802	Cw*0102	Cw*1505
A*0201	A*2603	B*0704	B*1522	B*39013	B*4901	Cw*0201	Cw*1601
A*0202	A*2604	B*0705	B*1523	B*39021	B*5001	Cw*02021	Cw*1602
A*0203	A*2901	B*0801	B*1524	B*39022	B*5101	Cw*02022	Cw*1603
A*0204	A*2902	B*0802	B*1525	B*3903	B*5102	Cw*0302	Cw*1701
A*0205	A*3001	B*1301	B*1801	B*3904	B*5103	Cw*0303	
A*0206	A*3002	B*1302	B*1802	B*3905	B*5104	Cw*0304	
A*0207	A*3003	B*1303	B*2701	B*39061	B*5105	Cw*0401	
A*0208	A*3004	B*1401	B*2702	B*39062	B*52011	Cw*0402	
A*0209	A*3005	B*1402	B*2703	B*3907	B*52012	Cw*0501	
A*0210	A*31011	B*1501	B*2704	B*40011	B*5301	Cw*0602	
A*0211	A*31012	B*1502	B*27052	B*40012	B*5401	Cw*0701	
A*0212	A*3201	B*1503	B*27053	B*4002	B*5501	Cw*0702	
A*0213	A*3301	B*1504	B*2706	B*4003	B*5502	Cw*0703	
A*0214	A*3302	B*1505	B*2707	B*4004	B*5601	Cw*0704	
A*0215N	A*3303	B*1506	B*2708	B*4005	B*5602	Cw*0801	
A*0216	A*3401	B*1507	B*2709	B*4006	B*5701	Cw*0802	
A*0217	A*3402	B*1508	B*3501	B*4007	B*5702	Cw*0803	
A*0301	A*3601	B*1509	B*3502	B*4101	B*5703	Cw*1201	
A*0302	A*4301	B*1510	B*3503	B*4102	B*5801	Cw*12021	
A*1101	A*6601	B*1511	B*3504	B*4201	B*5802	Cw*12022	
A*1102	A*6602	B*1512	B*3505	B*4402	B*5901	Cw*1203	
A*2301	A*68011	B*1513	B*3506	B*4403	B*67011	Cw*1301	
A*2402	A*68012	B*1514	B*3507	B*4404	B*67012	Cw*1401	
A*2403	A*6802	B*1515	B*3508	B*4405	B*7301	Cw*1402	
A*2404	A*6901	B*1516	B*3509	B*4406	B*7801	Cw*1403	
A*2405	A*7401	B*1517	B*3510	B*4501	B*8101	Cw*1501	
A*0406	A*8001	B*1518	B*3701	B*4601		Cw*1502	
A*2501		B*1519	B*3801	B*4701		Cw*1503	

Source: Adapted from Bodmer, J.G., Marsh, S.G., Albert, E.D., et al. Nomenclature for factors of the HLA system, 1995. *Tissue Antigens* 46:1-18. Used with permission.

TABLE 3.5 HLA DNA-based nomenclature for class II alleles

DRA*0101	DRB1*0421	DRB1*1314	DRB1*0811	DQB1*0603	DPB1*1601
DRA*0102	DRB1*0422	DRB1*1315	DRB1*09011	DQB1*0604	DPB1*1701
	DRB1*11011	DRB1*1316	DRB1*09012	DQB1*06051	DPB1*1801
DRB1*0101	DRB1*11012	DRB1*1317	DRB1*1001	DQB1*06052	DPB1*1901
DRB1*0102	DRB1*1102	DRB1*1318		DQB1*0606	DPB1*20011
DRB1*0103	DRB1*1103	DRB1*1319	DRB3*0101	DQB1*0607	DPB1*20012
DRB1*0104	DRB1*11041	DRB1*1320	DRB3*0201	DQB1*0608	DPB1*2101
DRB1*1501	DRB1*11042	DRB1*1321	DRB3*0202	DQB1*0609	DPB1*2201
DRB1*15021	DRB1*1105	DRB1*1322	DRB3*0203	DQB1*0201	DPB1*2301
DRB1*15022	DRB1*1106	DRB1*1401	DRB3*0301	DQB1*0202	DPB1*2401
DRB1*1503	DRB1*1107	DRB1*1402		DQB1*0301	DPB1*2501
DRB1*1504	DRB1*11081	DRB1*1403	DRB4*0101101	DQB1*0302	DPB1*26011
DRB1*1505	DRB1*11082	DRB1*1404	DRB4*0101102N	DQB1*03032	DPB1*26012
DRB1*1601	DRB1*1109	DRB1*1405	DRB4*0102	DQB1*0304	DPB1*2701
DRB1*1602	DRB1*1110	DRB1*1406	DRB4*0103	DQB1*0305	DPB1*2801
DRB1*1603	DRB1*1111	DRB1*1407		DQB1*0401	DPB1*2901
DRB1*1604	DRB1*1112	DRB1*1408	DRB5*0101	DQB1*0402	DPB1*3001
DRB1*1605	DRB1*1113	DRB1*1409	DRB5*0102		DPB1*3101
DRB1*1606	DRB1*1114	DRB1*1410	DRB5*0103	DPA1*0103	DPB1*3201
DRB1*03011	DRB1*1115	DRB1*1411	DRB5*0201	DPA1*0104	DPB1*3301
DRB1*03012	DRB1*1116	DRB1*1412	DRB5*0202	DPA1*02011	DPB1*3401
DRB1*0302	DRB1*1117	DRB1*1413	DRB5*0203	DPA1*02012	DPB1*3501
DRB1*0303	DRB1*1118	DRB1*1414		DPA1*02021	DPB1*3601
DRB1*0304	DRB1*1119	DRB1*1415	DQA1*0101	DPA1*02022	DPB1*3701
DRB1*0305	DRB1*1120	DRB1*1416	DQA1*01021	DPA1*0301	DPB1*3801
DRB1*0401	DRB1*1121	DRB1*1417	DQA1*01022	DPA1*0401	DPB1*3901
DRB1*0402	DRB1*1122	DRB1*1418	DQA1*0103		DPB1*4001
DRB1*0403	DRB1*1201	DRB1*1419	DQA1*0104	DPB1*01011	DPB1*4101
DRB1*0404	DRB1*12021	DRB1*1420	DQA1*0201	DPB1*01012	DPB1*4401
DRB1*0405	DRB1*12022	DRB1*1421	DQA1*03011	DPB1*02011	DPB1*4501
DRB1*0406	DRB1*12031	DRB1*0701	DQA1*0302	DPB1*02012	DPB1*4601
DRB1*0407	DRB1*12032	DRB1*0801	DQA1*0401	DPB1*0202	DPB1*4701
DRB1*0408	DRB1*1301	DRB1*08021	DQA1*05011	DPB1*0301	DPB1*4801
DRB1*0409	DRB1*1302	DRB1*08022	DQA1*05012	DPB1*0401	DPB1*4901
DRB1*0410	DRB1*1303	DRB1*08031	DQA1*05013	DPB1*0402	DPB1*5001
DRB1*0411	DRB1*1304	DRB1*08032	DQA1*0502	DPB1*0501	DPB1*5101
DRB1*0412	DRB1*1305	DRB1*08041	DQA1*0503	DPB1*0601	DPB1*5201
DRB1*0413	DRB1*1306	DRB1*08042	DQA1*0601	DPB1*0801	DPB1*5301
DRB1*0414	DRB1*1307	DRB1*0805		DPB1*0901	DPB1*5401
DRB1*0415	DRB1*1308	DRB1*0806	DQB1*0501	DPB1*1001	DPB1*5501
DRB1*0416	DRB1*1309	DRB1*0807	DQB1*0502	DPB1*11011	DPB1*5601
DRB1*0417	DRB1*1310	DRB1*0808	DQB1*05031	DPB1*11012	DPB1*5701
DRB1*0418	DRB1*1311	DRB1*0809	DQB1*05032	DPB1*1301	DPB1*5801
DRB1*0419	DRB1*1312	DRB1*0810	DQB1*0504	DPB1*1401	
DRB1*0420			DQB1*06011	DPB1*1501	
			DQB1*06012		
			DQB1*0602		

SOURCE: Adapted from Bodmer, J.G., Marsh, S.G., Albert, E.D., et al. Nomenclature for factors of the HLA system, 1995. *Tissue Antigens* 46:1-18. Used with permission.

sixth, and seventh digits in the allele designation in order to describe additional polymorphisms. The fifth digit, called a *silent mutation* or *silent substitution,* differentiates two alleles that encode the same HLA molecule but have slightly different DNA sequences. The sixth and seventh digits were added to describe alleles whose DNA differences lie outside of their coding regions. An example of this extended nomenclature system is shown in Figure 3.1. The fifth, sixth, and seventh digits in an HLA type are not thought to be important from a clinical standpoint and do not need to be considered in matching donors and recipients.

Structure and Function of the HLA Complex

Many genes are involved in the development of the immune system. There is, however, a set of closely linked genes that play a unique role in regulating the body's immune responses to immunological challenges presented by invasion of foreign organisms or tissue, such as in bone marrow transplantation. This set of closely linked genes is called the *Major Histocompatibility Complex (MHC).* It is often simply referred to as the *HLA complex* or *region.*

The MHC can be divided into three main regions: HLA class I, HLA class II, and HLA class III. Figure 3.2 illustrates schematically the organization of the HLA complex. The first region, HLA class I, includes HLA*A, *B and *C genes. The HLA class II region includes HLA*DRB1, *DRB3, *DRB4, *DRB5, *DQA1, *DQB1, *DPA1, and *DPB1 genes. The third region, HLA class III, is not as well understood as the other regions. It includes genes encoding proteins with known immune functions, such as the genes for some of the serum complement components (e.g., C2, C4), as well as other genes whose functions are currently unknown. For the purposes of this chapter, the discussion will focus only on the HLA class I and class II regions.

The genes in the class I and class II regions of the HLA complex encode HLA molecules expressed on cell surfaces. Class I HLA molecules are found on all nucleated cells of the body. Class II HLA molecules are found mainly on immune cells such as B lymphocytes, macrophages/monocytes, and dendritic cells. The HLA class I and II molecules are structurally similar. In general, each consists of a U-shaped complex (forming an antigen-binding groove in which to hold peptides) pro-

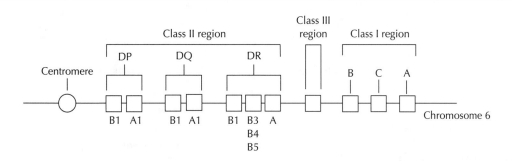

Figure 3.2 Organization of the HLA complex

truding from the cell membrane and a domain that crosses the cell membrane (Figure 3.3). The HLA molecule transports peptides, or small segments of protein, through the cell membrane for presentation in its binding groove to circulating T cells. The three-dimensional structure of class I and II HLA molecules is very important, because this structure defines how the HLA molecule interacts with the T cell.

The primary immunological function of HLA class I and II molecules is to present peptides to T cells for recognition. Most of the peptides are derived from the body's own proteins, but when the body is infected by an organism or foreign tissue is transplanted, the HLA molecules also pick up peptides derived from the broken-down proteins of the invader or foreign tissue. T cells are equipped with a receptor, referred to as the *T-cell receptor* (Figure 3.4), which recognizes a particular complex of HLA molecule plus peptide as self or nonself. It is believed that every antigen, foreign and self, is recognized by T cells only in conjunction with HLA molecules. T cells continually scan the surface of other cells, ignoring those displaying self peptides but locking on to those whose HLA molecules display non-self peptides. The T-cell receptor recognizes this assembly, the recognition activates lymphocytes and sets in motion a complex series of reactions aimed at destroying the invading cell and the foreign organism or tissue.

In the case of bone marrow transplant, host HLA molecules that have bound antigenic peptides elicit a response from the engrafted donor T cells, resulting in a graft-versus-host-disease (GVHD) reaction. In the other direction, when residual host T cells recognize the HLA molecules of the donor as foreign, the immune attack is then directed against the transplanted tissue, resulting in a process known as *rejection*. Rejection occurs far less frequently than GVHD in allogeneic bone marrow transplant because the pretransplant condi-

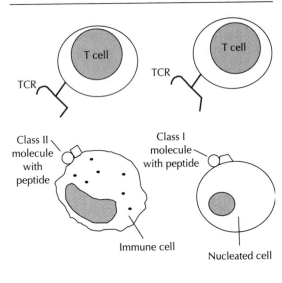

TCR = T–cell receptor

Figure 3.4 T-Cell recognition of processed antigen

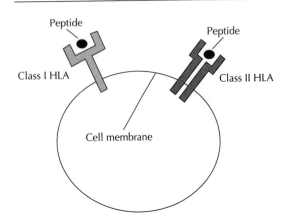

Figure 3.3 Class I and II HLA molecules

tioning regimen administered to the patient is intended to disable the marrow recipient's immune system.

Inheritance of HLA Types

The genes encoding HLA class I and II antigens are located very close to one another on the short arm of chromosome 6. These genes are tightly linked and inherited in blocks called *haplotypes.* A haplotype can be thought of as all the HLA genes inherited from one parent. An individual's HLA *phenotype,* the physical expression of his or her HLA type, is determined by both inherited haplotypes (Figure 3.5). All HLA genes are codominant, therefore both alleles of a given gene are expressed. Most people are heterozygous for each HLA gene, that is, they express two different HLA molecules or carry two different alleles for each gene (e.g., HLA-A2, A68). A person who inherits the same two alleles of a gene will be called homozygous for that gene (e.g., A2, A2).

Understanding the inheritance of HLA types is important when performing family typing studies to determine if there is a suitable marrow donor within the family. Each individual inherits one gene region or haplotype from his or her father and one from his or her mother. There are four possible haplotypes in each biological family (Figure 3.6). Consequently, each patient with a sibling has approximately a one in four chance (25%) that a sibling will have an identical HLA type, unless that sibling is an identical twin. In that case, the twin is a perfect genetic match for the patient. Marrow transplants performed using an identical twin as the donor are known as *syngeneic marrow transplants.*

In rare cases, the HLA genes can be separated by genetic recombination (i.e., crossover of genetic material between homologous chromosomes during meiotic division). This recombination occurs quite rarely (around 1% for

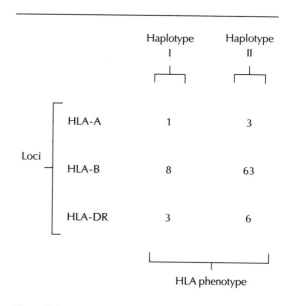

Figure 3.5 **Example of HLA phenotype**

HLA-A, -B), as established from testing large numbers of families. Recombination is evident when family typing studies are performed and greatly complicate the search for a marrow donor.

By mapping the HLA types of the parents and siblings, one can determine whether it is likely to find a match within the extended family by HLA typing grandparents, cousins, aunts, and uncles. Occasionally, a patient will possess one rare haplotype and one common haplotype. By tracing the origin of the rare haplotype, one can sometimes find a relative in the extended family who possesses the rare haplotype and by chance also possesses the common haplotype or at least shares some of the same common antigens within the common haplotype. When a match cannot be found within the immediate or extended family, patients and their families begin the search for an unrelated donor. That process is discussed later in this chapter.

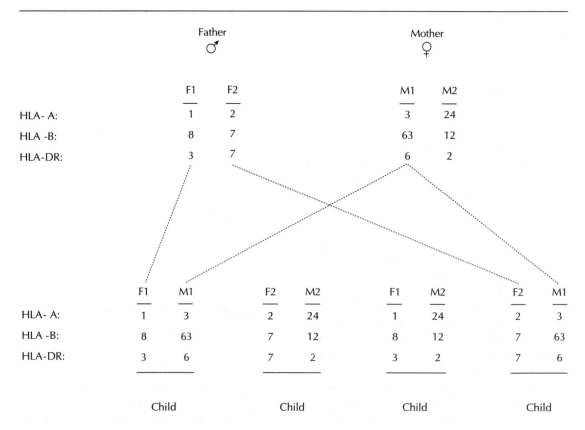

Figure 3.6 HLA inheritance

Certain combinations of HLA types are found more or less frequently than would be expected by random distribution. This phenomenon is known as *linkage disequilibrium*. Linkage disequilibrium can predict common combinations of HLA types. For example, the HLA type A1, B8, DR3 is a common HLA haplotype found in strong positive disequilibrium, meaning that it is found more frequently than would be expected by chance alone. If a donor were typed as A1, B8, it is quite likely that the HLA-DR type of that donor would be HLA-DR3 based on linkage disequilibrium. The cause of linkage disequilibrium is not known, but several hypotheses exist including a selective advantage of a given haplotype against disease, migration and admixture of two populations, and random drift of the gene pool.

Racial Distribution of HLA Types

It is frequently said that the best chance of finding a donor is to search within one's own race. In general, the frequency of specific HLA types differs or varies significantly among racial and ethnic groups, as does the pattern of linkage disequilibrium. Most HLA alleles occur in all ethnic groups, and only a very few, if any, HLA alleles are limited to a single ethnic group. The frequency of an HLA allele also varies within an ethnic group, sometimes depending on the geographic location of the population. Tables 3.6, 3.7, and 3.8 provide antigen frequencies by race, calculated from the donor registry of the National Marrow Donor Program (NMDP). From these tables, it is clear that some HLA types frequent within one race may be rare in other races.

HLA Typing

An individual's HLA type can be determined by using serological, cellular, and/or, molecular

TABLE 3.6 HLA Frequencies by race—locus A

HLA-A	African American	Asian/ Pacific Islander	Caucasian	Hispanic/Latino
1	6.1	5.2	15.3	7.6
2	19.7	24.7	28.6	28.6
3	8.9	2.9	13.6	8.4
9	13.7	22.8	11.4	16.5
10	7.5	6.4	6.4	5.1
11	1.6	17.5	6.2	4.9
19	30.2	18.4	14.0	19.8
23	10.6	0.4	1.9	3.0
24	3.1	22.4	9.5	13.6
25	0.5	0.1	2.2	1.2
26	3.0	4.8	4.0	3.4
28	10.3	2.0	4.5	8.9
29	3.4	1.3	3.6	4.6
30	13.8	2.5	2.6	4.8
31	1.8	3.5	2.8	4.8
32	1.7	1.2	3.8	2.8
33	7.2	9.9	1.2	2.7
34	3.8	1.5	0.2	0.5
36	1.9	0.0	0.0	0.2
43	0.0	0.0	0.0	0.0
66	0.2	0.0	0.0	0.1
68	9.1	1.7	4.2	8.1
69	1.2	0.3	0.3	0.8
74	2.3	.1	0.0	0.2
80	0.0	0.0	0.0	0.0

Note: Each broad antigen frequency is the sum of all its split antigens. Therefore, the frequencies within a race do not sum to 100%.

SOURCE: The National Marrow Donor Program, Minneapolis, Minnesota.

TABLE 3.7 HLA Frequencies by race—locus B

HLA-A	African American	Asian/ Pacific Islander	Caucasian	Hispanic/Latino
5	4.4	11.3	6.6	9.4
7	10.9	4.8	12.2	6.6
8	4.0	1.5	9.6	4.0
12	12.3	6.3	14.3	12.1
13	0.8	5.0	2.4	1.4
14	3.2	0.5	4.3	5.4
15	3.7	12.8	6.6	5.6
16	1.7	5.4	4.6	8.5
17	12.5	7.5	4.6	3.7
18	3.3	1.2	4.9	4.3
21	3.7	0.8	2.8	4.3
22	0.9	6.2	2.7	1.4
27	1.4	2.4	4.4	2.4
35	8.8	8.6	9.8	14.9
37	0.6	1.3	1.4	0.8
38	0.3	3.4	2.5	2.1
39	1.3	2.1	2.0	6.5
40	2.1	15.4	6.8	7.7
41	0.9	0.2	1.0	1.3
42	5.8	0.1	0.0	0.6
44	7.3	6.1	13.7	10.2
45	5.0	0.2	0.6	1.9
46	0.0	4.5	0.0	0.0
47	0.1	0.1	0.2	0.2
48	0.1	2.1	0.1	1.7
49	2.7	0.3	1.7	2.4
50	0.9	0.5	1.1	1.9
51	2.9	7.6	5.6	7.1
52	1.5	3.7	1.0	2.4
53	11.1	0.5	0.5	1.8
54	0.0	2.8	0.0	0.0
55	0.6	2.5	2.1	1.0
56	0.3	1.0	0.6	0.4
57	6.0	3.0	3.8	2.3
58	6.5	4.5	0.8	1.4
59	0.0	0.4	0.0	0.0
60	1.6	8.6	5.5	2.6
61	0.5	6.8	1.3	5.0
62	1.7	9.8	6.1	4.6
63	2.0	0.5	0.5	0.9
64	0.5	0.3	0.5	0.6

TABLE 3.7 *Continued*

HLA-A	African American	Asian/ Pacific Islander	Caucasian	Hispanic/Latino
65	2.7	0.3	3.8	4.8
67	0.0	0.2	0.0	0.0
70	7.5	1.0	0.4	1.8
71	1.1	0.4	0.1	0.5
72	6.4	0.5	0.2	1.3
73	0.0	0.0	0.0	0.0
75	0.0	2.2	0.0	0.1
76	0.0	0.1	0.0	0.0
77	0.0	0.1	0.0	0.0
78	0.2	0.0	0.0	0.0

Note: Each broad antigen frequency is the sum of all its split antigens. Therefore, the frequencies within a race do not sum to 100%.
SOURCE: The National Marrow Donor Program, Minneapolis, Minnesota.

TABLE 3.8 **HLA Frequencies by race—locus C**

HLA-A	African American	Asian/ Pacific Islander	Caucasian	Hispanic/Latino
1	7.2	3.6	11.2	8.7
2	16.3	18.7	15.4	11.4
3	13.4	4.9	11.0	8.0
4	5.7	15.4	16.9	20.7
5	17.1	16.9	12.5	10.6
6	19.1	14.2	14.8	17.8
7	10.1	7.7	13.4	10.7
8	6.3	6.7	2.9	9.8
9	2.9	9.6	1.1	1.1
10	1.9	2.5	0.9	1.4
11	12.0	4.7	10.3	8.3
12	5.2	12.2	2.2	2.3
13	17.1	7.3	11.9	10.9
14	2.0	6.9	2.9	6.9
15	15.2	17.2	14.4	9.0
16	1.2	1.5	0.9	2.4
17	7.0	4.8	10.8	7.0
18	6.4	0.1	0.3	1.0

Note: Each broad antigen frequency is the sum of all its split antigens. Therefore, the frequencies within a race do not sum to 100%.
SOURCE: The National Marrow Donor Program, Minneapolis, Minnesota.

(DNA-based) assays. Histocompatibility testing should only be carried out in an experienced laboratory that uses state-of-the-art reagents and methodologies and reports typing results according to the latest WHO Nomenclature report. The laboratory should be staffed with experts in the field of histocompatibility testing who understand the inheritance and distribution of HLA types as well as the currently accepted testing methodologies. Histocompatibility testing laboratories should be accredited by the American Society of Histocompatibility and Immunogenetics (ASHI). This organization inspects histocompatibility laboratories to ensure compliance with laboratory and testing standards established by ASHI and participation in external proficiency testing programs. These laboratories are an excellent resource for transplant nurses who have questions regarding a patient's HLA type or strategies to employ when searching for a marrow donor, either within the family or through unrelated donor registries.

Recently, the field of HLA typing has shifted from serologic and cellular-based typing methodologies to DNA-based methods. The difference between these approaches lies primarily with the determinant being characterized (Figure 3.7). In serologic methods, the HLA antigens expressed on the surface of white cells are identified by panels of antisera specific for HLA antigens, in much the same way that blood type antigens (ABO) expressed on the surface of red cells are identified in blood typing assays. By contrast, in DNA-based HLA typing methods, the target of identification is not the expressed HLA antigen, but rather the HLA allele that encodes the expression of those antigens. Figure 3.8 shows serologically defined HLA molecules and the corresponding genes identified by DNA-based typing methods.

There are several advantages to DNA-based HLA typing. The problems associated

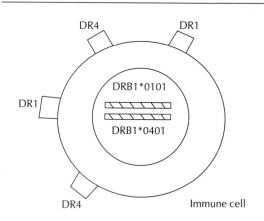

Figure 3.7   HLA typing uses antibodies or cellular reagents to identify HLA proteins (antigens) on the surface of the cell. DNA-based HLA typing identifies the gene that encodes the HLA antigens.

with serologic and cellular assays (including availability of quality typing reagents, poorly expressed antigens, low white cell count and cell viability—all of which profoundly impact the ability to define HLA types by serology or cellular methods) are eliminated with DNA-based methods. The accuracy of DNA-based typing methods far exceeds that which can be achieved by serologic or cellular assays. In addition, DNA-based typing methods can discern the primary structure of the HLA molecule, which is important in predicting how differences in HLA types will influence recognition of the HLA molecule by the T-cell receptor. A brief overview of each of the HLA typing methods in current use follows.

Serologic Methods

The standard method for serologic HLA typing has been the microcytotoxicity assay. In this

Serology	DR	DR52	DR53	DR51	DQ	DP	A	B	C
DNA	DRB1*	DRB3*	DRB4*	DRB5*	DQB1*	DPB1*	A*	B*	C*
					DQA1*	DPA1*			

Figure 3.8 Serology and DNA-based equivalents

NOTE: Outlined gene products are defined by cellular methods rather than by serology.

test, anti-HLA antibodies that are highly specific for different HLA antigenic determinants are used to characterize the patient's or donor's expressed HLA antigens. The microcytotoxicity assay requires live cells that express the target antigen. Sufficient numbers of these cells may be difficult to isolate from patients undergoing chemotherapy and/or radiation treatment or from patients with diseases such as aplastic anemia, where the number of cells is very low due to the nature of the disease. Blood samples must be received by the laboratory within 24 to 48 hours of collection or the viability of the cells may be compromised so as to prohibit accurate HLA typing.

Because HLA class I antigens are expressed on all nucleated cells of the body, a simple preparation of mononuclear cells from a peripheral blood sample is usually obtained to perform the class I serologic typing. Typing for class II antigens requires further separation of these mononuclear cells to enrich for B lymphocytes. Sera containing HLA antibodies are mixed with the isolated lymphocytes. The antibodies will bind only to their specific target antigens (e.g., anti-A2 antibody would only bind to a cell expressing HLA-A2 antigens).

When binding occurs, an antigen-antibody complex is formed on the cell surface. A reagent called *complement* is added to the antisera and cells, which causes cells with an attached antigen-antibody complex to die. A dye is added to the mixture. The dead cells absorb the dye, allowing quantitation of cell death by the laboratory. Cell death is considered a positive reaction. From the pattern of positive reactions with a specific panel of antisera, the serologic HLA type is discerned.

Most HLA typing sera are obtained from multiparous female blood donors, immunized to HLA through pregnancy. Since the sera is human derived, it is limited in quantity and difficult to standardize. Antisera required to HLA type minority patients or donors is often in short supply because of the small number of minority blood donors. More recently, monoclonal antibodies specific for certain HLA antigens have been developed for use in typing; however, these reagents have not been used widely because of the difficulty in interpreting the results and the lack of specificity of some of the monoclonal antibodies. Serologic reagents are unable to detect most HLA allelic variation; therefore, they provide only a broad definition

TABLE 3.9 Comparison of serology and DNA-based HLA typing

	Serology	DNA-based
Reagent supply	Poor	Excellent
Sensitivity	Fair	Excellent
Resolution	Fair	Excellent
Difficulty of interpretation	Easy to moderately difficult	Moderately difficult
Time	4 hours to 1 week	24 hours to 1 week
Cost	Low	Low to moderate
Failure rate	Moderate	Low

of an individual's HLA type. Table 3.9 shows the limitations of serologic typing and a comparison of this technique to DNA-based typing.

Cellular Methods

Some clinically relevant class II HLA antigens that can trigger the immune response are not readily detected by serologic methods. In the mid 1960s, it was shown that when lymphocytes from two different individuals were cultured together they could stimulate each other to proliferate, whereas when two populations of cells from HLA-identical individuals were mixed, the cells remained quiescent. This test is known as the *mixed lymphocyte reaction (MLR)* or *mixed lymphocyte culture (MLC)*. The lymphocytes' proliferation reaction was due to T cells' recognizing allelic differences in the class II HLA molecules expressed on the surface of the other cell population and reacting to those differences. Because highly specific class II antisera had been difficult to obtain, this assay became a routine test for HLA class II compatibility in marrow transplants and as an indicator for histoincompatibility between donor and recipient.

On the basis of MLC testing, class II antigens were originally described as a series of lymphocyte-activating determinants, products of the HLA-"D" gene (Dw1, Dw2, etc.). No HLA-D gene products have ever been isolated, although several distinct "HLA-D region" genes (DR, DQ, and DP) and their alleles have been identified. Formerly identified HLA-Dw, "antigens" are now considered to be immunogenic epitopes formed by combinations of HLA-D region determinants that were recognized by T cells.

There are major drawbacks associated with MLC tests, including the requirement for live, healthy cells, the sensitivity of the culture system to environmental factors, the length of time to complete the assay, and the difficulty in interpreting the test results. It is now known that this test is not predictive of GVHD; however, it is still considered valuable by some institutions and is used in conjunction with DNA-based typings for confirmation of histocompatibility of donor and recipient.

Molecular Methods

Recent developments in DNA-based techniques and their application to HLA typing have increased our ability to characterize HLA differences between patients and donors. The HLA alleles are currently defined by the presence of a unique sequence of nucleotides in the coding region of the individual HLA gene. The nucleotide sequence corresponds to specific amino acid residues in the expressed HLA molecules.

Therefore, the HLA phenotype of an individual can be extrapolated by direct determination of the nucleotide sequence for each of the HLA class I and II genes. These DNA-based methods do not require live cells, use manufactured rather than human-derived reagents, and can subdivide the HLA class II serologic types into allelic groups or allele-level typing, providing a higher resolution of HLA typing. DNA-based typing methods are highly accurate. In a large quality control study, the accuracy rate of one DNA-based typing method was greater than 99% for DRB1 and greater than 98% for DQB1 typing. (Ng et al., 1993.)

The development of the polymerase chain reaction (PCR) in the mid 1980s greatly improved the ability of laboratories to characterize HLA alleles. The PCR reaction generates billions of copies of the target strand of DNA in a process called *amplification* and can use very small samples. The most common PCR-based approach to HLA typing is a technique called *sequence-specific oligonucleotide probe (PCR-SSOP)*. This method uses short pieces of synthetic DNA (oligonucleotides) called *primers* to flank a specific region of the DNA to amplify. After the amplification step, the DNA is denatured (the double strand is separated into single strands by applying heat or adding a base), mixed with a panel of labeled oligonucleotide probes, and applied to a membrane. Each probe is designed to identify a specific nucleotide sequence in the DNA that is unique to a specific allele or group of alleles. If the probe has the sequence complementary to the target strand of DNA, it will anneal—or bind itself—to the target DNA in a reaction called *hybridization*. Given enough primers and probes, the PCR-SSOP can distinguish virtually all HLA alleles for a given HLA gene. This method is now used extensively, almost to the exclusion of serologic class II typing. Typing by PCR-SSOP has just recently been introduced for HLA class I typing.

Another common DNA-based typing approach is called *sequence-specific primer (PCR-SSP)* typing. This method uses selective amplification as a means of detecting the HLA type. A panel of primers, which includes at least one set of primers for each HLA type, is used for each sample. The specificity of the primers, rather than the probes, identifies the specific HLA alleles or allele groups. Amplification products are detected by gel electrophoresis. If the PCR reaction is negative, then the sample is assumed to lack the HLA allele or group of alleles specific for that primer. Although informative and relatively fast, this procedure requires many PCR reactions to obtain a complete typing and is not suited for high-volume HLA typing.

Another approach to DNA-based HLA typing is the *restriction-fragment length polymorphism (RFLP)* method. This method characterizes HLA types based on differences in restriction sites (or sites where DNA is cleaved by various restriction enzymes). HLA alleles exhibit unique cleavage patterns characteristic of a particular HLA allele or allele group. This method cannot distinguish all of the class II alleles and is not useful for class I typing because of the complexity of the resulting patterns. However, this method is still used in conjunction with other DNA-based typing techniques to obtain a high-resolution HLA typing.

Role of HLA in Matching for Transplantation

Histoincompatibility between a patient and donor can predispose the patient to graft failure, graft rejection, and GVHD. Patients who received transplants from an HLA phenotypically identical unrelated donor have an estimated 35% risk for development of severe acute GVHD, whereas those with a mismatch at a single HLA-A, -B or -DR locus have an approximate 50% risk (Martin, 1994). The three HLA genes thought to be most important to match for allogeneic bone marrow transplant are HLA*A, *B, and *DRB1. Most transplant centers require that a minimum of five out of six possible antigens or alleles match (two at HLA*A, two at HLA*B, and two at HLA*DRB1) with the donor before proceeding with an allogeneic marrow transplant. Although experience at a few institutions has indicated that haploidentical transplants (matching for one haplotype while mismatching for the other) between siblings or between a parent and a child can be performed successfully, only small numbers of these transplants have been performed and the data is not conclusive. Recent studies have also investigated the importance of other HLA genes, in particular HLA*C, *DQB1, and *DPB1, in the outcome of allogeneic marrow transplants; however, their contributions are not currently understood.

High-resolution DNA-based typing offers the opportunity to study the impact of HLA disparity beyond the level of serologic typing. The information gained from this level of HLA typing may result in a different evaluation of matching. For example, donors and patients thought to be matched by serology may be found to be mismatched when their samples are typed by high-resolution DNA-based methods. This newly identified mismatch may be a result of identifying HLA specificities with DNA-based methods that are often difficult to identify by routine serologic typing. It may also show that allele-level differences that result in a substitution of a particular amino acid residue in the HLA molecule may be more likely to impact peptide binding or recognition of the antigen by the T-cell receptor.

Based on the large number of HLA alleles identified, most patients will not find a complete molecular-matched donor. It is therefore critical to determine the relative importance of matching at an allele level and to determine whether all or only some HLA genes need to be

matched. In addition, it is important to determine whether there are permissive mismatches that can be tolerated without negatively affecting the outcome of the transplant. Studies involving retyping of donor and patient samples by DNA-based methods and correlating this new typing information with outcome data are being conducted by individual institutions and the National Marrow Donor Program to begin to answer these important questions.

DONOR ISSUES

Several common donor issues exist whether the donor is a relative or is unrelated to the patient. Confidentiality, informed consent, and the right to refuse donation rank high on the list of donor issues.

Unrelated Donor Registries

Before the mid 1980s, almost all allogeneic transplants were performed using marrow harvested from an HLA-identical sibling. Patients in need of a marrow transplant but lacking a family donor either did not receive a transplant, were forced to canvass the country searching independent small donor registries, or had to organize HLA typing drives themselves in hopes of identifying an unrelated donor.

In order to provide access to bone marrow transplantation for patients lacking a related donor, the U.S. Congress authorized establishment of a national registry of HLA-typed volunteers willing to donate marrow for an unrelated patient in need of a transplant. A contract was awarded to the National Marrow Donor Program in July 1986, and the first NMDP-facilitated unrelated donor transplant occurred in December 1987, just 3 months after the NMDP began operations. The NMDP is a network of member transplant, donor, and marrow collection centers that work together to provide patients in need of a bone marrow transplant access to unrelated volunteers willing to donate marrow for patients who have no family donor available. In its role as the U.S. National Bone Marrow Donor Registry, the NMDP has developed the world's largest computerized registry of volunteer marrow donors. As of January 1996, close to 2 million donors are listed on the NMDP's registry, with approximately 25,000 new volunteer donors added to the registry each month.

The success of the NMDP in building the unrelated donor registry can only be matched by its ability to identify potential donors for searching patients. As of January 1996, 70% of patient searches resulted in the identification of at least one HLA-A, -B, and -DR phenotypically identical unrelated donor. If a single HLA-A, -B, or -DR disparity were allowed by the transplant center, 95% to 99% of patients could identify at least one donor in this registry.

The NMDP has reached out internationally to provide patients access to as many donors as possible. The NMDP has cooperative search arrangements with registries in seven other countries: The Canadian Red Cross Society, France's Greffe de Moelle, the Australian Bone Marrow Donor Registry, the Austrian Bone Marrow Donor Registry, the Anthony Nolan Bone Marrow Trust in England, the Spanish Bone Marrow Donor Registry (REDMO), and the Swiss Bone Marrow Donor Registry. The NMDP is involved in ongoing discussions with other foreign registries to expand the international network and increase the number of available unrelated donors.

The NMDP Donor Search

The search for an unrelated donor involves several steps designed to ensure that the patient and donor are very closely matched and that the donor is healthy, informed, and willing to donate marrow. Searching for a potential unrelated donor can be a lengthy process, depending on the patient's HLA type and how representative that type is in the registry. Search time is also affected by the availability of donors and the speed at which the transplant center makes decisions at each step of the search process. Unfortunately, due to rare HLA types or disease progression, some patients never find a matched donor.

The search process begins with the preliminary search. The patient's HLA type is sent by the transplant center's physician, hematologist, or oncologist to the NMDP, where it is entered into the NMDP's STAR^{SM} (Search Tracking And Registry) computer system. A comparison of the patient's HLA type to the HLA types of the registered donors is performed. Within 24 hours of receipt of the search request, a report of potentially matched volunteers is electronically sent or mailed to the physician who requested it. The potential donors' identities are coded to maintain confidentiality and are listed in the order of best match. The NMDP does not list or provide access to donors who are mismatched for more than one HLA antigen. The preliminary search is free of charge and is intended to notify the physician and patient of the number of potential donors currently registered with the NMDP who are HLA compatible with the patient. HLA compatibility is the primary criterion to select donors; however, other criteria in addition to histocompatibility are considered by the transplant center. The nonhistocompatibility factors to consider in selection of donors include:

- Donor and patient sex match
- Donor parity
- Donor age
- Donor viral immunity (e.g., CMV, hepatitis, HIV)

If there is a decision to proceed with the donor search, donor activation or formalization of the search is requested by the patient's transplant center. Volunteer donors who are potential matches for a patient are selected by the transplant center's nurse or physician to undergo further histocompatibility testing. This testing may involve defining the volunteer donor's HLA-DRB1 type by DNA-based methods, if not previously defined, or confirming the patient's and volunteer's HLA-A, -B, and -DRB1 types to ensure compatibility. Testing for infectious disease is also performed on the donor's blood sample at this time.

When the transplant center determines that the donor and patient are indeed a match, a request is sent to the NMDP to arrange a donor information session and physical examination to determine that the donor is healthy, informed, and prepared to donate marrow. The NMDP works closely with the volunteer's donor center to coordinate this process. The potential donor is provided detailed information on the marrow collection procedure, including the risks associated with the anesthesia used during the procedure and the expected level of discomfort following the marrow collection. If the volunteer donor is interested in proceeding, he or she receives a thorough physical examination. The potential donor is also asked to donate one or more units of autologous blood to be stored in case the donor needs transfusion(s) during the marrow collection procedure. When the potential donor has been medically approved for marrow collection and has signed an informed consent, the transplant center is notified. The patient then begins pretransplant conditioning.

The donor's marrow is collected in an operating room at an NMDP-approved marrow collection center close to the donor's home. The collection is usually performed while the donor is under general anesthesia, although regional anesthesia can be used. Cells for marrow transplantation are obtained by aspirating marrow from the posterior iliac crests of the donor. Heparin is added as the anticoagulant, the marrow is filtered to remove bone particles and fat,

and the marrow is then transferred to two blood transfusion bags. Donors are surveyed by their donor centers repeatedly until they report a complete recovery. Typical symptoms reported after marrow donation are summarized in Table 3.10. Despite these symptoms, results of donor surveys indicate that 91% of donors would donate marrow again if asked, and less than 2% would decline future donations (Butterworth et al., 1993).

Immediately after the marrow is collected, a trained donor or transplant center representative transports the marrow to the transplant center. The patient receives the marrow intravenously, as he or she would receive a blood transfusion. The marrow cells migrate to the marrow cavity in the patient's bones where the cells begin to grow and reproduce.

The NMDP maintains communication with both the transplant center and the donor center

TABLE 3.10 Immediate postdonation experience

Symptom	Frequency of occurrence
Fatigue	79%
Pain at site of donation	73%
Pain with walking	67%
Low back pain	61%
Sore throat	58%
Pain with sitting	54%
Nausea	52%
Light-headedness	46%
Trouble climbing stairs	45%
Headache	33%
Vomiting	31%
Pain at site of IV	31%
Fever	29%
Pain from bandage	22%
Prolonged bleeding at site of donation	9%
Fainting	4%

SOURCE: Data from the National Marrow Donor Program, Minneapolis, Minnesota.

regarding the recipient's status and the donor's condition. Transplant centers send follow-up data on the recipient to the NMDP at 3 months, 6 months, and 1 year after transplant, and every year thereafter.

The identities of the donor and recipient remain confidential throughout the process. All communication between the donor center managing the donor and the transplant center managing the patient are conducted through the NMDP. The donor is only told minimal information about the recipient, such as the diagnosis, whether it is a child or an adult, and the chances for survival with and without the transplant. The patient is given no information about the donor. Only those staff at the NMDP, the transplant center, or the donor center with a need to know have access to the donor's or the recipient's identity. Donors and recipients are allowed to meet each other only if they have both expressed a strong desire to do so, and not until 1 year after the transplant.

Blood Cell Transplantation

Bone marrow progenitor cells, or stem cells, circulate in the peripheral blood in very low concentrations. These peripheral blood progenitor cells, collected via a series of apheresis procedures, have been a source of stem cells for autologous and more recently for allogeneic blood cell transplantation (BCT). If the donor is treated with a hematopoietic growth factor, such as recombinant human granulocyte colony-stimulating factor (G-CSF), the number of circulating progenitor cells is drastically increased (2 to 15 times) and only one or two apheresis procedures are required to collect an adequate number of cells for BCT. The advantages of peripherally derived stem cells over marrow cells in include the following:

- The collection of peripheral blood stem cells does not require the donor to undergo a sur-

gical procedure and eliminates risks associated with anesthesia.
- Recovery from marrow harvest takes approximately 2 weeks and significant complications can sometimes occur. Recovery from an uncomplicated apheresis collection is virtually immediate.
- Preliminary experience implies that peripherally derived stem cells may provide a more rapid engraftment of granulocytes and platelets than marrow-derived allogeneic stem cells.

There are some disadvantages to apheresis. Problems with venous access in the donor can occur and occasionally necessitate the placement of a central venous catheter to collect the product. The administration of G-CSF, although drastically reducing the number of apheresis procedures necessary to collect an adequate number of stem cells, has its own disadvantages. A very common side effect reported by persons receiving G-CSF is bone pain. Other common side effects include nausea, vomiting, and flulike symptoms such as headache, fatigue, and myalgias. The long-term risks of G-CSF administration in normal donors, although believed to be negligible, are not known. All of these issues need to be thoroughly discussed with the potential donor before the donor is asked to sign an informed consent and donate peripheral blood cells.

Umbilical Cord Blood

Another recently discovered source of stem cells is umbilical cord blood. This discovery led to the first successful umbilical cord blood transplant, performed in Paris in 1988 by Eliane Gluckman, for a patient with Fanconi's anemia. The transplant was successful and the patient was cured of his disease. The success of this transplant has served as an impetus for further investigation into the potential use of umbilical cord blood as a source of stem cells. As of the end of 1995, more than 100 umbilical cord blood transplants had been performed worldwide.

Cord blood is recovered through the umbilical vein just after delivery. Approximately 90 ml to 200 ml of cord blood are collected. Because blood clotting in umbilical cord and placental veins is relatively slow, a slight delay in retrieving the blood is permissible. Therefore, collection can be facilitated outside of the delivery room so as not to interfere with the delivery. The cord blood is stored frozen in a controlled rate freezer. Separate aliquots are stored for later HLA typing and testing for infectious disease.

Cord blood may be collected for use in transplanting a sibling or other family member or may be stored in a cord blood bank for an unrelated cord blood transplant. If the cord blood will be banked for use by an unrelated patient, the mother is surveyed regarding the child's ethnicity and risks of genetic and infectious diseases. A sample of the mother's blood is taken for infectious disease testing and possible HLA typing to help distinguish an ambiguous typing of the cord blood sample.

Cord blood is an attractive source of stem cells for transplantation because it is collected in a noninvasive manner and is a byproduct of normal deliveries. Its benefits include immediate availability of the product, absence of risk to donor, and low risk of transmissible infections such as those from cytomeglovirus and Epstein-Barr virus. A potential advantage umbilical cord blood transplants may have over unrelated donor marrow transplantation is that they are believed to carry a lower risk of GVHD, perhaps due to the naïveté of neonatal stem cells. Properties of the neonatal immune system that might account for the decreased capacity of umbilical

cord blood to mediate GVHD reaction are being explored.

There are some concerns about the use of umbilical cord blood in unrelated cord blood transplants. The newborns may carry undiagnosed genetic diseases that would have automatically excluded adult donors. Screening questions and some testing can minimize this risk to some extent; however, some of these diseases will not show up until later in the child's life, potentially after the cord blood is infused. The expense of collecting and storing a unit of umbilical cord blood that may never be used is substantial and has not yet been determined to be more cost effective than maintaining a registry of volunteer donors. There are also important unanswered questions at this time including:

- Will the number of stem and progenitor cells in umbilical cord blood be sufficient to engraft an adult? (Most of the transplants have been performed in children.)
- Will greater HLA disparities between donor and recipient be tolerated?
- Will the risk of leukemia relapse be greater if the risk of GVHD is lower?

The same issues of donor confidentiality exist in the cord blood setting, perhaps even to a greater extent than in the unrelated marrow donor setting. Currently, in existing cord blood banks, identifying information on donors is not maintained in order to protect the identities of the infant and mother.

Use of cord blood cells for transplantation purposes has raised questions of whether these cells should be stored for use later in life should the infant or his or her immediate family be in need of a stem cell transplant. Several commercial firms sell this service. The likelihood of use and the cost-effectiveness of this approach have not been established.

REFERENCES

Baxter-Lowe, L.A. 1994. Molecular techniques for typing unrelated marrow donors: potential impact of molecular typing disparity in donor selection. *BMT* 14(40 suppl):S42-S50.

Begovich, A.B., Erlich, H.A. 1995. HLA typing for bone marrow transplantation. *JAMA* 273(7):586-591.

Bodmer, J.G., et al. 1992. Nomenclature for factors of the HLA system, 1991. In Tsuji, T., Aizawa, M., Sasazuki, T. (Eds.) *HLA 1991*. Oxford: Oxford University Press, 17-31.

Bodmer, J.G., Marsh, S.G., Albert, E.D., et al. Nomenclature for factors of the HLA system, 1995. *Tissue Antigens* 46:1-18.

Butterworth, V.A., Simmons, R.G., Bartsch, G., et al. 1993. Psychosocial effects of unrelated bone marrow donation: Experiences of the National Marrow Donor Program. *Blood* 81(7):1947-1959.

Dupont, B., Yang S.Y. 1994. Histocompatibility. In Forman, S.J., Blume, K.G., Thomas, E.D. (Eds.) *Bone Marrow Transplantation*. Cambridge, MA: Blackwell Scientific, 22-40.

Juttner, C.F., Fibbe, W.E., Nemunaitis, J., et al. 1994. Blood cell transplantation: report from an International Consensus Meeting. *BMT* 14:689-693.

Klein, J., Takahata, N., Ayala, F. 1993. MHC polymorphism in human origins. *Sci Am* (Dec):78-83.

Lee, J. (Ed.) 1990. *The HLA System, A New Approach.* New York: Springer-Verlag.

Martin, P. 1994. Overview of transplant immunology. In Forman, S.J., Blume, K.G., Thomas, E.D. (Eds.) *Bone Marrow Transplantation*. Cambridge, MA: Blackwell Scientific, 16-21.

Ng, J., Hurley, C.K., Baxter-Lowe, L.A., et al. 1993. Large-scale oligonucleotide typing for HLA-DRB1/3/4 and HLA-DQB1 is highly accurate, specific and reliable. *Tissue Antigens* 42:473-479.

Perkins, H.A., Hansen, J.A. 1994. The U.S. National Marrow Donor Program. *Am J Pediatr Hematol Oncol* 16(1):30-34.

Petersdorf, E.W., Longton, G.M., Anasetti, C., et al. 1995. The significance of HLA-DRB1 matching on clinical outcome after HLA-A, B, DR identical, unrelated donor bone marrow transplantation. *Blood* 86(4):1606-1613.

Rodey, G.E. 1991. *HLA Beyond Tears.* Atlanta: De-Novo Inc.

Rubinstein, P., Rosenfield, R.E., Adamson, J.W., Stevens, C.E. 1993. Stored placental blood for unrelated bone marrow reconstitution. *Blood* 81(7):1679-1690.

Schwartz, B.D. 1991. The human major histocompatibility human leukocyte antigen (HLA) complex. In Stites, D., Terr, A.I. (Eds.) *Basic and Clinical Immunology.* Norwalk, CT: Appleton & Lange, 45-60.

Smith, B.R., Hansen, J.A., Rappeport, J.M. 1991. Bone marrow transplantation: selecting donors and diseases. *Am Soc Hematol Ed Progr* (Dec):104-111.

Thomas, E.D. 1995. Hematopoieitic stem cell transplantation. *Sci Am* (Sept-Oct):38-47.

Wagner, J.E., Kernan N.A., Steinbuch, M., et al. 1995. Allogeneic sibling umbilical-cord-blood transplantation in children with malignant and nonmalignant disease. *Lancet* 346:214-219.

4

Blood and Marrow Stem Cell Transplantation
Indications, Procedure, Process

Susan A. O'Connell, Kim Schmit-Pokorny

Marrow and blood stem cell transplantation are being used increasingly worldwide as treatments for selected malignant and nonmalignant disorders. Marrow and blood stem cell transplants enable patients to receive potentially lethal doses of chemotherapy or radiation therapy followed by hematopoietic rescue with marrow or blood stem cells. In recent years, there has been a dramatic increase in the number of transplants and transplant centers (Barrett, 1991; Bortin et al., 1992). According to the International Bone Marrow Transplant Registry (IBMTR), in 1994 more than 20,000 transplants were performed worldwide at more than 290 centers (see Figure 4.1).

The treatment processes of marrow and blood cell transplantation varies somewhat, but the common goal for most diseases is cure. The role of transplantation in nonmalignant diseases is to replace defective marrow; in malignant diseases, the goal of stem cell infusion is to rescue the marrow after the patient has received toxic doses of myelosuppresive therapy aimed at eradicating the underlying disease (Randolph, 1993; Treleaven and Barrett, 1995).

The concept of transplanting marrow and blood cells seems simple in theory. However, life-threatening side effects and toxicities make caring for the transplant patient extremely complex. It requires sophisticated technology and procedures, a highly specialized team of health-care workers, an adequately supportive environment, and many additional resources (Forman et al., 1994). Oncology nurses play a major role in the success of transplantation. Transplant scientists describe nurses' contribution this way.

> The nursing team in particular is responsible for the day-to-day care of patients. Nurses not only provide bedside management of complex protocol studies, but also bear the burden of emotional support through the difficult hospital period. They are the most readily available source of information for patients and families day and night. Without a strong nursing team, the entire BMT program is jeopardized. (Forman et al., 1994, p. xx)

As the field of marrow and blood cell transplantation evolves, so does transplant nursing.

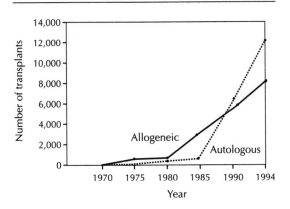

Figure 4.1 Annual number of transplants 1970–1994

SOURCE: Data presented here were obtained from the Statistical Center for the International Bone Marrow Transplant Registry, Milwaukee, Wisconsin. Used with permission.

The role of the transplant nurse is one of the most challenging oncology nursing specialties (Meyer, 1992).

Transplantation is defined as the transfer of living tissues or organs from one part of the body to another or from one individual to another. There are three major types of marrow and blood cell transplant: autologous, allogeneic, and syngeneic. Their names indicate the source of the marrow or blood cell that is transplanted, or infused, into the recipient.

Autologous

Autologous (self) marrow and blood cell transplantation involves the removal, storage, and reinfusion of the patient's own healthy marrow or blood stem cells. In essence, the autologous patient is his or her own donor. The use of autologous marrow as a source of regenerating

hematopoietic cells was first reported by Kurnick and colleagues (1958). They believed that increased intensity of treatment would permit the log kill of a tumor mass beyond the last viable cell. High-dose chemotherapy followed by autologous bone marrow transplantation (ABMT) appeared to offer the chance of curing malignancies in situations where myelosupression prevented the use of sufficient doses of chemotherapy without marrow rescue. The failure of early studies was due primarily to disease recurrence after inadequate doses of chemotherapy. During the last decade, interest in autologous BMT has skyrocketed as a result of new technology for marrow storage, cryopreservation, and purging as well as improvements in supportive care (Gale and Butturini, 1995). The major challenges still confronting autologous marrow and blood cell transplantation are major organ, nonhematologic, dose-limiting toxicities and relapse of disease. Three theories as to the cause of relapse following autologous transplant include tumor contamination of the marrow, inadequate treatment of minimal residual disease in the patient, and the lack of a graft-versus-leukemia effect (discussed later).

Allogeneic

In allogeneic transplantation marrow or blood stem cells are removed from a donor and infused into the patient (recipient). The donor can be related (other than identical twin) or unrelated. The ideal donor is human-leukocyte-antigen-identical (HLA-identical) to the patient. Commonly, the marrow is donated by a fully HLA-matched sibling. Because only about one in three patients eligible for a transplant has an HLA-identical sibling, partially matched family members or matched but unrelated donors from a volunteer registry have also been donors.

HLA typing involves testing leukocytes to identify genetically inherited antigens common to both donor and patient. It is important to obtain a full six-antigen match for a BMT whenever possible to prevent the donor marrow (specifically the T lymphocytes) from recognizing the recipient as foreign, leading to graft-versus-host disease (GVHD) (Freedman, 1988). GVHD is a unique complication of allogeneic transplant that can be a major impediment to successful transplantation (Buchsel, 1993). Alternatively, the patient's immune system can destroy the new bone marrow. This is referred to as *graft rejection.*

In the 1950s random donors were used to attempt to rescue patients with aplastic anemia or bone marrow failure that resulted from radiation accidents. These attempts were not successful except for patients receiving marrow from an identical twin (Pegg, 1966). The most frequent causes of death from the use of random donors were graft failure and GVHD. It was not until the advent of tissue typing and compatibility testing that patients began to benefit from marrow transplant.

During the 1970s clinical trials investigated the role of BMT in a wide variety of malignant and nonmalignant disorders. Standardized pretransplant conditioning regimens and GVHD prevention were developed. By 1980 allogeneic BMTs using matched sibling donors were achieving disease-free survivals in hematological malignancies in more than 50% of patients (Gee, 1991). During the last decade, application of biotechnology to clinical marrow and blood cell transplant has opened new research avenues in the prevention and treatment of GVHD with monoclonal antibodies and the use of hematopoietic growth factors and recombinant cytokines to promote hematopoietic and immune reconstitution. The major challenges that still face investigators are to reduce the high mortality rate due to GVHD, to develop more effective conditioning regimens, and to safely transplant stem cells across major histocompatibility barriers.

Syngeneic

Syngeneic marrow transplant involves harvesting stem cells from one identical twin and infusing them into the other. Identical twins have identical genetic types and are considered a perfect match. Syngeneic transplants, first attempted in the early 1960s to treat aplastic anemia, allowed investigators to learn that the hematopoietic system in humans could be replaced by that of a genetically identical donor (Whedon, 1991). This type of transplant has become relatively routine, with few complications. A higher incidence of leukemic relapse has been reported in syngeneic than in allogeneic marrow recipients because of the demonstrated antileukemic effect of graft-versus-host disease (Thomas, 1988). This is known as *graft-versus-leukemia effect,* and is discussed later in this chapter.

Blood Stem Cells

Stem cells obtained from the marrow or the peripheral blood are used in autologous or allogeneic transplants. Known by many names (e.g., progenitor cell, peripheral blood stem cell), the term *blood cell (BC)* has been chosen as the preferred term by an expert scientific consensus panel (Juttner, 1994).

Blood cell transplantation (BCT) is rapidly replacing bone marrow transplantation (BMT). BCT is associated with more rapid recovery of hematopoietic function than BMT and, therefore, less morbidity. Blood cells are now considered an appropriate source of hematopoietic support after intensive chemotherapy or radiotherapy in many situations (see Table 4.1). In autologous transplantation blood cells may be collected if there is marrow contamination or if the patient is unable to undergo general anesthesia. Blood cells are also used instead of bone marrow cells due to the accelerated hematopoietic engraftment following infusion. In allogeneic transplantation apheresis offers donors

TABLE 4.1 Considerations for sources of stem cells

Bone marrow	Blood cell	Umbilical cord blood
AUTOLOGOUS		
No marrow/bone involvement	Less risk of tumor contamination	
No marrow fibrosis	Immunologic effect	
Patient can undergo general or spinal anesthesia	No need for general anesthesia	
No prior pelvic irradiation		
Requires adequate marrow cellularity		
ALLOGENEIC		
Donor can undergo general or spinal anesthesia	Donor unable to undergo general or spinal anesthesia	Patient must be an infant or small child
	Need for a rapid engraftmen	Infant need not undergo general anesthetic

a less invasive method than traditional marrow harvests to collect the stem cells. It is hoped that the former may serve as an incentive for the general population to serve as unrelated donors. BCT also offers the possibility of immunologically tailored grafts with larger numbers of T lymphocytes and natural killer cells enabling an adoptive immunotherapeutic approach (Juttner et al., 1994).

Cord Blood Stem Cells

Umbilical cord blood is rich in hematopoietic stem cells and successful allogeneic engraftment has been achieved using this source (Forman, 1994). Cord blood can be HLA typed and cryopreserved, and can be a source of hematopoietic stem cells for HLA-matched unrelated individuals. However, the relatively small amount of cord blood may render such an approach impractical except as a source of stem cells to transplant to infants and small children. This new stem cell source prevents the need for marrow harvest under general anesthesia of infant donors.

Alternative sources of stem cells used experimentally and clinically include cadaveric and fetal liver. An attempt to transplant baboon marrow into an HIV-infected patient was made in 1995. Engraftment was not successful.

CLINICAL INDICATIONS

Malignant Diseases

According to 1994 data from the International Bone Marrow Transplant Registry, the most common indication for an allogeneic transplant is leukemia, and the most common indication for an autologous transplant is breast cancer (see Figure 4.2). Malignant diseases that are treated with marrow or blood stem cell transplantation include:

- Acute lymphocytic leukemia
- Acute myelogenous leukemia
- Chronic myelogenous leukemia
- Chronic lymphocytic leukemia
- Myelodysplastic syndrome ("preleukemia")

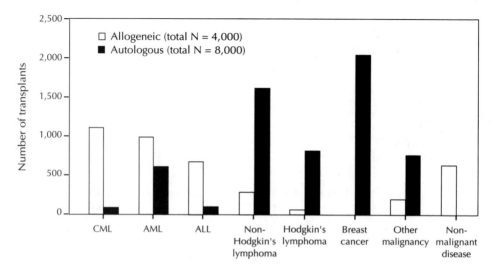

Figure 4.2   Indications for blood and marrow transplants in North America, 1994

SOURCE: Horowitz, M. 1995. *BMT Newsletter*, July 1995, vol. 2, no. 1. Used with permission.

- Monosomy 7 syndrome
- Non-Hodgkin's lymphoma
- Hodgkin's lymphoma
- Neuroblastoma
- Brain tumor
- Multiple myeloma
- Testicular germ cell tumors
- Breast cancer
- Lung cancer
- Ovarian cancer
- Melanoma
- Glioma
- Sarcoma
- Other solid tumors

Nonmalignant Diseases

Nonmalignant diseases, including congenital immunodeficiency diseases, were first treated with BMT in 1968 (Friedrich, 1994). Most of the transplants for nonmalignant diseases are done in children. Nonmalignant diseases that are treated with marrow or blood stem cell transplantation include:

- Hematologic Disorders
  Severe aplastic anemia
  Diamond-Blackfan anemia
  Fanconi's anemia
  Sickle cell anemia
  Beta thalassemia major
  Chediak-Higashi syndrome
  Chronic granulomatous disease
  Congenital neutropenia
  Reticular dysgenesis
- Congenital Immunodeficiences
  Severe combined immunodeficiency (SCID)
  Wiskott-Aldrich syndrome
  Functional T-cell deficiency
- Mucopolysaccharidoses
  Hurler's disease
  Hunter's disease

San Filippo syndrome
Morquios syndrome
- Lipidoses
Adrenoleukodystrophy
Methachromatic leukodystrophy
Gaucher's disease
- Miscellaneous
Osteopetrosis
Langerhan's cell histiocytosis
Lesch-Nyhan syndrome
Glycogen storage diseases

Bone Marrow Transplant Registries

The International Bone Marrow Transplant Registry receives information from more than 290 transplant centers in 44 countries and serves as a useful source of BMT statistics. Established in 1970, the database includes information for 40% of allogeneic transplants done between 1970 and 1994.

In 1991 the Autologous Blood and Marrow Transplant Registry–North America (ABMTR) began collecting data. More than 160 autotransplant centers participate in the ABMTR. This database includes about 50% of autotransplants done in North America between 1989 and 1994.

PATIENT ELIGIBILITY

Santos (1985) described several considerations for patient eligibility: (1) the malignancy is responsive to therapy, (2) the disease is in an early stage, (3) marrow toxicity is the only dose-limiting effect of the treatment, and (4) the source of stem cells is free of disease. These considerations have been modified over time as marrow purging and newer treatment modalities have become available. Overall medical condition, psychosocial well-being, age, and compliance are also concerns when evaluating a patient's eligibility for transplant.

Disease Status

Tumor bulk and sensitivity to chemotherapy and/or radiation must be considered when selecting a patient for transplant. Studies indicate that patients who have a low tumor burden and a disease responsive to chemotherapy experience an improved chance of disease-free survival following transplant (Crump et al., 1993; Jagannath et al., 1989).

The timing of a transplant in relation to disease status is integral to the overall outcome of the therapy. Outcomes of transplantation are best when the therapy is administered early in the course of the disease (Armitage and Gale, 1989). Controlled randomized studies are needed to further address this issue (Keating, 1995). Tables 4.2 and 4.3 present the likeli-

TABLE 4.2 Disease-free survival posttransplant in selected diseases

Disease	Disease phase	DFS 3 years
Hodgkin's disease (autologous transplants)	Never 1st CR	51 ± 16%
	1st relapse	56 ± 10%
	2d remission	57 ± 26%
Non-Hodgkin's lymphoma (autologous transplants)	1st CR	86 ± 13%
	1st relapse	62 ± 24%
	2d CR	63 ± 28%
Low-grade lymphoma	Never CR	59 ± 25%
Intermediate or immunoblastic lymphoma	1st CR	67 ± 19%
	1st relapse	37 ± 11%
	2d CR	64 ± 15%
	Never CR	30 ± 15%
Breast cancer (autologous transplants)	Stage 2	65 ± 15%
	Stage 3	68 ± 11%
	Inflammatory	57 ± 14%
	Metastatic	28 ± 3%

KEY: CR = complete remission, DFS = disease-free survival
SOURCE: Horowitz, IBMTR, 1995. Reprinted with permission.

TABLE 4.3 Five-year probabilities (95% confidence intervals) of LFS, survival, and relapse following HLA-identical sibling bone marrow transplants for ALL, AML, and CML according to disease state at transplant

Disease	State	N	Probabilities[b] of		
			DFS (%)	Survival (%)	Relapse (%)
ALL	Early[a]	699	50 (46–54)	52 (48–56)	29 (25–33)
ALL	Intermediate	728	38 (34–42)	39 (35–43)	45 (40–50)
ALL	Advanced	348	18 (14–23)	19 (15–24)	68 (61–74)
AML	Early	1515	54 (51–57)	56 (53–59)	24 (21–27)
AML	Intermediate	313	36 (30–42)	38 (32–44)	35 (28–43)
AML	Advanced	576	18 (14–22)	18 (14–22)	65 (60–70)
CML	Early	1782	52 (49–55)	57 (54–60)	19 (16–22)
CML	Intermediate	464	32 (27–37)	36 (31–41)	34 (28–41)
CML	Advanced	153	12 (6–24)	14 (8–24)	59 (47–70)

[a]Early leukemia refers to transplants performed in first complete remission of ALL or AML and first chronic phase of CML; intermediate leukemia refers to ≥ second complete remission of ALL or AML and ≥ second chronic phase or accelerated phase of CML; advanced leukemia refers to relapse of ALL or AML or blast phase of CML.

[b]All differences between disease states (within each disease) are significant at $p < 0.001$.

SOURCE: Data here were obtained from the Statistical Center for the International Bone Marrow Transplant Registry, Milwaukee, Wisconsin. Used with permission.

hood of 3 years of disease-free survival (DFS) by stage of disease at transplant for some common malignancies. In general, the earlier a patient receives a transplant, the greater the chance for longer disease-free survival.

Donor Availability

Tissue typing is usually performed on the patient's full siblings, parents, and children. If a matched related donor is identified, the transplant center will begin physical and psychological evaluations of the patient and potential donor. Patients without a matched related donor may be considered for an autologous transplant. If the patient's disease is not treatable

with an autologous transplant, an unrelated donor search may be initiated.

SELECTING A TRANSPLANT CENTER

The oncology nurse can play a critical role in assisting the patient and family to select a transplant center. Patients are usually overwhelmed with their diagnosis and are generally unfamiliar with treatment options. Table 4.4 outlines key questions the patient should ask when choosing a BMT center, although some patients may not have choices because of restrictions

TABLE 4.4 Selecting a transplant center

Location
Will I need to relocate? If so, for how long?
Does the center have adequate, affordable housing?
Will the center assist me in finding housing?
What will housing cost?

Experience
How long has the center's personnel been performing marrow or blood cell transplants?
How many transplants have they done in total?
What types of transplants are they currently performing?
How many transplants have they done for my disease?
What is their success rate with transplants for my disease?
How does their success rate compare with the national statistics?
What is their mortality rate associated with transplant for patients with my disease?
How does their mortality rate compare with the national mortality rate for my disease?
What complications have they experienced with transplants for my disease?
How do these complications compare with national statistics?
Am I at high risk for developing any complication? If so, what is their experience with this complication?

BMT Team
How many physicians are working with the program?
How much experience with transplant does each physician have?
Will I have a physician caring for me?
Are there specially trained BMT nurses and staff?
How much experience does the average BMT nurse have?
How many BMT nurse coordinators are there? Will there be one coordinator working with me during the transplant process?
Will a BMT clinical nurse specialist or nurse practitioner be working with me?

Who will be my primary medical professional in the hospital (resident, physician's assistant, nurse practitioner)? How much experience does he or she have in BMT?
Who are the consultants for various BMT complications (infectious disease, nephrology, cardiology, etc.)?
Will a social worker, psychologist, or psychiatrist support me emotionally during the transplant process?
Who are the other team members (pharmacist, dietitian, chaplain, volunteers, financial personnel, etc.)?

Treatment Plan
What is the proposed treatment plan?
Is this an investigational (research) study?
What is known to date about the treatment plan you are recommending for me?
Will my transplant be done on an outpatient basis? If so, what additional resources will I need (primary caregiver, etc.)? What percentage of outpatients are admitted for complication? Am I at any additional risk for complications?

Environment and Staffing
Do you have a designated BMT unit (or outpatient space/facility)?
How many BMT beds and outpatient slots do you have?
Will I be on a unit with other hematology or oncology patients?
What are the infection control practices (handwashing, use of gloves, masks, gowns, air filtering system, etc.)?
Do you have dedicated BMT nurses on your unit or in your clinic?
What is the nurse/patient ratio?
Will I have a primary nurse or case manager?
Are nurses with extensive experience in BMT supervising the BMT nursing staff?
If I should require critical care, will I be transferred to another unit? If so, how much training do the physicians and nurses in the Critical Care Unit have in BMT?

Continued

TABLE 4.4 Selecting a transplant center *Continued*

How would you describe the cleanliness of the BMT unit? Can I tour the BMT unit prior to making my decision?

Can my family and friends donate blood and platelets for me if we desire? Do you have a directed donor unit at your facility? Does your center have equipment for irradiating blood products?

Are there visitor restrictions?

Patient Education and Support Groups

Does your center offer classes for patients and family members?

Do you have written information about your BMT program?

Can I talk to one or two patients with my disease who have gone through BMT at your center?

Does your center have a support group for BMT patients and their families?

Finances

How much will my transplant cost?

Is there someone at your center who will help me obtain approval for insurance coverage?

Is there someone at your center who will help me with fundraising, if needed?

Other than hospital expenses, what other expenses can I expect (parking, travel, meals, housing, child care, medications, telephone, television, etc.)?

Follow-up Care

How long can I expect to be followed at your center?

To whom will my care be transferred after I leave this center? How much training in and experience with transplantation do they have?

---

imposed by their insurance companies (see Chapter 19).

A successful bone marrow transplant program has a team of highly skilled health-care professionals and volunteers working to provide the best possible care for the transplant recipient and his or her family. The team is usually comprised of administrators, physicians, physician's assistants, nurse practitioners, clinical nurse specialists, coordinators, staff nurses, pharmacists, social workers, psychologists or psychiatrists, dieticians, dentists, clergy, financial advisors, researchers, data management coordinators, laboratory technicians, and clerical staff. Many consultants and ancillary staff are also involved in this enormous team effort (see Figure 4.3). Some centers have volunteers who are former BMT recipients. After undergoing a training program provided by the center, they give information and support to the BMT patient and family.

The nursing team "is the most important single aspect of a successful BMT unit," according to the American Society of Clinical Oncologists and the American Society of Hematologists (ASCO/ASH, 1990). Nurses serve in many roles on the transplant team. Advanced practice nurses (e.g., clinical nurse specialist or nurse practitioner) are integral members of the transplant team. The clinical nurse specialist (CNS) functions as a consultant, educator, and researcher in the acute care and ambulatory care settings. The nurse practitioner (NP) works under a negotiated agreement with the institution to perform history and physical examinations and to order medications, blood products, and diagnostic studies. The NP may also perform bone marrow harvests, bone marrow biopsies and aspirations, skin biopsies, and lumbar punctures for instillation of intrathecal chemotherapy. Nurse coordinators or case managers plan and organize the pretransplant workup, harvest-

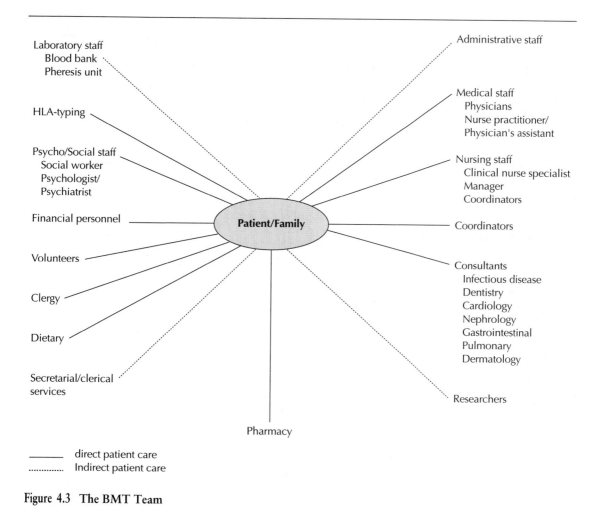

Laboratory staff
  Blood bank
  Pheresis unit

HLA-typing

Psycho/Social staff
  Social worker
  Psychologist/
  Psychiatrist

Financial personnel

Volunteers

Clergy

Dietary

Secretarial/clerical
services

Pharmacy

Patient/Family

Administrative staff

Medical staff
  Physicians
  Nurse practitioner/
  Physician's assistant

Nursing staff
  Clinical nurse specialist
  Manager
  Coordinators

Coordinators

Consultants
  Infectious disease
  Dentistry
  Cardiology
  Nephrology
  Gastrointestinal
  Pulmonary
  Dermatology

Researchers

———— direct patient care
·········· Indirect patient care

Figure 4.3 The BMT Team

ing of the marrow or blood cells, transplant phase, and follow-up care. Staff nurses provide direct nursing care to patients in acute care, ambulatory care, and home care settings. Nurse administrators and nurse managers facilitate the planning and development of the transplant program. It is imperative that nurses in these various roles work together closely to ensure quality and continuity of patient care (see Table 4.5).

TRANSPLANT PROCESS

Patient Evaluation

Patients undergo a variety of physiological and psychological assessments to determine if they are eligible for a transplant. Table 4.6 lists the common tests to evaluate a patient for marrow or blood stem cell transplant. A central venous

TABLE 4.5 Adult BMT patient care delivery process

Consultation phase →	*Pretransplant phase* →	*BMT workup* →
Referral Received Patient Care Coordinator (PCC) obtains basic information, completes referral form, makes appointments. Nurse Coordinator reviews summary letter of medical history; requests additional information. CNS/PA reviews summary letters prior to visit. **Consult Day** MD/CNS/PA reviews all medical information, performs H&P, reviews profile sheet completed by patient; initiates patient education, treatment options outlined, protocol consents provided; dictates letter to referring MD; completes intake form. Nurse Coordinator/Search Coordinator consults with pt. and donor regarding BMT process; initiates education, completes coordinator referral summary. **Eligibility Screening** BMT Team discuss eligibility at weekly meeting. Nurse Coordinator completes conference summary, verifies eligibility, completes checklist.	**Pretransplant Testing (pt. and donor)** Nurse Coordinator arranges pretransplant tests, reviews results, and communicates to physician/CNS/PA. Summary of patient eligibility and schedule sent to referring physician. Social Worker obtains baseline assessment of psychosocial needs, housing issues. Nurse Coordinator provides patient education class, tour of unit, introduction to nursing staff. Search Coordinator conducts search and updates pt., referring MD of progress; regular meetings with Medical Director to evaluate search process. **Pretransplant/Stem Cell Priming Chemotherapy** MD/CNS/PA on day of admission, writes chemo orders/admit note, communicates to inpatient staff, physician and protocol consents signed. Nurse Coordinator communicates with nursing staff, initiates critical pathway, discharge teaching, arranges follow-up, and sends referring physician summary; monitors diagnostics, labs, and pt. clinical condition post chemotherapy; communicates results to CNS/physician/PA/Blood Bank; schedules apheresis or harvesting.	**AUTOLOGOUS** **Bone Marrow Harvest** Pre-op Appointment MD/CNS/PA does ADP Visit (patient education regarding harvest, H&P, OR consent signed); protocol consents signed and patient update dictated. Nurse Coordinator does patient education and pre-op instructions. Harvest Procedure MD/CNS/PA performs harvest; writes post-op orders, completes discharge teaching, dictates OR note, discharges patient. Nurse Coordinator monitors pt./donor post harvest; schedules BMT admission if needed. **Stem Cell Apheresis** Pre-apheresis Appointment/HD Chemo Priming Admit See previous column regarding stem cell priming chemo admit. MD/CNS/PA evaluates disease response, H&P, bone marrow biopsies; protocol and apheresis consents signed; patient update dictated. Nurse Coordinator does patient education, calendar, prescriptions. Stem Cell Apheresis Procedures MD/CNS/PA evaluates patient during apheresis; places central line as needed; adjusts dose of growth factor. Nurse Coordinator develops schedule for BMT, continues education process, sends referring MD letter after completion of apheresis. **ALLOGENEIC** **Work-up Appointment** MD/CNS/PA evaluates patient and donor workup; dictates patient update; protocol consents signed; performs marrow biopsies, LPs as needed. Nurse Coordinator reviews BMT schedules, provides calendar, reviews and completes education record.

TABLE 4.5 *Continued*

Transplant phase →	Posttransplant phase
Transplant Admission Nurse Coordinator coordinates BMT admission: prepares admission orders, bedside packet and coordinator flowsheet (prior to admission); coordinates admission with unit staff, HOs, sends referring physician FAX update. Search Coordinator completes NMDP admission form. **Hospital Stay** Nurse Coordinator follows critical pathway, nursing care protocols, reinfusion, discharge teaching, sets up follow-up appointment, lab work, completes weekly summaries to referring physicians; communicates discharge plan to CNS/MD/PA. BMT Team—daily rounds Search Coordinator provides NMDP with recipient updates. Data Managers complete BMT discharge summary. **Discharge** Nurse Coordinator monitors labs prior to first clinic visit.	**Outpatient Follow-up** MD/CNS/PA Assesses patients through history and physical exams. Monitors laboratory values. Provides patient education and psychosocial support. Orders medication, blood products, hydration, diagnostic studies. Performs procedures (bone marrow biopsy and aspirate, spinal taps, skins biopsies, line removal, etc.) as needed. Follows up on outpatient clinical issues, test results. Communicates to referring physicians and BMT centers through telephone contact/letters. Communicates clinical findings and treatment plans to appropriate BMT members. Determines next clinic visit and orders blood to be drawn at that visit. Telephone follow-up with patients. Completes billing form. **100-Day & Annual Evaluation** PCC schedules 100-day, 1-yr, 2-yr, 3-yr, 4-yr, 5-yr testing and appointment. Nurse coordinator reviews anniversary appointment rest results, documents on flow in shadow chart. MD/CNS/PA—H&P; evaluates test results; sends letter to referring physician. Search Coordinator monitors completion of NMDP forms and provides NMDP with recipient updates.

SOURCE: The University of Michigan Health System and Comprehensive Cancer Center, Adult BMT Program, Ann Arbor, Michigan. Used with permission.

TABLE 4.6 Evaluation of a patient for marrow or
              blood stem cell transplant

Laboratory Tests

Complete blood count
Serum tests for major organ function (renal, hepatic, endocrine)
Hepatitis screen (A, B, C)
HIV
CMV
Herpes simplex virus
PT/PTT
ABO/Rh blood group typing
Pulmonary function tests
Chest x ray
MUGA/echocardiogram
ECG
Nutritional evaluation
Psychological evaluation
Social work evaluation
Dental exam

Staging Tests

Bone marrow aspirate and biopsy
Radiological tests (computerized tomography,
  magnetic resonance imaging, bone scans, x rays,
  gallium scans)
Tumor markers

**Additional Tests for Allogeneic Transplant
  Candidates**

ABO and Rh
  Histocompatible tissue typing
HLA typing (A, B, DR)
Sequence-specific probe (SSP) molecular typing
DNA fingerprinting (RFLP or VNTR)—Same sex
  matched donors

catheter is usually inserted prior to the administration of the high-dose therapy. During this work-up phase, which may last several days to one week, the patient and family are trying to learn about the transplant process. Nurses provide much of the information and education regarding the transplant and medical care.

Financial Issues

Early in the transplant process, determining financial coverage for the transplant is a necessity. Insurance benefits must be reviewed and authorization obtained. A professional, like the transplant coordinator or case manager, who understands the patient's history, the transplant process, and insurance terminology can assist with this process (Buchsel and Kapustay, 1995).

There is much variation in the costs of transplantation. Estimates range from $50,000 to $200,000, depending on the type (autologous or allogeneic) of transplant (Hillner, Smith, Desch, 1992) and whether it can be done as an outpatient or inpatient procedure. The Health Care Financing Administration (HCFA) guidelines approve transplant for patients with acute leukemia in remission, resistant non-Hodgkin's lymphoma, recurrent neuroblastoma, medulloblastoma, and advanced Hodgkin's disease. However, the efficacy of transplantation for patients with solid tumors is highly debated (Wodinsky, Dillman, MacDonald, 1994). Some patients have had to sue their insurance companies to obtain coverage for transplants (Wieseman, 1991; Wodinsky, Dillman, MacDonald, 1994). The Blue Cross and Blue Shield Association (BCBS) has supported a randomized, clinical trial comparing transplantation with standard care for patients with breast cancer (Hillner, Smith, Desch, 1992; Wieseman, 1991). Similar studies may also be supported by insurance companies in an effort to evaluate transplant versus standard therapy.

Obtaining insurance coverage or raising funds may delay the transplant procedure. During this delay, the patient's cancer may progress, making him or her physically ineligible for the transplant. Patients and their families may experience frustration over the delay in treatment.

Patient Education

Complete discussion of the entire transplant process can be conducted by the BMT coordinator, physician, and nurse practitioner during the initial evaluation or BMT interview. The patient usually receives a variety of educational materials (pamphlets, notebooks, videos, computer programs) that describe the transplant process. The initial interview may be quite overwhelming for the patient and family. During the evaluation and eligibility workup, reinforcement and frequent encouragement to ask questions are essential. The transplant coordinator is a primary, consistent contact during this phase. Outpatient nurses also provide much of the information regarding transplant. In addition to individual contact, patients and families may benefit from small group presentations and discussions. Prior to the start of the high-dose therapy, the main objective is clarifying and describing the transplant process.

Although informed consent for children is obtained from the parent, information should be given to the child in an age-appropriate manner (Abramovitz and Senner, 1995).

Donor Search

Approximately one in three patients has an HLA-identical sibling. This figure varies based on the ethnicity of the patient. Some ethnic groups are not well represented in the donor registry and therefore matches may be less likely. For the two thirds of patients who do not have a sibling match, a matched unrelated donor (MUD) search is performed. International searches are conducted among donor registries through the National Marrow Donor Program, established in 1986, the American Bone Marrow Donor Registry (ABMDR), and smaller registries throughout the world. In early 1996 there were approximately 2 million volunteers in the NMDP registry. In recent

years, there has been an increase in the use of marrow from unrelated donors. In 1988 unrelated donor marrow was used for 5% of allogeneic transplantations; by 1990 this figure had doubled to 10% (National Cancer Institute, 1994).

Tissue Typing

A critical component of allogeneic marrow or blood cell transplant is to determine the compatibility of the donor and the recipient. The degree of compatibility is determined by comparing their HLA typing. The HLA histocompatibility system includes at least six antigen groups that are located on the sixth chromosome: HLA-A, -B, -C, -DR, -DQ and -DP (Welte, 1994). This HLA code, or fingerprint, allows the body's immune system to differentiate self and nonself cells and to mount an immune reaction against non-self cells (Weinberg, 1991). Individuals inherit two sets of antigens, a maternal haplotype and a paternal haplotype. For marrow transplantation purposes, antigens are in two classes. Class I antigens are found on the surface of most nucleated body cells and are readily detected on leukocytes. They include antigens, or loci, A and B. They are identified or typed serologically or molecularly by a small blood sample (see Chapter 3). Class II antigens are less widely distributed in the body and are especially evident on B lymphocytes. They include DR, DQ, and DP antigens or loci. The most recent typing for class II antigens uses DNA technology to identify genes that specify antigens DR and DQ. Oligonucleotide probes are used to identify these genes. It is a very accurate typing method and can be performed from whole blood samples that have been frozen and stored, unlike serological typing that requires viable cells (Franklin-Barbajosa, 1992). The search for a compatible marrow donor involves comparing the HLA-A, -B, and, -DR antigens that are most involved in developing a response to graft-versus-host disease. The ideal donor is identical to the recipient at all three loci, resulting in a six-antigen match.

The mixed lymphocyte culture (MLC) mixes the lymphocytes of the donor and the recipient and cultures them together for a period of time. A strong reaction indicates differences in the HLA-D region antigens and indicates higher risk for GVHD. For many years the MLC was important in determining class II antigen compatibility of the donor and recipient. The MLC can be difficult to analyze or reproduce. It is especially difficult to interpret if the patient has a compromised immune system from the disease or treatment. Because of these limitations, the NMDP and many transplant centers no longer require the MLC test, but have confirmatory typing using DNA technology.

Donor Preparation

Once HLA typing has been reviewed to determine the most appropriate donor, education and medical evaluation of the transplant donor is conducted by the donor center. The standard physical evaluation of a donor includes:

- Medical history
- Physical exam
- Psychosocial evaluation
- Laboratory evaluation
  CBC with differential
  Serum tests for major organ function (renal, hepatic)
  Hepatitis screen (A, B, C)
  HIV
  CMV
  HSV
  ABO and Rh
  Histocompatible tissue typing (HLA typing A, B, DR, SSP, RFLP, VNTR)
- Electrocardiograph (BM donor only)
- Chest X ray (BM donor only)

Storage of autologous blood, which may be reinfused at the time of the bone marrow harvest, is done prior to the harvest. The blood will replace the blood lost during the bone marrow harvest, and may also decrease the donor's anxiety regarding exposure to viruses in the blood donation from the community (Dannie, 1991). A thorough description of the collection or harvesting procedure and the general transplant process is discussed. Assessment of the potential impact that stem cell collection or harvest may have on the donor's lifestyle and the relationship with the recipient should also be discussed. A social worker may also evaluate or follow up with the patient or family to help them to deal with stress related to the donation or concerns for the recipient.

Unrelated donors also receive counselling prior to the donation of stem cells. The healthcare provider must remember that the donor is a volunteer and should not be pressured into donating marrow or blood stem cells. The identity of an unrelated donor remains unknown to both the patient and the transplanting center.

Harvest Procedures

Stem cells may be harvested from circulating blood or bone marrow. The method depends on the patient's type of disease and the protocol.

Blood Cell Transplant
The use of blood stem cells is replacing marrow stem cells for both autologous and allogeneic transplant. Because there are fewer stem cells in the blood stream than in bone marrow, mobilizing or enhancing the number of stem cells in the blood by using chemotherapy and/or growth factors is a common practice.

Chemotherapy causes an increase in the number of circulating progenitor cells in the peripheral blood above the baseline level. During this increase, the stem cells are collected. Mobilizing stem cells with chemotherapy results in earlier engraftment (To et al., 1990). A single agent that has been used to mobilize stem cells is cyclophosphamide (Juttner et al., 1994). Using chemotherapy for mobilization has several disadvantages. Myelosuppressive chemotherapy may result in neutropenia and infection requiring antibiotic therapy (To et al., 1990). Also, stem cell mobilization does not occur until approximately 2 weeks following the myelosuppressive chemotherapy. If not enough stem cells are collected, the patient must undergo this chemotherapy again and continue the collections (Kessinger, 1993).

Hematopoietic growth factors are also used to mobilize stem cells (Socinski et al., 1988). Common growth factors used for mobilization are granulocyte-macrophage colony-stimulating factor (GM-CSF) and granulocyte colony-stimulating factor (G-CSF). Other growth factors that may mobilize stem cells which are currently in clinical trials are erythropoietin (EPO) and PIXY 321, a fusion molecule made from a combination of GM-CSF and interleukin 3 (IL-3).

An apheresis machine collects the stem cells from the peripheral blood. Usually the white blood count (WBC) is monitored to determine when to initiate the collection of stem cells. When growth factors are used for mobilization, collections may be started when the WBC reaches 10^9/liter. If chemotherapy is used for mobilization, the collections may begin when the WBC reaches 1^9/liter. The antecubital vein may be used, however if it is inadequate, the patient usually has a central venous catheter placed, most commonly in the subclavian vein. The apheresis machine centrifuges blood drawn from the patient, drawing the stem cell layer into a collection bag and returning the rest to the patient. Depending on the type of apheresis machine, the machine may process 7 to 15 liters of blood in 2 to 4 hours. The collection procedures are repeated daily until the target cell yield is obtained. The time to collect varies

from 1 to 7 days. Methods to determine an adequate collection of blood cells include evaluating the number of mononuclear cells (MNCs), colony-forming units-granulocyte and monocyte (CFU-GM), or CD34-positive cells. Assaying cells that express the CD34-positive antigen may help to predict engraftment, although the assay itself is not standardized and is variable from institution to institution (Juttner et al., 1994).

Side effects during the collection procedure are minimal and usually well tolerated by the patient (see Table 4.7). Small children may require blood products to prime the apheresis tubing to prevent removal of too much blood. Also, the overall collection time will be longer and a lesser amount of blood should be processed. Age-appropriate activities should also be available during the lengthy apheresis procedure.

Collecting stem cells from peripheral blood offers the donor a less invasive procedure than bone marrow harvesting (Juttner et al., 1994). Also, stem cells collected from a donor's blood may result in more rapid engraftment. Another potential advantage of collecting donor stem cells is that the product may contain natural killer cells, promoting an adoptive immunotherapeutic approach (Juttner et al., 1994).

The first allogeneic BCT was reported by Kessinger and colleagues (1989). Ten apheresis collections were obtained from the donor. The T lymphocytes were depleted to decrease graft-versus-host disease. Although the patient died from an infectious complication at approximately 1 month following the transplant, hematopoietic recovery was established. More recently, several centers are collecting stem cells from the donor. Usually the donor is mobilized with a growth factor, G-CSF. Approximately 100 allogeneic blood cell transplants were reported at the 1996 BMT symposiun in Keystone, Colorado. The data looked very encouraging, however it is too early to conclude that

TABLE 4.7 Some side effects of blood stem cell collection

Potential side effects	Etiology	Assessment	Intervention
Citrate toxicity	Hypocalcemia caused by citrate's binding of ionized calcium	Baseline serum calcium Patient age Paresthesias of the extremities or circumoral area during the procedure	Notify physician if low. Do not exceed 1.5 mg/kg/minute flow in pediatric patients. Slow flow rate and offer oral calcium. Increase calcium-containing foods. Give calcium supplements.
Hypovolemia	Extracorporeal volume greater than patient's tolerance	Baseline pulse and blood pressure, Hgb/Hct, and health history Brief physical assessment and vital signs every 5 minutes initially, gradually decreasing frequency as patient's tolerance is established. Assess for: Hypotension Tachycardia Light-headedness Diaphoresis Dysrhythmias	Notify physician of abnormal or unexpected findings before proceeding Interrupt the procedure until the patient is stable, then resume at a slower flow rate and minimal extracorporeal volume. Monitor physical status and vital signs closely. Notify physician if symptoms persist or progress. Administer blood products. Administer fluid.
Thrombocytopenia	Collection of platelets into product	Baseline platelet count Ascertain whether platelet-rich plasma will be returned at the procedure's completion	Notify physician if less than 50,000/mm³. Monitor for signs of postprocedure bleeding. Administer platelet products.
Miscellaneous Chilling	Cooling of blood while circulating in apheresis machine	Note any unusual response	Provide warmth (e.g., blankets, heating pad).
Severe headache	Intracranial metastases unique to patient with cancer		Treat the problem (e.g., analgesics for headache, transfusion support).
Prolonged cytopenia	Pediatric patients with less developed hematopoietic progenitor pool		Watch for patterns of emergencies in subsequent patients and report findings to the professional community.

SOURCE: Data from Hooper and Santas, 1993; Kessinger and Schmit-Pokorny, K., 1990. Used with permission.

BCT will replace BMT in allogeneic transplantation, as is occurring with autologous transplantation.

To and colleagues (1992) noted patients who received autologous BCTs recovered neutrophils and platelet counts and required less supportive care than patients who received an allogeneic or autologous BMT. This decrease in supportive care and inpatient length of stay translates into decreased cost of transplantation for patients who receive a BCT. Henon and colleagues (1992) noted more rapid granulocyte and platelet recovery following BCT. They also noted a decrease in the documented infections, transfusions, and length of hospitalization. Cost was reduced by 45% (Henon et al., 1992).

Bone Marrow Transplant

Bone marrow, which contains more stem cells than peripheral blood (McCarthy and Goldman, 1984), can be harvested as an inpatient or outpatient procedure, under general or spinal anesthesia. The patient is placed in a prone position and multiple needle aspirations from both posterior iliac crests are obtained. Marrow may also be aspirated from the anterior iliac crests and the sternum if the cell yield is not adequate from the posterior iliac crests. The amount of bone marrow or the number of nucleated cells necessary for transplant is not established; however, most institutions attempt to harvest a minimum of 1 to 2.5×10^8 nucleated cells per kilogram (Keating, 1995). The total fluid volume obtained is usually between 500 ml and 1000 ml. The entire harvest procedure usually takes 1 to 2 hours and the patient can be discharged following recovery. The bone marrow is filtered for removal of fat and bone particles and processed similarly to blood stem cells. Marrow obtained from a donor will be depleted of red cells or plasma if there is a major ABO incompatibility of donor and recipient.

Following the harvest and recovery, the donor may experience pain at the collection sites. Mild analgesics can be prescribed. The donor's body will replace the bone marrow cells that were removed in a few weeks. The risks involved with a bone marrow harvest are minimal.

Human Cord Blood

Collection of umbilical cord blood is not standardized among institutions. Often the cells are collected by the obstetrician or nurse midwife following delivery of the placenta. Wagner and colleagues (1995) reported that the median volume of cord blood harvested was 100 ml (range 42.1 to 282 ml).

Cryopreservation

Two methods of cryopreservation are commonly used to store stem cells from blood or bone marrow. The first method uses 10% by volume of dimethylsulfoxide (DMSO) followed by controlled-rate freezing and storage in a liquid nitrogen freezer. The second method uses 5% DMSO and 6% hydroxyethyl starch (HES). The cells are then stored in a −80°C or colder freezer (Kessinger, 1993).

Marrow Purging Techniques/ Positive Selection

If there is a concern that the autologous stem cell product contains malignant cells, removal is attempted by purging. Due to the loss of normal cells during the purging procedure, additional BM or stem cells may be collected when purging is anticipated (total = 1500 to 2000 ml) (Wallerstein and Deisseroth, 1993). Pharmacological methods to purge the stem cells of malignant cells include:

- 4-Hydroperoxycylophosphamide (4-HC)
- Mafosfamide
- Cisplatin
- VP-16
- Vincristine
- Methylprednisolone

- Merocyanine 540
- Immunologic methods
- Monoclonal antibodies and complement
- Immunotoxins
- Monoclonal antibodies and magnetic microspheres
- Toxins

Physical methods to purge stem cells include:

- Lectin agglutination
- Counterflow elutriation
- Photoactive agents
- Long-term bone marrow culture
- Positive selection for normal early progenitors

Residual tumor may be removed from the stem cell product, however, the stem cells may be harmed or depleted causing the patient to have slow engraftment. Shpall and colleagues (1995) suggest that although certain patients may benefit from purged stem cell products, randomized trials comparing purged and unpurged products are needed.

Ex Vivo Expansion of Stem Cells

Another approach to obtaining an adequate amount of stem cells for transplant is ex vivo expansion or growth of the cells in the laboratory following harvest or collection. Several growth factors are added to the stem cell cultures, followed by incubation to increase the number of cells.

Preconditioning Chemotherapy

Patients with bulky disease or high tumor burden may benefit from standard-dose chemotherapy prior to the high-dose chemotherapy to decrease tumor burden. It may also be given to test chemosensitivity. This chemotherapy (i.e., cyclophosphamide) may be combined with the process of blood cell collection and serve as a mobilizer for blood stem cells.

Preparative Regimens

Following the physical and psychological evaluations and harvesting of the blood or marrow cells, the patient receives the high-dose chemotherapy. The ideal preparative regimen is capable of eradicating malignancy, has tolerable morbidity without mortality, and has sufficient immunosuppressive effect in allogeneic marrow recipients to avoid graft rejection (Forman et al., 1994). Preparative regimens vary according to the disease and medical condition of the patient and the institution's protocol. The preparative regimen consists of high-dose chemotherapy with or without radiation therapy and is capable of eradicating the disease. No ideal preparative regimen has been determined; it is selected based on the chemosensitivity of the tumor. Determing appropriate antineoplastic transplant therapy has been the major focus of marrow transplant researchers for more than 20 years. Disease recurrence, treatment-related mortality, and graft failure all remain important causes of treatment failure.

High-dose chemotherapy is usually given over a course of 2 to 6 days. Table 4.8 is a general guide to the common chemotherapy agents. It lists examples of doses, toxicities, and methods of administration. For more detailed information, see Chapter 5.

Total body irradiation (TBI), total lymphoid irradiation (TLI), or total abdominal irradiation (TAI) can be used for immunosuppression of patients or to eradicate disease. In addition, localized irradiation may be used ("boost" treatment) for areas of presumed higher concentrations of malignant cells (Shank, 1994). If TBI is part of the preparative regimen, it may be given in one dose or in multiple doses over the course of several days (fractionated radiation therapy). Fractionated dosing schedules appear to minimize the risk of side effects and are generally preferred over single doses.

TABLE 4.8 Common high-dose chemotherapy agents

Drug	Common doses	Toxicity	Method of administration
BCNU	250 mg/m² 800 mg/m²	Neurologic, hepatic, pulmonary, renal	Dilute in supplied diluent, then in infusion fluid; IVI over 1–2 hours
Busulphan	12 mg/kg 14 mg/kg 16 mg/kg	Hepatic, pulmonary, seizures, mucositis, acute and chronic skin changes	Oral divided doses, usually over 4 days *Caution:* phenytoin cover
CCNU	200 mg/m² 500 mg/m²	Hepatic, renal, pulmonary	Oral
Cyclophosphamide	120 mg/kg 200 mg/kg 7.2 g/m²	HC, SIADH, cardiac	IVI over 1 hour in D5W, over 2–4 days *Caution:* HC prophylaxis
Cytosine arabinoside (ARA-C)	4 g/m² 24 g/m² 36 g/m²	Neurologic, ophthalmic, mucositis, pulmonary, skin rash	IVI (diluted) over 1–12 hours, over 1–6 days *Caution:* steroid eye drops
Cisplatin	150 mg/m²	Neurologic, auditory, renal, severe nausea, symptomatic hypomagnesemia	IVI (diluted) over 6–8 hours (cisplatin), over 0.5–1 hour (carboplatin)
Carboplatin	450 mg/m²		*Caution:* maintain good hydration
Daunorubicin	80 mg/m² 156 mg/m²	Cardiac, mucositis	IVI over 15–30 minutes in 100 ml infusion fluid
Doxorubicin	50 mg/m²		*Caution:* check previous total exposure (cardiac toxicity)
Etoposide (VP-16-213)	450 mg/m² 1 g/m² 2 g/m² 60 mg/kg	Hepatic, HC	IVI at 1 mg/m² (max) infusion fluid over 4 hours/liter *Caution:* precipitation of drug
Melphalan	140 mg/m² 180 mg/m²	Renal, mucositis	Dissolve in supplied diluent, further dilution; IVI over 30 minutes *Caution:* not diluted in D5W

KEY: IVI = intravenous infusion, D5W = 5% dextrose solution, HC = hemorrhagic cystitis, SIADH = inappropriate antidiuretic hormone secretion
SOURCE: Adapted with permission from Treleaven, J., Barrett, J. 1992. *Bone Marrow Transplantation in Practice.* New York: Churchill Livingstone, p. 249.

Considerations relevant to the effective therapy delivered include the nature of the radioactive source, source distance, patient positioning, total dose, and dose rate. Chapter 6 provides specific information on the use of radiation therapy in marrow and blood cell transplantation.

The preparative regimens may take place as an inpatient or outpatient. The patient may be admitted to a room on a unit designated for

TABLE 4.9 Some side effects of marrow and blood cell reinfusion (transplant)

Potential side effect	Etiology	Assessment	Intervention

Nausea
Vomiting
	DMSO	Evaluate amount and frequency.	Give antiemetics
			  Lorazepam (Ativan)
			  Diphenhydramine hydro-
			    chloride (Benadryl)
			  Ondansetron (Zofran)
			  Prochlorperazine (Compazine)

Hemoglobinuria
Elevated serum
  creatinine
Elevated serum bilirubin
	Lysis of RBCs
	DMSO
		Baseline creatinine and
		  bilirubin
		Hematest urine
			Hydration

Chest tightness
Cough
Dyspnea
Increased weight
Hypertension
Tachycardia
Tachypnea
	Volume of infusate	Vital signs every 15–30
		  minutes
		I/O hourly
			Decrease rate of infusion.
			Administer furosemide or
			  mannitol.
			Give oxygen.

Chills, fever	Coldness of product	Temperature every 15–30
		  minutes
			Provide warmth.
			Give meperidine hydro-
			  chloride.
			Give acetaminophen PRN.

Garlic taste or smell	DMSO	Ask patient if taste noticed	Provide mints or gum.

Anaphylactic reaction	DMSO	Notify physician for c/o
		  itching, wheezing, skin
		  rash or erythema.
			Stop infusion.
			Administer epinephrine.

Miscellaneous
  Diarrhea
  Headache
  Flushing
  Abdominal cramping
  Malaise
	DMSO	Evaluate frequency and
		  duration.
			Treat symptoms.
			Decrease rate of infusion.

transplant patients. Isolation techniques during transplantation include reverse isolation, or reverse isolation with special air handling systems, high efficiency particulate air (HEPA) filters, or laminar air flow (LAF) (Zerbe et al., 1994). Zerbe and colleagues (1994) reported that admitting patients to LAF caused more anxiety than simple reverse isolation. They concluded that these findings need to be replicated due to lack of research-based evidence to demonstrate efficacy of many reverse isolation techniques. Some institutions administer high-dose chemotherapy on an outpatient basis, admitting the patient to the hospital only if physical conditions necessitate. Some centers administer the high-dose chemotherapy on an inpatient basis, discharging the patient prior to the transplant or shortly after (Meisinger et al., 1996). Regardless of where the chemotherapy or radiation therapy is given, the patient is instructed in procedures of basic care including mouth care, incentive spirometry, skin care, handwashing, diet, neutropenic precautions, and activity.

Stem Cell Infusion

The day of the transplant or infusion of the stem cells is generally referred to as day 0. The patient is usually premedicated to lessen the side effects associated with cell infusion (transplant). Premedications may include lorazepam, diphenhydramine hydrochloride, meperidine hydrochloride, hydrocortisone, acetaminophen, furosemide, and methylprednisolone. The patient is usually hydrated prior, during, and following the infusion. The stem cells are thawed in a water bath at approximately 37°C until the product is liquid. The stem cells are then quickly infused via a central venous catheter, using a syringe or infusion pump (Kessinger, 1993). During the infusion and for several hours following, the patient may experience side effects associated with the dimethylsulfoxide preservative, volume of infusate, or amount of red blood cells infused (see Table 4.9). Kessinger and colleagues (1990) noted that patients who received larger volumes, containing greater number of red cells, had a larger number and greater severity of side effects. Children tend to tolerate complications associated with transplant better than adults (Shannon et al., 1987).

SUPPORTIVE CARE

Infections

Bacterial, viral, and fungal infections are common following BCT or BMT. Variables that contribute to the risk, type, and severity of infection include history of viral infections, type of transplant (allogeneic or autologous), use of central venous catheters, damaged oral or gastrointestinal mucosa, and degree and duration of neutropenia. Most centers prophylactically treat patients with antibiotics, although this practice may contribute to the development of antibiotic-resistant or overgrowth of pathogens (Wujcik et al., 1994). Patients receiving allogeneic transplants may have an increased risk of infection due to the need for immunosuppression following BMT or BCT (Wujcik et al., 1994).

Bacterial infections are the most common following high-dose therapy and engraftment (Wujcik et al., 1994). Normal flora that colonizes a patient can cause an infection when the patient becomes immunocompromised. Antibiotics administered to the patient also alter the normal flora, possibly causing an infection.

Mucositis caused by the high-dose therapy makes the gastrointestinal tract one of the most common sources of infection (Reed, 1993). Several bacterial infections that may originate from mucositis include staphylococci, streptococci, *E. coli, Klebsiella,* and *Pseudomonas* (Reed, 1993).

Bacterial infections can also affect the lungs, as in bacterial pneumonia. Right atrial catheters are also a source of infection. The most common organism is staphylococcus (Reed, 1993).

Despite prophylactic antibiotics, once a patient develops a fever, treatment involves a combination of an aminoglycoside, penicillin, and possibly vancomycin (Reed, 1993).

The most common viral infections during transplant are cytomegalovirus (CMV), herpes simplex viruses (HSV), Epstein-Barr virus (EBV), and varicella-zoster (VZV). Acyclovir is commonly administered prophylactically to prevent reactivation of the herpes simplex viruses and to treat some other herpes infections. Acyclovir-resistant HSV may also be treated with foscarnet (Wujcik et al., 1994).

Fungal organisms are part of the patient's normal flora. BMT or BCT treatment measures (antibiotics, catheters, total parenteral nutrition) can contribute to the development of fungal infections. Environmental factors such as nearby construction work can also contribute to the development of fungal infections. Detecting fungal infections is very difficult. Common fungal infections include *Candida, Aspergillus,* and *Pneumocystis carinii.* Supportive care includes prophylactic antifungal medications, such as amphotericin B and rooms with HEPA filters or laminar air flow.

Early detection of infections is a high priority for the nursing staff. Nurses should assess patients every 4 hours for infection. This assessment should include taking vital signs, assessing catheter sites, checking breath sounds, evaluating mental status, and assessing daily laboratory values.

Anemia and Thrombocytopenia

Following the high-dose therapy, the patient's platelet and red blood cell (RBC) counts will decrease. To prevent hemorrhage and anemia, the patient may require multiple transfusions of platelets and RBCs. All blood products should be irradiated to prevent graft-versus-host-disease from the blood transfusion. Leukocyte-reduction filters can remove white blood cells from the product thereby decreasing the number of transfusion reactions and reducing the likelihood of transmitting certain viruses attached to the white blood cell (i.e., CMV). HLA-matched platelets may be necessary for patients who become refractory to random platelet transfusions. Prevention of bleeding in the transplant patient is imperative. Bleeding may occur from the nose, mouth, gastrointestinal tract, cranium, bladder, and vagina. Petechiae and bruising may be noted. Transfusion of platelets usually occurs at a platelet count of less than 10,000/µl and less than 8.0 gm/dl of

hemoglobin, although centers vary in their threshold values.

Renal Toxicity

Renal impairment is identified as a common toxicity associated with BMT or BCT (King et al., 1992; Ballard, 1991). Acute renal failure (ARF) may develop during any stage of BMT/BCT (King et al., 1992). Nurses need to carefully assess the patient's fluid status (weight, input, and output), laboratory values, mental status, and medications to prevent ARF or to promote recovery following a diagnosis of ARF (Ballard, 1991). Management of ARF includes continued nursing assessments, use of diuretics or volume replacement, correcting electrolyte imbalances, reducing further nephrotoxins, managing infections, and providing emotional support (King et al., 1992; Ballard, 1991). Hemodialysis or continuous renal replacement therapy (CRRT) may be required to help correct ARF (King et al., 1992).

Hepatic Toxicity

Side effects following BCT or BMT that involve the liver include veno-occlusive disease (VOD), hepatic injury caused by medications and parenteral nutrition (McDonald 1993).

Veno-occlusive disease affects 10% to 60% of transplant patients and varies from a mild toxicity to liver failure and death (McDonald, 1993). Symptoms that determine the clinical diagnosis include jaundice, fluid retention, and hepatomegaly. Additional symptoms are increased liver size, liver tenderness, increased bilirubin, edema, and ascites. VOD is caused by cellular damage to the liver from chemotherapy (McDonald, 1993). A wide variance is noted among patients who develop VOD. Approximately 70% of patients recovery from VOD with supportive care only (McDonald, 1993). Treatment includes diuresis and managing sodium and water balance.

Bladder Toxicity

Acrolein, a metabolite of cyclophosphamide and ifosfamide, can cause hemorrhagic cystitis or bleeding from the bladder (Perry, 1995). Mesna (2-mercaptoethane sulfonate sodium) is an intravenous drug that may be given during the cyclophosphamide or ifosfamide administration that binds the acrolein and prevents damage to the bladder wall.

Patients who receive mesna but still develop bleeding from the bladder may receive aggressive intravenous hydration and/or bladder irrigation. Nurses need to carefully observe fluid status in these patients because the patient may retain fluid. Maintaining an adequate platelet level is also important to decrease bleeding (Ballard, 1991).

Infection may also cause bladder toxicity. Cytomegalovirus (CMV) and adenovirus are two common causes of bladder infection leading to bleeding, dysuria, and bladder pain.

Pulmonary Toxicity

Pulmonary complications following marrow or blood cell transplantation are a major cause of morbidity and mortality, affecting between 40% and 60% of patients (Height and Sheilds, 1995). Pneumothorax may be associated with pretransplant placement of a central line. Spontaneous pneumothorax may also occur in the acute phase of transplant. Predisposing factors include high-dose steroids, TBI, and poor nutrition with recent weight loss. Pulmonary edema can be seen in the first few days following marrow or blood cell transplant and is due to fluid overload. Previous exposure to anthracyclines and the use of cyclophosphamide and TBI during conditioning can exacerbate this complication (Hamilton and Pearson, 1986). Pulmonary hemorrhage is usually associated with infection and thrombocytopenia. More rarely, acute hemorrhagic pulmonary edema can occur and

is more common among matched unrelated transplant patients receiving high doses of cyclosporin (Sloane et al., 1983). This syndrome has a high mortality rate. Transient hypoxia may occur at the time of marrow infusion due to small particles of bone and fat in the marrow.

During the acute neutropenia phase following transplant, bacterial respiratory infections occur in 20% to 50% of individuals, particularly during neutropenia (Cordonnier et al., 1986). There may be few clinical or radiological signs. Oropharyngeal mucositis is a common complication and colonization by gram-positive or gram-negative organisms, particularly *Pseudonomas* species, *Klebsiella*, *Serratia*, and *Enterobacter* species, frequently occurs. Spread to the lungs may be direct by aspiration or indirect by bacteremia, leading to lower respiratory tract infection (Treleaven and Wiernik, 1995). Atypical organisms including mycoplasma pneumonia, legionella, and *Chlamydia* have also been implicated in the acute phase of transplant. Most antibiotic regimens are designed to cover both gram-negative and gram-positive organisms. Empiric treatment is usually initiated when patients become febrile. Early intervention results in resolution of most bacterial infections. If the patient does not respond to antibiotic therapy and exhibits signs of pulmonary infection, a bronchoscopy with bronchoalveolar lavage may be performed to attempt to identify the causative organism. Transbronchial biopsy or open lung biopsy are not routinely performed.

The herpes virus and cytomegalovirus (CMV) primarily account for the majority of posttransplant viral respiratory infections. Other herpes viruses are responsible for up to 7% of infectious pneumonitis (Chan et al., 1990). Herpes simplex pneumonitis occurs mainly in the first few weeks after transplant. Other respiratory viruses that have been implicated in episodes of posttransplant pneumonitis include respiratory syncytial virus (RSV), the parainfluenza viruses, and adenovirus.

Marrow and blood stem cell transplant patients are susceptible to respiratory fungal infections which are mainly due to *Aspergillus* species, *Candida* species, and occasionally *Cryptococcus neoformans*. During the acute phase, the risk of developing a fungal infection is directly related to the duration and severity of neutropenia. During the first 3 weeks, the risk of developing *Aspergillus* infection has been estimated at 1% per day, with the risk increasing to 4.3% per day after day 22 (Gerson et al., 1984). Even after recovery of neutrophils, the transplant patient remains at high risk for fungal infections due to the intensive preparative regimen and use of immunosuppressants.

Pneumocystis carinii (PCP) is an opportunistic organism that causes a desquamative alveolitis in immunocompromised patients with defective T-cell function. The peak time for posttransplant development of PCP is between 30 and 100 days, and the organism is implicated in up to 4% of cases of infectious pneumonitis (Hamilton and Pearson, 1986).

Interstitial pneumonitis occurs most frequently between 30 and 100 days following marrow transplantation in 20% to 65% of patients. In half of the cases, CMV infection is the responsible organism. The other half of the cases are due to other unidentifiable agents termed *idiopathic*. The risk factors for idiopathic pneumonia include the type of chemotherapy in the preparative regimen, pre-existing pulmonary abnormality, older age, TBI in the preparative regimen, methotrexate to prevent GVHD, and severe GVHD (Weiner et al., 1986). Occasionally patients respond to steroid treatment, but most do not. The mortality of marrow transplant patients with pneumonitis who require intubation and mechanical ventilation is greater than 90%. Bronchoalveolar lavage has become the "gold standard" for diagnosing pneumonitis following marrow trans-

plant. Open lung biopsy is very rarely used. Chapter 11 describes pulmonary toxicity associated with transplantation in detail.

Neurological Complications

Neurological complications can occur at any stage of marrow or blood stem cell transplantation. Table 4.10 lists causes of neurologic complications during the early post-BMT phase. Early clinical signs of neurological complications vary according to the causative factor. Although the patient may exhibit focal neurological signs, drowsiness or seizures are more usual (Kanfer, 1992). Routine neurologic assessments of the transplant patient should be performed in an effort to identify early neurologic changes and prevent long-term complications (Openshaw and Slatkin, 1994). Chapter 13 discusses neurological effects in more detail.

TABLE 4.10 **Causes of neurologic complications in early posttransplant phase**

Metabolic Causes
Respiratory failure—hypoxic encephalopathy of
  interstitial pneumonia
Hepatic failure—hepatic encephalopathy of VOD
  or GVHD
Renal failure—uremic encephalopathy

Infections
Bacterial—meningitis, gram-negative sepsis
Viral—CMV
Fungal—*Aspergillus, Candida albicans,*
  Cryptococcus
Protozoal—*Toxoplasma gondii*

Drug Toxicities
Chemotherapy, steroids, immunosuppressants,
  sedative-hypnotic drugs

Cerebrovascular Events
Infarction—ischemic stroke
Hemorrhage—intracranial bleeding

Gastrointestinal Complications

Most patients experience some degree of gastrointestinal (GI) complications including nausea, vomiting, anorexia, mucositis, and diarrhea during the acute phase of marrow or blood cell transplantation. The GI tract is affected by the preparative chemotherapy and total body irradiation (TBI). Chemotherapy acts on the midbrain vomiting centers, causing symptoms during the conditioning therapy (Chapko et al., 1989). The intensity of vomiting tends to be worse with higher dose regimens, but antiemetic therapy reduces the severity of symptoms. Patients remain mildly nauseated and anorexic for 3 to 6 weeks following the preparative regimen (Shuhart and McDonald, 1994). Mucositis causes swelling, pain, and in severe cases sloughing of the oropharyngeal epithelium, and may be worsened by superinfection and methotrexate therapy (Schubert et al., 1992). Mucositis pain can be effectively treated with opioids but can lead to gastric stasis, intestinal ileus, anorexia, and vomiting (Shuhart and McDonald, 1992).

Early gastrointestinal manifestations of acute GVHD include anorexia, nausea, vomiting, abdominal pain, and diarrhea. Endoscopic biopsy is often needed to confirm the diagnosis and rule out an infectious process.

Medications that the patient is receiving also contribute to nausea, anorexia, and diarrhea. Oral antibiotics (especially nystatin and trimethoprim sulfamethoxazole, amphotericin B given IV, and TPN have been associated with nausea, vomiting, and anorexia. Oral magnesium and nonabsorbable antibiotics (vancomycin, tobramycin, and nystatin) can cause mild diarrhea (Buchsel, 1993).

Infections of the GI system may also cause anorexia, vomiting, and diarrhea. Common infections of the GI system include CMV, HSV, Aspergillus, Toxoplasma, or viruses. Diarrhea associated with acute GVHD and infections is seen as early as day 7 in mismatched BMT patients (Hill et al., 1990).

Nursing care of the patient with gastrointestinal complications includes meticulous oral care, effective pain management, a good antiemetic program, adequate skin care, and nutritional assessment and support. See Chapter 10 for further information on gastrointestinal effects.

Acute Graft-versus-Host Disease

Acute GVHD is caused by donor T lymphocytes that attack the epithelium of the skin, gut, and liver in the marrow transplant patient (Wujcik et al., 1994). It occurs during the first 100 days post transplant. The incidence of acute GVHD ranges from 15% to 80% of patients undergoing allogeneic BMT (Kanfer, 1995). High risk factors for the development of acute GVHD include unrelated donor and HLA-mismatched donor, sex mismatching, donor parity, older age, and the type of GVHD prophylaxis. Table 4.11 shows the influences on incidence of GVHD. The median day of onset for acute GVHD is day 17 (Bortin et al., 1989). Clinical features of acute GVHD usually begin with a macropapular rash that may be pruritic or painful, red in color and initially involves the palm and soles. As the rash progresses, the cheeks, neck, and trunk are affected, often with papule formation. A "hyperacute" or severe form of GVHD includes fever, influenzalike symptoms, generalized erythroderma, and desquamation developing 7 to 14 days after transplant. A skin biopsy is performed to confirm the diagnosis.

Symptoms of intestinal GVHD include profuse diarrhea (several liters per day), gastrointestinal bleeding, crampy abdominal pain, and ileus. Some patients present with anorexia and dyspepsia and may not have lower tract involvement. Gastrointestinal endoscopy and biopsy are needed to confirm the diagnosis.

TABLE 4.11 Influences on incidence of GVHD

Degree of significance	Less GVHD	More GVHD
More Significant		
Donor-recipient relationship	Identical twins Self (autologous) Matched sibling	Mismatched relative Unrelated donor
Type of prophylaxis	T cell depletion MTX + CSP combined	None MTX alone CSP alone
Donor-recipient sex match	Male to male Male to female Nulliparous female to male	Parous female to male
Less Significant		
Age of recipient and donor	Younger	Older
BMT conditioning regimen	Less intensive	More intensive
Post-BMT viral infection (particularly cytomegalovirus)	No	Yes

SOURCE: Treleaven, J., Wiernik, P. 1995. *Color Atlas and Text of Bone Marrow Transplantation.* London: Mosby-Wolfe, p. 144. Used with permission.

Liver GVHD usually presents with elevated liver enzymes, liver tenderness, hepatomegaly, and eventual jaundice. Liver biopsy is usually not required if the patient already has documented skin or gut GVHD, but is useful in some cases.

Thrombocytopenia, anemia, leaky capillary syndrome, hemolysis, and ocular symptoms have been reported in patients with acute GVHD (Sullivan, 1994). Chapter 8 describes the clinical and pathological grading systems for acute GVHD that are commonly used.

Several methods are used to prevent the incidence and lower the severity of GVHD. Combination immunosuppressive agents (e.g., methotrexate, cyclosporin, steroids, cyclophosphamide), antibody treatment (IVIG, ATG, anti–T-cell monoclonal antibodies, anti-IL-2, anti-IL-1 and anti-TNF-alpha), and marrow T-cell depletion all show reduction in the incidence and severity of acute GVHD. New immunosuppressive agents being investigated in clinical trials include trimetrexate, succinylacetone, FK-506, rapamycin, thalidomide, and ultraviolet radiation (Sullivan, 1994). Steroids are used for the treatment of established GVHD. Chapter 8 discusses GVHD in more detail.

Cardiac Toxicity

Cardiac toxicity is a potentially fatal consequence of marrow transplant and is thought to be a side effect of cyclophosphamide conditioning (Kupariet et al., 1990). The life-threatening incidence is 5% to 10% of patients who receive regimens containing cyclophosphamide (Bearman et al., 1988). Severe cardiac toxicity is characterized by ECG voltage loss, progressive heart failure, or pericarditis with or without tamponade. These effects usually occur within several days to weeks of cyclophosphamide administration. Minor ECG changes, such as ST-T wave segment changes, supraventricular arrhythmias, or pericarditis without hemodynamically significant effusion develop in up to 90% of patients receiving cyclophosphamide-containing preparative regimens (Peterson and Bearman, 1994). Several studies have suggested that the dose of cyclophosphamide is a major factor in the development of cardiac toxicity. The contribution of prior anthracycline therapy, mediastinal radiotherapy, or TBI to the development of cardiac toxicity is unclear. Baseline MUGA scans are done to measure left ejection fraction prior to transplant. Some transplant centers exclude from transplantation patients whose resting left ejection fraction is less than 50%. In addition, most centers conduct daily ECGs prior to administration of cyclophosphamide.

Carmustine (BCNU) is another chemotherapeutic agent that is increasingly used in transplant preparative regimens and has been reported to be associated with cardiac toxicity (Kupari et al., 1990).

Treatment of severe cardiac toxicity consists of symptomatic pharmacological support and fluid management. Pericardiocentesis or placement of a pericardial window may be necessary for hemodynamically significant pericardial effusions (Peterson and Bearman, 1994).

Routine nursing assessment should include identifying high-risk patients, monitoring fluids, and monitoring cardiac behavior as needed.

ENGRAFTMENT AND RECOVERY

It takes approximately 14 to 21 days following the transplant for the cells to find their home ("homing") and begin to produce normal blood cells. Hematopoietic and immunological recovery of the transplant patient occur at variable speeds and are influenced by a number of factors including the nature and status of the primary disease, previously administered chemotherapy and radiation, the type of preparative regimen, the type of GVHD prophylaxis, viral complications (particularly CMV), and the use of antiviral agents (Messner and McCulloch, 1994).

The average length of hospital stay varies according to the patient's condition, type of transplant, and protocol. The advent of blood cell transplant and use of growth factors has dramatically reduced the length of hospital stay in recent years. Discharge planning should begin early in the course of the hospitalization. Transplant centers vary in their criteria for discharge from the acute-care setting. Common criteria for discharge following transplant include:

- Patient's absolute neutrophil count (ANC) is greater than 500/mm^3 for 2 consecutive days.
- Patient is afebrile and has been off antibiotics for 48 hours.
- Patient's oral intake is greater than 1000 Kcal per day.
- Nausea and vomiting is controlled.
- Diarrhea is less than 500 ml per day.
- Patient tolerance of oral medications has lasted at least 48 hours.
- Caregivers are able and willing to provide 24-hour care for as long as needed.
- The patient or caregiver is able to care for central venous catheter.

Discharge from the hospital is often a time of both excitement and anxiety for patients and their families. Patients looks forward to recuperating in their own homes, sleeping in their own beds, eating home-cooked foods, and resuming their previous lifestyles. At the same time, they are hesitant to "cut the cord" with the health-care team that has provided vigilant care in the hospital. Families may feel inadequate in providing the necessary care for the patients. It may also put an additional burden on families if someone must take time off from

Take your temperature twice a day (for the first month following discharge) or if you feel warm or have shaking chills. Notify the BMT nurse or physician if your temperature is 100.2°F or greater, or to report shaking chills. You may take acetaminophen after you have taken and recorded your temperature.

Other problems needing immediate attention and notification include:

- Headache, particularly if severe
- Nausea or vomiting
- Rash or small water-filled blisters
- Cough or any difficulty breathing
- Pain
- Bleeding
- Redness, tenderness, swelling, or drainage at central line exit
- Severe diarrhea and/or rectal pain

Avoid crowds, small children, people with colds or flulike symptoms.

Watch for bruises and bleeding. Avoid activity that might cause trauma. Avoid sharp objects (razors, knives, etc.).

Change central line dressing every Monday, Wednesday, and Friday, or as directed by your BMT nurse.

Follow dietary guidelines as recommended by your dietician. Keep a diary of the foods and fluids you take in and bring it with you on your first visit in the outpatient clinic.

Bring your medications and medication schedule with you for your first visit in the outpatient clinic.

For questions or problems call your BMT nurse or physician at _____ . If unable to reach him or her, call _____ and ask for the BMT physician on call.

Next appointment _____

Next blood count _____ (date)

_____ (location)

Medications to take at home:

_____

_____

_____

Figure 4.4   Home care for the blood cell or marrow transplant patient

work or change daily living patterns. It is important for the nurse to discuss these common feelings with patients and families when planning discharge. Patients need to be reassured that their discharge depends on competent caregivers and adequate supports and resources in the home. Additionally, the BMT team is available 24 hours a day, 7 days a week.

Self-Care and Home Care

It is critical that the BMT nurse provide verbal and written discharge instructions to patients and their families prior to discharge. These instructions should include signs and symptoms to report to the transplant center, bleeding precautions, infection control practices, central line care, dietary restrictions, medication instructions, dates of outpatient appointments and blood counts, and what to do in an emergency. Figure 4.4 illustrates common written discharge instructions given to marrow and blood stem cell transplant patients. It is not all-inclusive of written instructions given to the patients regarding follow-up care.

Follow-up Care

Follow-up care of the marrow or blood cell recipient for the first 100 days after transplant can be provided in an outpatient, ambulatory, or home-care setting. The focus of the health-care team is to prevent and treat complications and to assess engraftment and disease status in the post-BMT recipient. Major complications that may occur 30 to 100 days post-allogeneic transplant include acute GVHD, interstitial pneumonia (CMV and idiopathic), and disseminated fungal infection. Other complications that may occur during this phase are varicella-zoster virus, bacteremia, herpes simplex virus, and restrictive lung disease. Figure 4.5 illustrates the temporal sequence of major complications after allogeneic bone marrow transplan-

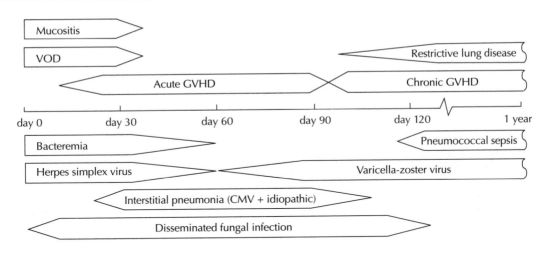

Figure 4.5 **Temporal sequence of major complications after allogenenic bone marrow transplantation on day 0**

SOURCE: Press, O.W., Schaller, R.T., Thomas, E.D.: *Complications of Organ Transplantation.* New York, Marcel Dekker, 1987. Reprinted courtesy of Marcel Dekker, Inc.

tation. Routine care includes thorough physical assessments, blood work, blood product transfusions, administration of TPN, antibiotics, immunoglobulin, and IV fluids, symptom management, skin biopsies, bone marrow biopsies and aspirations, spinal taps with the instillation of intrathecal chemotherapy, close monitoring of medication administration and drug levels, and care of the central venous catheter. Additionally, psychosocial support and physical therapy is continued during this posttransplant phase.

It is crucial that nurses working in the outpatient and home-care setting provide consistent care and communicate regularly. It is extremely beneficial for the home-care nurse to meet the patient and family prior to discharge. This will alleviate anxiety the patient and family may feel about the patient's going home.

Posttransplant Evaluation

Most centers evaluate disease status and major organ toxicity 100 days following transplant. Patients generally undergo the following tests: MUGA scan, pulmonary function test, liver function tests, and kidney function tests. Additional testing of tumor response is done individually for the particular disease and may include bone marrow biopsy and aspirate, tumor markers, CT scans, MRI, bone scans, and skeletal scans. Following this evaluation, patients are referred to their community physicians and nurses. Annual evaluations are recommended to examine the patient for transplant-related problems.

Delayed Complications after Transplant

The number of marrow and blood cell recipients is increasing rapidly. Most patients are able

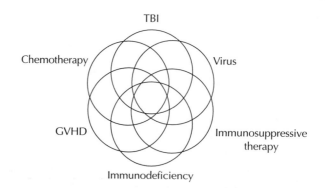

Figure 4.6
**Multifactorial etiology
of delayed posttransplant
complications**

SOURCE: Forman, S.J., Blume, K.G., Ponnall, T.E. 1994. *Bone Marrow Transplantation*. Boston: Blackwell Scientific Publications, 538. Used with permission.

to live a relatively normal productive life. Some, however, develop delayed or long-term complications that compromise quality of life. Common delayed complications following transplant include:

- Chronic graft-versus-host disease
- Pulmonary disease
- Neurologic complications
- Disease relapse
- Secondary malignancies
- Cataracts
- Sterility
- Growth and development disorders in children
- Psychosocial dysfunction
- Avascular necrosis
- Late infectious complications
- Dental problems
- Genitourinary dysfunction
- Chronic fatigue

Some delayed complications are transplant related (e.g., GVHD, immunodeficiency); others are due to the intensity of the preparative regimen (e.g., infertility, cataracts). Some of the delayed complications are related to the under-lying disease (e.g., recurrence of disease) and many are multifactorial in etiology (e.g., secondary malignancies, chronic pulmonary disease) (Deeg, 1994). Figure 4.6 shows multifactorial etiology of delayed posttransplant complications.

REFERENCES

Abramovitz, L., Senner, A. 1995. Pediatric bone marrow transplantation update. *Oncol Nurs Forum* 22(1): 107-115.

Armitage, J., Gale, R. 1989. Bone marrow autotransplantation. *Am J Med* 86:203-206.

ASCO/ASH. 1990. Recommended criteria for the performance of bone marrow transplantation. *Blood* 75(5): 1209.

Ballard, B. 1991. Renal and hepatic complications. In Whedon, M. (Ed.) *Bone Marrow Transplantation: Principles, Practice, and Nursing Insights.* Boston: Jones & Bartlett, 241-261.

Barrett, A.J. 1991. Worldwide bone marrow transplantation activity in the last decade. In Champlin, R.K., Gale, R.P. (Eds.) *New Strategies in Bone Marrow Transplantation.* New York: Wiley-Liss, 1.

Bearman, S.I., Appelbaum, F.R., Buckner, C.D., et al. 1988. Regimen-related toxicity in patients undergoing bone marrow transplantation. *J Clin Oncol* 6: 1562-1568.

Bortin, M.M., Horowitz, M.M., Rimm, A.A. 1992. Increasing utilization of allogeneic bone marrow transplantation. *Ann Intern Med* 116:505-512.

Bortin, M.M., Ringden, O., Horowitz, M.M., et al. 1989. Temporal relationships between the major complications of bone marow transplantation. *BMT* 4:339-334.

Buchsel, P. 1993. Bone marrow transplantation. In Groenwald, S., Frogge, M., Goodman M., et al. *Cancer Nursing: Principles and Practice,* 3d ed. Boston: Jones & Bartlett, 393-434.

Buchsel, P., Kapustay, P. 1995. Peripheral stem cell transplantation. *Oncol Nurs* 2(2):1-14.

Chan, C.K., Hyland, R.H., Hutcheon, M.A. 1990. Pulmonary complications following bone marrow transplantation. *Clin Chest Med* 11:323-332.

Chapko M.K., Syrjala, K.L., Schilter, I., et al. 1989. Chemotherapy toxicity during bone marrow transplantation: time course and variation in pain and nausea. *BMT* 4:181-186.

Cordonnier, C., Bernaudin, J.F., Bierling, P., et al. 1986. Pulmonary complications occurring after allogeneic bone marrow transplantation: a study of 130 consecutive transplanted patients. *Cancer* 58:1047-1054.

Crump, M., Smith, A., Brandwein, J., et al. 1993. High-dose etoposide, melphalan and autologous bone marrow transplantation for patients with advanced Hodgkin's disease: importance of disease status at transplant. *J Clin Oncol* 11(4):704-711.

Dannie, E. 1991. Assessment of bone marrow donors. *Nurs Stand* 5(32):28-31.

Deeg, J.H. 1994. Delayed complications after bone marrow transplantation. In Forman, S.J., Blume, K.G., Thomas, E.D. (Eds.) *Bone Marrow Transplantation.* Boston: Blackwell Scientific.

Forman, S.J., Blume K.G., Thomas, E.D. (Eds.) 1994. *Bone Marrow Transplantation.* Boston: Blackwell Scientific.

Franklin-Barbajosa, C. 1992. DNA profiling: the new science of identity. *Natl Geo* 181:112-24.

Freedman, S.E., 1988. An overview of bone marrow transplantation. *Semin Oncol Nurs* 4:3-8.

Friedrich, W. 1994. Marrow transplantation for primary immunodeficiency diseases. *Marrow Transplant Rev* 4(2):17-22.

Gale, R., Butturini, A. 1995. What is the best strategy for bone marrow and blood cell autotransplants in cancer? In Armitage, A., Antman, K. (Eds.) *High-Dose Cancer Therapy: Pharmacology, Hematopoietins, Stem Cells.* Baltimore: Williams & Wilkins, 117-119.

Gerson, S.L., Talbot, G.H., Hurwit, S. 1984. Prolonged granulocytopenia: the major risk factor for invasive pulmonary aspergillosis in patients with acute leukemia. *Ann Intern Med* 100:345-351.

Hamilton P.J., Pearson, A.D.J. 1986. Bone marrow transplantation and the lung. *Thorax* 41:497-502 (editorial).

Height, S., Sheilds, M. 1995. Problems following bone marrow transplantation. In Treleaven, J., Wiernik, P. (Eds.) *Color Atlas and Text of Bone Marrow Transplantation.* London: Mosby-Wolfe, 169-180.

Henon, P., Liang, H., Beck-Wirth, G., et al. 1992. Comparison of hematopoietic and immune recovery after autologous bone marrow or blood stem cell transplants. *BMT* 9:285-291.

Hill, H.H., Chapman, R.C., Kornell J.A., et al. 1990. Self-administration of morphine in bone marrow transplant patients reduces drug requirement. *Pain* 40:121-129.

Hillner, B., Smith, T., Desch, C. 1992. Efficacy and cost-effectiveness of autologous bone marrow transplantation in metastatic breast cancer. *JAMA* 267(15):2055-2061.

Hooper, P., Santas, E. 1993. Peripheral blood stem cell transplantation. *Oncol Nurs Forum* 20(8):1215-1221.

Horowitz, M. 1995. New IBMTR/ABMTR slides summarize current use and outcome of allogeneic and autologous transplants. *IBMTR Newsletter* 2(1):1-8.

Jagannath, S., Armitage, J., Dicke, K., et al. 1989. Prognostic factors for response and survival after high-dose cyclophosphamide, carmustine, and etoposide with autologous bone marrow transplantation for relapsed Hodgkin's disease. *J Clin Oncol* 7(2):179-185.

Juttner, C., Fibbe, W., Nemunaitis, J., et al. 1994. Blood cell transplantation: report from an international consensus meeting. *BMT* 14:689-693.

Kanfer, E. 1992. The diagnosis and management of early complications. In Treleaven, J., Barrett, J. (Eds.) *Bone Marrow Transplantation in Practice.* New York: Churchill Livingstone, 315-327.

Kanfer, E. 1995. Graft-versus-host disease. In Treleaven, J., Wiernk, P. (Eds.) *Color Atlas and Text of Bone Marrow Transplantation.* London: Mosby-Wolfe, 143-153.

Keating, A. 1995. Autologous bone marrow transplantation. In Armitage, A., Antman, K. (Eds.) *High-Dose Therapy: Pharmacology, Hematopoietins, Stem Cells.* Baltimore: Williams & Wilkins, 172-195.

Kessinger, A. 1993. Utilization of peripheral blood stem cells in autotransplantation. *Hematol Oncol Clin North Am* 7(3):535-545.

Kessinger, A., Schmit-Pokorny, K. 1990. Toxicities associated with cryopreserved autologous peripheral stem cell infusions: influence of purification methods. *J Clin Apheresis* 5:156.

Kessinger, A., Smith, D., Strandjord, S., et al. 1989. Allogeneic transplantation of blood derived, T cell-depleted hemopoietic stem cells after myeloablative treatment in a patient with acute lymphoblastic leukemia. *BMT* 4:643-646.

King, C., Hoffar, N., Murray, M. 1992. Acute renal failure in bone marrow transplantation. *Oncol Nurs Forum* 19(9):1327-1335.

Kupari, M., Violin, L., Suokas, A., et al. 1990. Cardiac involvement in bone marrow transplantation; electrocardiographic changes, arrhythmias, heart failure and autopsy findings. *BMT* 5:91-98.

Kurnick, N.B., Montano, A., Gerdes, J.C., et al. 1958. Preliminary observations on the treatment of post irradiation hemopoietic depression in man by the infusion of stored autologous bone marrow. *Ann Intern Med* 49:973.

McCarthy, D., Goldman, J. 1984. Transfusion of circulating stem cells. *CRC Crit Rev Clin Lab Sci* 20(1):1-24.

McDonald, G. 1993. Venoocclusive disease of the liver following marrow transplantation. *Marrow Transplant Rev* 3(4):49-54.

Meisinger, D., Sasse, S., Schmit-Pokorny, K. 1996. "Early discharge" autologous bone marrow or peripheral stem cell transplant patients: outcomes. *Oncol Nurs Forum* 23(2):328 (abstr).

Messner, H.A., McCulloch, E.A. 1994. Mechanisms of human hematopoiesis. In Forman, S.J., Blume, K.G., Thomas, E.D. (Eds.) *Bone Marrow Transplantation.* Boston: Blackwell Scientific, 41-71.

Meyer, C. 1992. The richness of oncology nursing. *AJN* 92(5):71-78.

National Cancer Institute Publication. 1994. Bone marrow transplantation and peripheral blood stem cell transplantation. *NIH Pub* 95-1178.

Openshaw, H., Slatkin, N.E. 1994. Neurological complications of bone marrow transplantation. In Forman, S.J., Blume, K.G., Thomas, E.D. (Eds.) *Bone Marrow Transplantation.* Boston: Blackwell Scientific, 482-496.

Pegg, D.E. 1966. Syngeneic bone marrow transplantation in man. In Pegg, D.E. (Ed.) *Bone Marrow Transplantation.* London: Lloyd-Luke, 102.

Perry, M. 1995. Genitourinary, gastrointestinal, endocrine, nervous system, and coagulation complications. In Armitage, A, Antman, K. (Eds.) *High-Dose Cancer Therapy: Pharmacology, Hematopoietins, Stem Cells.* Baltimore: Williams & Wilkins, 609-618.

Peterson, F.B., Bearman, S.I. 1994. Preparative regimens and their toxicity. In Forman, S.J., Blume, K.G., Thomas, E.D. (Eds.) *Bone Marrow Transplantation.* Boston: Blackwell Scientific, 96-113.

Press, O.W., Schaller, R.T., Thomas, E.D. 1987. *Complications of Organ Transplantation.* New York: Marcel Dekker.

Randolph, S. 1993. Home care of the bone marrow transplant recipient. *Home Healthc Nurse* 11(1):24-28.

Reed, E. 1993. Infectious complications during autotransplantation. *Hematol Oncol Clin North Am* 7(3):717-735.

Santos, G. 1985. Overview of autologous bone marrow transplantation. *Interl J Cell Cloning* 3:215-216.

Shank, B. 1994. Radiotherapeutic principles of bone marro transplantation. In Forman, S.J., Blume, K.G., Thomas, E.D. (Eds.) *Bone Marrow Transplantation.* Boston: Blackwell Scientific, 96-113.

Shannon, K., Cowan, M., Matthay, K. 1987. Pediatric bone marrow transplantation: intensive care management. *J Intensive Care Med* 2:328-344.

Shpall, E., Cagnoni, P., Gehling, U., et al. 1995. Bone marrow purging. In Armitage, A., Antman, K. (Eds.) *High-Dose Cancer Therapy: Pharmacology, Hematopoietins, Stem Cells.* Baltimore: Williams & Wilkins, 609-618.

Shubert, M.M., Williams, B.E., Lloid, M.E., et. al. 1992. Clinical assessment scale for the rating of oral mucosal changes following bone marrow transplantation. *Cancer* 69:2469-2477.

Shuhart, M.C., McDonald, G.B. 1994. Gastrointestinal and hepatic complications. In Forman, S.J., Blume, K.G., Thomas, E.D. (Eds.) *Bone Marrow Transplantation.* Boston: Blackwell Scientific, 454-481.

Sloane, J.P., Depledge, M.H., Powles, R.L. 1983. Histopathology of the lung after bone marrow transplantation. *J Clin Pathol* 36: 546-554.

Sobocinski, K.A., Horowitz, M.M., Rowlings, O.A., et al. 1994. Bone marrow transplantation—1994: a report from the International Bone Marrow Transplant Registry and the North American Autologous Bone Marrow Transplant Registry. *J Hematotherapy* 3:95-192.

Socinski, M., Cannistra, S., Elias, A., et al. 1988. Granulocyte-macrophage colony stimulating factor expands the circulating haemapoietic progenitor cell compartment in man. *Lancet* 1:1194.

Sullivan, K.M. 1994. Graft-versus-host disease. In Forman, S.J., Blume, K.G., Thomas, E.D. (Eds.) *Bone*

Marrow Transplantation. Boston: Blackwell Scientific, 339-362.

To, L., Roberts, M., Haylock, D., et al. 1992. Comparison of haematological recovery times and supportive care requirements of autologous recovery phase peripheral blood stem cell transplant, autologous bone marrow transplants and allogeneic bone marrow transplants. *BMT* 9(4):277-284.

To, L., Shepperd, K., Haylock., et al. 1990. Single dose of cyclophosphamide enable the collection of high numbers of hemapoietic stem cells from the peripheral blood. *Exp Hematol* 18:442.

Treleaven, J., Barrett, J. 1992. *Bone Marrow Transplantation in Practice.* New York: Churchill Livingstone.

Treleaven, J., Wiernik, P. 1995. *Color Atlas and Text of Bone Marrow Transplantation.* London: Mosby-Wolfe.

Wagner, J., Kernan, N., Steinbuch, M., et al. 1995. Allogeneic sibling umbilical-cord-blood transplantation in children with malignant and non-malignant disease. *Lancet* 346:214-219.

Wallerstein, R., Deisseroth, A. 1993. Use of blood and blood products. In DeVita, V., Hellman, S., Rosenberg, S. (Eds.) *Cancer: Principles and Practice of Oncology.* Philadelphia: J.B. Lippincott, 2262-2275.

Weinberg P.A. 1991. The human leukocyte antigen (HLA) system, the search for a matching donor, national marrow donor program development, and marrow donor issues. In Whedon, M. (Ed.) *Bone Marrow Transplantation: Principles, Practice, and Nursing Insights.* Boston: Jones & Bartlett, 105-131.

Weiner, R.S., Bortin, M.M., Gale, R.P. 1986. Interstitial pneumonitis after bone marrow transplantation. *Ann Intern Med* 104:168-175.

Welte, K. 1994. Matched unrelated transplants. *Semin Oncol Nurs* 10(1):20-27.

Whedon, M.B. 1991. *Bone Marrow Transplantation: Principle, Practice, and Nursing Insights.* Boston: Jones & Bartlett.

Wieseman, T. 1991. Suing insurers: litigation over autologous bone marrow transplants and breast cancer. *Oncol Issues* 6(2):7-12.

Wodinsky, H., Dillman, R., MacDonald, S. 1994. Assessing peripheral stem cell transplant technology. *J Oncol Manage* 3(4):22-27.

Wujcik, D., Ballard, B., Camp-Sorrell, D. 1994. Selected complications of allogeneic bone marrow transplantation. *Semin Oncol Nurs* 10(1):28-41.

Zerbe, M., Parkerson, S., Spitzer, T. 1994. Laminar air flow versus reverse isolation: nurses' assessments of moods, behaviors, and activity levels in patients receiving bone marrow transplants. *Oncol Nurs Forum* 21(3):565-568.

5

Pharmacologic and Biologic Agents

Suzanne P. Dix, Gary C. Yee

Patients who undergo bone marrow transplantation receive a wide variety of medications from cytotoxic agents to medications to prevent or treat adverse effects of cytotoxic therapy. Many medications commonly used in other oncology patients are also used in patients who receive bone marrow transplantation, but often in higher doses or on different schedules. Allogeneic bone marrow transplantation patients also require at least 6 months of immunosuppressive therapy, which puts them at risk for complications that often require additional pharmacologic interventions. More recently, the use of high-cost biotechnology products, such as colony-stimulating factors, has become standard care. Prudent and rational use of pharmacologic and biologic agents including chemotherapy, immunosuppressive agents, and other supportive care medications is integral to the success of BMT.

Comprehensive knowledge of the rationale for selection of various drug therapies and the unique aspects related to dosing, administration, and monitoring of medications given to BMT patients is essential. In addition, staff who care for this population of patients must be able to recognize common toxicities associated with these medications and know how to prevent or treat them.

CHEMOTHERAPY

Preparative Regimens

The ideal preparative regimen for BMT requires four main properties (the 4 *A*s), which are outlined in Table 5.1. The aim of the preparative regimen varies depending on the type of transplant, autologous or allogeneic, and the indication for BMT, malignant or nonmalignant disease. The goals of preparative regimens for allogeneic BMT for malignant diseases are to eradicate residual malignancy, suppress the patient's immune system to prevent graft rejection, and ablate the host bone marrow to allow space for the donor bone marrow. In autologous BMT, immunosuppression is not needed because the source of bone marrow is the host, which eliminates the risk for graft rejection or GVHD. Thus, antitumor and ablative effects are the main goals of a preparative regimen for autologous BMT. In BMT for nonmalignant diseases such as aplastic anemia, the need to eradicate malignancy is eliminated, leaving immunosuppressive and ablative effects as the main properties of the preparative regimen.

Knowing the ideal properties of a preparative regimen helps one understand the design and evolution of various BMT preparative regi-

TABLE 5.1 Ideal properties of BMT preparative regimens

	Allogeneic for malignant disease	Allogeneic for nonmalignant disease	Autologous for malignant disease
Immunosuppress (Antigraft rejection)	Yes	Yes	No
Eradicate malignancy (Antitumor)	Yes	No	Yes
Make space for new marrow (Ablation)	Yes	Yes	Yes
Avoid/minimize overlapping toxicity	Yes	Yes	Yes

mens. The first BMTs were performed in patients undergoing allogeneic BMT for hematologic malignancies. Total body irradiation alone was one of the first strategies to prepare these patients for allogeneic BMT. Although TBI is capable of producing all three desired properties (immunosuppression, ablation, and antitumor effects), TBI lacks sufficient antileukemic effects to eradicate residual leukemia or prevent relapse. Additional trials with cyclophosphamide alone showed insufficient antitumor response while demonstrating adequate immunosuppressive and ablative effects. Given this history, TBI and cyclophosphamide were combined and resulted in excellent response rates in patients undergoing BMT for hematologic malignancies, thus becoming the "gold standard" of preparative regimens. Subsequently, busulfan was substituted for TBI in hopes of reducing TBI-associated toxicity and for convenience because of the lack of adequate TBI facilities in some centers. A comparison of the combination of busulfan and cyclophosphamide to the standard combination of cyclophosphamide and TBI reported equivalency, but varying toxicity profiles. Thus, busulfan and cyclophosphamide became the first standard combination chemotherapeutic regimen for

allogeneic BMT. In an effort to enhance antitumor effects and reduce relapse rates, investigators have subsequently evaluated the addition of other drugs to TBI or to the combination of TBI and cyclophosphamide or busulfan and cyclophosphamide.

For autologous BMT, current preparative regimens vary substantially from the initial regimens for allogeneic BMT. Autologous preparative regimens are designed to maximize cytotoxic effects against specific malignancies and avoid or minimize overlapping nonhematologic toxicities. Because hematologic toxicity does not hamper dosing in the BMT setting, many studies in the autologous BMT setting have evaluated escalating doses of single drugs or combinations of drugs. In these studies, previously unknown nonhematologic dose-limiting toxicities have been recognized (see Table 5.2). Common preparative regimens and their doses, therapeutic roles, and toxicities are outlined in Table 5.3.

Cyclophosphamide

Pharmacology
Cyclophosphamide, an alkylating agent, is a cyclic phosphamide ester of mechlorethamine.

TABLE 5.2 Single agent high-dose chemotherapy

Drug	Total dose	Nonhematologic dose-limiting toxicity	Other nonhematologic toxicities
Cyclophosphamide	50–200 mg/kg (5–7.2 gm/m²)	Cardiac	Hemorrhagic cystitis, N/V/D, SIADH, nasal congestion, metallic taste
Busulfan	16 mg/kg	Hepatic	Seizures, mucositis, hyperpigmentation, cataracts
Etoposide	2.4–3.5 gm/m²	Mucositis	Dermatologic, N/V/D, hemorrhagic cystitis
Melphalan	40–200 mg/m²	Mucositis	N/V/D
Thiotepa	135–1575 mg/m²	Mucositis, Neurologic	Dermatologic
Carboplatin	800–1600 mg/m²	Hepatic	Renal, otic, N/V/D, electrolyte wasting
Cisplatin	100–250 mg/m²	Renal	N/V/D, otic, peripheral neuropathy
Cytarabine	1.5–24 gm/m²	Neurologic	Ocular, capillary leak syndrome, flulike syndrome, dermatologic, N/V/D, mucositis
Carmustine	1050–1350 mg/m²	Pulmonary Hepatic	N/V, flushing, hypotension
Ifosfamide	7.5–16.0 gm/m²	Renal	Cardiac, neurologic

KEY: N/V/D = nausea, vomiting, and/or diarrhea

Following administration, cyclophosphamide is rapidly metabolized by hepatic microsomal enzymes to the intermediate metabolite 4-hydroxycyclophosphamide (4-HC) (Dorr and Von Hoff, 1994). Then 4-HC is further metabolized to ultimately yield phosphoramide mustard and acrolein, as well as other inactive metabolites. Phosphoramide mustard acts as the major alkylating component by forming crosslinks with DNA strands, which lead to cell death. Acrolein does not possess antitumor effects but is toxic to bladder epithelial cells and results in hemorrhagic cystitis. Sulfhydryl-containing compounds such as mesna are capable of preventing hemorrhagic cystitis without inhibiting cytotoxic effects by selective inactivating acrolein. Cyclophosphamide, like other alkylating agents, is non–cell-cycle specific, but tends to work most effectively on rapidly dividing cells. Cyclophosphamide also exhibits potent immunosuppressive activity.

Therapeutic Use

Given its antitumor and immunosuppressive activity, cyclophosphamide serves as the foundation of many BMT preparative regimens used in a variety of malignant and nonmalignant diseases. Cyclophosphamide in combination with TBI or busulfan is considered the standard preparative regimen for patients undergoing allogeneic BMT for acute or chronic myelogenous leukemia (Champlin and McGlave, 1994; Long and Blume, 1994). Due to its potent immunosuppressive effects, cyclophosphamide alone or in combination with low-dose TBI or total lymphoid irradiation is standard

TABLE 5.3 Common preparative regimens

	Dose/route[a]	Common disease/ transplant type	Nonhematologic noninfectious toxicities
CY/TBI			
Cyclophosphamide	120–200 mg/kg IV	AML/CML/AA	Mucositis, N/V/D, hemorrhagic cystitis,
Total body irradiation	8–16 Gy fractionated	allo/auto	hepatic/VOD, idiopathic interstitial pneumonitis, chronic lung disease, hypothyroidism, cataracts, growth deficiencies
BU/CY			
Busulfan	14–16 mg/kg po	AML/CML	Mucositis, N/V/D, VOD, hemorrhagic
Cyclophosphamide	120–200 mg/kg IV	allo/auto	cystitis, seizures, dermatologic toxicity, cataracts, chronic lung disease
VP-16/TBI			
Etoposide	60 mg/kg IV	ALL/allo/auto	Mucositis, N/V/D, dermatologic
Total body irradiation	12–13.2 Gy fractionated		toxicity, idiopathic interstitial pneumonitis
BU/CY/VP-16			
Busulfan	16 mg/kg po	NHL/HD/MM	Mucositis, N/V/D, hemorrhagic cystitis,
Cyclophosphamide	120 mg/kg IV	Allo/auto	VOD, dermatologic toxicity, seizures
Etoposide	30 mg/kg IV		
BEAM			
Carmustine	300 mg/m^2 IV	NHL/HD	Mucositis, N/V/D, idiopathic interstitial
Etoposide	400–800 mg/m^2 IV	Allo/auto	pneumonitis, chronic lung disease
Cytarabine	800–1600 mg/m^2 IV		
Melphalan	500 mg/m^2 IV		
BCV			
Carmustine	600 mg/m^2 IV	NHL/HD	Hepatic/VOD, mucositis, N/V,
Cyclophosphamide	7200 mg/m^2 IV	Allo/auto	hemorrhagic cystitis, pericarditis,
Etoposide	2400 mg/m^2 IV		idiopathic interstitial pneumonitis, chronic lung disease
BCC			
Carmustine	600 mg/m^2 IV	Breast	N/V/D, mucositis, renal, hepatic/
Cisplatin	165 mg/m^2 IV	Auto	VOD, hypertension, congestive heart
Cyclophosphamide	5625 mg/m^2 IV		failure, pulmonary
TCC (STAMP V)			
Thiotepa	500 mg/m^2 IV	Breast	Mucositis, N/V/D, dermatologic
Cyclophosphamide	6000 mg/m^2 IV	Auto	toxicity, hemorrhagic cystitis, renal,
Carboplatin	800 mg/m^2 IV		hepatic, transient congestive heart failure
ICE			
Ifosfamide	1500 mg/m^2 IV	NHL/HD/solid tumors	Mucositis, N/V/D, renal, hepatic,
Carboplatin	1000 mg/m^2 IV	Auto	cardiac, neurologic
Etoposide	1250 mg/m^2 IV		

[a] Doses represent total dose. The total dose is often divided over several days. Doses also vary depending on the protocol and BMT center.

among preparative regimens for allogeneic BMT for aplastic anemia (Storb, 1994). More recently designed preparative regimens add other drugs to standard busulfan/cyclophosphamide or TBI/cyclophosphamide combinations in an attempt to increase antileukemia activity. Because of the broad spectrum of activity among solid tumors, cyclophosphamide has also been incorporated into many autologous BMT preparative regimens. In preparative regimens for breast cancer, cyclophosphamide is combined with either carmustine and cisplatin or thiotepa with or without carboplatin (Antman et al., 1990; Eder et al., 1988; Peters et al., 1990). Cyclophosphamide is often given with etoposide and busulfan or carmustine in various preparative regimens for autologous BMT for Hodgkin's or non-Hodgkin's lymphoma (Reece et al., 1991; Wheeler et al., 1990; Zander et al., 1987). Cyclophosphamide is also used in high single doses to mobilize stem cells into the peripheral blood for use as autologous rescue.

Toxicities

High-dose cyclophosphamide regimens are often complicated by toxicities similar to those observed with lower dose regimens including nausea and/or vomiting, diarrhea, and hemorrhagic cystitis. Nausea and/or vomiting, which may be severe, usually begin 6 to 12 hours after a dose and subside within 24 hours. With high-dose cyclophosphamide, hemorrhagic cystitis occurs more frequently and with greater severity than with lower dose regimens due to higher concentrations of the bladder toxin, acrolein, a metabolite of cyclophosphamide. Hyperhydration or mesna, an agent that binds to acrolein, is effective in preventing this complication. The onset may be acute or delayed from 24 hours to weeks after therapy. Micro- or macroscopic hematuria may occur and is usually transient. Persistent gross hematuria is typically managed with intravenous hydration, but may require more aggressive therapy including bladder irrigations, cystoscopy with cauterization or formalin instillation, or cystectomy. A syndrome of inappropriate antidiuretic hormone (SIADH) has also been described with high-dose regimens. Other adverse effects associated with high-dose cyclophosphamide include nasal congestion and a metallic taste during the infusion.

The dose-limiting toxicity of high-dose cyclophosphamide is cardiotoxicity characterized by endothelial damage producing hemorrhagic necrosis. (Gottdiener et al., 1981) Cardiotoxicity occurs in as many as 20% of patients receiving high-dose cyclophosphamide with an associated mortality rate of 10% (Steinherz et al., 1981; Gottdiener et al., 1981) Cardiac abnormalities usually manifest with symptoms characteristic of congestive heart failure including pulmonary edema or pericardial effusions. Cardiac dysfunction may be ameliorated by continuous infusion or twice-daily infusions rather than single, high-dose short infusions (Braverman et al., 1991).

Dosing, Administration, and Monitoring

Doses for high-dose cyclophosphamide regimens range from total regimen doses of 5 to 7.2 g/m^2 or 50 to 200 mg/kg. The maximum tolerated total dose in BMT patients is 200 mg/kg. Doses are typically administered intravenously as short infusions (1 to 2 hours) or as a continuous infusion for 2 to 4 consecutive days. Daily doses do not usually exceed 1.5 g/m^2 or 60 mg/kg, but higher daily IV doses have sometimes been used to mobilize peripheral blood stem cells. To decrease the risk of hemorrhagic cystitis, aggressive hydration, bladder irrigations or mesna uroprotection should begin prior to and continue for 24 to 72 hours following cyclophosphamide. Doses of mesna range from 100% to 150% of the cyclophosphamide dose and are given in divided doses or by continuous infusion. Antiemetic regimens such as those used for highly emetogenic chemotherapy agents like cisplatin should be given. Frequent monitoring of serum or urine chemistries is helpful, particularly in patients receiving aggressive hydration regimens, to prevent electrolyte wasting or to recognize SIADH.

Busulfan

Pharmacology

Busulfan is a bifunctional alkylating agent that exerts its cytotoxic effect by interfering with DNA interstrand crosslinking and to a greater extent, DNA-protein crosslinking. In low doses, busulfan selectively inhibits growth of granulocytes, but inhibits all hematopoietic cell lines when administered in high-dose regimens before BMT (Dorr and Von Hoff, 1994; Buggia et al., 1994). Although the exact bioavailability of oral busulfan is unknown, it is reportedly well absorbed following oral administration despite its poor solubility. Absorption behavior is highly variable in BMT patients, and there are no clear data on the effect of food on busulfan bioavailability. Being a small, lipophilic molecule, busulfan readily crosses the blood-brain barrier producing CSF concentrations similar to that in plasma. Busulfan is extensively metabolized by enzymatic pathways to at least 12 noncytotoxic metabolites. The pharmacokinetic profile of high-dose busulfan is age dependent. Total body clearance is two to four times higher in children than in adults receiving high-dose busulfan due to differences in bioavailability, elimination rate, and/or volume of distribution. Some data also suggest the busulfan disposition undergoes circadian variation with higher busulfan clearance rates in the evening. Busulfan possesses minimal immunosuppressive activity and is used prior to BMT for its myeloablative and antitumor activity.

Therapeutic Use

Busulfan is most frequently used in combination with cyclophosphamide in both adult or pediatric patients undergoing allogeneic or autologous BMT for myeloid malignancies. Several randomized trials report equivalency between the standard preparative regimen of cyclophosphamide/TBI and the busulfan/cyclophosphamide regimen in patients undergoing allogeneic BMT for AML or CML (Santos et al., 1984). Other cytotoxic agents may be added to the standard busulfan/cyclophosphamide regimen to enhance antitumor activity, particularly in patients with lymphoid or other malignancies.

Toxicities

The toxicity profile for high-dose busulfan is different from that of chronic low-dose busulfan. Unlike low-dose regimens, high-dose busulfan is often associated with mild to moderate nausea and vomiting. Mucositis, which is often severe, occurs in up to 70% of patients receiving busulfan-containing preparative regimens (Dorr and Von Hoff, 1994). Seizures have also been observed during high-dose busulfan regimens and are dose dependent in children (Vassal et al., 1990). Tonic-clonic seizures without focal neurologic findings typically occur on the third or fourth day of therapy and may be preceded by visual changes or nonspecific involuntary muscle movements (Murphy et al., 1992). Phenytoin or clonazepam is effective prophylaxis against busulfan-associated neurotoxicity. Dermatologic toxicity described as a "busulfan tan" may also occur and is characterized by generalized hyperpigmentation of the body occurring 2 to 4 weeks following busulfan therapy.

Hepatotoxicity, specifically veno-occlusive disease, is the dose-limiting toxicity of preparative regimens containing busulfan alone or in combination with cyclophosphamide (Peters et al., 1987; Santos et al., 1984). Increased busulfan exposure as measured by the area under the concentration-versus-time curve has been correlated with an increased risk for VOD (Grochow et al., 1989). In one report, reduced doses of busulfan based on individualized pharmacokinetic monitoring significantly decreased the incidence of VOD in patients with initial high busulfan exposures (Grochow, 1993). Others suggest that increased busulfan exposure is merely a marker for decreased hepatic function and associated increased risk for VOD (Buggia et al., 1994).

Dosing, Administration, and Monitoring

Because busulfan is a poorly water soluble drug, it is currently available only in oral form, although intravenous preparations are under investigation. The most common dosing regimen in adult BMT patients is 16 mg/kg (total dose), given in doses of 1 mg/kg every 6 hours over 4 days. Because of altered pharmacokinetic parameters, children receiving doses on a mg/kg basis often exhibit less toxicity and therapeutic benefit than adults receiving similar regimens due to decreased exposure, or area under the curve (AUC), to busulfan. Currently, several pediatric regimens determine dosage of busulfan according to body surface area at a total regimen dose of 600 mg/m² over 4 days as single or multiple daily doses and report similar busulfan AUCs and associated toxicity as seen in adults doses on a mg/kg basis (Yeager et al., 1992; Shaw et al., 1994).

Because busulfan is only available in tablets of 2 mg in the United States, many tablets are required for one dose. To facilitate administration, busulfan tablets are often packed into clear gel caps to reduce the number of pills to be swallowed. Recipes for a busulfan suspension have also been developed in some centers for patients unable to tolerate the pills. Because absorption of agents administered by the oral route is essential, many centers have adopted standard procedures to administer repeat doses of busulfan to patients who vomit shortly after a dose (Table 5.4). Antiemetics for moderately emetogenic chemotherapeutic agents such as

phenothiazenes or oral ondansetron are usually sufficient to prevent vomiting after a dose.

Given the risk for neurotoxicity, anticonvulsant prophylaxis is initiated within 24 hours prior to the first dose of busulfan. Phenytoin is frequently administered orally as 15 to 18 mg/kg loading dose divided into 4 doses followed by a daily dose of 5 to 8 mg/kg during and up to 24 hours after busulfan therapy. As more centers adopt an individualized dosing approach, numerous blood draws may also be required following the first or repeated doses of busulfan in order to calculate patient-specific pharmacokinetic parameters.

Etoposide

Pharmacology

Etoposide is in the mitotic inhibitor class of antineoplastic agents. It is a semisynthetic epipodophyllotoxin exerting its cytotoxic effect mainly via inhibition of DNA topoisomerase II enzymes. Cytotoxic effects of etoposide are cell-cycle specific with maximal effects demonstrated in the G_2 phase and some activity also evident in the late S phase.

Therapeutic Use

Etoposide exhibits broad antitumor effects including marked activity against leukemias, lymphoid malignancies, small cell lung cancer, and refractory multiple myeloma. Etoposide has been used alone or in combination before both allogeneic and autologous BMT. As a single agent, etoposide has been evaluated in phase I/II trials in patients undergoing autologous BMT for refractory or advanced solid tumors. In the allogeneic setting, etoposide is most commonly used for additional cytotoxic effect and combined with TBI to treat advanced hematologic malignancies, particularly acute lymphocytic leukemia (Blume et al., 1987). For autologous BMTs, etoposide is frequently combined with

TABLE 5.4 Template for busulfan dosing guidelines

1. Within 24 hours prior to first dose of busulfan, begin phenytoin _____ (4 mg/kg) po q 6h x 4 doses, then (5 mg/kg per day) _____ q 8h. Obtain phenytoin level prior to A.M. dose on the second and third day of busulfan therapy. Discontinue phenytoin in A.M. on _____ (at least 24 hours after last dose of busulfan).
2. On ___/___/___ (day -___) at 0900 begin busulfan _____ (1 mg/kg/dose) po q 6h x 16 doses. Give doses at 0300, 0900, 1500, 2100 on ___/___ , ___/___ , ___/___ , ___/___ . Last due at 0300 on ___/___.
   a. If patient vomits within 30 min of administration of busulfan and has tablets or tablet fragments in vomitus, repeat 100% of busulfan dose.
   b. If patient vomits within 30 minutes of administration of busulfan and has NO tablets or tablet fragments in vomitus, repeat 50% of busulfan dose.
   c. If patient vomits 30 to 60 min after administration of busulfan, repeat 50% of busulfan dose.
3. Draw busulfan levels with first dose as follows:
   a. Draw levels in 10 ml green top tube.
   b. Label all tubes with "busulfan level," patient name, medical record number, date, and time drawn.
   c. Draw baseline level immediately prior to first dose, then 30, 60, 90, 120, 180, 240, 300, 360 min after first dose.
   d. Batch samples and deliver to chemistry lab.
   e. Please complete bedside data sheet and deliver to lab with samples.
   f. Keep patient NPO from 0700 to 1500 on day of busulfan levels.
4. Please document all repeat doses of busulfan required on MAR. Write order for repeat doses (and amount) required.

NOTE: If busulfan area under the curve (AUC) is greater than 1500 $\mu mol \times min/L$, then decrease busulfan dose proportionally to achieve an AUC = 1200 $\mu mol \times min/L$.

cyclophosphamide and busulfan or carmustine to treat patients with lymphoma (Jagannath et al., 1989; Reece et al., 1991; Wheeler et al., 1990). Another common regimen combines etoposide with carmustine, cytarabine, and melphalan (Gaspard et al., 1988).

Toxicities

Aside from myelosuppression, common toxicities observed with high-dose etoposide include mucositis, nausea and/or vomiting, hepatitis, hemorrhagic cystitis, and dermatologic reactions. Mucositis is often severe and has been the dose-limiting toxicity in phase I studies with etoposide alone before BMT (Postmus et al., 1984). Dose-dependent reversible hepatitis has been reported in patients receiving high-dose

etoposide alone at doses greater than 6 gm/m² (Wolff et al., 1983). When etoposide is used in combination with TBI, hemorrhagic cystitis occurs frequently in patients not receiving aggressive hydration (Blume et al., 1987). Dermatologic reactions to high-dose etoposide include a Stevens-Johnson type syndrome over the trunk and neck and an often painful rash on the palms, soles, underarms, or groin that usually resolves in 1 to 3 weeks. There are rare reports of etoposide-associated hypersensitivity reactions including steroid- or antihistamine-responsive bronchospasm.

Dosing, Administration, and Monitoring

Total doses of etoposide as a single agent before BMT range from 2.4 to 3.5 g/m². In combination with TBI, its optimal dose is 60 mg/kg. Etoposide doses range from 160 to 1250 mg/m^2 when combined with various chemotherapeutic agents. Etoposide has been administered in a variety of schedules, but most commonly as long intravenous infusions over at least 4 hours due to the large volume required for dilution and to prolong exposure. Due to its relative instability in saline, etoposide doses must often be prepared just prior to administration to decrease the risk of precipitation. Undiluted infusions of etoposide, which avoid the need for high volumes of saline, have also been used but can be associated with cracking of plastic pump cassettes. Because hemorrhagic cystitis can be a complication of high-dose etoposide, large volumes of saline may actually be beneficial.

Melphalan

Pharmacology
Melphalan is a bifunctional alkylating agent with significant activity against multiple myeloma. Melphalan also exhibits high single-agent activity against testicular and ovarian carcinoma as well as certain sarcomas. The cytotoxic activity is generally described as non–cell-cycle specific, although some data suggest greater activity in cycling cells. In animal models, melphalan has also demonstrated immunosuppressive properties.

Therapeutic Use
Melphalan has been used alone or in combination with other chemotherapeutic agents most frequently before autologous BMT for refractory or advanced malignancies. However, due to its immunosuppressive properties, regimens containing melphalan have more recently been used before allogeneic BMT (Van Besien et al., 1995) Combination regimens include melphalan with carmustine/etoposide/cytarabine, busulfan/cisplatin/cyclophosphamide, or TBI (Gaspard et al., 1988). Melphalan-based regi-

mens have been frequently used in BMTs both for solid tumors including breast, testicular, ovarian, and melanoma cancer, and for hematologic malignancies including acute myelogenous leukemia, lymphomas, and multiple myeloma.

Toxicities
Primary nonhematologic toxicities associated with melphalan-based combination preparative regimens include mucositis, nausea, vomiting, and diarrhea. Mucositis is the nonhematologic dose-limiting toxicity with a maximal tolerated dose 225 mg/m^2. In phase I/II trials to evaluate the addition of melphalan to a standard combination of cyclophosphamide/cisplatin/carmustine, unexpected nephrotoxicity was observed and may be due to melphalan's interaction with cisplatin or carmustine (Peters et al., 1986). After carmustine was removed from the regimen, nephrotoxicity was still evident but less severe, which suggests poorly tolerated overlapping toxicities when these four drugs are used in combination. Rare cases of SIADH, hepatotoxicity, vasculitis, interstitial pneumonitis, and secondary leukemias have also been reported following the use of melphalan with BMT.

Dosing, Administration, and Monitoring
In the BMT setting, melphalan is routinely administered intravenously as short infusion over 15 to 30 minutes. Doses range from 40 to 200 mg/m^2 given usually over 1 to 2 days.

Thiotepa

Pharmacology
Thiotepa, a polyfunctional alkylating agent, is converted to TEPA and other ethylenimine metabolites, which account for the majority of its cytotoxic activity. Thiotepa is non–cell-cycle specific and considered to be a true stem cell toxin. Some experimental data suggest cross-resistance between thiotepa and other alkylat-

ing agents; however, other studies suggest tumor resistance may be overcome with dose escalation.

Therapeutic Use

Initially, thiotepa was noted to have activity against a variety of malignancies including breast, ovarian, Hodgkin's disease, and leukemia (Dorr and Von Hoff, 1994). Modest antitumor activity has also been demonstrated with melanoma, testicular cancer, and pediatric tumors (Wolff et al., 1990). Due to its lack of significant extramedullary toxicity despite dose escalation beyond myelotoxic doses and its wide array of cytotoxic activity, thiotepa has been used alone and in combination prior to autologous BMT most frequently, but also allogeneic BMT more recently. As a single agent, total doses greater than 180 mg/m^2 necessitate stem cell rescue to overcome myelotoxicity. When tested in combination, thiotepa and cyclophosphamide show marked synergy in cultured human breast cancer cells (Antman et al., 1992). One of the more common combination regimens for BMTs for breast cancer includes continuous infusion thiotepa in combination with cyclophosphamide and carboplatin (STAMP V).

Toxicities

In phase I trials evaluating thiotepa alone before autologous BMT, central nervous system toxicity was dose limiting and characterized as an organic brain syndrome with impaired cognitive function, confusion, somnolence, forgetfulness, and inappropriate behavior (Wolff et al., 1990) Following high-dose thiotepa alone or in combination, mucositis is common and can be severe. Dermatologic reactions are dose dependent and occur in up to 60% of patients receiving maximal doses. Dermatologic toxicity is manifested as either acute erythroderma affecting the palms or soles, which may be maculopapular

and desquamating, or a more generalized rash consisting of total body hyperpigmentation or bronzing, which may persist for several months. With high-dose thiotepa, mild to moderate nausea and/or vomiting occur frequently, but typically respond to antiemetic therapy. With single-agent high-dose thiotepa, there has been one report of fatal hepatotoxicity.

Dosing, Administration, and Monitoring

As a single agent before BMT, total doses of thiotepa range from 135 to 1575 mg/m^2 with a maximally tolerated dose of 1125 mg/m^2. In combination before BMT, total doses are typically in the range of 350 to 900 mg/m^2. In most preparative regimens, total regimen doses of thiotepa are divided daily over 2 to 4 days. In BMT, thiotepa is administered intravenously as short infusions over 1 to 2 hours or as continuous infusions given over several days. In the setting of breast cancer, continuous infusions of thiotepa and carboplatin are superior to bolus administration (Teicher et al., 1989) Laboratory studies report the presence of significant amounts of active metabolites in the urine 24 to 48 hours following high-dose thiotepa, which decrease substantially over the next 24 hours. Given this persistence of alkylating activity, many preparative regimens including thiotepa incorporate a prolonged chemotherapy-free period (rest days) before infusion of stem cells. For example, the STAMP V regimen that includes a 4-day continuous infusion of thiotepa requires a 3-day washout following completion of the thiotepa before stem cells are infused.

Carboplatin

Pharmacology

As a platinum analogue, carboplatin's mechanism of action is similar to that of cisplatin and is typically classified as an alkylating agent. Although the exact mechanism of these agents is not known, data suggest activated carboplatin metabolites form DNA-DNA and DNA-protein crosslinks leading to cell death. Cytotoxic effects of carboplatin are not cell-cycle specific; however, response may be maximized when carboplatin is exposed to cells in S phase.

Therapeutic Use

Ovarian cancer is the primary tumor for which carboplatin has demonstrated its greatest cytotoxic activity. Carboplatin has equivalent, if not superior, activity to cisplatin in the treatment of ovarian cancer with the highest response rates seen early in the treatment schema before platinum resistance develops. Other solid tumors for which carboplatin has demonstrated cytotoxicity include testicular cancer, breast cancer, non–small-cell lung cancer, and head and neck cancer. Carboplatin was incorporated into a common preparative regimen (STAMP V) for breast cancer consisting of cyclophosphamide and thiotepa for additive cytotoxicity but also to decrease the emergence of drug resistance (Antman et al., 1992).

Toxicities

In the study of phase I dose escalation to evaluate carboplatin with marrow support, hepatotoxicity was the dose-limiting toxicity. The hepatotoxic profile varied from that described for veno-occlusive disease and was characterized by biliary stasis with transient but sometimes prolonged bilirubin elevations without associated abdominal tenderness or ascites. The hepatotoxicity was not fatal, but did appear dose related and associated with failure of other organ systems at escalating doses. Ototoxicity was also observed and dose related with a trend toward greater toxicity in patients who had received previous cisplatin therapy. Of the platinum analogues, carboplatin is less nephrotoxic than cisplatin when given in conventional doses. Interestingly, non–dose-related nephrotoxicity

occurred in 30% of patients participating in this phase I study within a few days of completing therapy. Other severe toxicities observed included one case of interstitial pneumonitis and optic neuritis. When escalating doses of carboplatin were combined with cyclophosphamide and etoposide, the dose-limited toxicity was nephrotoxicity (Shea et al., 1989). Neutropenic enterocolitis and intestinal perforation have also been reported with carboplatin-containing preparative regimens (Mehta et al., 1992). Use of high-dose carboplatin alone or in combination is also associated with nausea, vomiting, and electrolyte wasting, all of which are more severe effects than that described with conventional dose therapy.

Dosing, Administration, and Monitoring

Before BMT, total carboplatin doses usually range from 800 to 1600 mg/m^2 with 2000 mg/m^2 being the maximally tolerated dose when used alone. Doses higher than 1200 mg/m^2 typically require marrow or stem cell rescue. Regimens are most commonly administered as a continuous infusion to enhance cytotoxicity and potentially decrease gastrointestinal and renal toxicity, which may be exacerbated with bolus administration (Antman et al., 1992). With use of high-dose carboplatin, include frequent monitoring of electrolytes and urine output as well as daily assessment of auditory function.

Cisplatin

Pharmacology

As a platinum compound and alkylating agent, cisplatin's primary mechanism of action is through binding to DNA, producing intrastrand crosslinks, and DNA adducts. Recent interest has arisen in cisplatin's interaction with other components of the cell such as glutathione. Cisplatin's activity is not cell-cycle specific.

Therapeutic Use

Cisplatin possesses a broad spectrum of antitumor activity and has been associated with great advances in the management of previously non-responsive malignancies. In conventional dosing, cisplatin has substantial activity against ovarian cancer. Cisplatin has been combined with other chemotherapeutic agents and used for a variety of solid tumors including small-cell and non–small-cell lung, bladder, head and neck, breast cancer, and gastrointestinal malignancies. Although myelosuppression occurs infrequently with conventional doses, profound myelosuppression is observed with high-dose cisplatin (≥ 200 mg/m^2). Given this phenomenon and its antitumor activity, cisplatin has been incorporated into some BMT preparative regimens. Cisplatin has been combined with various agents such as cyclophosphamide with carmustine or etoposide in preparative regimens for autologous BMT for metastatic or high-risk breast cancer (Peters et al., 1990). There has been little interest in incorporating cisplatin into preparative regimens for allogeneic BMT due to its lack of immunosuppressive and antileukemia effects as well as the potential additive nephrotoxicity when given before cyclosporin or tacrolimus.

Toxicities

Toxicities associated with cisplatin in combination with other agents before BMT include those seen at conventional dosing, particularly nephrotoxicity, ototoxicity, and neurotoxicity. When escalating doses of cisplatin were combined with cyclophosphamide and etoposide, nephrotoxicity was dose limiting (Somlo et al., 1994). In addition, one patient required a long-term hearing aid and two patients experienced symptomatic peripheral neuropathies. In one study, the incidence of cisplatin-associated nephrotoxicity increased with older age, prolonged neutropenia, and use of amphotericin, both not with use of aminoglycoside (Cooper et al., 1993). As with conventional dose therapy, severe nausea and/or vomiting and hypomagnesiumia are associated with high-dose cisplatin therapy.

Dosing, Administration, and Monitoring

Before autologous BMT, total cisplatin doses range from 100 to 250 mg/m^2 with the upper limit defined as the maximal tolerated dose due to dose-limiting nephrotoxicity. Cisplatin doses are often divided over 2 to 5 days as short infusions. Maintenance of adequate hydration and urine flow before and 24 hours after therapy is essential. Measures such as pre- and posttreatment saline infusions with or without mannitol are often used. In addition, patients should be given aggressive prophylactic antiemetic regimens and monitored for ototoxicity and peripheral neuropathies.

Cytarabine

Pharmacology

Cytarabine, an antimetabolite, is cell-cycle specific and exerts its cytotoxic effects against cells in S phase (i.e., dividing cells) and has no effect on nonproliferating cells. The cytotoxic activity of cytarabine depends on its intracellular phosphorylation to Ara-CTP, which acts as a competitive inhibitor of DNA polymerase and serves as a chain terminator following incorporation into DNA. Although cytarabine has been shown to block both humoral and cellular immune responses, its immunosuppressive capacity compared to cyclophosphamide is small.

Therapeutic Use

Cytarabine is primarily active against hematologic malignancies of both myeloid and lymphoid origin. Low-dose cytarabine in combination with an anthracycline is standard therapy for acute myelogenous leukemia. Regimens of high-dose cytarabine have been used for aggressive induction and consolidation for AML. Being one of the single most active drugs against leukemic cells, high doses of cytarabine have been incorporated into various preparative regimens for patients undergoing BMT for hematologic malignancies (Peterson et al., 1989; Ridell et al., 1988). Although cytarabine is immunosuppressive, the addition of TBI or cyclophosphamide is necessary to obtain sufficient immunosuppression for allogeneic BMT. Another common regimen before autologous BMT incorporates cytarabine in combination with carmustine, etoposide, and melphalan (BEAM) (Gaspard et al., 1988).

Toxicities

Adverse effects associated with cytarabine in BMT vary depending on the schedule of administration. Given in high doses as short infusions every 12 hours, toxicities are similar to those seen in standard high-dose consolidation regimens and include neurotoxicity and ocular toxicity. Neurotoxicity occurring in up to 10% of patients manifests as cerebellar dysfunction composed of ataxia, dysarthria, nystagmus, and slurred speech (Rudnick et al., 1979). The risk for associated central nervous effects increases with older age, underlying renal dysfunction, and cumulative cytarabine dose. Cerebellar dysfunction is frequently reversible if therapy is discontinued once detected, although rarely central nervous damage is permanent and requires long-term rehabilitation. Ocular toxicity occurs in the form of a chemical conjunctivitis with excessive tearing, photophobia, pain, and blurred vision. Symptoms typically resolve within a few days, but visual acuity may take weeks to resolve. Unlike frequent bolus injections, when cytarabine is administered as a prolonged infusion, a capillary leak syndrome

progressing to noncardiogenic pulmonary edema and respiratory failure has been observed (Haupt et al., 1981). Respiratory compromise may be acute or delayed up to 3 weeks after therapy and usually consists of tachypnea and hypoxia with diffuse interstitial pulmonary infiltrates. Other adverse events occurring with both schedules of cytarabine include a flulike syndrome accompanied by fevers, chills, and arthralgias and skin rashes. With intermittent dosing, gastrointestinal toxicity, particularly nausea and vomiting, can be severe and dose limiting. Dermatologic reactions include acral erythema on the palms and soles, which may progress to bullae formation, and desquamation as well as more generalized nonspecific rashes on the neck, chest, or other areas.

Dosing, Administration, and Monitoring

Due to its cell-cycle specificity, dosing regimens designed to maximize exposure of malignant cells to cytarabine are most commonly employed in BMT preparative regimens. Like high-dose induction or consolidation regimens, schedules of frequent short infusions of 2 to 3 g/m² every 12 hours for 8 to 12 doses are standard. More recently, investigators have evaluated the use of lower dose (1500 mg/m²) continuous infusion cytarabine in preparative regimens for acute and chronic myeloid leukemia. When cytarabine is given intermittently, daily neurologic evaluations should be performed to detect any cerebellar dysfunction. With continuous infusion regimens, care should be taken to avoid fluid overload during and up to 3 weeks after therapy. Maintaining strict input and output (I/O) and adequate diuresis helps preventing respiratory compromise. To prevent conjunctivitis, corticosteroid eye drops should be started within 24 hours before high-dose regimens (> 200 mg/m² per day) and continue for several days after therapy. Acetaminophen or mild narcotics may help ameliorate flulike symptoms.

Carmustine

Pharmacology

As a nitrosourea, carmustine is an alkylating agent whose metabolites inhibit several enzymatic pathways involved in DNA synthesis. Carmustine possesses crossresistance similar to other alkylating agents. Although carmustine is not typically considered cell-cycle specific, some investigators have noted differences in the degree of cytotoxicity based on the phase of the cell cycle, particularly increased activity in cells in the G_1, G_2, or S phase.

Therapeutic Use

For conventional therapy, carmustine is most frequently used for brain cancers and has significant activity against glioblastoma. Carmustine also has activity against refractory lymphomas and multiple myeloma. High-dose carmustine-based combination regimens with autologous bone marrow or stem cell support have demonstrated responses in breast cancer, neuroblastoma, gliomas, and malignant lymphomas (Gaspard et al., 1988; Peters et al., 1990; Reece et al., 1991; Wheeler et al., 1990; Zander et al., 1987).

Toxicities

Pulmonary and hepatic toxicity are the dose-limiting toxicities for high-dose carmustine and have been fatal in 15% to 20% of cases (Takvorian et al., 1983). Pulmonary toxicity is characterized by severe interstitial pneumonitis with frequent opportunistic infections such as cytomegalovirus. Frequently symptoms, which may not develop until months after therapy, are consistent with obstructive lung disease and often responsive to corticosteroids. Pulmonary toxicity has been correlated with increased exposure to carmustine as measured by the AUC in women with breast cancer who receive high-dose carmustine in combination with cyclophosphamide and cisplatin before BMT

(Jones et al., 1992). Hepatotoxicity manifests as a doubling of hepatic enzymes within a week of therapy in up to 90% of patients. Veno-occlusive disease also occurs in up to 20% of patients and may be minimized with fractionated doses instead of single high-dose infusions. (Ayash et al., 1990). In patients with CNS tumors who receive high-dose carmustine, neurotoxic effects including seizures and encephalopathy as well as hypothyroidism and prolactinemia have been observed. In the majority of patients, high-dose carmustine therapy is also complicated by nausea which usually begins 2 hours after therapy and lasts for 4 to 6 hours. Facial flushing and hypotension during the infusion have been reported and are more common with rapid injections.

Dosing, Administration, and Monitoring

Doses of high-dose carmustine followed by autologous stem cell rescue vary depending on whether it is used alone or in combination with other chemotherapeutic agents. Used alone for glioblastomas, doses of carmustine usually range from 1050 to 1350 mg/m². Fatal hepatic necrosis was observed at doses greater than 2000 mg/m²; thus, typical doses are limited to 1200 mg/m² (Herzig et al., 1981). Used in combination for various malignancies, doses range from 450 to 900 mg/m². Carmustine may be given as a single intravenous infusion or divided into two infusions separated by 12 hours. Carmustine should be infused no faster than 3 mg/m² per minute to avoid facial flushing and hypotension. Typical infusion durations are at least 2 hours. When carmustine is used for CNS tumors, mannitol or dexamethasone may prevent cerebral edema.

Ifosfamide

Pharmacology

Like cyclophosphamide, ifosfamide must undergo activation by microsomal enzymes before exerting its alkylating cytotoxic activity. The ifosforamide mustard metabolite is responsible for much of the inhibition of DNA activity, while the metabolite, acrolein, binds to bladder epithelial cells resulting in hemorrhagic cystitis. Ifosfamide is not cell-cycle specific.

Therapeutic Use

Ifosfamide possesses a wide range of antitumor activity including activity against both hematologic malignancies and solid tumors. Substantial cytotoxic activity is demonstrated with ifosfamide-based regimens when used for Hodgkin's disease, refractory lymphomas, advanced testicular, sarcoma, ovarian, and breast cancers. Ifosfamide also has demonstrated activity against acute and chronic leukemias. In the BMT setting, ifosfamide is used most often in combination with carboplatin and etoposide (ICE) for autologous BMT in patients with refractory or relapsed germ cell tumors, malignant lymphomas, and other solid tumors (Lotz et al., 1991).

Toxicities

The predominant toxicity in ifosfamide-based preparative regimens is nephrotoxicity. In phase I/II studies of ifosfamide in combination with carboplatin and etoposide, irreversible renal failure, cardiac failure, and neurotoxicity limited further dose escalation (Wilson et al., 1992). In other studies evaluating ifosfamide in similar combinations, renal toxicity and mucositis were common but tolerable (Barnett et al., 1993). Patients with germ cell tumors who receive extensive prior cisplatin-based therapy experience more severe nephrotoxicity when receiving ifosfamide-based preparative regimens and are able to tolerate only 60% of the common ifosfamide dose (Broun et al., 1991). At doses below the maximally tolerated dose, renal toxicity most often manifests as acute, mild, and transient elevations in serum creatinine

peaking the day after completion of ifosfamide. However, nephrotoxicity can be severe and results in permanent loss of 50% of renal function in about 10% of patients (Wilson et al., 1992). Central nervous system toxicity as manifested by lethargy and confusion often correlates with declining renal function. In studies attempting to escalate doses of combinations of carboplatin and ifosfamide, both of which are associated with renal dysfunction when given in high doses alone, nephrotoxicity was the dose-limiting toxicity, which suggests overlapping toxicities of these two agents (Lotz et al., 1991). Ifosfamide therapy is complicated by hemorrhagic cystitis if appropriate preventive measures such as mesna uroprotection are not taken. Nausea or vomiting lasting up to 3 days is common, but often preventable, and may be more severe with rapid injection.

Dosing, Administration, and Monitoring

Total doses of ifosfamide for BMT range from 7.5 to 16.0 g/m^2 with maximal tolerated doses varying depending on the combination of drugs and previous cisplatin therapy. Standard combinations of ifosfamide with carboplatin and etoposide (ICE) report a maximally tolerated total dose of 16 g/m^2 for ifosfamide (Wilson et al., 1992). In patients who receive extensive prior cisplatin, the maximally tolerated dose of ifosfamide was 10 g/m^2 (Broun et al., 1991). Because large single doses of ifosfamide are associated with greater toxicity than fractionated or continuous infusions, ifosfamide-based preparative regimens typically administer total ifosfamide doses over 4 to 5 days. Short infusions are well tolerated but continuous infusions of ifosfamide have also been used in the BMT setting. Adequate hydration and uroprotection with mesna are recommended for patients receiving ifosfamide. Hydration should begin within 24 hours before and continue for approximately 72 hours after ifosfamide therapy. Administering conventional doses of ifosfamide commonly involves two mesna regimens: 60% of the ifosfamide dose in three divided doses 0, 4, and 8 hours after ifosfamide or 100% of the ifosfamide dose as 6- to 24-hour infusions. High-dose ifosfamide-based preparative regimens have used higher doses of mesna and usually call for mesna doses equalling 125% to 160% of the ifosfamide dose either fractionated or as a continuous infusion. Mesna can be conveniently admixed in the same bag as ifosfamide. Given ifosfamide's nephrotoxic potential, intravenous hydration may be beneficial up to 7 days after stem cell infusion, but fluid status should be monitored carefully and adequate diuresis maintained to avoid congestive heart failure or pulmonary edema.

IMMUNOSUPPRESSIVE AGENTS

Cyclosporin

Pharmacology

Cyclosporin is a cyclic undecapeptide isolated from the fungus *Tolypocladium inflatum Gams*. Cyclosporin's immunosuppressive effects are mediated through specific and reversible inhibition of immunocompetent lymphocytes. Although the precise mechanism of action is not clearly defined, cyclosporin's inhibition of interleukin-2 synthesis and other lymphokines, which ultimately blocks the normal immune cascade, serves as the basis for much of its immunosuppressive effects. Much of cyclosporin's immunosuppressive activity is mediated through binding to specific cytoplasmic immunosuppressant-binding proteins or immunophilins. The complex of bound cyclosporin inhibits calcineurin, an intergral component of signal transduction pathways mediated by T-cell receptors. Cyclosporin is not lymphocytotoxic or myelosuppressive, but rather suppresses the lymphocytic response to alloantigens. Cyclo-

sporin is extensively metabolized by the cytochrome P-450 III-A, enzyme system primarily in the liver but also in the gastrointestinal tract and kidney. Numerous metabolites have been identified, however both the biologic and toxic effects of cyclosporin are mainly attributable to activity of the parent drug. Following oral administration, absorption of cyclosporin is erratic, incomplete, and dependent on the formulation. Elimination of cyclosporin is primarily through the biliary route and the terminal elimination half-life is about 9 hours.

Therapeutic Use

Cyclosporin is most frequently used to prevent acute GVHD, but is also used to treat chronic GVHD (Sullivan, 1994). As a prophylactic agent, cyclosporin has been used alone or in combination (Table 5.5). A standard regimen developed by the Seattle group consists of cyclosporin with low doses of intravenous methotrexate given on days 1, 3, 6, and 11 after marrow infusion (Storb et al., 1986). Other combination regimens may omit the dose of methotrexate on day 11. Regimens with cyclosporin alone often use high intravenous doses of cyclosporin initially, and then taper to maintenance doses, which are continued for several months (Tutschka et al., 1983; Deeg et al., 1985). In a study comparing similar doses of cyclosporin alone or in combination with methotrexate, the combination was found to be superior and associated with a significant reduction in grade II to IV GVHD (Storb et al., 1986). Cyclosporin has also been used in combination with corticosteroids with or without methotrexate to prevent GVHD (Chao et al., 1993).

In the treatment of high-risk chronic GVHD, the combination of cyclosporin alternating daily with corticosteroids has been associated with a higher response and lower infection rates than non–cyclosporin-based

TABLE 5.5 Regimens to prevent GVHD

Single-Agent Therapy		
Cyclosporin	5 mg/kg CIV	Days −2–2
	3.75 mg/kg IV	Days 3–15
	1.25 mg/kg IV q 12 h	Day 15 −[a]
	5 mg/kg po q 12 h	[a]–day 50
	3.75 mg/kg po q 12 h	Days 50–170
Double Combination Therapy		
Cyclosporin	1.5 mg/kg IV q 12 h	Day −1–[a]
	6.25 mg/kg po q 12 h	[a]–day 50
	Decrease 5% per week	Days 50–180
Methotrexate	15 mg/m^2	Day 1
	10 mg/m^2	Days 3, 6, 11
Triple Combination Therapy		
Cyclosporin	5 mg/kg/d IV	Days −2–3
	3 mg/kg/d IV	Days 4–14
	3.75 mg/kg/d IV	Days 15–35
	10 mg/kg/d PO	Days 36–83
	8 mg/kg/d PO	Days 84–97
	6 mg/kg/d PO	Days 98–119
	4 mg/kg/d PO	Days 120–180
Methotrexate	15 mg/m^2	Day 1
	10 mg/m^2	Days 3, 6
Methylprednisolone	0.5 mg/kg/d IV	Days 7–14
	1.0 mg/kg/d IV	Days 15–28
	0.8 mg/kg/d IV	Days 29–44
	0.5 mg/kg/d IV	Days 43–56
	0.2 mg/kg/d IV	Days 57–119
	0.1 mg/kg/d IV	Days 120–180

[a]Oral therapy is initiated when the patient begins to eat or can tolerate oral medications.

regimens (Table 5.6) (Sullivan et al., 1988). Although cyclosporin is considered first line therapy for high-risk chronic GVHD, it has a limited, if any, role in the treatment of established acute GVHD that develops on cyclosporin prophylaxis. Cyclosporin has been associated with objective response rates similar to that of methylprednisolone in patients who develop acute GVHD on non–cyclosporin-based prophylactic regimens (Kennedy et al., 1985).

Toxicities

Toxicities associated with use of cyclosporin in patients who undergo BMT are similar to those described in patients who receive solid organ transplants and include nephrotoxicity, hypertension, hypomagnesiumia, and neurotoxicity (Table 5.7). In the randomized trial comparing cyclosporin to the combination of cyclosporin and methotrexate, approximately 50% of patients in both arms experienced a doubling of

TABLE 5.6 Treatment of chronic GVHD

	Low risk	High risk
Treatment		
Prednisone[a]	1 mg/kg qod	1 mg/kg qod
Cyclosporin (oral)	none	6 mg/kg q 12 h qod
Infection Prophylaxis[b]		
Trimethoprim/Sulfamethoxazole (Bactrim®, Sulfa®)	DS po bid daily	DS po bid daily

[a]For long-term corticosteroid therapy, initiate H_2 receptor antagonist to prevent peptic ulcer disease.
[b]If unable to tolerate trimethoprim/sulfamethoxazole, substitute aerosolized pentamidine 300 mg per month and penicillin 250 mg po bid.

TABLE 5.7 Toxicities of immunosuppressive agents

Cyclosporin	Tacrolimus	Methotrexate	Corticosteroids	ATG
Nephrotoxicity	Nephrotoxicity	Mucositis	Hyperglycemia	Infection risk
Hypertension	Hypertension	Delayed engraftment	Muscle wasting	Fever, chills
Hypomagnesiumia	Hypomagnesiumia	Hepatotoxicity	Infection risk	Dermatologic
Tremor (hand)	Tremor		GI hemorrhage	reactions
Neurotoxicity	Neurotoxicity		Hypertension	Hypersensitivity
Hyperkalemia	Hyperkalemia			Serum sickness
Hirsutism	HUS			
HUS				

KEY: HUS = hemolytic uremic syndrome, ATG = antithymocyte globulin

serum creatinine over baseline. Nephrotoxicity is typically reversible with subsequent reduction of cyclosporin doses, but may necessitate hemodialysis in 10% to 15% of patients (Storb et al., 1986). Both an acute and chronic form of nephrotoxicity have been described. Acute nephrotoxicity due to renal vasoconstriction and ischemia is usually reversible and associated with reduced glomerular filtration, increased proximal tubular reabsorption, oliguria, and hyperkalemia. Chronic toxicity is rare, typically not reversible, and results in interstitial fibrosis and loss of nephrons. The risk for nephrotoxicity may be increased with the use of other nephrotoxins such as amphotericin and aminoglycosides.

Hypertension has been reported in up to 50% of marrow graft patients who receive cyclosporin. Elevations in both the systolic and diastolic blood pressures usually begin within weeks of initiating therapy and may be mediated through renal vasoconstrictive effects. Although reducing the dose may decrease the blood pressure, antihypertensive therapy is preferred for sustained hypertension due to the risk for GVHD with reduced cyclosporin. A fine tremor in the hands, usually mild in severity, is the most common form of neurotoxicity reported in allograft patients receiving cyclosporin. Tremors may resolve despite continued therapy or resolve with dose reduction. Seizures have also been reported during cyclosporin therapy and may be associated with concurrent corticosteroid use, hypomagnesemia and/or hypertension. A severe form of typically reversible neurotoxicity manifested as cortical blindness, quadraplegia, seizures, and/or coma with associated white matter changes on head CT or MRI has also occurred in BMT patients who received cyclosporin.

Dosing, Administration, and Monitoring

Table 5.5 summarizes multiple regimens in which cyclosporin is used to prevent GVHD. Cyclosporin is usually initiated by the intravenous route beginning 1 or 2 days before marrow infusion. Initial intravenous doses range from 2.5 to 7.5 mg/kg per day given as slow infusions over 4 to 6 hours in two divided doses or as continuous 24-hour infusions (Parr et al., 1991). One report suggests no difference between techniques of administration in the incidence of GVHD or nephrotoxicity, but notes a greater frequency of paresthesias and flushing if intermittent doses are given over 1 hour or less (McGuire et al., 1988). Once patients are able to tolerate oral medications, cyclosporin is converted to the oral route using either capsules or oral suspension. Ratios for converting the dose from intravenous to oral vary among institutions; most centers use a 1:3 to 1:5 conversion factor in order to maintain similar blood levels between intravenous and oral dosing. Oral cyclosporin is available as soft gelatin capsules or an oral solution. Recently approved, a new mi-

croemulsion formulation (Neoral®) was developed to provide increased bioavailability. Because this new formulation has increased bioavailability, the standard formulation (Sandimmune®) and microemulsion formulation (Neoral®) are not considered bioequivalent and should not be used interchangeably on an equivalent dose basis.

Methods of discontinuation of cyclosporin vary among centers, but discontinuation usually occurs around 6 months after BMT if there is no evidence of GVHD. Some centers opt to taper cyclosporin therapy and others do not. To treat chronic GVHD, cyclosporin is administered orally to high-risk patients as 12.5 mg/kg per day in two divided doses alternating daily with corticosteroid therapy (Table 5.6). The duration of therapy in the chronic GVHD depends on the patient's response and tolerance.

Monitoring cyclosporin concentrations continues to be controversial and is less well defined for BMT than for solid organ transplants. Variations in reported cyclosporin concentrations based on the use of whole blood or plasma and on assay methodology detecting only parent drug (monoclonal) or parent plus metabolites (polyclonal) complicate this issue. Several studies report a correlation between cyclosporin concentration and the risk for GVHD. One study suggests patients with low cyclosporin concentrations are at greater risk for GVHD than those with higher concentrations (Gluckman et al., 1984). Other studies suggest low cyclosporin concentrations are predictive of GVHD only during the first week after BMT or during the week prior to development GVHD (Santos et al., 1987; Yee et al., 1988). In addition, toxicity is not easily correlated with cyclosporin concentrations. While one study reports a more rapid onset of renal dysfunction in patients with high cyclosporin concentrations, other studies suggest the

TABLE 5.8   Drug interactions with cyclosporin

Decreased cyclosporin concentrations	Increased cyclosporin concentrations	Additive nephrotoxicity
Phenytoin	Erythromycin	Amphotericin
Phenobarbital	Ketoconazole	Aminoglycosides
Carbamazepine	Itraconazole	Melphalan
Rifampin	Fluconazole	NSAIDs
Nafcillin	Diltiazem	Tacrolimus
Octreotide	Verapamil	
Sulphonamides	Nicardipine	
and trimethoprim	Tacrolimus	

KEY: NSAIDs = Non-steroidal anti-inflammatory drugs

majority of patients will develop renal dysfunction even if cyclosporin concentrations are low (Kennedy et al., 1985). Even more important, cyclosporin levels that have been reported to preserve renal function are below those reported to prevent GVHD. Thus, while routine in many institutions, the need for frequent monitoring of cyclosporin concentrations is questionable. One option for monitoring would be to measure cyclosporin once weekly, increasing doses only if levels are below the lower end of therapeutic range based on the institution's standards, and decreasing doses only in the setting of significant toxicity such as nephrotoxicity.

One situation in which measurement of cyclosporin concentrations may be more crucial is that of changing the administration route from intravenous to oral. Given the erratic absorption of cyclosporin, trough concentrations obtained before changing to oral and after a few oral doses are often helpful to determine if oral dosing regimens are achieving concentrations similar to those achieved with intravenous regimens.

Other routine monitoring of BMT patients receiving cyclosporin should include frequent measurements of electrolytes and blood pressure. Cyclosporin is also associated with a number of clinically significant drug interactions (Table 5.8). Concomitant use of cyclosporin with these medications may require more frequent monitoring of concentration or alteration of dose. Other medications with additive nephrotoxicity have also been identified and should be avoided or minimized in patients receiving cyclosporin (Table 5.8).

Methotrexate

Pharmacology

Methotrexate's primary cytotoxic mechanism of action is through inhibition of dihydrofolate reductase, the enzyme responsible for reduction of folic acid to tetrahydrofolic acid. This inhibition ultimately leads to a lack of purine and pyrimidine synthesis, adversely affecting DNA and RNA synthesis. The immunosuppressive actions of methotrexate are less well defined, but are partially due to inhibition of lymphocyte proliferation. Folinic acid (leucovorin calcium), a derivative of tetrahydrofolic acid, can often block the adverse effects of methotrexate if given shortly after administration while preserving the rapid onset of immunosuppressive effects.

Therapeutic Use

Methotrexate is primarily used to prevent GVHD both alone and in combination with other immunosuppressive agents (Table 5.5). Animal GVHD models indicate the critical time for methotrexate administration is within the first 2 weeks after BMT, but also note toxicity correlates with increased or daily exposure (Lochte et al., 1962). Therefore, most regimens using methotrexate opt to give infrequent doses during the first 2 weeks after BMT typically on days 1, 3, 6, and 11 after marrow infusion. Used alone for prophylaxis, methotrexate therapy is continued weekly until approximately day 100. Combined with other immunosuppressive agents such as cyclosporin or more recently tacrolimus, methotrexate therapy is not continued beyond day 11. In a study comparing methotrexate alone and a short course of methotrexate combined with a 180-day course of cyclosporin in leukemia patients, the combination was found to be superior in terms of reduction of GVHD and overall survival (Storb et al., 1986). Likewise, the addition of a short course of methotrexate to a regimen of intermediate doses of cyclosporin until day 180 resulted in a decreased incidence of GVHD compared to cyclosporin alone, but also increased toxicity including mucositis and delayed engraftment (Storb et al., 1986). Of interest, reports validate the influence of methotrexate and indicate a greater risk for GVHD in patients unable to receive the full prescribed course of methotrexate compared to those receiving all four prescribed doses. In prophylactic regimens incorporating more immunosuppressive agents than just cyclosporin and methotrexate, short courses of methotrexate have been modified to include only three doses on day 1, 3, and 6 after marrow infusion.

Toxicities

Toxicities associated with low doses of methotrexate in the BMT include mucositis, hepatotoxicity, and delayed engraftment (Table 5.7). In comparisons of cyclosporin alone to cyclosporin plus methotrexate, a significantly higher number of patients receiving the combination experienced more severe mucositis than those not receiving methotrexate (Storb et al., 1986). Methotrexate prophylaxis has also been associated with an increased risk for veno-occlusive disease. In a study comparing GVHD prophylaxis with cyclosporin and methylprednisolone or methotrexate, the incidence of VOD, particularly fatal VOD, was significantly higher in the group receiving methotrexate (Essel et al., 1992). Folinic acid rescue has been investigated in an attempt to decrease the incidence of regimen-related toxicity when using methotrexate prophylaxis (Nevill et al., 1992). The incidence of grade II-IV mucositis and hepatotoxicity were significantly reduced by administering folinic acid rescue beginning 12 to 24 hours after administration of methotrexate and continuing for 12 to 24 hours. The incidence of GVHD was not adversely affected by the administration of folinic acid rescue. Methotrexate has also been associated with significant increases in the time to achieve an ANC over $500/\mu l$ and typically prolongs this period by 5 days when compared to regimens without methotrexate (Storb et al., 1986). Delayed engraftment associated with methotrexate prophylaxis is particularly evident in patients undergoing BMT from matched unrelated donors.

Dosing, Administration, and Monitoring

Short courses of methotrexate typically administer doses of 15 mg/m^2 slow IVP on day 1 and 10 mg/m^2 on days 3, 6, and 11 (Table 5.5). Extended courses of methotrexate continue the 10 mg/m^2 dosing weekly to day 102 post stem cell infusion. Not all centers routinely administer folinic acid rescue following methotrexate injections. One published regimen initiates folinic acid, two doses of 15 mg/m^2 IV or oral every 6 hours beginning 12 hours after the day 1 dose of methotrexate and 6 to 8 doses of 10 mg/m^2 every 6 hours beginning 24 hours after the day 3, 6, and 11 doses. Modified regimens and reduced doses of folinic acid may also be beneficial. Care should be taken to avoid having folinic acid present during the administration of methotrexate. Most regimens opt to begin folinic acid at least 12 hours, and often 24 hours, after the methotrexate.

Although some centers routinely monitor methotrexate blood levels 24 hours after a dose, available data suggest concentrations often do not correlate with toxicity. In one report 68% of the methotrexate concentrations obtained were at or below the detectable limit of the assay (Nevill et al., 1992). Despite these low concentrations of methotrexate, patients still benefited from folinic acid rescue, which supports a lack of correlation between concentrations and toxicity. Other data confirm these observations and suggest that, given assay limits, routine monitoring of methotrexate concentrations in the BMT setting is not necessary (Dix et al., 1995). However, it is reasonable to monitor concentrations of methotrexate in patients at risk for prolonged methotrexate elimination (i.e., renal impairment or third spacing due to ascites or pleural effusions).

Tacrolimus

Pharmacology
Formerly known as FK506, tacrolimus is a macrolide immunosuppressive agent produced by *Streptomyces tsukubaensis*. Tacrolimus suppresses both humoral and cellular immune responses through mechanisms similar to that of cyclosporin. Tacrolimus inhibits T-cell or lymphocyte activation and binds to a specific cytoplasmic immunophilin, FKBP-12. The complex of bound tacrolimus inhibits calcium-dependent signal transduction pathways in T cells and ultimately blocks synthesis of lymphokines such as interleukin-2. Like cyclosporin, the absorption of tacrolimus following oral administration is highly variable with an average bioavailability of 20% to 30%. Being highly lipophilic, tacrolimus undergoes extensive tissue distribution. Tacrolimus is metabolized by the liver, but unlike cyclosporin, less than 1% of the drug is excreted unchanged in the bile or urine. Thus, impaired hepatic function is associated with prolonged elimination and higher plasma concentrations of tacrolimus.

Therapeutic Use
Tacrolimus has been most extensively studied in the setting of liver transplantation. Recently, however several phase II trials have evaluated the role of tacrolimus for prophylaxis of acute GVHD in BMT patients (Nash et al., 1995; Devine, Geller et al., 1994; Fay, Pirjeiro et al., 1994). These trials, in both sibling and matched unrelated donor allografts, suggest tacrolimus in combination with methotrexate or methylprednisolone is comparable to cyclosporin-based combinations in terms of development of grade II-IV GVHD and overall survival. The superiority of either cyclosporin or tacrolimus remains to be determined, although data from a randomized trial are forthcoming.

Toxicities
Although tacrolimus was developed with the hope for less toxicity than cyclosporin, reports in both solid organ and marrow transplant patients suggest their toxicity profiles are similar (Table 5.7). Like cyclosporin, nephrotoxicity has been the most common and prob-

lematic adverse event. In a phase II study combining tacrolimus with methotrexate or methylprednisolone, nephrotoxicity occurred in 78% of patients with 22% of patients requiring hemodialysis (Nash et al., 1995). In patients who did not require dialysis, nephrotoxicity occurred late after transplant and resolved with dose reduction. Other predominant adverse events observed in this trial included veno-occlusive disease, hypertension, and hyperglycemia. Of interest, the majority of patients reported a burning discomfort in their hands and/or feet or severe headache during the infusion. These symptoms improved with a slower rate of infusion or after changing to oral tacrolimus. As with cyclosporin, there have been rare reports of hemolytic uremic syndrome and neurotoxicity characterized by white matter changes on head CT or MRI with or without cortical blindness in BMT patients receiving tacrolimus. Other adverse effects similar to those reported with cyclosporin have also been reported in patients with liver allografts who receive tacrolimus; they include hyperglycemia, hyperkalemia, hypomagnesemia, tremor, and headache.

Dosing, Administration, and Monitoring

Because it is approximately 100 times more potent that cyclosporin, tacrolimus doses are typically 100 times lower than cyclosporin doses. Continuously infused intravenous doses of 0.03 mg/kg per day are initiated the day before marrow infusion and subsequently converted to twice-daily oral doses totaling 0.12 mg/kg per day, when patients can tolerate oral medications. Food does not appear to alter the absorption of tacrolimus. Monitoring parameters similar to those discussed with cyclosporin also apply for tacrolimus. Like cyclosporin, tacrolimus has been associated with several pharmacokinetic and pharmacodynamic drug interactions (Table 5.9).

Corticosteroids

Pharmacology

The mechanism of the immunosuppressive effects of corticosteroids is not clearly understood. Possible mechanisms include potent inhibition of interleukin-1 production, inhibition of T-cell migration, inhibition of RNA and

TABLE 5.9 Drug interactions with tacrolimus

Decreased concentrations of tacrolimus	Increased concentrations of tacrolimus	Additive nephrotoxicity
Phenytoin	Clotrimazole	Amphotericin
Phenobarbital	Ketoconazole	Aminoglycosides
Carbamazepine	Itraconazole	Cisplatin
Rifampin	Fluconazole	Cyclosporin
	Diltiazem	
	Methylprednisolone	
	Metoclopramide	
	Erythromycin	
	Clarithromycin	
	Bromocriptine	

DNA, and prevention of interaction between lymphocytes and monocytes. In addition to the benefits of steroid-induced immunosuppression, problematic secondary effects are also observed, specifically increased suspectibility to infection.

Therapeutic Use

In the BMT setting, the most frequently administered corticosteroids are methylprednisolone and prednisone, both of which are cornerstones in the treatment and prophylaxis of acute GVHD (Table 5.5, Figure 5.1). Corticosteroids

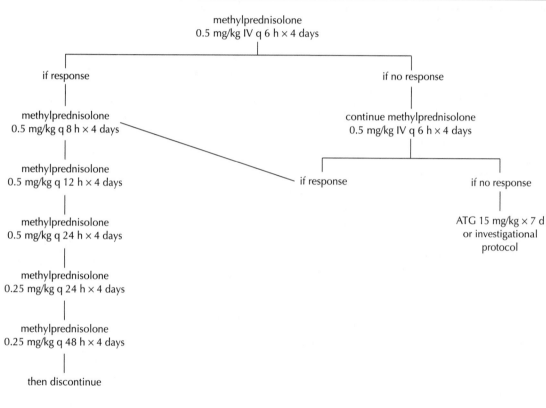

RECOMMENDATIONS:
 When patient is tolerating oral intake, convert methylprednisolone from IV to po (1:1).
 Obtain blood cultures qod while patient remains in hospital.
 If GVHD flares, increase methylprednisolone dose to previous level.

Figure 5.1 **Treatment of acute GVHD in patients receiving cyclosporin or tacrolimus prophylaxis**

are also first-line therapy for treatment of chronic GVHD (Sullivan, 1994) (Table 5.6). To treat acute GVHD, courses of methylprednisolone are typically administered over several days and then tapered over several weeks in order to avoid a flair of GVHD. In steroid-based prophylactic regimens, corticosteroids are usually initiated on day +7 and continued on a tapering schedule for several weeks following BMT (Chao et al., 1993). Prolonged, high-dose courses of corticosteroids are often used to treat chronic GVHD and continued or tapered based on the patient's response.

Toxicities

BMT patients receiving extended courses of corticosteroids are at risk for typical corticosteroid-induced complications including infection, peptic ulcer disease with GI hemorrhage, hyperglycemia, muscle atrophy, and an Addison-like syndrome, among others (Table 5.7). Numerous reports document a significantly increased risk of infection and infection-related mortality in BMT patients with GVHD requiring long-term steroids. Infections caused by *Aspergillus* or cytomegalovirus are particularly virulent in BMT patients who receive prolonged therapy with corticosteroids.

Dosing, Administration, and Monitoring

Dosing regimens of corticosteroids in BMT patients vary substantially among centers or protocols. To treat acute GVHD, methylprednisolone is most frequently initiated intravenously at doses of 2 to 10 mg/kg/day, then changed to oral administration and tapered over several weeks, once response is documented (Figure 5.1). To treat high-risk chronic GVHD, often prednisone is initiated at doses of 1 mg/kg daily with cyclosporin on alternate days and then continued on every other day based on the patient's response and toxicity (Table 5.6). In low-risk chronic GVHD patients, 1 mg/kg of

prednisone on alternate days is often sufficient to control GVHD. Lower doses of corticosteroids are usually employed as prophylaxis. One recently published study initiated intravenous methylprednisolone, 0.5 mg/kg per day on day 7, and then increased the dose to 1 mg/kg per day on day 15. At day 29, oral prednisone was substituted for methylprednisolone and gradually tapered over several weeks.

When corticosteroids are being administered, frequent measurements of blood glucose and blood pressure should be obtained particularly at initiation or during higher dose regimens. When extended courses of corticosteroids are anticipated, the addition of antacid medications such as ranitidine or famotidine should be strongly considered in order to prevent or lessen complications of peptic ulcer disease. Due to the high risk of infection and potential to mask fevers with corticosteroids, frequent blood cultures should also be obtained during therapy. Patients should be followed closely for osteoporosis or signs of muscle or bone atrophy and doses minimized or discontinued if these complications are detected. As a general rule, corticosteroids can be toxic for BMT patients and doses and duration of therapy should be minimized.

Antithymocyte Globulin

Pharmacology

Antithymocyte globulin (ATG), also known as lymphocyte immune globulin, is a lymphocyte-selective immunosuppressant. ATG is now the only commercially available polyclonal preparation of antilymphocyte antibodies. ALG, antilymphoctye globulin, is no longer commercially available. ATG works by binding to peripheral lymphocytes, which are then excreted. Through this action, ATG ultimately blocks many humoral and cellular immune responses. ATG is an immune globulin purified from the sera of animals immunized with human thymocytes. The commercially available product, Atgam®, is purified from horse serum. Some academic centers have purified other forms of ATG from animals other than horses and made them available to patients allergic to horses or unable to tolerate the horse serum preparation.

Therapeutic Use

Presently, ATG is most used for the treatment of acute GVHD (Figure 5.1). Initial promising studies showed ATG was effective in controlling acute GVHD; however, subsequent comparative studies show no benefit of ATG over corticosteroids as initial treatment for acute GVHD (Storb et al., 1974; Doney et al., 1981). In some cases patients receiving ATG failed therapy more often than patients receiving either methylprednisolone or cyclosporin. Given these results, most centers reserve ATG therapy for patients with steroid refractory acute GVHD. ATG has also been used to prevent GVHD; however, studies do not suggest additional benefit over conventional prophylactic regimens. ATG is not typically administered in the setting of chronic GVHD.

Toxicities

Fever and chills are the most common adverse effects occurring during ATG therapy and may decrease in severity after the first few doses (Table 5.7). Serum sickness may also occur at any time during or after therapy and is characterized by fever, malaise, arthralgia, lymphadenopathy, and cutaneous eruptions. Patients receiving ATG may also experience a drop in their neutrophil and platelet counts. Due to the immunosuppressive effects of ATG, infection remains a major cause of morbidity and mortality of patients who received it. These patients tend to be susceptible to viral infections caused by herpes simplex virus and cytomegalovirus as well as Epstein-Barr virus. Dermatologic reac-

tions may occur in up to 25% of patients receiving ATG including if infused through a peripheral vein, a chemical phlebitis. Although uncommon, hypersensitivity reactions are reported in patients receiving ATG presumably due to allergic reactions against the animal sera.

Dosing, Administration, and Monitoring

To treat GVHD, ATG is usually administered at a dose of 15 mg/kg every other day for 7 days (Figure 5.1). Even though the risk for anaphylaxis is extremely low, most institutions administer an intradermal or epicutaneous skin test and a saline control to evaluate potential hypersensitivity. The predictive value of these tests is certainly not 100%; patients with negative tests may demonstrate hypersensitivity and patients with positive tests have been reported to tolerate subsequent infusions of ATG (Bielory et al., 1988). To prevent infusion-associated fever and chills, antipyretics such as acetaminophen or corticosteroids and antihistamines are routinely administered before the infusion. Infusions are typically administered over 4 to 8 hours through an inline filter. Patients should be checked frequently during the infusions for signs of hypersensitivity.

ANTIBACTERIALS

Bacterial infections are associated with substantial morbidity and mortality during the initial recovery following BMT and can be problematic up to several months after BMT depending on the patient's clinical status. During the initial neutropenic period following BMT, the management of infection can be divided into empiric and treatment strategies as well as preventive strategies. As with other febrile, neutropenic patients, BMT patients require broad-spectrum, empiric antibacterial regimens at the time of first neutropenic fever. In most BMT centers, empiric regimens are designed to offer

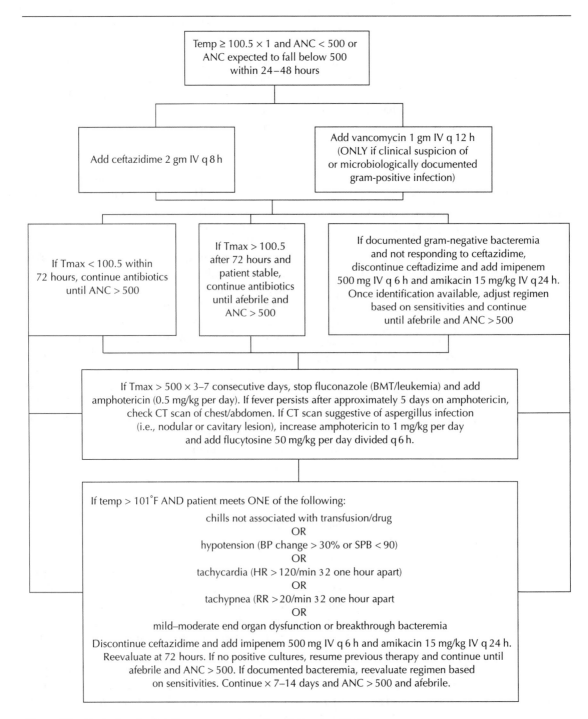

Figure 5.2 Algorithm for febrile neutropenic patient following BMT

Source: Bone Marrow Transplant/Leukemia Program, Emory University Hospital, Atlanta, Georgia. Used with permission.

a broad spectrum of activity focusing on gram-negative coverage including *Pseudomonas aeruginosa* and may also include gram-positive coverage. Examples of effective monotherapy regimens are a third-generation, antipseudomonal cephalosporin such as ceftazidime or a carbapenem such as imipenem. Combination regimens are also often used and typically include an antipseudomonal, extended-spectrum penicillin such as ticarcillin ± clavulanate or piperacillin ± tazobactam along with an aminoglycoside such as gentamicin, tobramycin, or amikacin. If the suspicion of gram-positive infection is high due to severe mucositis or indwelling central venous catheter, then vancomycin may be started initially with these empiric regimens. If gram-positive prophylaxis is being used or the concern for severe gram-positive infection is low, then vancomycin is often withheld and initiated if there is no response to the empiric regimen.

Due to the high predictability of which types of bacterial infection tend to occur early following BMT, in addition to the morbidity and mortality associated with infection, many centers have investigated and adopted strategies with prophylactic antibiotics to prevent bacterial infections during neutropenia. Both absorbable and nonabsorbable regimens have prevented infection. Nonabsorbable regimens historically included gram-negative coverage with agents like oral gentamicin or polymixin and gram-positive coverage with agents like vancomycin. These regimens were given orally to sterilize the GI tract, were often poorly tolerated, and thus ineffective when compared to current strategies. Randomized, placebo-controlled clinical trials report that selective decontamination of the gut with norfloxacin or systemic prophylaxis with cotrimoxazole or ciprofloxacin significantly decreased the incidence of serious gram-negative bacteremia following BMT or during prolonged neutropenia (Gualtieri et al., 1983; Karp et al., 1987;

Winston et al., 1987). In general these regimens are well tolerated, initiated within the week of BMT and continued until neutrophil recovery, and not associated with emergence of resistant gram-negative organisms. Because of an increasing incidence of streptococcal infections, specifically *Strep. viridans*, and the associated morbidity and mortality in BMT patients, some centers routinely initiate gram-positive prophylaxis during neutropenia following BMT (Villablanca et al., 1990). Regimens that have been efficacious include penicillin, vancomycin, rifampin, and some macrolide antibiotics such as clarithromycin (Attal et al., 1991; Gilbert et al., 1994). As with any prophylactic regimen, the potential emergence of resistant organisms must be weighed against the potential benefit of prevention of infection. Because of the concern of the emergence of vancomycin-resistant enterococcal organsims, some centers are eliminating vancomycin as a prophylactic agent and reserving its use for clinically or microbiologically documented gram-positive infection. Examples of prophylactic and empiric regimens are outlined in Figures 5.2 and Table 5.10.

ANTIFUNGALS

As with management of bacterial infections early following BMT, management of fungal infections can be divided into prophylactic, empiric, and treatment strategies. Many BMT centers initiate some form of fungal prophylaxis early following BMT; although, some centers are avoiding the need for fungal prophylaxis as new technologies such as peripheral blood stem cell transplantation or hematopoietic growth factors are being used to decrease the duration of neutropenia. Fluconazole is commonly used to prevent fungal infections early after BMT and is generally well tolerated. A large, multicenter randomized trial reports patients who receive fluconazole prophylaxis following BMT

TABLE 5.10 Antibiotic prophylaxis for BMT patients

Patient type	Start day	Drug	Dose/route/regimen	Stop day
All patients	Day −1	Norfloxacin	400 mg po bid	Afebrile & ANC > 500 × 1–2 days
All patients	Day −1	Fluconazole	400 mg po/IV qd	Afebrile & ANC > 500 × 2 days or when amphotericin started
All patients	Day −1	Clarithromycin	500 mg po q 12 h	Afebrile & ANC > 500 × 1–3 days
HSV+ patients	Day 0	Acyclovir	62.5 mg IV q 4 h	ANC > 500 × 1–3 days
All patients	Prior to discharge or after engraftment	TMP/SMX	1 DS tab po bid twice weekly	Day 180
Patients with CMV+ blood culture/PCR	Day of positivity	Ganciclovir	5 mg/kg q 12 h × 1–2 weeks then 5 mg/kg qd	Day 100

SOURCE: Bone Marrow Transplant/Leukemia Program, Emory University Hospital, Atlanta, Georgia. Used with permission.

experience significantly fewer superficial and systemic fungal infections than patients who receive placebo (Goodman et al., 1992). Additionally, mortality due to fungal infections is lower in fluconazole-treated patients. Of concern, however, are reports of increasing incidences of fluconazole-resistant organisms such as *Candida krusei* or *glabrata* in patients receiving fluconazole prophylaxis (Wingard et al., 1991). Fortunately, these organisms respond to amphotericin.

Other approaches to antifungal prophylaxis include topical antifungals such as oral nystatin or inhaled or intranasal amphotericin. These approaches may be complicated by poor patient tolerance and compliance. Itraconazole, an antifungal agent that acts against some *Candida* species and, more important, against *Aspergillus* species, is an attractive agent for the prevention of fungal infection in patients

with prolonged periods of neutropenia and patients requiring long-term, aggressive immunosuppression. Currently, itraconazole is only available in a capsular oral formulation requiring an acidic medium for absorption; thus, compliance or the achievement of adequate serum concentrations may be problematic in BMT patients. Of note, however, a suspension and intravenous formulation of itraconazole are under development.

Regardless of the prophylactic strategy, systemic amphotericin therapy is still considered the standard for patients with documented fungemia during neutropenia or prolonged fevers on broad-spectrum antibacterial coverage. Generally, from 0.5 to 1.0 mg/kg of amphotericin is initiated empirically after 5 to 7 days of persistent fever on empiric antibacterial therapy. Higher doses (1.0–1.5 mg/kg per day) of amphotericin are often required when treating fluconazole-resistant organisms such as *Candida krusei* or *glabrata* or *Aspergillus* infections. In BMT patients, therapy with amphotericin is often complicated by infusion-related-adverse effects including high fevers and chills, which might be ameliorated by premedicating infusions with antipyretics such as acetaminophen and/or hydrocortisone and antihistamines such as diphenhydramine. Due to its inherent toxicity and the need for frequent, concomitant use of nephrotoxic agents such as acyclovir, aminoglycosides, and cyclosporin or tacrolimus, amphotericin therapy is also complicated by nephrotoxicity, which can be severe. Various attempts to reduce nephrotoxicity have been evaluated in small trials, including saline loading and renal dose dopamine, with only moderate, if any, success. Various liposomal formulations of amphotericin are under development with the hope of maintaining antifungal efficacy while minimizing or eliminating nephrotoxicity and infusion-related adverse effects.

In 1995 the FDA approved one of these products, amphotericin B lipid complex (ABELECT™), for treatment of *Aspergillus* infections in patients intolerant to conventional amphotericin. While this agent provides an attractive alternative to conventional therapy in BMT patients, its benefit must be weighed against its cost. Currently, this product is 20 times more expensive than conventional amphotericin. No data is yet available from large, randomized trials in BMT patients to demonstrate a greatly increased efficacy or decreased toxicity that would offset the tremendously increased cost. Thus, amphotericin B lipid complex should be used judiciously and only in BMT patients intolerant of conventional amphotericin therapy. In addition to amphotericin, oral antifungals such as fluconazole or itraconazole can be considered in suspectible systemic or superficial *Candida* or *Aspergillus* infections, respectively, that occur after engraftment.

ANTIVIRALS

Acyclovir

Pharmacology

Acyclovir selectively inhibits the replication of many viruses of the Herpesvirus family, specifically herpes simplex virus 1 (HSV-1) and 2 (HSV-2), varicella-zoster virus (VZV), and Epstein-Barr virus (EBV). To exert its antiviral activity, acyclovir must be initially converted to its monophosphate form by a viral-encoded thymidine kinase, which is not present in uninfected cells. Following this initial conversion, acyclovir is ultimately converted to its triphosphate form by cellular enzymes. The triphosphorylated form of acyclovir inhibits viral DNA synthesis by competitive inhibition with a substrate for viral DNA polymerase. In terms of antiviral activity, acyclovir is most active against HSV-1, HSV-2, and VZV, with higher concentrations required to prevent replication of HSV-2 and even higher for VZV. Because cytomegalovirus (CMV) lacks the viral-encoded thymidine kinase required for acyclovir activation, CMV is generally considered resistant to acyclovir (Whitley and Gnann, 1992).

Therapeutic Use

Acyclovir is commonly used to treat HSV-1 and HSV-2 infections following autologous and allogeneic BMT. Numerous studies of BMT patients and other immunocompromised patients document the ability of intravenous acyclovir to successfully treat mucocutaneous HSV infections (Mitchell et al., 1981; Wade et al., 1982; Meyers et al., 1982). In general, these trials report shorter periods of viral shedding, decreased duration of pain, and accelerated healing of viral lesions in patients receiving intravenous acyclovir compared to those receiving placebo. Initial studies focused on the use of intravenous acyclovir due to acyclovir's poor bioavailability when administered orally, 15% to 20%, particularly in a population with severe mucositis and nausea/vomiting such as BMT patients. However, one randomized study of patients who developed HSV infection following BMT reports that oral acyclovir, 400 mg po 5 times a day, was more effective than placebo and similar in efficacy to previously published studies of patients who received intravenous acyclovir (Shepp et al., 1985). Of note, however, in this study the median time to development of the HSV infection was 28 days following BMT, which may represent a time when mucositis or other GI toxicity was resolving and afforded greater patient compliance with this oral regimen.

The majority of HSV seropositive patients will reactivate the HSV infection usually in the second or third week following BMT. Due to the predictability of this reactivation of infection, acyclovir has also been evaluated in numerous trials as an agent to prevent HSV infection. In these trials, intravenous acyclovir given in multiple daily doses effectively prevented reactivation of HSV infection when compared to placebo (Saral et al., 1981; Hann et al., 1983; Lundgren et al., 1985). Other trials have also reported successful prevention of HSV infection when administration of oral acyclovir followed BMT (Wade et al., 1984; Gluckman et al., 1983). Of note, in many of these prophylactic trials, infections recurred frequently after discontinuation of acyclovir.

Some clinicians, concerned about emergence of resistance and cost, question the need for prophylactic acyclovir in BMT patients. Acyclovir-resistant HSV strains are documented with the resistance most often mediated by lack of the viral-encoded thymidine kinase required for activation of acyclovir. In general, infections due to acyclovir-resistant strains of HSV are mild and resolve without therapy, although these infections can be associated with

severe consequences such as esophagitis and pneumonia (Ljungman et al., 1990; Sacks et al., 1989). Of note, however, analyses of large numbers of BMT patients who received prolonged courses of prophylactic acyclovir report only rare cases of acyclovir-resistant HSV strains (Burns, 1994). In contrast, repeated courses of acyclovir in BMT patients have been associated with progressively increasing rates of acyclovir-resistant HSV strains (Wade et al., 1983). Although economics are an issue with any prophylactic therapy, in the BMT setting, this argument can be countered by reviewing the consequences of HSV infections. Increased severity of mucositis and risk of superinfection may both require more intravenous and costly medications and prolonged hospitalization.

Intravenous acyclovir is the current treatment of choice for VZV infections following BMT (Balfour et al., 1983; Meyers et al., 1984; Shepp et al., 1986). To adequately suppress VZV infections, higher concentrations and thus higher doses of acyclovir are required. One study does suggest oral acyclovir is as effective as IV acyclovir in treating VZV infections following BMT, although the sample size of the study is small (Ljungman et al., 1989). Because of the need for high concentrations and the concern about erratic bioavailability, use of oral acyclovir therapy for VZV infections should be cautioned in this group of immunocompromised patients until data from larger, randomized trials are available.

Toxicities

Acyclovir therapy is generally well tolerated in BMT patients. Nephrotoxicity has been associated with the administration of higher doses of acyclovir as rapid infusions or in dehydrated states. This nephrotoxicity, most often due to crystallization of acyclovir within the renal tubules, is reversible upon discontinuation of therapy, and can be minimized or prevented by adequate hydration during acyclovir therapy. Infrequent, reversible neurotoxicity including disorientation, hallucinations, tremors, ataxia, lethargy, agitation, and seizures has also been reported in patients receiving intravenous acyclovir.

Dosing, Administration, and Monitoring

Various dosing regimens have been given to BMT patients, for both prophylaxis and treatment. In general, the intravenous route of administration is preferred to prevent or treat HSV infections, although the oral route may be an alternative if mucositis or GI toxicity is or is expected to be mild. To treat HSV infection, the recommended dose of acyclovir is 250 mg/m² or 5 mg/kg IV every 8 hours for 7 days. An oral regimen of 400 mg 5 times a day for 10 days has been shown to be effective in a group of patients who developed HSV infections late after BMT. To prevent HSV infection, effective doses range from 250 mg/m² IV every 8 hours to 62.5 mg/m² IV every 4 hours. In one study which tried to minimize administration of IV acyclovir, the reactivation of HSV infection was not significantly decreased by once-daily administration when compared to placebo, which suggests multiple daily doses are required in order to suppress reactivation (Shepp et al., 1985). Oral regimens have been effective in some studies of prophylaxis and range from 200 to 400 mg 4 to 5 times a day. Prophylactic acyclovir therapy is typically continued through the period of neutropenia and may be prolonged in order to prevent recurrent infections.

The intravenous route is recommended when treating VZV infections and the recommended dose is 10 mg/kg or 500 mg/m² IV every 8 hours for 7 days. Adequate hydration with oral intake or intravenous fluids should be maintained during high-dose acyclovir therapy in order to prevent nephrotoxicity.

Ganciclovir

Pharmacology

Ganciclovir is a synthetic nucleoside analogue that inhibits replication of several members of the Herpesvirus family including cytomegalovirus (CMV), herpes simplex virus-1 and -2 (HSV), human herpes virus-6 (HHV-6), Epstein-Barr virus (EBV), and varicella-zoster virus (VZV). To exert its antiviral activity, ganciclovir must be converted to a triphosphate form. In cells infected with HSV, conversion occurs through a viral thymidine kinase. In CMV-infected cells, cellular kinases are responsible for phosphorylation and activation of ganciclovir. Levels of ganciclovir-triphosphate are higher in CMV-infected cells than in uninfected cells, indicating preferential phosphorylation of ganciclovir in CMV-infected cells. Following phosphorylation, the antiviral activity of ganciclovir is mediated through inhibition of DNA synthesis by either competitive inhibition of DNA polymerase or direct incorporation into viral DNA leading to chain termination.

Therapeutic Use

Although ganciclovir possesses activity against other members of the Herpesvirus family, therapeutic use in BMT patients has been limited to CMV infection. Ganciclovir is used both to treat and prevent CMV disease, particularly CMV interstitial pneumonitis (CMV-IP) (Table 5.11). Prior to the use of ganciclovir, mortality from CMV-IP was about 90%. With the combination of ganciclovir and immunoglobulin, the mortality rate has been reduced to less than 50% (Emanuel et al., 1988; Reed et al., 1988; Schmidt et al., 1988). The benefit of the combination is thought to be due to the antiviral activity of ganciclovir and the additional immunomodulatory effects of intravenous immunoglobulin. Interestingly, ganciclovir alone does not substantially effect the natural progression

TABLE 5.11 Strategies to treat or prevent CMV infection

	Treatment of CMV-IP	*Preemptive therapy*	*Prophylactic therapy*
Regimen	Ganciclovir 5 mg/kg IV q 12 h × 21 d, then 5 mg/kg 5x/week & IVIg 500 mg/kg qod x 21 d, then 500 mg/kg per week	Ganciclovir 5 mg/kg IV q 12 h x 7 d, then 5 mg/kg qd through day 100	Ganciclovir 5 mg/kg IV q 12 h x 5 d, then 5 mg/kg qd through day 100
Patient Population	CMV-IP	Asymptomatic CMV infection	CMV seropositive patient or donor
Initiation of Therapy	At time of BAL or lung tissue diagnosis	At time of CMV-positive blood, urine, throat, or BAL culture after BMT	At engraftment
Incidence of CMV Infection			Decreased
Incidence of Disease		Decreased	Decreased
Survival Advantage	Yes	Yes	No

of CMV-IP. Ganciclovir is also used alone or in combination to treat CMV-associated enteritis in BMT patients. During ganciclovir therapy, patients with CMV enteritis no longer excrete the virus; however, gastrointestinal symptoms often persist despite 2 weeks of therapy (Reed et al., 1990).

Due to the high mortality rate associated with CMV-IP, ganciclovir and other antivirals are frequently used in allogeneic BMT patients at risk for CMV disease to prevent progression to CMV-IP. Given prophylactically to CMV-seropositive patients or those with seropositive donors, ganciclovir decreases the incidence of CMV-asymptomatic infection and CMV disease including CMV-IP and enteritis, but does not significantly decrease mortality when compared to placebo (Atkinson et al., 1991; Goodrich et al., 1993; Winston et al., 1993). Ganciclovir has also been given to patients with asymptomatic CMV infection as determined by positive surveillance cultures of blood, urine,

throat, or bronchoaveolar lavage fluid following allogeneic BMT (Goodrich et al., 1991; Schmidt et al., 1991). Given in this preemptive fashion, ganciclovir significantly decreased the incidence of CMV-IP; and in one study, mortality was also decreased (Goodrich et al., 1991).

Toxicities

The most problematic adverse effect of ganciclovir in BMT patients is hematologic toxicity (Table 5.12). Neutropenia occurs in approximately one third of BMT patients receiving ganciclovir and frequently causes interruption of therapy. Neutropenia may occur at any time but typically occurs during the first or second week of therapy and resolves within 1 week of discontinuation of ganciclovir. Thrombocytopenia with platelet counts of less than 25,000/mm^3 have also been reported in up to one third of patients receiving ganciclovir. Nephrotoxicity, manifested by elevated serum creatinine, has been reported in up to 20% of

TABLE 5.12 Toxicities of ganciclovir and foscarnet reported from clinical trials in BMT patients

	Ganciclovir	*Foscarnet*
MAJOR	Neutropenia, nephrotoxicity (?)	Nephrotoxicity, anemia, neutropenia, hypocalcemia, hypo/hyperphosphatemia, hypomagnesiumia, hepatotoxicity
MINOR	Headache, tremor, cardiovascular effects	Hypokalemia, nausea, vomiting, parasthesia, skin rash

patients in some studies; although other studies report no difference in the degree of creatinine elevation when compared to placebo. Adverse effects on the central nervous system (CNS) that include abnormal dreams, confusion, agitation, seizures, tremor, trismus, and ataxia have also been reported in approximately 5% of patients receiving ganciclovir.

Dosing, Administration, and Monitoring

In the BMT setting, ganciclovir is routinely given through the intravenous route. An oral formuation of ganciclovir was recently released, although data on its use in BMT patients is not available and may be limited due to poor bioavailability. Various dosing schedules of ganciclovir have been evaluated based on the premise for use (Table 5.11). In general, regimens involve a course of induction therapy over 1 to 3 weeks followed by maintenance therapy until day 100 to 120 following BMT to prevent reactivation of infection. The maximal single dose of ganciclovir to be administered is 6 mg/kg over 1 hour. Larger doses or more rapid infusions result in increased toxicity.

Due to the risk of hematologic toxicity, complete blood counts should be checked frequently during ganciclovir therapy, particularly in patients with preexisting neutropenia. Numerous guidelines are available in terms of dosing recommendations during neutropenia or thrombocytopenia; but in general ganciclovir

therapy should not be initiated when the ANC is less than 500/µl or the platelet count is less than 25,000/mm³. If neutropenia (ANC less than 1000/µl) or thrombocytopenia occurs during therapy, ganciclovir should be temporarily withheld and resumed upon recovery of desired blood counts. If the potential benefit of therapy outweighs the risk, as in the case of CMV-IP, myeloid growth factors such G-CSF or GM-CSF should be considered to try to overcome neutropenia. Because ganciclovir is renally excreted, serum creatinine levels or creatinine clearance should also be assessed frequently during therapy. Doses and schedules must be adjusted in the setting of renal dysfunction in order to avoid accumulation and increased toxicity.

Reconstituted solutions of ganciclovir have a high pH (alkaline) and despite further dilution can cause pain or phlebitis at the injection site. Thus, ganciclovir should only be infused into peripheral veins with adequate blood flow or into central venous lines. Guidelines issued for handling or disposing of cytotoxic drugs should be followed due to the alkalinicity of the ganciclovir solution and its potential for carcinogenecity. Adequate hydration should also be maintained during ganciclovir therapy in order to avoid accumulation.

Ganciclovir has been associated with several clinically significant drug interactions. When ganciclovir is used in combination with other drugs that inhibit replication of rapidly dividing cells such as amphotericin, dapsone, flucytosine, pentamidine, trimethoprim-sulfamethoxazole, or cytotoxics, increased hematologic toxicity may occur; thus, the benefits of these drugs in combination must be weighed against the risks. When combined with imipenem-cilastatin, a greater risk for generalized seizures may be present. Concomitant use of ganciclovir and didanosine (DDI) or zidovudine (AZT) results in decreased exposure to ganciclovir and increased exposure to didanosine or zidovudine.

Foscarnet

Pharmacology

Foscarnet, or phosphonoformic acid, inhibits replication of members of the Herpesvirus family. Its antiviral activity is mediated through selective inhibition of the pyrophosphate binding site on virus specific DNA polymerases and reverse transcriptases. Foscarnet does not require activation through thymidine kinase or other virally encoded enzymes; thus, viral strains resistant to acyclovir or ganciclovir may be sensitive to foscarnet.

Therapeutic Use

Although approved by the FDA only to treat CMV retinitis, foscarnet is frequently used in BMT patients in a variety of ways. In general, foscarnet is used as second-line therapy in patients with viral infections refractory to conventional therapy including infections due to acyclovir-resistant HSV or ganciclovir-resistant CMV (Razis et al., 1994; Safrin et al., 1991). Foscarnet may also be substituted for ganciclovir in patients with ganciclovir-induced or preexisting pancytopenia. Foscarnet has also been investigated to prevent CMV infection, but results are not comparable or superior to those reported with ganciclovir regimens (Reusser et al., 1992).

Toxicities

Nephrotoxicity is the major complication associated with foscarnet therapy and occurs to some degree in the majority of patients (Table 5.12). Elevations in serum creatinine appear most commonly during the second week of therapy, but may occur at any time. Recovery of renal function usually occurs within 1 week after discontinuation of foscarnet, but can sometimes take weeks to occur. Changes in doses based on the manufacturer's nomograms are necessary if renal function is decreased at initiation or occurs during therapy.

Along with nephrotoxicity, foscarnet may cause severe mineral and electrolyte imbalances. Hypocalcemia is the most frequent effect, but hypomagnesiumia, hypokalemia, and hypo- or hyperphosphatemia may also occur. Foscarnet causes a dose-related transient decrease in ionized calcium most likely due to chelation of available calcium. Onset of symptomatic hypocalcemia or other electrolyte disturbances may be acute and associated with neurologic or cardiac abnormalities such as seizures or arrhythmias. Hematologic abnormalities have also been reported in patients receiving foscarnet. Anemia may occur in up to one third of patients, but is typically manageable with transfusion. Neutropenia is reported in approximately 15% of patients, but rarely requires discontinuation of therapy. Other reported adverse effects occurring in greater than 5% of patients are outlined in Table 5.12.

Dosing, Administration, and Monitoring

In patients with normal baseline renal function, foscarnet is typically administered for induction therapy as 40 to 60 mg/kg every 8 hours and maintenance therapy as 90 mg/kg once daily in the setting of CMV-IP. Foscarnet should not be administered by rapid injection because toxicity may be increased with excessive plasma levels. Typical infusion rates are over 1 hour through a central or peripheral line. Undiluted foscarnet

(24 mg/ml) may be administered through a central line, but for peripheral administration foscarnet must be further diluted to 12 mg/ml to avoid irritation. Due to the risk for nephrotoxicity and electrolyte disturbances, baseline serum chemistries including calcium and creatinine should be obtained and monitored at least twice weekly during induction and every 1 to 2 weeks during maintenance therapy. Upon initiation of therapy, patients should be monitored closely for signs of electrolyte wasting such as numbness, tingling in extremities, and muscle cramps. Careful adjustments of dose based on renal function and replacement of electrolytes are essential to avoid excessive toxicity. The use of other nephrotoxic drugs such as amphotericin, aminoglycosides, and IV pentamidine should be avoided or minimized during foscarnet therapy.

New Antiviral Agents

In 1995 the FDA approved two new oral antivirals, famciclovir and valacyclovir, for the treatment of VZV infection in immunocompetent adults. Famciclovir is a prodrug of penciclovir, an antiviral agent whose spectrum and mechanism of action are similar to that of acyclovir, but that has a higher affinity for the viral-encoded thymidine kinase required for activation. In normal hosts with VZV infection, famciclovir demonstrated similar efficacy to that of acyclovir with a significantly shorter duration of zoster-associated pain (Portnoy, 1994). Due to its long intracellular half-life, famciclovir has the advantage of less frequent dosing than oral acyclovir, 3 times daily and 5 times daily, respectively. Valacyclovir is a prodrug of acyclovir and has a greater oral bioavailability than oral acyclovir, thus resulting in high concentrations of acyclovir in the body or infected cells. Studies in immunocompetent patients with VZV infection report similar efficacy of acyclovir, 800 mg orally 5 times daily, and valacyclovir, 1 gm orally 3 times daily, but note a statistically significant difference or trend toward decreased duration of pain in valacyclovir-treated patients.

To date, no comparative trials in BMT or immunocompromised patients have been published using famciclovir or valacyclovir for the treatment of VZV infection, although trials are under way. As with oral high-dose acyclovir for the treatment of VZV infection after BMT, caution should be exercised with famciclovir or valacyclovir in these patients until results from randomized trials are available. Soruvidine (BV-ara-U), another new antiviral agent not yet approved by the FDA, has been evaluated in immunocompromised patients with herpes zoster who failed or were intolerant to standard therapy. In this small study of patients with AIDS or hematologic malignancies, soruvidine was well tolerated and the majority of patients with cutaneous VZV infection responded to soruvidine (Brennan et al., 1995).

MISCELLANEOUS

Intravenous Immunoglobulin

Pharmacology

Intravenous immunoglobulin (IVIg) contains approximately 5% immune globulins, or antibodies. Several products are commercially available and contain similar levels of IgG, but may vary in the presence of antibodies other than IgG and antibody titers to various organisms. To prepare IVIg products, samples of plasma are obtained from paid or volunteer donors, then pooled, purified, and standardized. IVIg's mechanism of action is based on the passive replacement of antibody in patients who have an impaired ability to form antibodies (i.e., alterations in humoral immunity or B-cell–mediated production of immunoglobulins). IVIg has also been associated with immunoregulatory effects such as increased suppressor T-cell function with associated decreased autoantibody production and the provision of antiidiotypic antibodies. These immunomodulatory effects may prevent GVHD or other autoimmune reactions.

Therapeutic Use

Immunoglobulin therapy is standard treatment of hypogammaglobulinemia, but is also effective in other immunodeficiency disorders. In the setting of BMT, IVIg has been used in a number of ways but most frequently to boost treatment of infection and to prevent infection or GVHD (Sullivan et al., 1990). IVIg in combination with ganciclovir is considered standard first-line therapy for CMV-IP (Zaia, 1994). The premise for the use of prophylactic IVIg is to provide passive immunization and to serve as a nonspecific immune modulator rather than to provide specific anti-infective effects. Early studies of IVIg evaluated its ability to prevent CMV infection in seronegative patients. Results from trials are conflicting on IVIg's sole ability to prevent CMV infection, particularly, CMV-IP. The largest placebo-controlled trial evaluating conventional IVIg notes a lower rate of interstitial pneumonitis in CMV-seropositive patients receiving IVIg; but overall mortality was no different between IVIg- and placebo-treated patients (Sullivan et al., 1990). Many centers have replaced the routine use of prophylactic IVIg with other effective methods to prevent CMV infection such as modified blood product support or ganciclovir preemptive therapy. The role of IVIg to prevent other infections or GVHD remains controversial. Data from several trials suggest IVIg prophylaxis may decrease the risk of gram-negative infection and acute GVHD in certain subsets of patients.

Toxicities

In most cases, IVIg is well tolerated in BMT patients. Systemic adverse effects occur in less than 10% of patients and are typically due to infusion rate, activation of complement, or anaphylactic reactions to a component of the product (Wordell, 1991). Immunodeficient patients are at greatest risk for reactions due to complement activation, particularly those who have not received IVIg before or within the last month. Patients may infrequently experience itching, angioedema, chills, flushing, nausea, vomiting, fever, syncope, hypotension, hypertension, myalgia, leg cramps, or mild chest, joint, or back pain during the infusion. Most adverse effects appear to be related to the rate of infusion and may be relieved by slowing or temporarily discontinuing the infusion. Anaphylaxis to IVIg has been rarely reported and is related to IgA levels in the IVIg product. Another concern with IVIg is the risk of viral transmission through the IVIg preparation. Given new purification techniques and screening tests for all plasma products, the risk of viral transmission with IVIg products is very low.

Dosing, Administration, and Monitoring

The dosing and schedule of IVIg varies depending on the indication. For hypogammaglobulinemia, doses of 100 to 200 mg/kg are administered monthly. To treat CMV-IP, regimens involving an induction course followed by maintenance therapy are outlined in Table 5.11. Used prophylactically, IVIg doses range from 400 to 500 mg/kg given weekly early after transplant, then monthly during the period of immune reconstitution. One standard prophylactic regimen administers IVIg, 500 mg/kg, once weekly until day 90, then monthly until day 360. Patients should be monitored closely during IVIg infusions for adverse effects, and the infusion slowed or temporarily discontinued if patients complain of chest or other pain, flushing, wheezing, or other outlined infusion-related adverse effects. If symptoms are severe, acetaminophen, an antihistamine, or hydrocortisone may be administered. If the infusion is discontinued, it should then be resumed at a slower rate following resolution of symptoms. Each IVIg product has guidelines for infusion rates; in general, they recommend beginning the infusion slowly for the first 30 minutes and then increasing the rate, if no adverse effects are noted. Most IVIg infusions require 2 to 6 hours to complete. With proper patient education, IVIg infusions have been safely administered in the outpatient or home setting.

Hematopoietic Growth Factors

Pharmacology

Hematopoietic growth factors (HGFs) (also referred to as *colony-stimulating factors*) are endogenous glycoproteins that are essential components of the microenvironment of the hematopoietic system. HGFs regulate the proliferation and differentiation of hematopoietic cells and in some cases increase the functional activity of mature hematopoietic cells (Yee and Stanley, 1994). HGFs can be classified according to their activity on specific hematopoietic cells—either early, intermediate, or late-acting. Early acting HGFs act on pluripotent stem cells, and late acting HGFs act on committed progenitor cells and may increase the activity of mature cells. Intermediate acting HGFs act on both uncommitted and committed progenitor cells. Although individual HGFs have demonstrated activity on hematopoiesis, a combina-

tion of endogenously administered early, intermediate, and late acting HGFs is necessary to reproduce and significantly impact hematopoiesis.

Numerous HGFs including interleukins have been recognized and prepared by recombinant DNA technology through varying production sources. The commercially available colony-stimulating factors in the United States are granulocyte colony-stimulating factor (G-CSF), granulocyte-macrophage colony-stimulating factor (GM-CSF), and epoetin (EPO). Other products available in Europe or under investigation are outlined in Table 5.13.

Epoetin

Pharmacology

Epoetin alfa, a biosynthetic form of the endogenous glycoprotein erythropoietin, is a late acting HGF that stimulates the maturation of erythroid progenitor cells into mature red blood cells and maintains their function. Erythopoietin is an important factor in the feedback system responsible for regulating the circulating red cell mass and its oxygen-carrying capacity.

Therapeutic Use

While only approved for anemias in patients with chronic renal failure, zidovudine-treated HIV-infected patients, and chemotherapy patients with nonmyeloid malignancies, epoetin has also been evaluated in the BMT setting.

TABLE 5.13 Recombinant forms of CSFs

Molecule	Generic name	Trade name	Manufacturer	Source
G-CSF	Filgrastim	Neupogen	Amgen	Bacteria
G-CSF	Lenograstim	Neutrogin	Chugai	Chinese hamster ovary cell
GM-CSF	Sargramostim	Leukine	Immunex	Yeast
GM-CSF	Molgramostim	Leucomax	Schering/Sandoz	Bacteria
GM-CSF	Regramostim		Sandoz, Chugai	Chinese hamster ovary cell
GM-CSF	Ecogramostim			Chinese hamster ovary cell

Data suggest autologous BMT patients possess an adequate erythropoietic response following BMT and allogeneic patients have a defective response. The majority of trials administering EPO following autologous BMT either alone or combined with other HGFs demonstrate no difference in transfusion requirements when compared to patients not receiving EPO. Although some randomized trials in allogeneic BMT patients have been more promising and report decreased requirements of red blood cell transfusion along with more rapid erythroid recovery in patients receiving EPO compared to no EPO, other studies have demonstrated no positive impact of EPO following allogeneic BMT (Steegmann et al., 1992; Klaesson et al., 1994; Biggs et al., 1995). Enhanced erythropoiesis following administration of EPO has been noted in allogeneic patients with GVHD and in those receiving cyclosporin and methotrexate prophylaxis (Klaesson et al., 1994; Biggs et al., 1995). One study reports an economic advantage for allogeneic patients receiving EPO compared to control patients because they require fewer transfusions and shorter hospitalization (Klaesson et al., 1995).

Toxicities

Although EPO has been associated in some patient populations with mild to moderate toxicity including worsening or development of hypertension, thrombocytosis, hyperkalemia, increased blood urea nitrogen concentrations, iron deficiency, and flulike symptoms, it has been well tolerated by BMT patients and devoid of such side effects. Of note, in one study, 12% of BMT patients who received EPO discontinued EPO because of joint pain (Klaesson et al., 1994).

Dosing, Administration, and Monitoring

The recommended dose of EPO in cancer patients is 150 U/kg subcutaneously 3 times a week for 8 weeks followed by a doubled dose (300 U/kg 3 times per week) if adequate response is not achieved. This starting dose and doses up to 200 U/kg daily have been evaluated following BMT. As of yet, the optimal dose or proven benefit of EPO following BMT is yet to be determined. In other patient populations, EPO is not recommend for patients with grossly elevated pretreatment endogenous erythropoietin levels (> 200 mU/ml). EPO levels have been less well correlated with response in BMT patients, thus the value of pretreatment levels is questionable.

Filgrastim and Sargramostim

Pharmacology

Both filgrastim and sargramostim can be referred to as myeloid growth factors given their restricted effects on the growth of cells of myeloid origin. Filgrastim primarily regulates the production and proliferation of neutrophils. Sargramostim has a slightly broader range of activity; it regulates production and proliferation of neutrophils, eosinophils, and monocytes. Both agents have demonstrated enhancement of the activity of mature neutrophils and for sargramostim, also the effects of monocytes and macrophages. Filgrastim (G-CSF) is prepared by an *Escherichia coli* production system and sargramostim (GM-CSF) by a yeast (*Saccaromyces cerevisiae*) production system.

Therapeutic Use

Although these agents have different FDA-approved indications, they have generally been used to enhance neutrophil recovery following autologous BMT in patients with nonmyeloid malignancies. Randomized placebo-controlled trials of either filgrastim or sargramostim following autologous BMT report a significantly shorter duration of neutropenia when compared to placebo (Nemunaitis et al., 1991;

Schmitz et al., 1995; Stahel et al., 1994). Other more pertinent endpoints related to the duration of neutropenia such as decreased duration of hospitalization, intravenous antibiotics, and incidence of infection have also been reported in some, but not all, of these trials (Gilmore and Dix, 1995). In terms of relapse or overall mortality, no advantageous or detrimental effects due to the use of these agents have been reported. Two pharmacoeconomic studies of sargramostim following autologous BMT note a significant reduction in either overall cost or the inpatient cost of BMT when compared to placebo (Gulati et al., 1992; Luce et al., 1994).

The use of CSFs following allogeneic BMT remains more controversial. Both agents have been shown to be safe in patients receiving marrows from sibling donors in that higher rates of GVHD or relapse have not occurred in patients receiving CSFs (Masoaka et al., 1989; Nemunaitis, Rosenfield, et al., 1995; Schriber et al., 1994). The cost-effectiveness of these agents in the allogeneic (sibling) BMT setting remains open to debate because only one randomized trial of sargramostim has demonstrated an impact on pertinent clinical endpoints such as a shorter duration of hospitalization and decreased incidence of mucositis or infection (Nemunaitis et al., 1995). In matched unrelated donor transplants, two reports note a higher, although unexplained, mortality rate in patients receiving either filgrastim or sargramostim (Anasetti et al., 1993; Schriber et al., 1994).

CSFs, particularly sargramostim, have also been used effectively to treat graft failure following BMT (Nemunaitis et al., 1990). They may also ameliorate drug-induced neutropenia such as that which occurs with ganciclovir. CSFs are also frequently used to mobilize peripheral blood stem cells and increase the cell yield during harvesting of peripheral blood stem cells.

Toxicities

In general, the commercially available CSFs are well tolerated. The most commonly reported adverse effect is medullary bone pain particularly in the lower back. Other adverse effects have been reported, but occur at a similar rate in patients receiving CSFs or placebo. These nonspecific adverse effects include fever, myalgias, fatigue, headache, rash, nausea, and vomiting. Peripheral edema and pericardial effusions have been reported in patients receiving sargramostim and occur at a slightly higher rate than placebo-treated patients.

The adverse effects of GM-CSF vary depending on the preparation. Significant first-dose reactions involving hypotension, pulmonary edema, and respiratory compromise have been reported with the *E. coli*-derived GM-CSF product, but have not occurred with sargramostim, the yeast-derived commercially available product.

Dosing, Administration, and Monitoring

The FDA-approved dosing regimens for filgrastim and sargramostim are outlined in Table 5.14. Lower filgrastim doses of 5 µg/kg have also been used successfully after transplant. Used prior to BMT to mobilize peripheral blood stem cells, filgrastim is typically given in daily doses of 5 to 10 µg/kg or higher. Both agents can be administered by subcutaneous or intravenous route, but most centers prefer subcutaneous administration for convenience and decreased cost. In patients with preexisting skin rashes, persistent thrombocytopenia, or peripheral edema, the intravenous route may be preferred. Each agent has specific recommendations for discontinuation of therapy, but in general most centers either stop or taper therapy when ANC recovery is sustained. One method is to stop CSF therapy when the ANC is greater than 1500/µl for 1 to 3 days. Significant and rapid drops in the ANC may occur

TABLE 5.14 Guidelines for use of CSFs following BMT

	GM-CSF (Sargramostim)	G-CSF (Filgrastim)
Indication		
FDA-approved indication	Following autologous BMT for non-myeloid malignancies[a]	Following BMT for nonmyeloid malignancies
Clinical practice use	Following autologous and allogeneic BMT[b] for nonmyeloid and myeloid malignancies[b]	Following autologous and allogeneic BMT[b] for nonmyeloid and myeloid malignancies[b]
Dose		
FDA-approved dose	250 µg/m² per day	10 µg/kg per day
Clinical practice use	250 µg/m² per day	5–10 µg/kg per day
Route		
FDA-approved route	IV over 2 hours	Continuous IV or SC
Clinical practice use	SC, IV infusion	SC, IV/SC infusion
Duration of therapy		
FDA-approved	From day 0 to day 21 after BMT	From day 0; when ANC > 1000/µl × 3 d, taper dose to 5 µg/kg/d; when ANC > 1000/µl × 3 more days, discontinue
Clinical practice use	From day 0 until ANC > 1500/µl × 1–3 d	From day 0 until ANC > 1500/µl × 1–3 d

[a]Also FDA approved for graft failure following BMT.

[b]Use following allogeneic BMT and following BMT for myeloid malignancies is still controversial.

following discontinuation and CSF therapy may need to be resumed if the ANC falls below 500/µl. Complete blood counts should be monitored frequently during and following discontinuation of CSF therapy.

Investigational HGFs

Clinical Experience

Numerous HGFs, most of which are early acting, are under development and investigation in both preclinical and clinical trials (Table 5.15). One major area of investigation is to evaluate the potential of new HGFs, either alone or in combination, to enhance trilineage hematologic recovery after BMT, more specifically, to reduce duration and severity of thrombocytopenia. The gene for the greatly sought-after factor that regulates megakaryocytopoiesis, thrombopoeitin, was recently discovered and cloned (Kaushansky, 1995). Thrombopoieitin, also known as megakaryocyte growth and development factor (MGDF) or the ligand to the c-Mpl receptor, initiates the proliferation and maturation of megakaryocyte progenitors and regulates further platelet production. Preclinical data conclude that pegylated human MGDF regulates platelet production and function and results in a dose-dependent thrombocytosis and megakaryocyte hyperplasia. In mice, MGDF reversed carboplatin-induced thrombocytopenia in a dose-dependent manner by increasing the number of megakaryocytes in the marrow and circulating platelets (Ulich et al., 1995). Initial results from phase I clinical trials suggest platelet counts rise from baseline following

TABLE 5.15 **Investigational HGFs in BMT patients**

				Hematopoeitic activity	
HGF	*WBC*	*Plts*	*RBC*	*Areas of research*	*Toxicities*
MGDF/TPO	−	+++	−	Hematologic recovery	Thrombocytosis
IL-1	+	+	?	Hematologic recovery Graft failure	Fever, chills, headache, tachycardias, myalgias, hypotension (dose-limiting)
IL-2	−	−	−	Hematologic recovery Immune modulation	
IL-3	+	+++	?	Hematologic recovery Graft failure Immune modulation PSBC mobilization	Fever, headache, urticaria, neck stiffness, local erythema, rash, flulike symptoms
IL-6	−	+	?	Hematologic recovery	Fever, chills, rigors, rash, headache, fatigue, hepatotoxicity (dose-limiting)
IL-11	−	+	?	Hematologic recovery	Flulike symptoms, mild anemia, edema
PIXY 321	+	+++	?	Hematologic recovery PBSC mobilization	Local erythema ± tenderness, pruritis, flulike symptoms, headache, bone pain
SCF	+	+	?	Hematologic recovery PBSC mobilization	Rash, angioedema, dyspnea, allergic/ anaphylactoid reactions, injection-site reactions

Source: Adapted from Yee and Stanley, 1994.

administration of pegylated human MGDF (rHuMGDF). Additional phase I/II trials of rHuMGDF after high-dose chemotherapy and peripheral blood stem cell transplantation in breast cancer patients are ongoing. IL-1 has been studied following BMT to evaluate its hematopoietic and immunomodulatory effects. In a phase I/II trial in lymphoma patients, higher doses of IL-3 ($\geq$ 3 μg/m^2 per day) administered for 7 days after autologous BMT were associated with enhanced neutrophil recovery and decreases in red blood cell and platelet transfusions, as well as a decrease in the number of hospital days and charges while lower doses had no significant impact on hematologic recovery (Weisdorf et al., 1994).

Another phase I/II trial in lymphoma patients undergoing autologous BMTs notes enhanced neutrophil recovery, a decreased incidence of infection, and a survival advantage in patients receiving IL-1 (Nemunaitis et al., 1994).

Interleukin-3 has also been evaluated alone or in combination with other HGFs in patients undergoing autologous BMT. Compared to historical controls receiving no HGFs following autologous BMT, the administration of IL-3 resulted in accelerated recovery of neutrophils and platelets (Nemunaitis et al., 1993). However, compared to control autologous BMT patients receiving GM-CSF, the rate of myeloid recovery was similar. Simultaneous administration of GM-CSF and IL-3 following BMT has failed to enhance hematologic recovery. However, one study reports a reduction in the need for platelet transfusions in autologous BMT patients receiving sequential administration, 5 to 10 days of IL-3 followed by GM-CSF, when compared to historical control patients receiving no HGF, GM-CSF alone, or G-CSF alone (Fay et al., 1994). Enhancement of hematologic recovery by sequential administration is most likely due to IL-3's proliferative effects on progenitor cells, leading to increased numbers of target cells for later acting HGFs like G-CSF or GM-CSF.

Another early acting HGF, PIXY 321 is a yeast-derived fusion protein of GM-CSF and IL-3 developed with the goal of combining the granulocyte- and macrophage-enhancing effects of GM-CSF with the multilineage, specifically thrombopoietic, effects of IL-3. Phase II trials in BMT patients also suggest that the IV dose of PIXY 321 $\geq$ 125 μg/m^2 per day significantly accelerates recovery of neutrophils and platelets (Vose et al., 1993). However, in a phase III trial in autologous BMT patients, comparing GM-CSF and PIXY 321 resulted in similar neutrophil and megakaryocytic recovery (Vose et al., 1995).

Interleukin-6 (IL-6), a multifunctional HGF affecting megarkaryocyte growth and development, myeloid cell differentiation, T-cell stimulation, and acute-phase reactant responses, has also been evaluated both alone or in combination with either GM-CSF or G-CSF following autologous BMT. Administered alone, IL-6 has yet to make a significant impact on hematologic recovery following autologous BMT (Lazarus et al., 1993). One trial evaluating the combination of IL-6 and GM-CSF following autologous BMT reported more promising results, suggesting the combination is well tolerated and may accelerate both neutrophil recovery and the time to platelet transfusion independence (Fay et al., 1993). In a randomized trial, both neutrophil and platelet recovery rates were similar in a trial comparing G-CSF alone to the combination of G-CSF and IL-6 administered following autologous BMT for breast cancer (Devine et al., 1994).

Interleukin-11 (IL-11), an early acting HGF that enhances megakaryocyte growth in vitro, is also being evaluated in a phase I trial in combination with G-CSF following autologous BMT (Champlin and McGlave, 1994). Many of these investigational early acting HGFs are also being evaluated as peripheral-blood progenitor-mobilizing agents and immune modulators.

Stem cell factor (SCF), also known as c-*kit* ligand, steel factor, or mast cell growth factor, represents one of the earliest acting HGFs in development, but has little effect on hematopoiesis when administered alone in tolerable doses. However, when administered in low doses combined with G-CSF, SCF doubles progenitor cell yields and may increase platelet recovery when these collected cells are administered following high-dose chemotherapy (Glaspy et al., 1994).

In terms of immune modulation, some data suggest lymphoma patients receiving IL-1 after autologous BMT may have an increase in cytolytic function, although the impact of this finding on the decreasing relapse is yet to be determined (Katsanis et al., 1994). Interleukin-2 (IL-2) with or without lymphokine-activated killer cells (LAK) is being administered in clinical trials to evaluate the potential to prevent relapse following BMT for hematologic malignancies (Benyunes et al., 1993). IL-2's immunomodulatory effects are mediated through stimulation of the generation and proliferation of killer cells in the bone marrow and peripheral blood. Preclinical studies and some clinical studies suggest IL-2 with or without LAK cells may decrease rate of relapse following both autologous and allogeneic BMT by stimulating a response similar to that described as the graft-versus-leukemia (GVL) effect. IL-2 is also been investigated as an immunologic purging agent with the hopes of eliminating leukemia cell contamination of autologous bone marrow and to mediate cultured marrow growth of cytotoxic T lymphocytes (Klingemann et al., 1994; Heslop et al., 1989).

Toxicity

While trials with many of these investigational HGFs have been promising, some of these agents have been associated with moderate to severe toxicity in BMT patients.

PEG-rHuMGDF. In the initial phase I studies evaluating escalating doses of subcutaneously administered PEG-rHuMGDA, or placebo, the study drug has been well tolerated with no dose-limiting toxicities noted. In a blind study, one patient receiving 1.0 µg/kg per day of the drug developed thrombocytosis, but this adverse effect did not result in serious complications.

IL-1. Trials in BMT patients evaluating the high doses of IL-1 required for its hematopoietic effects have been haunted by dose-limiting severe hypotension that required fluid or pressor support. Other reported serious toxicities following administration of IL-1 include renal failure, arrhythmias, and a pulmonary capillary leak syndrome. Some trials suggest severe toxicity lessened by administering IL-1 as short IV infusions instead of continuously (Yee and Stanley, 1994). The majority of patients receiving IL-1 experience fever, chills, myalgias, headache, fatigue, nausea, vomiting, and anorexia.

IL-2. Side effects of IL-2 following BMT have been dose dependent and related to the time of administration following BMT (Klingemann and Phillips, 1995). IL-2 infusions are more tolerable if initiated several weeks after rather than immediately following BMT. Severe toxicities including life-threatening hypotension and pulmonary edema have been reported in patients receiving IL-2 early after transplant. Fever has also been reported and can be severe enough to require discontinuation of the drug.

Other toxicities, which typically do not require discontinuation, include fatigue, rash, nausea, vomiting, diarrhea, and weight gain.

IL-3. Common toxicities in BMT patients receiving IL-3 alone or in combination with other HGFs include fever and headache, which can be dose limiting, and a flulike syndrome (Nemunaitis et al., 1993). The incidence and severity of adverse effects is dose related and also increased in patients undergoing autologous BMT (Yee and Stanley, 1994). Dermatologic reactions can occur frequently and include facial flushing, rash, urticaria, and mild erythema at the injection site. IV infusions of IL-3 appear to be more toxic than SC injections. In addition, several trials note high rates of dose reduction or drug discontinuation in patients receiving IL-3.

IL-6. Administration of IL-6 has been associated with a flulike syndrome, headache, nausea, vomiting, and anorexia. Some patients developed transient, mild elevations in transaminases, alkaline phosphatase, creatinine, and fasting blood glucose levels, as well as an increase in acute-phase reactants. In non–BMT patients, dose-limiting toxicities of atrial fibrillation and hepatotoxicity occurred at 30 µg/kg per day. In BMT patients, the maximum tolerated dose appears to be much lower than in other patient populations. Transient hypotension requiring pressor support following the first dose of IL-6 occurred in two patients who received 1-hour IV infusions, but did not recur with subsequent doses. One trial notes dose-limiting hepatotoxicity following IV infusions in patients with metastatic breast cancer who underwent autologous BMT; another randomized trial comparing G-CSF alone to the combination of G-CSF and IL-6 was stopped due to a higher incidence of veno-occlusive disease than in historic controls.

PIXY 321. PIXY 321 is generally well tolerated, but can commonly produce local skin reactions including erythema, tenderness, and pruritis following subcutaneous injection. Flulike symptoms including fever, headache, malaise, and myalgia have also been reported. Approximately 25% of PIXY-321-treated patients experienced bone pain. Adverse effects appear to be more common at higher doses (≥ 250 lg/m^2 per day) and with continuous IV infusion than with SC administration.

IL-11. IL-11 has generally been well tolerated in the low doses in BMT patients. SCF, like the other early acting HGFs, has been associated with an increase in constitutional symptoms and also with symptoms of mast cell activation including mild to moderate injection reactions as well as systemic symptoms of angioedema, dermatographia, dyspesia, and hypotension (Crawford et al., 1993).

REFERENCES

Anasetti, C., Anderson, G., Appelbaum, F., et al. 1993. Phase III study of rhGM-CSF in allogeneic marrow transplantation fromunrelated donors. *Blood* 82:454a (abstr).

Antman, K., Ayash, L., Elias, A., et al. 1992. A phase II study of high-dose cyclophosphamide, thiotepa, and carboplatin with autologous marrow support in women with measurable advanced breast cancer responding to standard-dose therapy. *J Clin Oncol* 10:102-110.

Atkinson, K., Downs, K., Golenia, M., et al. 1991. Prophylactic use of ganciclovir in allogeneic bone marrow transplantation: absence of clinical cytomegalovirus infection. *Br J Hematol* 79:57-62.

Attal, M., Schlaifer, D., Rubie, H., et al. 1991. Prevention of gram-positive infections after bone marrow transplantation by systemic vancomycin: a prospective, randomized trial. *J Clin Oncol* 9:865-870.

Ayash, L., Hunt, M., Antman, K. 1990. Hepatic occlusive disease in autologous bone marrow transplantation of solid tumor and lymphomas. *J Clin Oncol* 8: 1699-1706.

Balfour, H., Bean, B., Laskin, O., et al. 1983. Acyclovir halts progression of herpes zoster in immunocompromised patients. *N Engl J Med* 308:1448-1453.

Barnett, M., Coppin, C., Murray, N., et al. 1993. High-dose chemotherapy and autologous bone marrow transplantation for patients with poor prognosis nonseminomatous germ cell tumors. *Br J Cancer* 68(3):594-598.

Bielory, L., Wright, R., Nienhuis, A., et al. 1988. Antithymocyte globulin hypersensitivity in bone marrow failure patients. *JAMA* 260(21):3164-3167.

Benyunes, M., Massumoto, C., York, A., et al. 1993. Interleukin-2 with or without lymphokine-activated killer cells as consolidative immunotherapy after autologous bone marrow transplantation for acute myelogenous leukemia. *BMT* 12:159-163.

Biggs, J., Atkinson, K., Booker, V., et al. 1995. Prospective randomised double-blind trial of the in vivo use of recombinant human erythropoietin in bone marrow transplantation from HLA-identical sibling donors. *BMT* 15:129-134.

Blume, K., Forman, S., O'Donnell, M., et al. 1987. Total body irradiation and high-dose etoposide: a new preparatory regimen for bone marrow transplantation in patients with advanced hematologic malignancies. *Blood* 69(4):1015-1020.

Braverman, A., Antin, J., Plappert, M., et al. 1991. Cyclophosphamide cardiotoxicity in bone marrow transplantation: a prospective evaluation of new dosing regimens. *J Clin Oncol* 9(7):1251-1223.

Brennan Rowe, N., Collins, D., Miner, R., et al. 1995. Open-label soruvidine (BV-ara-U) in the treatment of cutaneous varicella-zoster virus (VZV) in immunocompromised adults who failed or were intolerant of standard therapies. 35th Annual Interscience Conference on Antimicrobial Agents and Chemotherapy, San Francisco, Sept. 17–20 (abstr H97).

Broun, E., Nichols, C., Tricot, G., et al. 1991. High-dose carboplatin/VP-16 plus ifosamide with autologous bone marrow support in the treatment of refractory germ cell tumors. *BMT* 7(1):53-56.

Buggia, I., Locatelli, F., Regazzi, M., et al. 1994. Busulfan. *Ann Pharmacother* 28:1055-1062.

Burns, W. 1994. Herpes simplex virus. In Forman, S., Blume, K., Thomas, E. (Eds.) *Bone Marrow Transplantation.* Oxford: Blackwell Scientific, 404-411.

Champlin, R., McGlave, P. 1994. Allogeneic bone marrow transplantation for chronic myeloid leukemia. In Forman, S., Blume, K., Thomas, D. (Eds.) *Bone Marrow Transplantation.* Boston: Blackwell Scientific, 595-606.

Chao, N., Schimdt, G., Niland, J., et al. 1993. Cyclosporin, methotrexate, and prednisone compared with cyclosporin and prednisone for prophylaxis of acute graft-versus-host disease. *N Engl J Med* 329:1225-1230.

Cooper, B., Creger, R., Soegiarso, W., et al. 1993. Renal dysfunction during high-dose cisplatin therapy and autologous hematopoiesis stem cell transplantation: effect of aminoglycoside therapy. *Am J Med* 94:497-504.

Crawford, J., Lau, D., Erwin, R., et al. 1993. A phase I trial of recombinant methionyl human stem cell factor in patients with advanced non-small cell lung carcinoma. *Proc Am Soc Clin Oncol* 12:338a.

Deeg, H., Storb, R., Thomas, E., et al. 1985. Cyclosporin as prophylaxis for graft-versus-host disease: a randomized study in patients undergoing marrow transplantation for acute nonlymphoblastic leukemia. *Blood* 65:1325-1334.

Devine, S., Geller, R., Holland, K., et al. 1994. FK506-based immunosuppression for prevention of graft-versus-host disease after matched unrelated donor marrow transplantation. *Blood* 84:341a.

Devine, S., Winton, E., Holland, H., et al. 1994. Simultaneous administration of interleukin-6 (rhIL-6) and Neupogen (rhG-CSF) following autologous bone marrow transplantation (ABMT) for breast cancer. *Blood* 84:343a.

Dix, S., Devine, S., Geller, R., et al. 1995. Lack of clinically significant interaction between low-dose methotrexate and tacrolimus or cyclosporin in bone marrow transplant patients. *J Natl Canc Inst* 87:1641-1642.

Doney, K., Weiden, P., Storb, R., et al. 1981. Treatment of graft-versus-host disease in human allogeneic marrow graft recipients: a randomized trial comparing antithymocyte globulin and corticosteroids. *Am J Med* 11:1-8.

Dorr, R., Von Hoff, D. 1994. *Cancer Chemotherapy Handbook*, 2d ed. Norwalk, Conn: Appleton & Lange.

Eder, J., Antman, K., Elias, A., et al. Cyclophosphamide and thiotepa with autologous bone marrow transplantation in patients with solid tumors. *J Natl Canc Inst* 80: 1221-1226.

Emanuel, D., Cunningham, I., Jules-Elysee, K., et al. 1988. Cytomegalovirus pneumonia after bone marrow transplantation successfully treated with the combination of ganciclovir and high-dose intravenous immune globulin. *Ann Intern Med* 109:777-782.

Essel, J., Thompson, J., Harman, G., et al. 1992. Marked increase in veno-occlusive disease of the liver associated with methotrexate use for graft-versus-host disease prophylaxis in patients receiving busulfan/cyclophosphamide. *Blood* 79:2784.

Fay, J., Collins R., Pineiro, L., et al. 1993. Concomitant administration of interleukin-6 (rhIL-6) and leucomax

(rhGM-CSF) following autologous bone marrow transplantation—a phase I trial. *Blood* 82:1707a.

Fay, J., Lazarus, H., Herzig, R., et al. 1994. Sequential administration of interleukin-3 (rhIL-3) and granulocyte-macrophage colony-stimulating factor after autologous bone marrow transplantation for malignant lymphoma: a phase I/II trial multicenter trial. *Blood* 84:2151-2157.

Fay, W., Pirjeiro, L., Collins, R., et al. 1994. FK506-based immunosuppression for prevention of graft-versus-host disease after unrelated marrow donor transplantation. *Blood* 84:708a.

Gaspard, M., Maraninichi, D., Stoppa, A., et al. 1988. Intensive chemotherapy with high doses of BCNU, etoposide, cytosine arabinoside, and melphalan (BEAM) followed by autologous bone marrow transplantation: toxicity and antitumor activity in 26 patients with poor-risk malignancies. *Cancer Chemother Pharmacol* 22: 256-262.

Gilbert, C., Meisenberg, B., Vredenburgh, J., et al. 1994. Sequential prophylactic oral and empiric once-daily parenteral antibiotics for neutropenia and fever after high-dose chemotherapy and autologous bone marrow support. *J Clin Oncol* 12:1005-1011.

Gilmore, C., Dix, S. 1995. Cytokine therapy following bone marrow transplantation: review of GM-CSF and G-CSF. *Pharmacother Pharmacotherapy* 16:593-608.

Gimema Infection Program. 1991. Prevention of bacterial infection in neutropenic patients with hematologic malignancies: a randomized multicenter trial comparing norfloxacin with ciprofloxacin. *Ann Intern Med* 115:7-12.

Glaspy, J., McNiece, I., LeMaistre, F., et al. 1994. Effects of stem cell factor (rh-SCF) and filgrastim (rhG-CSF) on mobilization of peripheral blood progenitor cells (PBPC) and on hematological recovery posttransplant: early results from a phase I/II study. *Proc Am Soc Clin Oncol* 13:76a.

Gluckman, E., Lokeic, F., Devergie, A., et al. 1984. Pharmacokinetic monitoring of cyclosporin in allogenic bone marrow transplants. *Transplant Proc* 17:500-501.

Gluckman, E., Lotsberg, J., Devergie, A., et al. 1983. Oral acyclovir prophylactic treatment of herpes simplex infection after bone marrow transplant. *J Antimicrob Chemother* 12(suppl B):161-167.

Goodman, J., Winston, D., Greenfield, R., et al. 1992. A controlled trial of fluconazole to prevent fungal infections in patients undergoing bone marrow transplantation. *N Engl J Med* 326:845-851.

Goodrich J., Bowden, R., Fisher, L., et al. 1993. Prevention of cytomegalovirus disease after allogeneic bone marrow transplant by ganciclovir prophylaxis. *Ann Intern Med* 118:173-178.

Goodrich, J., Mori, M., Gleaves, C., et al. 1991. Early treatment with ganciclovir to prevent cytomegalovirus disease after allogeneic bone marrow transplant. *N Engl J Med* 325:1601-1607.

Gottdiener, J., Appelbaum, F., Ferrans, V., et al. 1981. Cardiotoxicity associated with high-dose cyclophosphamide. *Arch Intern Med* 141:758-763.

Grochow, L. 1993. Busulfan disposition: the role of therapeutic monitoring in bone marrow transplantation induction regimens. *Semin Oncol* 20(4, suppl 4):18-25.

Grochow, L., Jones, R., Brundrett, R., et al. 1989. Pharmacokinetics of busulfan: correlation with veno-occlusive disease in patients undergoing bone marrow transplantation. *Cancer Chemother Pharmacol* 25: 55-61.

Gualtieri, R., Donowitz, G., Kaiser, D., et al. 1983. Double-blind randomized study of prophylactic trimethoprim-sulfamethoxazole in granulocytopenic patients with hematologic malignancies. *Am J Med* 74: 934-940.

Gulati, S., Bennett, C. 1992. Granulocyte-macrophage colony-stimulating factor (GM-CSF) as adjunct therapy in relapsed Hodgkin's disease. *Ann Intern Med* 116: 177-182.

Hann, I., Prentice, H., Blackbock, H., et al. 1983. Acyclovir prophylaxis against herpes virus infections in severly immunocomprised patients: a randomized double-blind trial. *BMJ* 287:384-388.

Haupt, H., Hutchins, G., Moore, G., et al. 1981. Ara-C lung: non-cardiogenic pulmonary edema complicating cytosine arabinoside therapy of leukemia. *Am J Med* 70: 256-261.

Haas, R., Ehrhardt, R., Witt, B., et al. 1993. Autografting with peripheral blood stem cells mobilized by sequential administration interleukin-3/granulocyte-macrophage colony-stimulating factor following high-dose chemotherapy in non-Hodgkin's lymphoma. *BMT* 12: 643-649.

Herzig, G., Phillips, G., Herzig, R., et al. 1981. High-dose nitrosourea (BCNU) and autologous bone marrow transplantation: a phase I study. In Prestayko, A., Crooke, S., Baker, L., et al. (Eds.) *Nitrosoureas: Current Status and New Developments.* New York: Academic Press, 337-341.

Heslop, H., Gottlieb, D., Bianchi, A., et al. 1994. In vivo induction of gamma interferon and tumor necrosis factor by interleukin-2 following intensive chemotherapy or autologous marrow transplantation. *Blood* 74: 1374-1380.

Jagannath, S., Armitage, J., Dicke, K., et al. 1989. Prognostic factors for response and survival after high-dose cyclophosphamide, carmustine, and etoposide with autologous bone marrow transplantation for relapsed Hodgkin's disease. *J Clin Oncol* 7(2):179-185.

Jones, R., Matthes, S., Shpall, E., et al. 1992. BCNU plasma exposure (AUC) correlates with the risk of non-infectious pulmonary injury following cyclophosphamide, cisplatin, and BCNU with autologous bone marrow support. *Proc Am Soc Clin Oncol* 11:132.

Karp, J., Merz, W., Hendrickson, C., et al. 1987. Oral norfloxacin for prevention of gram-negative bacterial infections in patients with acute leukemia and granulocytopenia. *Ann Intern Med* 106:1-7.

Kaushansky, K. 1995. Thrombopoeitin: the primary regulator of platelet production. *Blood* 86:419-431.

Katsanis, E., Weisdorf, D., Xu, Z., et al. 1994. Infusions of interleukin-1 after autologous transplantation for Hodgkin's disease and non-Hodgkin's lymphoma induce effector cells with antilymphoma cytolytic activity. *J Clin Immunol* 14:205-211.

Kennedy, M., Deeg, H., Storb, R., et al. 1985. Treatment of acute graft-versus-host disease after allogeneic marrow transplantation: randomized study comparing steroids and cyclosporin. *Am J Med* 78:978-983.

Kennedy, M., Yee, G., McGuire, T., et al. 1985. Correlation of serum cyclosporin concentration with renal dysfunction in marrow transplant recipients. *Transplantation* 40:249-253.

Klaesson, S., Ringden, O., Ljungman, P., et al. 1994. Reduced blood transfusion requirements after allogeneic bone marrow transplantation: results of a randomised, double-blind study with high-dose erythropoeitin. *BMT* 13:397-402.

Klingemann, H., Eaves, M., Barnett, M., et al. 1994. Transplantation of patients with high-risk acute myeloid leukemia in first remission with autologous marrow cultures in interleukin-2 followed by interleukin-2 administration. *BMT* 14:389-396.

Klingemann, H., Phillips, G. 1995. Is there a place for immunotherapy with interleukin-2 to prevent relapse after autologous stem cell transplantation for acute leukemia? *Leuk Lymphoma* 16:397-405.

Lazarus, J., Winton, E., Williams, S., et al. 1993. Phase I study of recombinant human interleukin-6 (IL-6) after autologous bone marrow transplant (ABMT) in patients with poor-prognosis breast cancer. *Blood* 82:677a.

Lochte, H., Levy, S., Guenther, D., et al. 1962. Prevention of delayed foreign marrow reaction in lethally irradiated mice by early administration of methotrexate. *Nature* 196:1110-1111.

Long, G., Blume, K. 1994. Allogeneic bone marrow transplantation for acute myeloid leukemia. In Forman, S., Blume, K., Thomas, D. (Eds.) *Bone Marrow Transplantation*. Boston: Blackwell Scientific, 607-617.

Lotz, J., Machover, D., Malassagne, B., et al. 1991. Phase I-II study of two consecutive courses of high-dose epipodophyllotoxin, ifosfamide, and carboplatin with autologous bone marrow transplantation for treatment of adult patients with solid tumors. *J Clin Oncol* 9(10): 1860-1870.

Ljungman, P., Ellis, M., Hackman, R., et al. 1990. Acyclovir-resistant herpes simplex virus causing pneumonia after marrow transplantation. *J Infect Dis* 162: 244-248.

Ljungman, P., Lonnqvist, B., Ringden, O., et al. 1989. A randomized trial of oral versus intravenous acyclovir for treatment of herpes zoster in bone marrow transplant recipients. *BMT* 4:613-615.

Luce, B., Singer, J., Weschler, J., et al. 1994. Recombinant human granulocyte-macrophage colony-stimulating factor after autologous bone marrow transplantation for lymphoid cancer. *Pharmacoeconomics* 6:42-48.

Lundgren G., Wilczek, H., Lonnovist, B., et al. 1985. Acyclovir prophylaxis in bone marrow transplant recipients. *Scand J Infect Dis* 47(suppl):137-144.

Masoaka, T., Takaku, F., Kato, S., et al. 1989. Recombinant human granulocyte colony-stimulating factor in allogeneic bone marrow transplantation. *Exp Hematol* 17:1047-1050.

McGuire, T., Tallman, M., Yee, G., et al. 1988. Influence of infusion duration on the efficacy and toxicity of intravenous cyclosporin in bone marrow transplant patients. *Transplant Proc* 20:501-504.

Mehta, J., Nagler, A., Or, R., et al. 1992. Neutropenic enterocolitis and intestinal perforation associated with carboplatin-containing conditioning regimens for autologous bone marrow transplantation. *Acta Oncologia* 31:591.

Meyers, J., Wade, J., Mitchell, C., et al. 1982. Multicenter collaborative trial of intravenous acyclovir for treatment of mucocutaneous herpes simplex virus infections in the immunocompromised host. *Am J Med* 73A: 229-235.

Meyers, J., Wade, J., Shepp, D., et al. 1984. Acyclovir treatment of varicella-zoster virus infection in the compromised host. *Transplantation* 37:571-574.

Mitchell C., Gentry, S., Boen, J., et al. 1981. Acyclovir therapy for mucocutaneous herpes simplex infections in immunocompromised patients. *Lancet* Jun 27: 1389-1392.

Murphy, C., Harden, E., Thompson, J. 1992. Generalized seizures secondary to high-dose busulfan therapy. *Annals Pharmacother* 26:30-31.

Nash, R., Etzioni, R., Storb, R., et al. 1995. Tacrolimus (FK506) alone or in combination with methotrexate or methylprednisolone for the prevention of acute graft-versus-host disease after marrow transplantation from HLA-matched siblings: a single center study. *Blood* 85(12):3746-3753.

Nemunaitis, J., Appelbaum, F., Lilleby, K., et al. 1994. Phase I study of recombinant interleukin-1 beta in patients undergoing autologous bone marrow transplant for acute myelogenous leukemia. *Blood* 83:3473-3479.

Nemunaitis, J., Appelbaum, F., Singer, J., et al. 1993. Phase I trial with recombinant human interleukin-3 in patients with lymphoma undergoing autologous bone marrow transplantation. *Blood* 84:2151-2157.

Nemunaitis, J., Lilleby, K., Buckner, C., et al. 1992. Phase I study of recombinant interleukin-1 beta in patients with bone marrow failure. *Blood* 80:418a.

Nemunaitis, J., Rabinowe, S., Singer, J., et al. 1991. Recombinant granulocyte-macrophage colony-stimulating factor after autologous bone marrow transplantation for lymphoid cancer. *N Engl J Med* 324:1773-1778.

Nemunaitis, J., Rosenfield, C., Ash, R., et al. 1995. Phase III randomized, double-blind placebo-controlled trial of rhGM-CSF following allogeneic bone marrow transplantation. *BMT* 15:949-954.

Nemunaitis, J., Singer, J., Buckner, C., 1990. Recombinant human granulocyte-macrophage colony-stimulating factor in graft failure after bone marrow transplantation. *Blood* 76:245-253.

Nevill, T., Tirgan, M., Deeg, H., et al. 1992. Influence of post-methotrexate folinic acid rescue on regimen-related toxicity and graft-versus-host disease after allogeneic bone marrow transplantation. *BMT* 9:349-354.

Parr, M., Messino, M., McIntyre, W. 1991. Allogeneic bone marrow transplantation: procedures and complications. *Am J Hosp Pharm* 48:127-137.

Peters, W., Henner, W., Bast, R., et al. 1986. Novel toxicities associated with high-dose combination alkylating agents in autologous agents in autologous bone marrow support. In Dicke, K., Spitzer, G., Zander, A. (Eds.) *Autologous Bone Marrow Transplantation: Proceedings of the First International Symposium*. Houston: University Texas Cancer Center, M.D. Anderson Hospital, 231-235.

Peters, W., Henner, W., Grochow, L., et al. 1987. Clinical and pharmacologic effects of high-dose single agent busulfan with autologous bone marrow support in the treatment of solid tumors. *Cancer Res* 47:6402-6406.

Peters, W., Shpall, E., Jones, R., et al. 1990. High-dose combination alkylating agents with bone marrow support as initial treatment for metastatic breast cancer. *J Clin Oncol* 6:1368-1376.

Peterson, F. Appelbaum, F., Bigelow, C., et al. 1989. High-dose cytosine arabinoside, total body irradiation and marrow transplantation for advanced malignant lymphoma. *BMT* 4:483-488.

Portnoy, J. 1994. Famciclovir in the treatment of herpes zoster infection. Seventh International Conference on Antiviral Research, Charleston, SC, Feb 27–Mar 4.

Postmus, P., Mulder, N., Sleijfer, D., et al. 1984. High-dose etoposide for refractory malignancies: a phase I study. *Cancer Treat Rep* 68(12):1471-1474.

Razis, E., Cook, P., Mittelman, A., et al. 1994. Treatment of ganciclovir-resistant cytomegalovirus with foscarnet: a report of two cases occurring after bone marrow transplantation. *Leuk Lymphoma* 12:477-480.

Reece, D., Barnett, M., Connors, J., et al. 1991. Intensive chemotherapy with cyclophosphamide, carmustine, and etoposide followed by autologous bone marrow transplantation for relapsed Hodgkin's disease. *J Clin Oncol* 9:1871-1879.

Reed, E., Bowden, R., Dandliker, P., et al. 1988. Treatment of cytomegalovirus pneumonia with ganciclovir and intravenous cytomegalovirus immunoglobulin in patients with bone marrow transplants. *Ann Intern Med* 109:783-788.

Reed, E., Wolford, J., Kopecky, K., et al. 1990. Ganciclovir for the treatment of cytomegalovirus gastroenteritis in bone marrow transplant patients—a randomized, placebo-controlled trial. *Ann Intern Med* 112:505-510.

Reusser, P., Gambertoglio, J., Lilleby, K., et al. 1992. Phase I–II trial of foscarnet for prevention of cytomegalovirus infection in autologous and allogeneic marrow transplant recipients. *J Infect Dis* 166:473-479.

Ridell, S., Appelbaum, F., Buckner C., et al. 1988. High-dose cytarabine and total body irradiation with or without cyclophosphamide as a preparative regimen for marrow transplantation for acute leukemia. *J Clin Oncol* 6:576-582.

Rudnick, S., Cadmnan, E., Capizzi, R., et al. 1979. High dose cytosine arabinoside (HDAARAC) in refractory acute leukemia. *Cancer* 44:1189-1193.

Sacks, S., Wanklin, R., Reece, D., et al. 1989. Progressive esophagitis from acyclovir-resistant herpes simplex. Clinical roles for DNA polymerase mutants and viral heterogeneity? *Ann Intern Med* 111:893-899.

Safrin, S., Crumpacker, C., Chatis, P., et al. 1991. A controlled trial comparing foscarnet with vidarabine for acyclovir-resistant mucocutaneous herpes simplex in the acquired immunodeficiency syndrome. *N Engl J Med* 325:551-555.

Santos, G., Tutschka, P., Brookmeyer, R., et al. 1984. Marrow transplantation for acute nonlymphocytic leukemia after treatment with busulfan and cyclophosphamide. *N Engl J Med* 309:1347-1352.

Santos, G., Tutschka, P., Brookmeyer, R., et al. 1987. Cyclosporin plus methylprednisolone versus cyclophosphamide plus methylprednisolone as prophylaxis for graft-versus-host disease: a randomized double-blind study in patients undergoing allogeneic marrow transplantation. *Clin Transplant* 1:21-28.

Saral, R., Burns, W., Laskin, O., et al. 1983. Acyclovir prophylaxis of herpes-simplex-virus infections: a randomized, double-blind, controlled trial in bone marrow transplant recipients. *N Engl J Med* 305:63-67.

Schmidt, G., Horak, D., Niland, J., et al. 1991. A randomized, controlled trial of prophylactic ganciclovir for cytomegalovirus pulmonary infection in recipients of allogeneic bone marrow transplant patients. *N Engl J Med* 324:1005-1011.

Schmidt, G., Kovacs, A., Zaia, J., et al. 1988. Ganciclovir/immunoglobulin combination therapy for the treatment of human cytomegalovirus-associated interstitial pneumonia in bone marrow allograft recipients. *Transplantation* 46:905-907.

Schmitz, N., Dreger, P., Zander, A., et al. 1995. Results of a randomized, controlled, multicentre study of recombinant human granulocyte colony-stimulating factor (filgrastim) in patients with Hodgkin's disease and non-Hodgkin's lymphoma undergoing autologous bone marrow transplantation. *BMT* 15:261-266.

Schriber, J., Chao, N., Long, G., et al. 1994. Granulocyte colony stimulating factor after allogenic bone marrow transplantation. *Blood* 84:1680-1684.

Shaw, P., Scharping, C., Brian, R., et al. 1994. Busulfan pharmacokinetics using a single daily high-dose regimen in children with acute leukemia. *Blood* 84(7):2357-2362.

Shea, T., Flaherty, M., Elias, A., et al. 1989. A phase I clinical and pharmacokinetic study of carboplatin and autologous bone marrow support. *J Clin Oncol* 1(10):651-661.

Shepp, D., Dandliker, P., Flournoy, N., et al. 1985. Once-daily intravenous acyclovir for prophylaxis of herpes simplex virus reactivation after marrow transplantation. *J Antimicrob Chemother* 16:389-395.

Shepp, D., Dandliker, P., Meyers, J. 1986. Treatment of varicella-zoster virus infection in severely immunocompromised patients: a randomized comparison of acyclovir and vidarabine. *N Engl J Med* 314:208-212.

Shepp, D. Newton B., Dandliker P., et al. 1985. Oral acyclovir therapy for mucocutaneous herpes simplex virus infections in immunocompromised marrow transplant recipients. *Ann Intern Med* 102:783-785.

Somlo, G., Doroshow, J., Forman, S., et al. 1994. High-dose cisplatin, etoposide, and cyclophosphamide with autologous stem cell re-infusion in patients with responsive metastatic or high-risk primary breast cancer. *Cancer* 73:125-134.

Stahel, R., Jost, L., Cerny T., et al. 1994. Randomized study of recombinant human granulocyte colony-stimulating factor after high-dose chemotherapy and autologous bone marrow transplantation for high-risk lymphoid malignancies. *J Clin Oncol* 12:1931-1938.

Steegmann, J., Lopez, J., Otero, M., et al. 1992. Erythropoietin treatment in allogeneic BMT accelerates erythroid reconstitution: results of a prospective controlled randomized trial. *BMT* 10:541-546.

Steinherz, L., Steinherz, R., Mangiacasale, D., et al. 1981. Cardiac changes with cyclophosphamide. *Med Pediatr Oncol* 9:417-422.

Storb, R. 1994. Bone marrow transplantation for aplastic anemia. In Forman, S., Blume, K., Thomas, D. (Eds.) *Bone Marrow Transplantation.* Boston: Blackwell Scientific, 583-594.

Storb, R., Deeg, H., Farewell, V., et al. 1986. Marrow transplantation for severe aplastic anemia: methotrexate alone compared with a combination of methotrexate and cyclosporin for prevention of acute graft-versus-host disease. *Blood* 68:119-125.

Storb, R., Deeg, H., Whitehead, J., et al. 1986. Methotrexate and cyclosporin compared with cyclosporin alone for prophylaxis of acute graft-versus-host disease after marrow transplantation for leukemia. *N Engl J Med* 314:729-735.

Storb, R., Gluckman, E., Thomas, E., et al. 1974. Treatment of established human graft-versus-host disease by antithymocyte globulin. *Blood* 44:57-75.

Sullivan, K. 1994. Graft-versus-host disease. In Forman, S., Blume, K., Thomas, D. (Eds.) *Bone Marrow Transplantation.* Boston: Blackwell Scientific, 339-362.

Sullivan, K., Kopecky, K., Jocom, J., et al. 1990. Immunomodulatory and antimicrobial efficacy of intravenous immunoglobulin in bone marrow transplantation. *N Engl J Med* 323:7-13.

Sullivan, K., Witherspoon, R., Storb, R., et al. 1988. Alternating-day cyclosporin and prednisone for treatment of high-risk chronic graft-v-host disease. *Blood* 72(2):555-561.

Takvorian, T., Parker, L., Hochberg, F., et al. 1983. Autologous bone marrow transplantation: host effects of high-dose BCNU. *J Clin Oncol* 1:610-620.

Teicher, B., Holden, S., Eder, J., et al. 1989. Influence of schedule on alkylating agent cytotoxicity in vitro and in vivo. *Cancer Res* 49:6994-6998.

Tutschka, P., Beschorner, W., Hess, A., et al. 1983. Cyclosporin-A to prevent graft-versus-host disease: a pilot study in 22 patients receiving allogeneic marrow transplantation. *Blood* 61:318-325.

Ulich, T., Castillo, J., Yin, S., et al. 1995. Megakaryocyte growth and development factor ameliorates carboplatin-induced thrombocytopenia in mice. *Blood* 86:971-976.

Van Biesen, K., Demuyneb, H., Lemaistre, C., et al. 1995. High-dose melphalan allows durable engraftment of allogeneic bone marrow. *BMT* 15:321-323.

Vassal, G., Deroussent, A., Hartmann, O., et al. 1990. Dose-dependent neurotoxicity of high-dose busulfan in children: a clinical and pharmacological study. *Cancer Res* 50:6203-6207.

Villablanca, J., Steiner, M., Kersey, J., et al. 1990. The clinical spectrum of infections with viridans streptococci in bone marrow transplant patients. *BMT* 6:387-393.

Vose, J., Anderson, J., Bierman, P., et al. 1993. Initial tiral of PIXY321 (GM-CSF/IL-3 fusion protein) following high-dose chemotherapy and autologous bone marrow transplantation (ABMT) for lymphoid malignancy. *Proc Am Soc Clin Oncol* 12:1237a.

Wade, J., McLaren, C., Meyers, J., et al. 1983. Frequency and significance of acyclovir-resistant herpes simplex virus isolated from marrow transplant patients receiving multiple courses of treatment with acyclovir. *J Infect Dis* 148:1077-1082.

Wade, J., Newton, B., Flournoy, N., et al. 1984. Oral acyclovir for prevention of herpes simplex virus reactivation after marrow transplantation. *Ann Intern Med* 100:823-838.

Wade, J., Newton, B., McLaren, C., et al. 1982. Intravenous acyclovir to treat mucocutaneous herpes simplex virus infection after marrow transplantation. *Ann Intern Med* 96:265-269.

Weisdorf, D., Katsanis, E., Verfaille, C., et al. 1994. Interleukin-1 alpha administered after autologous transplantation: a phase I/II clinical trial. *Blood* 84:2044-2049.

Wheeler, C., Antin, J., Churchill, W., et al. 1990. Cyclophosphamide, carmustine, and etoposide with autologous bone marrow transplantation in refractory Hodgkin's disease and non-Hodgkin's lymphoma: a dose-finding study. *J Clin Oncol* 8:648-656.

Whitley, R., Gnann, J. 1992. Acyclovir: a decade later. *N Engl J Med* 327:782-789.

Wilson, W., Jain, V., Bryant, G., et al. 1992. Phase I and II study of high-dose ifosfamide, carboplatin, and etoposide with autologous bone marrow rescue in lymphomas and solid tumors. *J Clin Oncol* 10(11): 1712-1722.

Wingard, J., Merz, W., Rinaldi, M., et al. 1991. Increase in *Candida krusei* infection among patients with bone marrow transplantation and neutropenia treated prophylactically with fluconazole. *N Engl J Med* 325: 1274-1277.

Winston, D., Ho, W., Bartoni, K., et al. 1993. Ganciclovir prophylaxis of cytomegalovirus infection and disease in allogeneic bone marrow transplant recipients. *Ann Intern Med* 118:179-184.

Winston, D., Ho, W., Champlin, R., et al. 1987. Norfloxacin for prevention of bacterial infection in granulocytopenic patients. *Am J Med* 82(suppl B):40-46.

Wolff, S., Fer, M., McKay, C., et al. 1983. High-dose VP-16-213 and autologous bone marrow transplantation for refractory malignancies: a phase I study. *J Clin Oncol* 1(11):701-705.

Wolff, S., Herzig, R., Fay, J., et al. 1990. High-dose N,N',N"-triethylenethiophosphoramide (thiotepa) with autologous bone marrow transplantation: phase I studies. *Semin Oncol* 17(1, suppl 3):2-6.

Wordell, C. 1991. Use of intravenous immune globulin therapy: an overview. *DICP Ann Pharmacother* 25: 805-817.

Yeager, A., Wagner, J., Graham, M., et al. 1992. Optimization of busulfan dosage in children undergoing bone marrow transplantation: a pharmacokinetic study of dose escalation. *Blood* 80(9):2425-2428.

Yee, G., Self, S., McGuire, T., et al. 1988. Serum cyclosporin concentration and risk of acute graft-versus-host disease after allogeneic marrow transplantation. *N Engl J Med* 319:60-65.

Yee, G., Stanley, D. 1994. Investigational hematopoietic growth factors. *Highlights on Antineoplastic Drugs* 12: 32-43.

Zaia, J., 1994. Cytomegalovirus infection. In Forman, S., Blume, K., Thomas, D. (Eds.) *Bone Marrow Transplantation.* Boston: Blackwell Scientific, 376-403.

Zander, A., Culbert, S., Jagannath, S., et al. 1987. High dose cyclophosphamide, BCNU, and VP-16 (CBV) as a conditioning regimen for allogeneic bone marrow transplantation for patients with acute leukemia. *Cancer* 59:1083-1086.

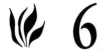

6

Radiation Therapy in Transplantation

Roberta Anne Strohl

Total body irradiation (TBI) is a complex treatment technique used in preparation for bone marrow transplantation. The delivery of high doses of radiation to the entire body requires considerable planning and meticulous technique. Acute and late toxicities occur in multiple organ systems. All of the nurses involved in the care of the individual receiving total body irradiation must understand the treatment technique and anticipated reactions in order to adequately prepare the extremely anxious patient for this rigorous therapy.

RATIONALE

When X rays are absorbed in biological material, a chain of events is initiated starting with the conversion of photon energy into a fast-moving electron and culminating with the breaking of chemical bonds and the production of biological effect. Radiation has DNA as its target of activity within the cell. The energy produced by ionizing radiation is sufficient to pull apart the weak covalent bonds that hold DNA together. The energy from X rays is not absorbed uniformly and results in localized effect in charged particles. In addition to direct effect on DNA, the ionization that occurs within cellular water produces powerful oxidizing agents and free radicals, which further damage DNA. The result is that cells lose their capacity for proliferation. Cellular death caused by radiation is mitotically linked. Cells function but die when division is attempted because the altered DNA cannot replicate. The rate at which cells die when exposed to radiation is linked to their mitotic rate. Cells that divide more rapidly are more quickly damaged by radiation. This is true for both tumor and normal cells (Withers, 1992).

In conventional radiation treatment the local field includes the tumor and surrounding lymph nodes. Cancer cells with their loss of proliferation control are damaged and eventually destroyed by radiation because they are unable to repair damage from radiation. Normal tissues within the field are also affected by the radiation but as long as the dose is within tolerable limits, repair and repopulation can occur (Withers, 1992).

In TBI for bone marrow transplantation the therapeutic goal is causing an immunosuppressive effect on hematopoietic tissue. Eradication of malignant cells and cell populations with genetic disorders may also be accomplished with TBI (Shank, 1994).

TREATMENT

Bone marrow transplantation requires a conditioning regimen to eliminate immune competent cells in order to facilitate engraftment. TBI may be included as a part of the preparatory regimen. Most recently, concerns about late effects of combined modality treatment has led to conditioning regimens of high-dose chemotherapy alone. Improved survival has increased concern about both acute and late complications. The advantages of TBI in conditioning are that there is no sparing of sanctuary sites such as the testes, dose homogeneity is independent of blood supply, no cross-resistance occurs with other agents, there are not issues with excretion of drugs, and dose distribution can be tailored by shielding and/or boosting (Shank, 1994).

TECHNIQUE

The conventional treatment setup of the patient lying on the table under the head of the ma-

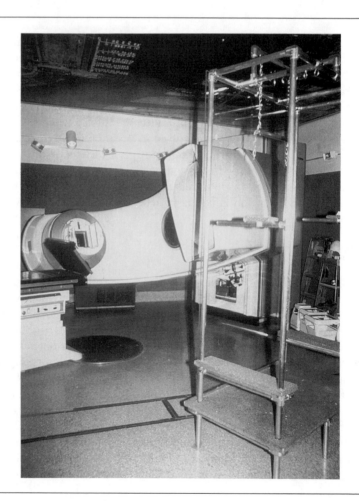

Figure 6.1
This treatment device for TBI allows positioning and distance from the source of radiation.

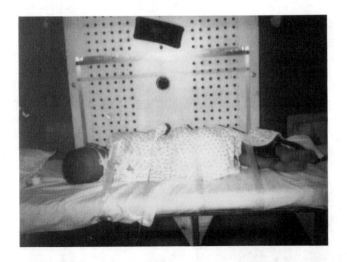

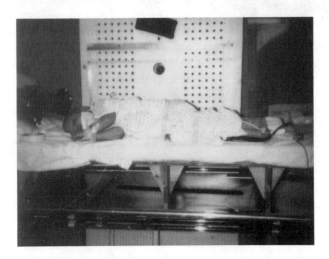

Figure 6.2
Patient in two different positions for TBI on stretcher

chine is not possible in TBI. In order to achieve a field large enough to encompass the entire body, the distance from the source of the radiation to the patient must be increased (Figure 6.1). Patients can be treated while they lie on a stretcher (Figure 6.2) or stand in a device made specifically for TBI therapy (Figure 6.3) (Lin and Drzymala, 1992).

The therapy is given in a fractionated fashion of either two or three treatments per day to a total dose of 1200 to 1500 cGy. Twice-daily treatment at 200 cGy per treatment is the most common fractionated regimen. TBI is very effective in leukemic cell kill while minimizing normal tissue effects. Fractions are given at least 4 to 6 hours apart for maximum normal

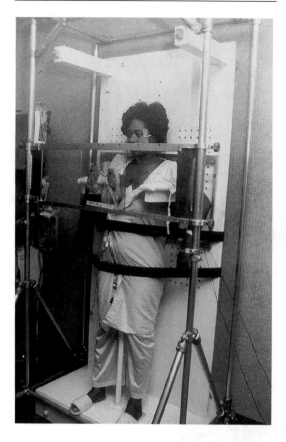

Figure 6.3   Patient in standing position for TBI

tissue repair between treatments (Shank, 1983; Kim, Gerbi, Lo, 1992).

If the patient is treated while he or she is in the standing position, custom-made blocks are designed to shield the lung to minimize interstitial pneumonitis (Figure 6.4). The rib area, which is under the lung block, can be boosted with superficial radiation in the form of electrons (Figure 6.5). When the patient is treated in the lying position the hands are crossed over the chest to shield the lungs (Dutreix et al., 1986; Cosset et al., 1989).

Measurements are taken in order to determine the physics plan for therapy. The computer-generated plan uses measurements of distance and patient thickness to calculate the dose distribution (Table 6.1).

During therapy solid-state diodes are placed on the patient during each treatment to verify the calculated dose. Dosimeters may also be placed on the eye in order to estimate the dose to the lens (Table 6.2). Testicular boosting may be added with superficial electrons in order to decrease testicular relapses. The entire treatment including setting up the field and checking films may take 45 minutes to 1 hour (Kim, Gerbi, Lo, 1992).

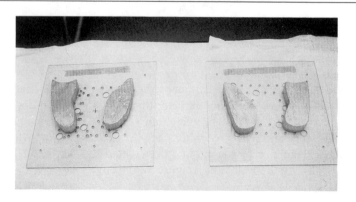

Figure 6.4   Lung blocks for TBI

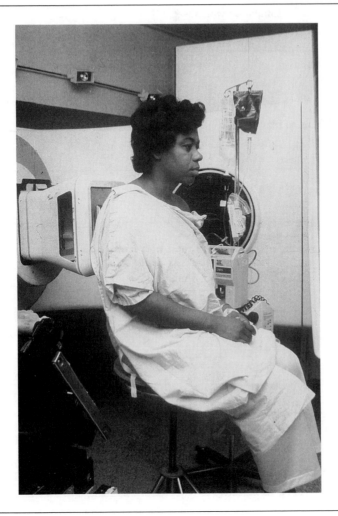

Figure 6.5
This woman is receiving
electron boost for her ribs.

ACUTE SIDE EFFECTS

As a general principle, it has been found that most acute side effects are higher with single doses of TBI than with fractionated regimens.

Nausea and Vomiting

Nausea and vomiting can actually occur while treatment is being delivered in the inadequately medicated patient. The highly proliferative gas-

tric mucosa exhibits an early reaction to radiation mediated by the large number of serotonin receptors located in the gut. The treatment technique needs to be known before determining the antiemetic regimen. If the patient is treated in the standing position, regimens that cause drowsiness may be contraindicated. Syncopal episodes have occurred when patients are treated standing. In this author's experience they have been more common when the patient is standing and facing into the treatment device

TABLE 6.1 Clinical physics: total body simulation worksheet

	Anterior field	*Posterior field*
Field size	_____	_____
Collimator angle	_____	_____
Gantry angle	_____	_____
TSD to umbilicus	_____	_____
Distance from anterior umbilicus to film board	_____	_____

Distance along long axis of patient		*Patient thickness*		
			AP/PA	*Lateral*
Top of head to neck	_____			
Neck to hip	_____	Forehead	_____	_____
Hip to feet	_____	Neck	_____	_____
Total length of patient	_____	Chest with arms	_____	_____
Forehead to neck	_____	Chest without arms	_____	_____
Neck to chest	_____	Umbilicus	_____	_____
Chest to umbillicus	_____	Hip	_____	_____
Umbilicus to hip	_____	Knee	_____	_____
Hip to knee	_____	Ankle	_____	_____
Knee to ankle	_____		_____	_____

TABLE 6.2 Dose delivery

DOSE DELIVERY: DECTOR-TYPE—MACHINE

Date	Site	*Ant. diode reading*	*Post. diode reading*	*Total reading*	*Percentage of dose*
____	Umbilicus	_____	_____	_____	_____
____	Midchest	_____	_____	_____	_____
____	Apex ____ lung	_____	_____	_____	_____
____	Lower lobe ____ lung	_____	_____	_____	_____
____	Center ____ lung	_____	_____	_____	_____
____	Cranium	_____	_____	_____	_____
____	Eye	_____	_____	_____	_____
____	Neck	_____	_____	_____	_____
____	Testes	_____	_____	_____	_____

for the posterior field. It seems that staring into the blank device provides little visual orientation and when combined with phenothiazines, anxiety, and anemia, syncope can occur. It must be the undivided responsibility of a single individual to monitor the standing patient for signs of syncope. Patients are instructed to call out or raise a hand if they feel faint.

Antiserotonin agents are effective in controlling emesis during TBI. Single dosing each morning prior to the first treatment with rescue medication ordered for breakthrough vomiting is beneficial. Patients who have had previous difficulties with nausea and vomiting during cancer treatment and those who are extremely anxious about therapy are particularly vulnerable. Antianxiety agents may be ordered with consideration of their timing relative to treatment for the standing regimens (Spitzer et al., 1994; Tiley et al., 1992).

Immunosuppression

Immunosuppression is obviously a therapeutic goal in TBI. Being able to achieve a higher total dose with fractionation results in fewer relapses. In animal studies engraftment is dependent on TBI dose. Higher doses are needed as the genetic disparity between donor and host increase (Deeg, 1983; Anasetti et al., 1989).

Diarrhea

Mild to moderate diarrhea may occur within the first 48 hours of therapy and usually subsides quickly upon completion of TBI. The contribution of chemotherapeutic agents to the diarrhea needs also to be considered. Antispasmodic and antidiarrheal agents are given to minimize diarrhea (Deeg, 1983).

Fever, Chills, Parotitis

Fever and chills occurring after treatment have been reported. They are usually self-limiting and most patients become afebrile after 24 hours. The fever may be related to the release of soluble mediators from leukemic and normal cells. During this period a swelling of the parotid glands may occur with resolution expected in 2 to 3 days. Persistent fever should not be dismissed as related to radiation (Deeg, 1983).

Skin Reactions

Mild erythema is noted in the first few days following TBI in patients who received high-dose cyclophosphamide prior to radiation. If busulfan was a part of the conditioning regimen moist erythema may develop over the elbows, heels, and finger tips. The conventional measures for skin care are recommended (Deeg, 1983).

Mucositis

Patients may complain of dry mouth during therapy and develop mucositis 5 to 7 days after treatment. Chemotherapeutic agents included in the conditioning regimen obviously contribute to oral discomfort. Oral care before and after meals is essential in the immunocompromised host to prevent serious sequelae (Deeg, 1983).

Alopecia

Reversible alopecia occurs about 2 weeks after TBI.

DELAYED EFFECTS

Interstitial Pneumonitis

Interstitial pneumonitis is an important side effect because it plays a prominent role in mortality after BMT. Pneumonitis occurs in 20% of BMT patients even when TBI is not given. Pneumonitis may be fatal in up to two thirds of patients who develop it. The median time from treatment cessation to diagnosis is about 2 months.

Preexisting lung disease, diagnosis of CML, total radiation dose and dose rate, chemotherapy, prior splenectomy, viruses (CMV, herpes simplex), fungi (aspergillus), *Pneumocystis carinii,* and graft compatibility and graft-versus-host disease are all factors that contribute to pneumonitis (Granena et al., 1993; Shank, 1983).

Rates of pneumonitis are higher with single-fraction TBI. Early decline in diffusion capacity is seen in those individuals who develop pneumonitis. At 3 years after TBI, Deeg (1983) reports an improvement of diffusion capacity and lung capacity over baseline.

Shank found that treatment of 120 cGy three times per day using partial lung blocks had an incidence of 33% pneumonitis compared with 70% for a single dose of 1000 cGy (Shank, 1994).

Cataracts

Cataracts are also common in patients receiving TBI in a single fraction. The incidence at 5 years is 80% with single-dose and 19% with fractionated TBI. It is reported that 18% of marrow transplant patients treated with chemotherapy alone as a preparatory regimen develop cataracts. The use of steroids increases the possibility of cataract formation. Cataracts are treated surgically (Shank, 1994).

Hepatic Disorders

Chronic hepatitis is increased in individuals with abnormal SGPT prior to transplant. The time course for development of increased liver enzymes is in the range of 20 to 40 days after transplant (Locasciulli et al., 1989).

Veno-occlusive disease is defined by hepatomegaly, weight gain, and jaundice. Elevated alanine aminotransferase (ALT) prior to trans-

plant is a significant risk factor (McDonald, 1993; Baglin, 1994).

Renal Dysfunction

Characteristics of renal changes after TBI include increased serum creatinine and decreased creatinine clearance, increased BUN, decreased glomerular filtration rate, anemia, hypertension, and peripheral edema. Pathologically one sees extreme subendothelial widening of the glomerular basement membranes, anterior intimal thickening, and atrophic tubules. Contributing factors include cytosine arabinoside and busulfan. Partial renal blocking using renal ultrasound to localize the kidneys may be employed to decrease renal toxicity (Lawton et al., 1994).

Neuroendocrine Function

Thyroid
Children who receive TBI as a part of the conditioning regimen have an increased incidence of decreased thyroid function. Single treatments result in a higher incidence of overt hypothyroidism (13%) than do treatments in those who receive fractionated TBI (3%) (Sanders, 1990).

Growth
Growth velocity is decreased in TBI regimens. Subnormal growth hormone levels are noted in 87% of children who receive cranial irradiation and TBI, and in 42% of children who receive TBI alone. Administration of growth hormone results in some improvement although the response is not as significant as in children who have deficiencies of growth hormone but have not received radiation (Sanders, 1990).

Dental Abnormalities
Children under 6 years who receive TBI exhibit arrested root development, premature apical

closure, enamel hypoplasia, and macrodontia. Children older than 7 have only arrested root development. Facial growth is arrested in vertical development of the lower third of the face (Sanders, 1994).

Puberty

Primary gonadal failure is evident in children who receive TBI, requiring supplements of the appropriate sex hormone to promote pubertal development (Sanders, 1990).

Fertility

Amenorrhea occurs in 100% of women receiving TBI. In one study, women younger than 26 years old who received chemotherapy alone recovered ovarian function at 3 to 42 months, median 6 months. Women older than 26 years developed primary ovarian failure. Recovery may occur after primary failure. In a TBI study, 372 of 380 patients had recovery at 3 to 7 years. Men receiving chemotherapy alone recover testicular function with normal gonadotropin and testosterone levels and spermatogenesis. Recovery is unrelated to age. Most patients receiving TBI have preservation of Leydig cell function with normal testosterone and serum leutenizing hormone. Spermatogenesis is absent and Sertoli cell function is abnormal. Recovery is rare (Sanders, 1994).

Central Nervous System

Structural and functional changes are noted following cranial irradiation and intrathecal medications. Cognitive changes are seen in children with leukemia. Younger children (under 8) show lower IQ scores, visual-motor deficits, and problems with abstract thinking. Andykowski and colleagues (1990) identified increasing cognitive dysfunction with increasing TBI dose. Kramer and colleagues (1992) did not identify significant IQ or adaptive behavior changes. Long-term follow-up is needed to further document this effect.

Second Malignancies

The major risk factors for second malignancies in patients receiving TBI are immunosuppression related to the radiation and graft-versus-host disease. In one report, 116 second cancers were identified in 9732 patients. Leukemias and lymphomas are most common. There have been few reports of malignancies in human marrow transplant patients though meticulous long-term follow-up is needed as survival from BMT increases (Shank, 1994).

The rationale for continuing to include TBI in BMT conditioning in spite of the significant acute and late toxicities is related to studies that demonstrate better treatment results. Conflicting reports exist and one could also cite studies that show little or no difference between busulfan or cyclophosphamide alone and inclusion of TBI. Inoue and colleagues (1993) found overall survival and relapse rates significantly better in regimens containing TBI.

PATIENT EDUCATION AND EMOTIONAL SUPPORT

Preparing patients for TBI requires ongoing educational and emotional support. Even individuals who have previously received radiation are anxious about receiving this extensive treatment. The thought of the entire body being exposed to what is, without transplantation, a lethal dose of radiation leads to a significant amount of appropriate anxiety. The knowledge that should transplant not be successful therapeutic options are limited also promotes fear. King and colleagues (1985) found that information that helped prepare patients for stressful events included sensory and temporal descriptions of what would happen. Patients' anxiety can be reduced by providing them an accurate understanding of the sights, sounds, smells, tactile dimensions, and tastes of the event as well as the sequence of activities.

Nurses involved in the care of the patient receiving TBI should familiarize themselves with the sensations and plan of the procedure in order to effectively teach patients and families. Side effects, both acute and late, are numerous. Acute effects should be emphasized before therapy, and presented with a plan for their management. Late effects are described in the informed consent process but also must be revisited after treatment and at each follow-up visit. Young children who survive transplantation will need ongoing assistance in coping with late effects because reactions to sequelae change as the children mature. How one feels about being infertile at the age of 9 years is quite different from confronting and mourning this loss at age 20.

SUMMARY

Total body irradiation is a complex treatment that results in multiorgan system sequelae. Caring for these patients and their families requires knowledge and understanding of the treatment plan and the physiologic effects of radiation. Ongoing support and guidance are essential to assist patients and families in coping with both acute and late reactions.

REFERENCES

Anasetti, C., Amos, D., Beatty, P., et al. 1989. Effect of HLA compatibility on engraftment of bone marrow transplantation in patients with leukemia or lymphoma. *N Engl J Med* 320(4):197-204.

Andrykowski, M.A., Altmaier, E.M., Barnett, R.T., et al. 1990. The quality of life in adult survivors of allogeneic bone marrow transplantation. *Transplantation* 50(3): 399-406.

Baglin, T.P., 1994. Veno-occlusive disease of the liver complicating bone marrow transplantation. *BMT* 13(1): 1-5.

Cosset, J.M., Baume, D., Pico, J.L., et al. 1989. Single dose versus hyperfractionated total body irradiation before allogeneic bone marrow transplantation: a nonrandomized comparative study of 54 patients at the Institute Gustave-Roussy. *Radiother Oncol* 15(2):151-160.

Deeg, H.J., 1983. Acute and delayed toxicities of total body irradiation. *Int J Radiat Oncol Biol Phys* 9(12): 1933-1939.

Dutreix, J., Janoray, P., Bridier, A., et al. 1986. Biologic and anatomic problems of lung shielding in whole body irradiation. *J Natl Canc Inst* 76(6):1333-1336.

Granena, A., Carreras, E., Rozman, C., et al. 1993. Interstitial pneumonitis after BMT: 15 years experience in a single institution. *BMT* 11(6):453-458.

Inoue, T., Ikeda, H., Yamazaki, H., et al. 1993. Role of total body irradiation as based on the comparison of preparation regiments for allogeneic bone marrow transplantation for acute leukemia in first complete remission. *Strahlentherapie und Onkologie* 169(4):250-255.

Kim, T., Gerbi, B., Lo, J. 1992. Total body irradiation for bone marrow transplantation. In Levitt, S. (Ed.) *Levitt and Tapley's Technological Basis of Radiation Therapy*, 2d ed. Philadelphia: Lea & Febiger, 382-397.

King, K., Nail, L., Kreamer, K., et al. 1985. Patients' descriptions of the experience of receiving radiation therapy. *Oncol Nurs Forum* 12(4):49-55.

Kramer, J., Crittenden, M., Halberg, F., 1992. A prospective study of cognitive functioning following low-dose cranial radiation for bone marrow transplantation. *Pediatrics* 90(37):447-450.

Latini, P., Aristei, C., Aversa, F., et al. 1991. Lung damage following bone marrow transplantation after hyperfractionated total body irradiation. *Radiother Oncol* 22(2):127-132.

Lawton, C.A., Fish, B., Malder, J., 1994. Effect of nephrotoxic drugs on the development of radiation nephrotoxicity after bone marrow transplantation. *Int J Radiat Oncol Bio Phys* 28(47):883-889.

Lin, H., Drzymala, R., 1992. Total-body and hemi-body irradiation. In Perez, C., Brady, L., (Eds) *Principles and Practice of Radiation Oncology*, 2d ed. Philadelphia: Lippincott, 256-265.

Locasciulli, A., Bacigalupo, A., Albert, A., 1989. Predictability before transplantation of hepatic complication following allogeneic bone marrow transplantation. *Transplantation* 48(1):68-72.

McDonald, G.B., Hinds M.S., Fisher, L.D., 1993. Veno-occlusive disease of the liver and multiorgan failure after bone marrow transplantation: a cohort study of 355 patients. *Ann Intern Med 118* (4):255-67.

Sanders, J.E., 1990. Late effects in children receiving total body irradiation for bone marrow transplantation. *Radiother Oncol* (suppl 1):82-87.

Sanders, J.E., 1994. Late effects in Forman, S., Blume, K., Thomas, E. (Eds). *Bone Marrow Transplantation.* Boston: Blackwell Scientific, 527-537.

Shank, B. 1983. Techniques of magna-field irradiation. *Int J Radiat Oncol Biol Phys* 9(12):1925-1933.

Shank, B., 1994. Total body irradiation for bone marrow transplantation. 36th Annual Meeting American Society for Therapeutic Radiation and Oncology, Reston, VA, Refresher Course.

Spitzer, T., Bryson, J., Cirenza, E., et al. 1994. Randomized double-blind, placebo-controlled evaluation of oral ondansetron in the prevention of nausea and vomiting associated with fractionated total-body irradiation. *J Clin Oncol* 12(11):2432-2438.

Tiley, C., Powles, R., Catalono, J., et al. 1992. Results of a double blind placebo controlled study of ondansetron as an antiemetic during total body irradiation in patients undergoing bone marrow transplantation. *Leuk Lymphoma* 7(4):317-321.

Withers, H., 1992. Biologic basis of radiation therapy. In Perez, C., Brady, L. (Eds.) *Principles and Practice of Radiation Oncology,* 2d. ed. Philadelphia: Lippincott, 64-97.

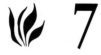

7

Genetics and Gene Therapy

Jean Jenkins

Advances in the realm of basic science as the result of biotechnological progress have facilitated the understanding of the role that genes play in human health and illness. As knowledge is gained about how genes function, greater opportunity exists to prevent, treat, or perhaps cure diseases caused by malfunctioning genes. Gene therapy has the potential to be successful in diseases with common single deficient genes such as sickle cell anemia and thalassemia. However, most of the current studies of gene therapy focus on more complex polygenic diseases (e.g., cancer) that arise from the interaction of two or more improperly functioning genes (Wivel, 1994). Although gene therapy is experimental, the impact of adding another treatment option has created excitement and hope for future health care. The role that nurses play in caring for patients receiving gene therapy is evolving. As research progresses, nurses must assess the impact of this new treatment modality. Planning the best way to educate and care for patients undergoing gene therapy is essential to the successful implementation and evaluation of this new treatment modality.

THE HUMAN GENOME INITIATIVE

Proteins create the body's structure and function (Miller, 1992). The body determines what proteins to make by the sequence of the genetic code—adenine (A), thymine (T), cytosine (C), guanine (G)—within a gene. This coding also regulates when cells are active by regulating gene expression telling them to turn on or off. Genes are composed of segments of deoxyribonucleic acid, or DNA. As scientists decode the ways DNA is organized within the gene, normal and abnormal genes can be identified. The abnormal genes then become the target for future gene therapy. There are several ways that genetic abnormalities can cause disease (Table 7.1). Heredity or environmental factors may effect the gene structure resulting in changes or mutations that affect gene function.

The Human Genome Project is a comprehensive, collaborative research effort to decode the human genome or all the genetic instructions in the human body (Collins and Galas, 1993). The advances in understanding the normal codes for the more than 100,000 human genes will provide a foundation for determination of sites for application of gene therapy. However, the success of the clinical application of such knowledge rests on the understanding of gene expression or how the gene's coded information results in structure and function and whether illness results from the gene alone or in combination with other factors.

162

TABLE 7.1 Genetic abnormalities

Abnormality	Result	Example of disease
Alterations in a critical gene code	Nonfunctional gene(s) where product is limited, not available, or abnormal	Sickle cell, ADA
Abnormal regulatory gene	Amount of gene product is more than needed for function	Thalassemia
Abnormal cell growth control genes	Rate of cell growth uncontrolled	Cancer
Abnormal signaling	Intracellular and extracellular communication pathway, defective response to external stimuli	Major histocompatibility II deficiency
Abnormal intercellular communication	Inaccurate cellular communication, defective response	Charcot-Marie-Tooth disease
Abnormal DNA repair	Hypersensitivity to external factors that damage DNA	Ataxiatelangiectasia

SOURCE: Data from Culver, K. 1994.

GENE THERAPY

Gene therapy, or gene transfer, is the actual delivery of normal genes into a patient to repair, replace, or compensate for defective genes (Lyon and Corner, 1995). There are four potential types of gene therapy: (1) somatic cell gene transfer, (2) enhancement gene transfer, (3) eugenics gene transfer, and (4) germline therapy (Table 7.2). Currently the only type of gene therapy approved for clinical trials is somatic cell gene transfer in which corrected genetic materials are placed in the body's cells (e.g., bone marrow cells or fibroblasts) for correction of the nonreproductive cells. These clinical trials are investigating gene therapy for the treatment of patients with incurable disease (Anderson, 1992).

Society will need to resolve whether there are valid reasons to utilize other types of gene transfer. Discoveries such as the obesity gene provide the opportunity to assess whether enhancement gene therapy or gene transfer to improve upon a desirable trait should be permitted. Eugenics gene therapy or the engineering of genes to favor certain characteristics elicits strong emotions and fear of revisiting historical mistakes and injustices (Penticuff, 1994). Germline therapy makes alterations to reproductive cells thereby passing on all genetic changes to future generations (Danks, 1994). Only somatic cell gene transfer is currently being used in clinical trials.

Application of gene therapy depends on delivery of the corrected genes to the malfunctioning sites in the body. A number of methods are being researched to assess the efficiency and effectiveness of gene augmentation or addition of normal copies of the gene to a cell with defective copies (Afione, Conrad, Flotte, 1995).

In Vitro Method

The in vitro method of gene transfer is the method most widely used for ongoing clinical trials. It involves removal of target cells from the

TABLE 7.2 Types of gene therapy

Somatic cell gene transfer	Insertion of a gene to correct a genetic defect in the somatic cells of the body (nonreproductive)
Enhancement gene transfer	Insertion of a gene(s) to enhance a known characteristic such as intelligence or abilities
Eugenics gene transfer	Attempt to improve upon human traits through gene transfer and improve upon desirable qualities in society
Germline therapy	Insertion of a gene into the reproductive tissue (sperm or egg) to correct a disorder in both patient and offspring

body to be altered genetically and then reinfused. The cells must be accessible, able to tolerate manipulation, and able to engraft and survive for a long time (Blaese and Culver, 1991). This method has been utilized with lymphocytes, peripheral CD34-positive blood cells, hepatocytes, skin fibroblasts, and bone marrow cells. The disadvantage of this method is that nondividing cells such as kidney, liver, or brain cells are not easily grown in vitro and it is difficult to reimplant them in sufficient numbers.

In Vivo Method

The in vivo gene transfer approach involves direct instillation of the altered gene into the patient. This approach offers the greatest opportunity for directly affecting disease sites, decreasing risks, and diminishing the expense of the procedure (Culver, 1994). Clinical trials using in vivo gene transfer include cystic fibrosis and melanoma (Crystal et al., 1994; Plautz et al., 1994).

Vectors

Both in vitro and in vivo approaches to gene transfer require a vector or a vehicle that transfers the corrected genes into the cells. There are many possible modes of action for the gene that is to be delivered into the body, and that desired action might also influence the type of vector selected (Jolly, 1994). A good delivery system or vector has several characteristics: (1) it can be easily produced in large quantities, (2) it can easily deliver the gene to the desired tissue and penetrate the target cells, (3) it induces cellular uptake of the DNA, (4) it has a long level of expression or ability to convert the DNA blueprint into its gene product, and (5) it must be safe (Holzman, 1995). The two categories of vector are viral and nonviral (Table 7.3).

Viral Vectors

Most gene transfer trials use a disabled mouse retrovirus to deliver the healthy genes. The viral genes required for replication are removed to prevent runaway infection. Retroviruses are efficient for putting corrected genes into rapidly dividing cells such as bone marrow cells. One potential disadvantage of retroviral vectors is that they integrate randomly into the host cell and might cause insertional mutagenesis (IM), initiating cancer, or causing other damage. This has not been observed clinically but does provide rationale for laboratory and animal safety testing programs prior to initiation of clinical studies (Gunter, Khan, Noguchi, 1993).

The adenovirus vector has an affinity for the respiratory tract since it commonly causes benign respiratory tract infections in humans. Trials have used this gene transfer method administered through nasal and bronchial passage

TABLE 7.3 Methods of gene transfer

Type	Examples	Safety issues
Viral	Retroviral vector	Insertion of gene in wrong place, insertional mutagenesis (IM) initiating cancer, potential for immune reaction
	Adenovirus	IM, inflammatory response resulting from immune reaction
	Adeno-associated viral vector	IM
	Herpes simplex vector	IM, virulence questionable
	Human immunodeficiency virus (HIV)	Not known, potential for virus/vector recombination
	Vaccinia vector	Dangerous in immunosuppressed with risk of infection
Nonviral		
Chemical calcium-phosphate transfection		Not yet known
Physical microinjection, electroporation, bombardment		Repeated administrations needed increasing chance of hypersensitivity
Fusion	Liposomes	Repeated administrations needed increasing chance of hypersensitivity
Receptor-mediated endocytosis	DNA-protein complexes or viral envelop/capsid-DNA complexes	Not yet known

SOURCE: Modified from Culver, K., 1994, and Jolly, D., 1994.

aerosolization for cystic fibrosis (Afione, Conrad, Flotte, 1995). An advantage of the adenovirus vector is that it works efficiently in dividing or nondividing cells. A disadvantage is that it has limited integration and expression in the cells and creates an immune reaction that results in inflammation at the site of gene transfer (Simon et al., 1993).

Adeno-associated virus type 2, a human parvovirus, has been developed as a vector to improve gene transfer to the lungs for cystic fibrosis. Additionally, this vector seems to work well in hematopoietic cells and is being tested in human immunodeficiency virus (HIV) infection and thalassemia.

Future prospects for viral vectors are being explored. Herpes simplex (HSV) vectors for central nervous system disease, *Vaccinia* vectors and HIV vectors to treat HIV, polio, hepatitis B, and other vectors are under development to try to improve the safety and efficacy of viral vectors for clinical applications.

Nonviral Vectors

Nonviral methods of gene transfer include chemical techniques, mechanical techniques, membrane fusion-mediated transfer, and direct DNA uptake or receptor-mediated DNA transfer (Morgan and Anderson, 1993). Examples of nonviral gene methods of transfer are listed in Table 7.3. One of the biggest advantages of this type of vectors is that they are less expensive to develop than viral vectors. Viral vectors must go through extensive and expensive FDA-approved quality-control safety testing to ensure clinical-grade vectors (Anderson, 1994c). A disadvantage of nonviral vectors is that repeated administrations may be necessary if continued gene expression is needed. Further development of nonviral vectors that target specific types of cells will facilitate the clinical application of gene transfer in expanded settings.

Candidate Diseases for Gene Therapy

It is probable that every disease is influenced by genetic makeup (Anderson, 1994a). Therefore, the potential for application of gene transfer as a therapy is immense. However, the rate of development of gene therapy applications depends on gene isolation, sequencing, and availability of feasible gene transfer methods. An understanding of what intervention is needed to correct the genetic defect will improve as technologic capability and clinical testing increases.

Candidate diseases for human gene therapy include classic genetic diseases as well as complex and acquired genetic diseases. The number of clinical protocols continues to increase with more than 100 in progress at the end of 1994 (Anderson, 1994b). Approved studies primarily focus on cancer, as well as genetic diseases, HIV, and others (Table 7.4). Concern expressed has been that the availability of a commercial market for treatments might be driving current clinical trial resources (Meyers, 1994). The expense of gene transfer studies is in obtaining clinical-grade quality vectors and implementing the clinical protocol itself (Anderson, 1994c). There is greater support from companies to evaluate gene products that might offer a profit, such as gene products that affect large populations, than for products for rare classical genetic diseases. These financial considerations might be affecting the availability of gene product and the types of clinical trials implemented, which in turn may be a limiting factor to complete evaluation of this treatment modality.

TABLE 7.4 Types and frequency of clinical protocols

Disease	Type	% Total trials
	Marker studies	25
	Clinical therapy trials	75
Cancer	Melanoma, renal cell, ovarian, neuroblastoma, brain, lung, breast, colon, mesothelioma, hematologic malignances	69
Genetic Diseases	Cystic fibrosis, Gaucher disease, ADA deficiency, familial hypercholesterolemia, alpha-1-antitrypsin deficiency, Fanconi's anemia, and Hunter syndrome	19
AIDS		8
Other Diseases	Rheumatoid arthritis, peripheral vascular disease	4

SOURCE: Abstracted from Anderson, W., 1994b and 1994d.

Clinical Trials in the Transplant Setting

The assessment of gene therapy techniques and treatment outcomes applies to genetic diseases and others treatable by bone marrow transplantation (Krauss, 1992). The first trials assessed the feasibility and outcome of genetically altered lymphocytes in cancer patients. Gene marking studies allow tracking of a labeled gene as a method to identify where the target cell goes. In these early studies, the marker gene allowed scientists to track the destination of tumor-infiltrating lymphocytes in the body (Rosenberg, 1992). Results indicated that these modified cells could survive for long periods of time, thus providing a method to assess how long these genetically modified cells exist once reinfused into the patient.

Another question that gene therapy methods have helped address is, What cell populations are present in harvested marrow? Initial investigation of techniques assessing genetically modified gene incorporation involved marking marrow and peripheral blood progenitor cells prior to autologous transplantation to track the reinfused cells (Brenner, 1995). Results indicate autologous marrow harvested from patients in apparent clinical remission may still have tumorigenic cells in the purged marrow which contribute to relapse (Brenner, 1993). Use of marker genes to determine the source of relapse are in progress. A second series of clinical studies are assessing the efficacy of different methods of marrow purging (Brenner et al., 1994).

Marker studies also indicated that gene transfer into hematopoietic progenitor and stem cells has some difficulties to be addressed to improve clinical application of gene therapy (Dunbar and Emmons, 1994). Low levels of incorporation of the corrected genes into the individual's cells occurred. This means that after treatment with gene therapy there were insufficient cells with the corrected gene in the patient. The desired result that the modified gene would correct the genetic defect was limited by the lack of expression or proper functioning of the corrected gene (Apperley, 1993). Techniques that assess and diminish difficulties that result from the difference between the use of genetically altered bone marrow cells and peripheral blood stem cells in engraftment, durability, and hematopoietic recovery may offer important biological answers about conditions that enhance gene transfer and expression in hematopoietic tissue (Bjorkstrand et al., 1994). Another source of stem cells, the umbilical cord blood, shows promise for both transplantation and gene therapy (Thompson, 1995).

Table 7.5 lists examples of gene transfer to modulate immunocyte function in the treatment of autoimmune conditions, infectious disease, and cancer (Brenner, 1995). The first clinical trial of gene therapy was in the immunodeficiency disorder adenosine deaminase deficiency (Culver, Anderson, Blaese, 1991). The alteration of T lymphocyte and macrophage functions are targets of gene therapy for HIV infection. Trials evaluating the use of gene transfer in the prophylaxis and treatment of graft-versus-host disease may soon be implemented.

Carcinogenesis appears to offer several distinct approaches to genetic applications for treatment. Two examples of immunotherapeutic approaches to increase specificity of treatment to tumor cells include targeting antigens expressed on tumor cells and targeting genes essential for tumor growth or survival (Hwu, 1995). A trial testing injection of plasmids carrying an HLA gene into a tumor mass hopes to induce an immune response to the cancer (Anderson, 1995).

Generating tumor vaccines from genetic modification of tumor cells isolated from bone marrow may enhance immune recognition of the neoplastic cells or make cells more effective in destroying tumors. Sixteen clinical trials of

TABLE 7.5 Bone marrow transplant protocols using gene transfer

Categories of protocol	Disease studied	Institution
GENE THERAPY		
Cancer (nonvaccine)	Advanced cancer	NIH, U. Michigan
	Brain tumors	NIH, Iowa Methodist, CHLA, Columbia U., St. Jude, U. Pennsylvania
	Mesothelioma	U. Pennsylvania
	NHL, NSCLC	M.D. Anderson
	Ovarian	M.D. Anderson
	Breast	Columbia U., NIH, M.D. Anderson, Vanderbilt U.
	Leptomeningeal carcinomatosis	NIH
	Colorectal	Mayo Clinic, U. Alabama
	Melanoma	Arizona Cancer Ctr
Cancer (vaccine)	with tumor necrosis factor	NIH
	with IL-2	NIH
	with IL-4	U. Pittsburgh
	Ovarian	U. Rochester
	Neuroblastoma	St. Jude, UCLA
	Melanoma, renal	MSKCC, U. Illinois, UCLA, U. Michigan
	Renal	Johns Hopkins
	Melanoma	Duke U., NIH
	Glioblastoma	Case Western Reserve, SDRCC
	Breast, H/N, T cell	U. Pittsburgh
	SCLC	U. Miami
	Prostate	Johns Hopkins
	Breast	Duke U.
	Cancer	SDRCC
HIV		U. Washington Shared Med. Res. Foundation, U. Michigan, USC, U. Cal. at San Diego, NIH
Inherited Genetic Disorder	Severe combined immune deficiency	NIH
	Hypercholesterolemia	U. Pennsylvania
	Alpha-1 antitrypsin deficiency	Vanderbilt U.
	Cystic fibrosis	Rockefeller U., U. Pennsylvania, U. Michigan, HHMI, Childrens Hosp. Ohio, U. North Carolina, U. Alabama, U. Washington, Johns Hopkins, New England Medical Center
	Fanconi's anemia	NIH
	Gaucher disease	U. Pittsburgh, NIH, FHCRC
	Hunter syndrome	U. Minnesota
Other	Rheumatoid arthritis	U. Pittsburgh
	Peripheral artery disease	New England Medical Center

Table 7.5 *Continued*

Categories of protocol	Disease studied	Institution
GENE MARKING		
Bone Marrow Cells	AML, neuroblastoma, CML, ALL	St. Jude, M.D. Anderson, Indiana U.
Bone Marrow/PB	CML	M.D. Anderson
	Multiple myeloma	NIH
	Breast, CML, HIV	NIH
	Solid tumors	FHCRC
	CLL, NHL	M.D. Anderson
BMSC	Pediatric malignancies	St. Jude
CTL	Leukemia	St. Jude
Hepatocytes	Acute hepatic failure	Baylor
PBSC	Lymphoid malignancies	FHCRC
TIL	Advanced cancer	NIH
	Melanoma	U. Pittsburgh
	Renal cell	UCLA
	Ovarian	M.D. Anderson

KEY: ALL = acute lymphocytic leukemia, AML = acute myelogenous leukemia, BMSC = bone marrow stem cells, CHLA = Children's Hospital Los Angeles, CLL = chronic lymphocytic leukemia, CTL = cytotoxic T lymphocytes, CML = chronic myelogenous leukemia, HHMI = Howard Hughes Medical Institute, HIV = human immunodeficiency virus, MSKCC = Memorial Sloan-Kettering Cancer Center, NHL = non-Hodgkin's lymphoma, NIH = National Institutes of Health, NSCLC = non-small cell lung cancer, PB = peripheral blood cells, PBSC = peripheral blood stem cells, SCLC = small cell lung cancer, SDRCC = San Diego Regional Cancer Center, TIL = tumor infiltrating lymphocytes, U = university, UCLA = University of California at Los Angeles, USC = University of Southern California.

this approach have been proposed (see Table 7.5). Data to date indicates stable disease response in several patients with melanoma and renal cell cancers. Side effects noted have ranged from none to induration at vaccine site, erythema, pruritus, pain, fatigue, fever, nausea, vomiting, and abdominal pain.

Another focus of gene therapy in cancer is the use of drug-resistant genes to enable the bone marrow to tolerate aggressive chemotherapy (Banerjee et al., 1994). The multidrug resistance gene (MDR) found in many cancer cells decreases toxicity from high-dose chemotherapy by actively pumping these drugs out of the cell (Zhang and Fang, 1995). Although multidrug resistance is a major obstacle in treating cancer with chemotherapy, chemoprotection of drug-sensitive cells may be desired. Trials in progress are evaluating whether the insertion of MDR genes into bone marrow progenitor cells can provide significant protective tissue effects to permit administration of higher dosages of chemotherapy needed to eradicate the cancer.

The application of gene therapy to hematologic disorders has been the focus of years of laboratory work. Gene transfer may be possible for diseases such as thalassemia and sickle cell anemia as more is learned about regulatory complexities within the gene (Krauss, 1992). The full potential of clinical application of gene therapy for hematologic disorders will be realized when there is greater ability to generate vectors that are targeted, efficient, and safe, and systemic regulation of genes is better understood.

SAFETY AND ETHICS

Scientific Safeguards

Gene therapy is a rapidly developing clinical field. This progress has been decades in the making with laboratory and animal safety and feasibility testing (Ostrove, 1994). All experimentation in humans must proceed with great caution. Experiments that manipulate, modify, or characterize the building blocks of our humanness require even greater oversight, at least initially, to assure appropriate techniques for clinical application (Anderson, 1994a, d). The Recombinant DNA Advisory Committee (RAC) was created in 1976 to promote public discussion and safety with regard to any experimentation with recombinant DNA (Post, 1994). Guided by the "Points to Consider" document, all federally funded gene therapy researchers must address this body which consists of diverse members representing the interests of patients and society (Culver, 1994). Approval for gene therapy studies must also include evaluation by an institutional review board and the U.S. Food and Drug Administration (FDA) (Kessler et al., 1993). As with any clinical trial, the risk versus the benefit of the study must be assessed prior to approval.

Staff Safety

New technology must also be assessed for risks to health-care providers who develop or administer gene therapy to patients. Although every aspect of quality control in vector development has been assured, there are no data on risks of repeated exposure of staff to genetically altered products. Just as with chemotherapy, many unknown risks are associated with handling these agents. Gene products have not yet been evaluated for effects on laboratory or health-care personnel. Theoretically, the risk of exposure to the corrected DNA product might cause a hypersensitivity to the retroviral vector, resulting in inflammation at the exposure site. This would only happen if accidental exposure to large amounts of vector occurred. It is important to make sure that guidelines, standards, and procedures for gene therapy consider risks to assure safe handling of these products.

Patients' Safety

Adequacy of resources to create a safe environment for clinical trial implementation is necessary. This includes both laboratory and clinical support staff who are knowledgeable about the physical, ethical, and social implications of this treatment modality (McGarrity, 1992). Training of staff must be ongoing to maintain competency in addressing patients' and families' questions and concerns. At present, minimal adverse physical effects of gene therapy have been reported (ORDA, 1994). Extensive and long-term monitoring for physical effects, as well as to evaluate the adequacy of health-care resources to promote patient safety, will be needed.

Ethical concerns include acquisition, development, and utilization of genetic information so that patients' rights are protected. The anxiety, potential stigmatization, or discrimination resulting from diagnosis of a genetic condition may increase the psychological burden of the patient and family considering gene therapy. The patient's choice to undergo gene therapy must be determined after receiving sufficient information about the treatment and other available options.

Societal implications of gene therapy include consideration of the costs of developing and providing access to genetic therapies; impact on future generations; unavailability of knowledgeable resources to provide counseling and manage genetics health care; and need for development of legal and health policy that balances the technology capabilities with the values of society.

Public Acceptance

It is essential that society understand the physical, philosophical, and theoretical possibilities of gene therapy. Greater education and opportunity for multidisciplinary forums enhances decision making and public approval (Gustafson, 1994). Results of two public surveys (March of Dimes Birth Defects Foundation, 1992; Macer, 1992) indicate that the public is aware of benefits such as improvement or cure of disease as well as the risks of side effects from gene therapy. Although the techniques for administration of gene therapy are difficult to understand, the public opinion of this modality to benefit humanity is favorable. Whether this acceptance and approval of genetic engineering will extend from treatment of disease into germline therapy, which involves manipulation of reproductive cells within the body that affect future offspring requires ongoing evaluation (Hamilton, 1994).

Moral Considerations

Genetic knowledge unleashes many exciting possibilities, but also many dilemmas (Andrews et al., 1994). Potential dilemmas include risk of knowing too much or too little as a result of genetic testing; being able to predict illnesses but not having effective treatments; and having the ability to make reproductive decisions based on genetic information. Critical values, cultural influences, and ethical philosophies provide a backdrop to ongoing conflict, con-frontation, and decisions that influence the health-care options of the future (Engelking, 1995). The potential for use and abuse of genetic knowledge requires that nurses be active members in personal and professional activities that examine and set policies to direct the conduct of developing genetic science. The exact manner in which gene therapy will evolve to benefit humankind can be influenced by nurses.

IMPLICATIONS FOR NURSING

Education

The nursing profession must be proactive in planning curriculum changes in both undergraduate and graduate programs. They must begin by preparing faculty to incorporate genetic and molecular biology terminology, scientific concepts, and implications for patient care. Consideration of additional required courses in genetics or molecular biology is crucial for preparation of nurses who will be implementing genetics health care (George, 1992). Continuing educational programs to give updates of the progress in the Human Genome Project and results of gene transfer clinical trials will be needed for nurses to meet patients' expectations. The media has created a method for society to be aware of this progress, creating a challenge for health-care professionals to do the same.

Specific educational preparation of nurses to care for patients undergoing gene therapy must include information about the disease, where the genetic defect is, and how gene therapy will correct the problems resulting from the malfunctioning gene. Background understanding of the laboratory and preclinical work facilitate an understanding of effects that might be expected and indicate important systems to monitor. No effects have been noted in the BMT population who received gene therapy that differ from those that have been noted in patients who have BMT alone. Understanding the rationale, techniques, and potential effects of gene therapy will give nurses a foundation from which to begin educating patients and families.

Educational materials for patients and families must be designed to provide information about genetics, genetic testing, and gene therapy. Much work has been accomplished in the prenatal and early childhood settings that offer examples of such educational materials (Forsman, 1994). Videos and computers could complement written material to provide several methods to reinforce this complex information.

Clinical

Nurses provide direct care to patients experiencing the confusion, concern, and excitement that accompany new clinical trials. Nurses often administer or assist with the delivery of the experimental treatments and provide support, education, and evaluation of effects. Most gene-altered cells are administered intravenously like BMT infusions, although other routes are under investigation (Wheeler, 1995). The actual treatment is often simpler than the usual BMT therapies because less preconditioning may be required and the accompanying chemotherapy and radiation may be less aggressive. Careful assessment and documentation of treatment administration and effects are essential to the ongoing progress and safety of clinical protocols. Signs and symptoms to watch for in terms of acceptance or rejection of the gene transfer treatment are the same as those to monitor with BMT. Effective follow-up for patients who receive gene therapy to determine long-term clinical implications is important (Ledley, 1995). Many times patients are treated in an investigational treatment facility and then need referral and follow-up care at a local site. Collaboration, coordination, and communica-

tion among health-care professionals are critical to successful outcomes of the treatment and follow-up. Prospective registration and tracking of patients are desirable to obtain adequate patient numbers to determine long-term consequences of gene transfer.

Research

Nurses are in an ideal situation to observe and monitor the effectiveness of nursing interventions in gene therapy. Substantial toxicity or complications can prevent wide application of new treatments. Nursing research on how best to address issues of concern (e.g., education, nursing care, administration of treatment) should be considered for any new treatment modality. Nursing research that complements research from biomedical trials can offer an opportunity for a team approach to effectively anticipate and meet patients' needs.

Other

Gene therapy is an evolving treatment that will offer many challenges to health-care professionals. The potential is there to revolutionize the way health is defined. The role of nurses in health-care delivery can be modeled to incorporate genetic health care as advances in diagnosing, preventing, and treating illness emerge (Scanlon and Fibison, 1995).

FUTURE DIRECTIONS

Realistic expectations are necessary when discussing the future of gene transfer as a routine medical treatment that is offered at the bedside (Verma, 1994). The goal of gene therapy is to offer patients therapeutic options that are superior in efficacy, safety, quality, and cost (Ledley, 1995). This requires even greater collaboration of biotechnology companies and scientists/physicians to develop technology that assures quality control at an affordable price. Realistic expectations of this investigational treatment modality is important. Development and testing of new drugs often spans 8 to 10 years. Gene therapy options may evolve more quickly as technological capabilities and discoveries permit. Nurses can seize the opportunity to develop models of care that keep pace with this discovery of knowledge and can create an environment for the safe, ethical application of genetic knowledge.

REFERENCES

Afione, S., Conrad, C., Flotte, T. 1995. Gene therapy vectors as drug delivery systems. *Clin Pharmacokinetics* 28(3):181-189.

Anderson, W.F. 1992. Human gene therapy. *Science 8:* 808-813.

Anderson, W.F. 1994a. Genetic engineering and our humanness. *Human Gene Therapy* 5:755-760.

Anderson, W.F. 1994b. End-of-the-year potpourri—1994. *Human Gene Therapy* 5:1431-1432.

Anderson, W.F. 1994c. Yes, Abbey, you are right. *Human Gene Therapy* 5:1199-1200.

Anderson, W.F. 1994d. Human gene marker/therapy clinical protocols. *Human Gene Therapy* 5:1537-1551.

Anderson, W.F. 1995. Gene therapy for cancer. *Human Gene Therapy* 5:1-2.

Andrews, L., Fullarton, J., Holtzman, N., Motulsky, A. (Eds.) 1994. *Assessing Genetic Risks: Implications for Health and Social Policy.* Washington, DC: National Academy Press.

Apperley, J. 1993. Bone marrow transplant for the haemoglobinopathies: past, present and future. *Bailliere's Clin Haematol* 6:299-325.

Banerjee, D., Zhao, S., Li, M., et al. 1994. Gene therapy utilizing drug resistance genes: a review. *Stem Cells 12:* 378-385.

Bjorkstrand, B., Gahrton, G., Dilber, M., et al. 1994. Retroviral-mediated gene transfer of CD34-enriched bone marrow and peripheral blood cells during autologous stem cell transplantation for multiple myeloma. *Human Gene Therapy* 5:1279-1286.

Blaese, R.M., Culver, K. 1991. Progress toward the application of gene therapy. In Nance, S. (Ed.) *Clinical and Basic Science Aspects of Immunohematology.* Rosland, VA: American Association of Blood Banks, 1-11.

Brenner, M. 1993. Gene marking to trace origin of relapse after autologous bone marrow transplantation. *Lancet* 341:85-86.

Brenner, M. 1995. Human somatic gene therapy: progress and problems. *J Intern Med* 237:229-239.

Brenner, M., Krance, R., Heslop, H., et al. 1994. Assessment of the efficacy of purging by using gene marked autologous marrow transplantation for children with AML in first complete remission. *Human Gene Therapy* 5:481-499.

Collins, F., Galas, D. 1993. A new five-year plan for the U.S. Human Genome Project. *Science* 262(5130):43-46.

Crystal, R., McElvaney, N., Rosenfeld, M., et al. 1994. Administration of an adenovirus containing the human CFTR cDNA to the respiratory tract of individuals with cystic fibrosis. *Nature Genetics* 8:42-51.

Culver, K. 1994. *Gene Therapy: A Handbook for Physicians.* New York: Mary Ann Liebert.

Culver, K., Anderson, W, and Blaese, R. 1991. *Human Gene Therapy* 2:107-109.

Danks, D. 1994. Germline gene therapy: no place in treatment of genetic disease. *Human Gene Therapy* 5: 151-152.

Deeg, H. 1994. Prophylaxis and treatment of acute graft-versus-host disease: current state, implications of new immunopharmacologic compounds and future strategies to prevent and treat GVHD in high risk patients. *BMT* 14:S56-S60.

Dunbar, C., Emmons, R. 1994. Gene transfer into hematopoietic progenitor and stem cells: progress and problems. *Stem Cells* 12:563-576.

Engelking, C. 1995. Genetics in cancer care: confronting a pandora's box of dilemmas. *Oncol Nurs Forum* 22: 27-34.

Forsman, I. 1994. Evolution of the nursing role in genetics. *J Obstet Gynecol Neonatal Nurs* 23:481-486.

George, J. 1992. Challenges for nursing education. *J Pediatr Nurs* 7(1):5-8.

Gunter, K., Khan, A., Noguchi, P. 1993. The safety of retroviral vectors. *Human Gene Therapy* 4:643-645.

Gustafson, J. 1994. A Christian perspective on genetic engineering. *Human Gene Therapy* 5:747-754.

Hamilton, M. 1994. Genetics and heavenly intervention. *Human Gene Therapy* 1:1433-1435.

Holzman, D. 1995. Gene therapy depends on finding the right vector. *J Natl Canc Inst* 87(6):406-410.

Hwu, P. 1995. The gene therapy of cancer. *PPO Update* 9:1-13.

Jolly, D. 1994. Viral vector systems for gene therapy. *Cancer Gene Therapy* 1(1):51-64.

Kessler, D., Siegel, J., Noguchi, P. 1993. Regulation of somatic-cell therapy and gene therapy by the Food and Drug Administration. *N Engl J Med* 329:1169-1173.

Krauss, J. 1992. Hematopoietic stem cell gene replacement therapy. *Biochemica et Biophysica Acta 1114*: 193-207.

Ledley, F. 1995. After gene therapy: issues in long-term clinical follow-up and care. *Adv Genetics* 32:1-16.

Lyon, J., Corner, P. 1995. *Altered Fates.* New York: Norton.

Macer, D. 1992. Public acceptance of human gene therapy and perceptions of human genetic manipulations. *Human Gene Therapy* 3:511-518.

March of Dimes Birth Defects Foundation. 1992. *Genetic Testing and Gene Therapy: National Survey Finding.* White Plains, NY.

Miller, J. 1992. The ABCs of DNA. *Threads of Life, UCSF Magazine* Sept:4-11.

Morgan, R., Anderson, W. 1993. Human gene therapy. *Ann Rev Biochem* 62:191-217.

Meyers, A. 1994. Gene therapy and genetic diseases: revisiting the promise. *Human Gene Therapy* 5:1201-1202.

McGarrity, G. 1992. Resource needs for institutional programs in human gene therapy. *Human Gene Therapy* 3:279-284.

ORDA. 1994. Recombinant DNA Advisory Committee Data Management Report. *Human Gene Therapy* 6: 535-546.

Ostrove, J. 1994. Safety testing programs for gene therapy viral vectors. *Cancer Gene Therapy* 1:125-131.

Penticuff, J. 1994. Ethical issues in genetic therapy. *J Obstet Gynecol Neonatal Nurs* 23(6):498-501.

Plautz, G., Nabel, E., Fox, B., et al. 1994. Direct gene transfer for the understanding and treatment of human disease. *Ann NY Acad Sci USA* 716:144-153.

Post, L. 1994. RAC's review of gene therapy: it's time to move on. *Human Gene Therapy* 5:1311-1312.

Rosenberg, S. 1992. Gene therapy for cancer. *JAMA* 268:2417-2419.

Scanlon, C., Fibison, W. 1995. *Managing Genetic Information: Implications for Nursing Practice.* Washington, DC: ANA.

Simon, R., Engelhardt, J., Yang, Y., et al. 1993. Adenovirus-mediated transfer of the CFTR gene to lung of nonhuman primates: toxicity study. *Human Gene Therapy* 4:771-780.

Thompson, C. 1995. Umbilical cords: turning garbage into clinical gold. *Science* 268:805-806.

Verma, I. 1994. Gene therapy: hopes, hypes, and hurdles. *Molecular Medicine* 1(1):2-3.

Wheeler, V. 1995. Gene therapy: current strategies and future applications. *Oncol Nurs Forum* 22(2):20-26.

Wivel, N. 1994. Gene therapy molecular medicine of the 1990s. *Int J Tech Assess Health Care* 10(4):655-663.

Zhang, W., Fang, X. 1995. Gene therapy strategies for cancer. *Expert Opinion on Investigational Drugs* 4: 487-514.

PART II
Acute Effects

8

Graft-versus-Host Disease

Kathryn Ann Caudell

Graft-versus-host disease (GVHD) is a significant complication of allogeneic bone marrow and peripheral blood cell transplantation. Despite advances in immunosuppressive drug therapy, GVHD continues to be a major contributor to transplant-related deaths. GVHD occurs when immunocompetent cells are transplanted from a donor to a recipient who expresses tissue antigens not present in the donor and who cannot mount a response that is effective in destroying the transplanted cells (Billingham, 1966; Deeg, 1994). The probability of GVHD tends to increase with the degree of mismatch between the donor and the recipient. This type of response can also occur after transplants of organs that contain lymphoid tissue or stem cells, unirradiated blood-product transfusions in immunoincompetent individuals, and unirradiated blood-product transfusions in immunocompetent individuals whose donors are homozygous for one of the recipient's HLA haplotypes (Anderson and Weinstein, 1990; Grishaber, Birney, Strauss, 1993)

Graft-versus-host disease primarily affects the liver, skin, gastrointestinal tract, and immune system. However, there is ample documentation that mucous membranes including the mouth and conjunctivae, airways, and bone marrow can also be involved (Deeg, 1994). Interventions to reduce the risk of developing GVHD include (1) limiting marrow

transplantation donors to those who have an HLA genotypical identical sibling (Beatty et al., 1985), (2) infusing T-cell–depleted bone marrow (Mitsuyasu et al., 1986; Hale and Waldmann, 1994; Antin et al., 1991), (3), and administering immunosuppressive agents prophylactically (Weaver et al., 1994). Current prophylaxis for GVHD centers around in vivo posttransplant immunosuppression, the most widely used protocol consisting of methotrexate (MTX) and cyclosporin-A (CsA). Unfortunately, this combination prophylaxis protocol and administering T cell-depleted bone marrow are both associated with a higher risk of relapse (Weaver et al., 1994; Ringden et al., 1993; Aschan et al., 1994).

INCIDENCE

The incidence of GVHD varies widely depending on the type of transplant and on the degree of HLA mismatch between the donor and the recipient. GVHD generally does not occur in syngeneic transplants, those in which the donor and recipient are identical twins, because the siblings are completely matched for all of the histocompatibility complex and for all genetic loci. Nor is it likely to occur in autologous transplants, those in which the patient serves as his or her own source of marrow. Hood and colleagues (1987), however, summarized several reports of GVHD-like phenomena (primarily skin rashes, vesicles, and bullae) in both autologous and syngeneic transplants, and reported nine additional cases from their institution. Although the histologic and clinical evidence supporting the occurrence of GVHD in these groups is compelling, the authors also concluded that a drug-related etiology could not be entirely ruled out (Hood et al., 1987).

Evidence exists that CsA administered for GVHD prophylaxis can induce a T-lymphocyte–dependent autoaggression syndrome disorder (SGVHD) following syngeneic and/or autologous bone marrow transplantation (Fischer et al., 1995). This syndrome has been observed to occur 14 to 28 days after CsA therapy is discontinued and is basically identical to GVHD in terms of the histopathologic lesions and organs affected. CsA alters differentiation of T cells and inhibits clonal deletion in the thymus (Gao et al., 1989; Jenkins et al., 1988). Although the grade of SGVHD may be II or III, this disorder is not life-threatening and usually resolves quickly upon administration of glucocorticoids (Ferrara and Deeg 1991).

In allogeneic HLA genotypically identical sibling transplants, the occurrence of grades II to IV acute GVHD has ranged from 40% to 59% (Weaver et al., 1994; Aschan et al., 1994).

Despite immunosuppressive therapy with CsA either alone or in combination with MTX, several studies have shown that acute GVHD (including grades II to IV defined in Table 8.1) still develops in 20% to 45% of HLA-matched bone marrow transplant patients (Weisdorf et al., 1990) although combination immunosuppressive therapy has resulted in a reduced incidence of and mortality from acute GVHD (Ringden et al., 1993; Storb et al., 1986). Earlier clinical trials from several European institutions revealed a decreased incidence and improved patient survival when CsA was administered prophylactically (Powles et al., 1980; Haus et al., 1981; Barrett et al., 1982; Gratwohl et al., 1983).

Incidence of GVHD in allogeneic transplants mismatched for 2 or 3 HLA antigens reaches 80% and the risk of graft failure is 20% (Przepiorka et al., 1994). T-cell–depleted marrow transfusions or increased immunosuppressive therapy have not produced beneficial responses in these patients (Ash et al., 1991; Anasetti et al., 1991). Several research groups are examining the effects of IL-2 on the incidence of GVHD in both human (Przepiorka et al., 1994) and murine populations (Szebeni et al., 1994; Fowler et al., 1994). Data from these study groups reveal that IL-2 administration limits GVHD to mild to moderate severity in

TABLE 8.1   Clinical stages of acute graft-versus-host disease

Stage	Skin	Liver	Gut
I	Maculopapular rash < 24% body surface	Bilirubin 2–3 mg/dl	Diarrhea 500–1000 ml/day
II	Maculopapular rash 25–50% body surface	Bilirubin 3–6 mg/dl	Diarrhea 1000–1500 ml/day
III	Generalized erythroderma	Bilirubin 6–15 mg/dl	Diarrhea > 1500 ml/day
IV	Desquamation and bullae	Bilirubin > 15 mg/dl	Pain or pileus

SOURCE: H.J. Deeg, et al. 1984. Graft-versus-host disease: pathophysiological and clinical aspects. *Annual Review of Medicine* 35:11-24. Reproduced with permission.

2-antigen mismatched marrow recipients, reduces the histopathologic tissue damage, and prolongs survival.

Several risk factors have been identified that may predispose the patient to GVHD. These include a donor-recipient sex mismatch (an increased incidence is noted with female donors to male recipients), increased age of the patient, the cumulative number of blood transfusions (Weisdorf et al., 1990), the number of T cells transfused, the prophylaxis protocol (Ferrara and Deeg, 1991), and the intensity of the conditioning regimen (Deeg, 1994).

Blood cell transplantation (BCT) is a promising new procedure to treat selected leukemias and several types of solid tumors. Most of these transplants are autologous; however, a few allogeneic BCTs have been performed. Due to a larger ratio of donor T cells present in peripheral blood cell transfusions, it is speculated that GVHD may be a more severe problem in this patient population than in allogeneic bone marrow transplants (Buchsel and Kapustay, 1995). Because of the small number of allogeneic BCTs performed thus far, it is difficult to predict the incidence of and degree of severity of GVHD in this population.

Chronic GVHD occurs more than 100 days after BMT and may be an extension of acute GVHD, may occur after a disease-free period following a GVHD episode, or may occur with no history of the disease (Ferrara and Deeg, 1991). Its incidence ranges from 25% to 60% and the risk increases with increasing patient and donor ages, previous acute GVHD, infusion of nonirradiated donor buffy coat cells or marrow, previous CMV infection, and positive donor CMV serology (Ferrara and Deeg, 1991; Quiquandon et al., 1994).

It is unclear why GVHD develops in some patients and not in others despite prophylactic therapy with immunosuppressive agents. Subtherapeutic serum concentrations of the immunosuppressive drugs may be one reason. Serum concentration variability among patients receiving the same drug dose is another possible explanation (Yee et al., 1988). Blood-product transfusion from a donor who is homozygous for one of the recipient's haplotypes may also explain the variability of incidence (Anderson and Weinstein, 1990; Ferrara and Deeg, 1991; Grishaber et al., 1993).

PATHOPHYSIOLOGY

Acute GVHD

In the last several years, understanding of the pathophysiological mechanisms causing acute GVHD have evolved. Previously, it was thought that GVHD was initiated by the donor's immunocompetent T lymphocytes reacting against the immunoincompetent recipient's issues. This resulted in donor-lymphocyte–mediated damage to the recipient's target cells or organs (Tsoi, 1982). In the last several years however, the role of the lymphokines interleukin-2 (IL-2) and interferon gamma (IFNγ) and monokines such as interleukin-1 (IL-1) and interferon alpha (INFα) have emerged as critical mediators in GVHD. When T cells become activated, they secrete IL-2 and IFNγ which in turn activate monocytes and macrophages to secrete the inflammatory monokines IL-1 and INFα. The new paradigm of GVHD pathophysiology includes the following: (1) T cells are involved in critical antigen recognition and activation roles which take place in the afferent phase of GVHD, and (2) monocytes and non-T cells mediate the efferent phase of GVHD during which time the inflammatory monokines and other substances cause target destruction (Ferrara, 1994).

The immunopathogenesis of the afferent phase of acute GVHD is a multistep process that includes antigen presentation, T-cell activation, and proliferation and differentiation of the activated T cells. This phase peaks at approximately 5 days and is completed within the week following transplantation. In one murine model, the clinical signs of epithelial GVHD were not evident until week 2 following transplantation, during which time systemic IL-2 levels had decreased considerably. Furthermore, the IL-2 mRNA was produced solely in the spleen and not in the epithelium. Given these observations, it appears that the T-cell response with subsequent IL-2 production is distinctly separate, both in time and in tissue distribution, from the efferent phase (Ferrara, 1994).

When donor marrow enters the recipient, the mature donor T cells recognize the recipient's alloantigens. This is accomplished by a process called *antigen recognition*. Donor antigen presenting cells (APCs) that are naturally contained in bone marrow such as mononuclear phagocytes and B cells recognize the proteins of the host as foreign. These cells envelop the alloantigen proteins, digest them, and display fragments of the proteins on their cell surfaces. The fragments are at that point recognized by T cells initiating T-cell activation (Ferrara and Deeg, 1991). When T cells become activated, they produce and secrete IL-2, which acts as an autocrine growth factor as well as an activator of other lymphocytes. In response to IL-2, the T cells subsequently proliferate and differentiate into multiple clones and memory cells.

The importance of IL-2 and IFNγ in the afferent phase has become more evident in recent years. As mentioned, donor T cells recognize alloantigens in the host and are subsequently activated, secreting IL-2 and IFNγ. IFNγ in turn activates the newly engrafted mononuclear cells such as macrophages, which then secrete IL-1, tumor necrosis factor alpha (TNFα) and additional IFNγ. Holler and colleagues (1990) discovered that TNFα levels peaked shortly after the completion of the BMT

conditioning regimen and were elevated on the average of 25 days before the diagnosis of GVHD. Ninety percent of the patients who demonstrated abnormally elevated TNFα levels during their conditioning regimes developed severe acute GVHD and less than 30% had long-term survival. The patients who exhibited elevated levels of TNFα between day +1 and day +90 had a 50% survival; those who had normal TNFα levels up to day +90 had an 80% survival. Additional support for this hypothesis comes from a murine study in which single injections of anti-TNFα antibodies were injected in mice prior to recipient irradiation and allogeneic BMT. GVHD-related mortality rates decreased from 58% to 17% in the mice that received the antibodies (Holler et al., 1993).

In the efferent phase, the activated mononuclear cells begin secreting the inflammatory monokines IL-1, TNFα, and IFNγ. It is thought that endotoxin may provide a secondary stimulatory signal for the macrophages that were primed in the afferent phase. Several lines of evidence support this hypothesis. Allogenically transplanted germ-free mice selectively contaminated with bacteria such as *Staphylococcus epidermidis* or *Lactobacillus* do not exhibit worsened GVHD. When contaminated with gram-negative rod bacteria, however, they experience fatal acute GVHD (Antin and Ferrara, 1992). Patients with aplastic anemia who are assigned to laminar air flow rooms during transplantation and who receive gut and skin decontamination experience less acute GVHD than those who are treated in conventional rooms (Storb et al., 1983). Finally, clinical trials indicate that individuals who receive high-dose gammaglobulin exhibit a reduced risk of acute GVHD (Sullivan et al., 1990).

The use of microbial-free environments through the use of laminar air flow (LAF) rooms, gut and skin sterilization, antibiotics, and sterile food is the clinical attempt to eliminate the initiation or enhancement of GVHD through bacterial mechanisms. Despite problems of patient compliance with such strict regimens, they appear to provide a beneficial effect by decreasing the frequency of acute GVHD (Deeg, 1988).

Graft-versus-Leukemia Effect

Strategies for preventing GVHD focus on interfering with the afferent phase of the response in that they try to eliminate donor T cells or block activation responses. Although these methods have reduced the severity of GVHD, they are associated with higher rates of graft failure and incidence of relapse. This relapse is thought to be related to a graft-versus-leukemia effect by which leukemia cells are considerably reduced during periods of acute GVHD (Ferrara and Deeg, 1991). Graft-versus-leukemia is highly associated with the occurrence of graft-versus-host disease. In fact, there appears to be an inverse relationship between the occurrence of GVHD and relapse. In allogeneic bone marrow recipients with GVHD grades II through IV the relapse rate is 2.5 times lower than in syngeneic recipients or in allogeneic recipients without GVHD (Weiden et al., 1979). Furthermore, this risk is considerably higher in patients with chronic myelogenous leukemia than other forms of leukemia (Deisseroth et al., 1993).

The cellular mechanisms that mediate the graft-versus-leukemia reaction are not well understood. For instance, it is unclear if the same or different cell populations mediate both graft-versus-leukemia and graft-versus-host disease. It is thought that CD8-positive cytotoxic T lymphocytes are the primary effector cells in the graft-versus-leukemia reaction. Support for this hypothesis was produced in a study in which selective depletion of CD8-positive cells in combination with posttransplant CsA yielded a significant reduction of acute GVHD, but an increased rate of leukemia relapse occurring in 11% of the sample (Champlin et al., 1990).

Patient survival has unfortunately been similar between patients who receive allogeneic transplants and those who receive syngeneic transplants since the lower leukemia relapse rate in allogeneic transplants is offset by higher mortality from complications of GVHD. In an effort to reduce leukemia relapse, some studies have attempted to produce GVHD by administering additional donor T cells. This approach has had many limitations because control and prediction of the course of GVHD is currently very difficult (Thomas, 1988).

Chronic GVHD

Chronic GVHD has characteristics similar to the naturally occurring autoimmune collagen-vascular diseases such as scleroderma, systemic lupus erythematosus, and rheumatoid arthritis. Fibrosis and atrophy of one or more organs occurs. The fibrotic and inflammatory changes in chronic GVHD are quite pronounced and are of longer duration than the processes occurring in acute GVHD. Chronic GVHD normally develops approximately 3 months following transplantation, but has been reported to occur as long as 2 years after transplant (Wingard et al., 1989). Occasionally, necrosis and fibrosis can be present at the same time, leading to a diagnosis of acute and chronic GVHD. Chronic GVHD may also occur in the absence of acute GVHD. However, more typically, chronic GVHD occurs following an incidence of acute GVHD.

Chronic GVHD is characterized by a complicated immunopathogenesis involving the interaction of alloimmunity and immune dysregulation, which produces severe immunodeficiency and autoimmunity. During chronic GVHD, T cells secrete unusual patterns of cytokines, particularly IL-4 and IFNγ (but not IL-2), that have the ability to stimulate the production of collagen by fibroblasts. Thus, these T cells are considered to have autoreactive characteristics (Ferrara and Deeg, 1991). Under normal circumstances, developing T cells that are autoreactive are deleted in the thymus gland. This naturally occurring process facilitates self-tolerance, one of the fundamental properties of the immune system (Abbas et al., 1994). It is thought that the thymus gland may become damaged during the conditioning regimen or acute GVHD, leading to an inability of the thymus to delete the autoreactive T cells. Two dominant factors associated with the development of chronic GVHD are prior acute GVHD and increasing patient age (Storb et al., 1986; Sullivan, 1986).

CLINICAL MANIFESTATIONS

Clinical manifestations of acute and chronic GVHD differ. They are described below and are summarized in Table 8.2.

Acute GVHD

The median onset of GVHD is approximately 25 days after transplant although it can occur within days in poorly HLA-matched recipients or those who have not received prophylaxis (Ferrara and Deeg, 1991; Champlin and Gale, 1984). As mentioned previously, GVHD primarily affects the immune system, skin, liver, and gastrointestinal tract. Acute GVHD leads to necrosis of epithelial cells. In addition to these systems, GVHD has also been reported to occur in the conjunctivae, airways, bone marrow (Deeg, 1994), and nervous system (Liedtke et al., 1994).

Skin

The most common initial presenting manifestation is a maculopapular rash involving the palms, soles, trunk, and ears (see Figure 8.1). Bullae, ulcerations, and epidermal necrosis may occur, progressing to a generalized desquamation of the skin in severe cases. Hair follicles are

injured and occasionally destroyed as well (Ferrara and Deeg, 1991).

Gastrointestinal System

Patients who experience gastrointestinal GVHD usually experience skin and/or liver GVHD. Presenting symptoms of gut GVHD include nausea and vomiting, abdominal pain, anorexia, and paralytic ileus. Watery hemenegative diarrhea usually develops, progressing to hemepositive diarrhea as more of the intestinal mucosa begins to slough (Ford and Ballard, 1988). Several liters of diarrhea may be produced daily resulting in severe hypoalbuminemia and fluid and electrolyte imbalances. The severity of

TABLE 8.2 Clinical manifestations of acute and chronic graft-versus-host disease

Affected organ	Acute	Chronic
Skin	Erythematous rash	Lichen planuslike eruption
	Exfoliation	Scleroderma
	Bullous eruption	
	Toxic epidermal necrolysis	
Gastrointestinal tract	Diarrhea	Malabsorption
	Abdominal cramps	
	Vomiting	
Liver	Abnormalities of function	Chronic active hepatitis
Other	Fever	Recurrent infection
	Malaise	Prolonged impaired immunity
	Weight loss	
	Eosinophilia	
	Lymphopenia	
	Positive direct Coombs' test	

SOURCE: Lucas, C.F., and Barrett, A.J. 1982. Bone Marrow Transplantation. *Update* p. 2403, with permission.

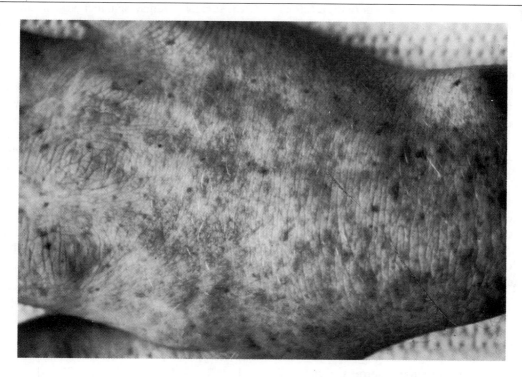

Figure 8.1 **The most common initial presenting manifestation is a maculopapular rash.**

GVHD and the patients's response to treatment often are quantitated by measuring stool volumes (Sullivan, 1983).

Liver
Liver function abnormalities that appear with GVHD include elevated alkaline phosphatase and bilirubin levels. The serum glutamic oxaloacetic transaminase (SGOT) may increase, but somewhat slower than the alkaline phosphatase and bilirubin levels (Sullivan, 1983). Coagulation values may be abnormal as well. Right upper-quadrant pain, hepatomegaly, and jaundice may be exhibited (Ford and Ballard, 1988) with ascites and encephalopathy in more severe cases. The clinical manifestations of liver

GVHD and veno-occlusive disease, another common side effect of BMT, are similar with the exception of weight gain and right upper-quadrant pain in GVHD (Ferrara and Deeg, 1991).

Immune System
Delayed immunologic recovery and prolonged severe immunoincompetence occur during episodes of acute GVHD. In vitro studies in which leukocytes from unrelated donors are mixed with leukocytes from allogeneic BMT patients experiencing GVHD show that cell-mediated lympholysis (CML) against the donor leukocytes is severely impaired. The addition of IL-2 to the mixed leukocyte culture (MLC) corrects

this impairment, which suggests that defects in helper cells or cooperation between the helper T cells and the APCs may be present (Brkic et al., 1985). Other evidence supporting CML impairment is provided by studies that show in vivo impaired immunity against viral infections. Regardless of the cytomegalovirus (CMV) serological status prior to transplant, the incidence of acute GVHD was found to increase significantly the risk of subsequent CMV infection and CMV interstitial pneumonia (Meyers et al., 1986). This GVHD-produced immunoincompetence in addition to that produced by immunosuppressive therapy increase susceptibility to infections (Ferrara and Deeg, 1991). In fact, the majority of GVHD related mortalities usually result from infectious complications than from organ failure.

Chronic GVHD

Chronic GVHD is a complex syndrome whose clinical manifestations resemble naturally occurring collagen vascular disorders. Figure 8.2 provides a visual representation of the incidence of various clinical manifestations observed in chronic GVHD.

Skin

The skin is the most frequently affected system with greater than 95% of patients experiencing alterations in this organ (Deeg et al., 1984a). Inflammatory changes occur early in the pathological course and fibrotic changes are seen later. Pruritis and erythema in the malar area are early symptoms. This erythema then spreads to other integumentary areas. Patchy alopecia and mucous membrane and nail abnormalities may occur. Integumentary lesions have been found to occur usually in sun-exposed areas, although they have occurred occasionally in non–sun-exposed areas. Insidious pigmentary changes might occur in some patients; in others, patchy hyper- or hypopigmentation might develop only in the periorbital

area, sites of trauma, or undergarment area. A mottled appearance of the skin with faint, blotchy macular erythema has been observed. Hyperkeratotic, flat-topped perifollicular papules might also develop (see Figure 8.3).

Approximately 6 to 18 months after transplantation, the skin becomes progressively indurated and adheres to the underlying fascia. The dermis becomes thickened. Progressive skin involvement resembles scleroderma in which bronze-colored hyperpigmentation, hide-bound skin, pressure-point ulcerations, and joint contractures occur (Shulman et al., 1980) (see Figure 8.4).

Lichenoid reactions with concurrent destruction of the epidermal basal layer and pilar

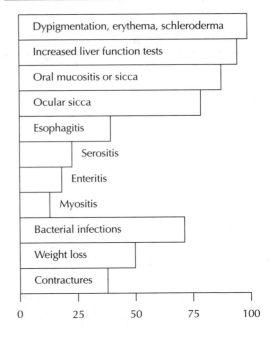

Figure 8.2 Incidence of clinical manifestations in patients with extensive chronic GVHD

SOURCE: H.J. Deeg, et al. 1984. Bone marrow transplantation: a review of delayed complications. *British Journal of Haematology* 57:185, with permission.

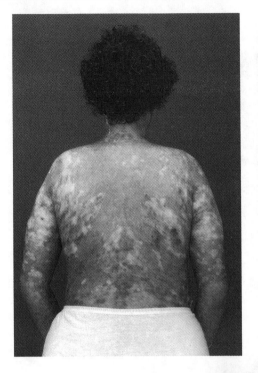

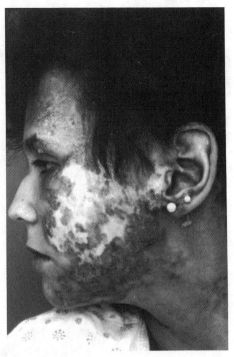

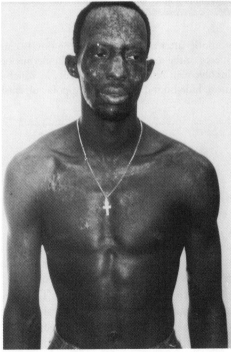

Figure 8.3
Chronic skin GVHD may
begin with an erythema in
the malar area spreading to
other areas. Integumentary
lesions have been found
to occur usually in sun-
exposed areas, although
they occasionally have occurred in non–sun-exposed
areas. Insidious pigmentary
changes may occur in some
patients. In others patchy
hyperpigmentation, some-
times only in the periorbital
area, sites of trauma, or undergarment area, may de-
velop. A mottled appear-
ance of the skin with faint,
blotchy macular erythema
has been observed. Hyper-
keratotic, flat-topped perifollicular papules may also
occur.

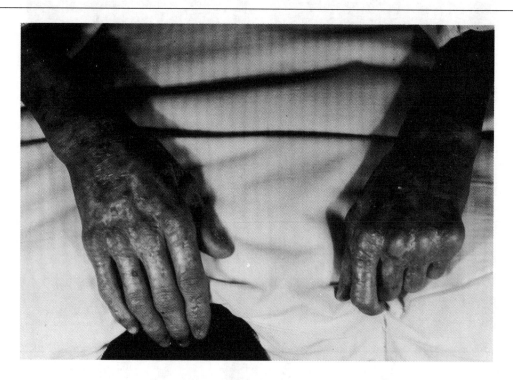

Figure 8.4   Approximately 6 to 18 months after transplantation, the skin becomes progressively indurated and adheres to the underlying fascia. The dermis becomes thickened. Progressive skin involvement resembles scleroderma in which bronze-colored hyperpigmentation, hide-bound skin, pressure-point ulcerations, and joint contractures occur.

units are frequent in chronic GVHD. The destructive fibrosing inflammatory reactions occur around the eccrine coils, deep dermal nerves, and in the subcutaneous fat (see Figure 8.5). Approximately 80% of patients with chronic GVHD exhibit skin alterations that resemble widespread lichen planus with papulosquamous dermatitis, plaques, desquamation, and dyspigmentation. Alopecia is also frequently present. As chronic epidermal GVHD progresses and becomes more severe, it resem-

bles scleroderma and includes induration, joint contractures, atrophy, and chronic skin ulcers (Ferrara and Deeg, 1991).

A localized, self-limiting variant form of chronic GVHD occurs in 20% of the patients, specifically in those patients with no history of acute GVHD. This form is characterized by clusters of small lesions or large areas of induration, hyper- or hypopigmentation, and epidermal atrophy. The inflammatory changes range from absent to mild and the deep reticu-

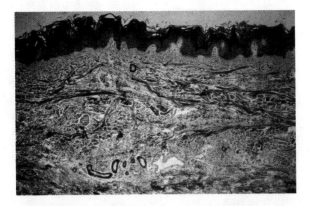

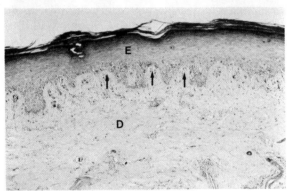

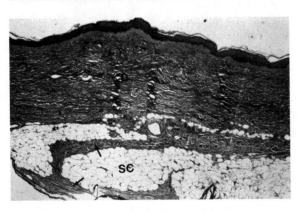

Figure 8.5
Top photo shows normal skin. E = epidermis, D = dermis, A = adnexal structures, SC = subcutaneous tissue. Center and bottom photos show progressive changes that occur with chronic GVHD. Lichenoid reactions with concurrent destruction of the epidermal basal layer (indicated by arrows on center photo) and pilar units are frequent in chronic GVHD. The destructive fibrosing inflammatory reactions occur around the eccrine coils, deep dermal nerves, and in the subcutaneous fat. Skin biopsies demonstrate fibroplasia that may advance to epidermal flattening and atrophy, loss of cell dermal appendages, and fibrous remodeling of the reticular dermis with expansion into the subcutaneous fat (bottom photo).

lar dermis demonstrates nodular fibrous re-modeling. The lesions may expand and cause extensive depigmentation and scarring before they resolve (Shulman and Sullivan, 1988).

Sicca Syndrome

Sicca syndrome, or dry gland syndrome, oc-curs in approximately 80% of patients with chronic GVHD. It is characterized by the devel-opment of lymphoplasmacytic infiltrates in-itially around the ductal structures of glands such as the lacrimal glands, salivary glands, and submucosal glands, subsequently resulting in fi-brous destruction. The most frequently in-volved organs are the eyes, nose, mouth, air-ways, and vagina. The presenting symptoms include dry mucous membranes of the conjunc-tiva, mouth, esophagus, urethra, and vagina (Sale et al., 1981).

Gastrointestinal Tract

The gastrointestinal clinical manifestations of chronic GVHD differ considerably from those of acute GVHD. Lichenoid inflammation with subsequent destruction of the mucosa and sub-mucosal glands occurs more frequently in the esophageal area than in the stomach, intestine, and colon (McDonald et al., 1981). If the mu-cosal damage is severe and ulcerations pene-trate the muscularis mucosa, inflammatory polyps may develop. In an attempt to limit the depth and area of ulceration, the muscularis contracts and thickens, thereby producing a protrusion of the intervening mucosa into the lumen (Galati et al., 1993). Bloody diarrhea, which frequently occurs in patients with acute GVHD, is rarely seen in chronic GVHD (McDonald et al., 1986).

Eighty percent of the patients with chronic GVHD exhibit involvement of the mouth (Schubert and Sullivan, 1990). The patients most frequently complain of pain, particularly

if eating hot or warm foods, and of dry mucous membranes. Lichen planus-type lesions are commonly found on the buccal mucosa appear-ing as fine white reticular striae on the buccal mucosa, and large plaques on the buccal sur-face and lateral aspect of the tongue (see Figure 8.6). Dental caries and periodontitis may occur due to xerostomia. Histopathological altera-tions observed include atrophy, necrosis of squamous cells, and mononuclear cell infiltra-tion (Klingemann, 1988).

Eyes

Approximately 65% to 80% of patients with extensive chronic GVHD experience ocular in-volvement. Insufficient tear production occurs as a result of sicca syndrome. The patients may complain of dryness, grittiness, pain, burning, and photophobia. Keratitis and scarring may also result from the ocular sicca (Klingemann, 1988; Calissendorff et al., 1989).

Lungs

In 5% to 10% of patients with chronic GVHD, acquired obstructive small airway disease devel-ops. It is characterized by the development of bronchiolar lesions which results in fibrous obliteration of the lumen (see Figure 8.7). The obstructive airway may be the result of de-pressed mucosal immunity and repeated infec-tions compounded by aspiration from simulta-neously occurring esophageal disease (Shulman and Sullivan, 1988).

Vagina

Inflammation, sicca, adhesions, and stenosis of the vagina may occur in severe cases of chronic GVHD (Corson et al., 1982). If any of these occur, systemic immunosuppressive therapy is recommended, and surgery might be required. If these symptoms occur in the absence of chronic GVHD, lack of use or long-term com-

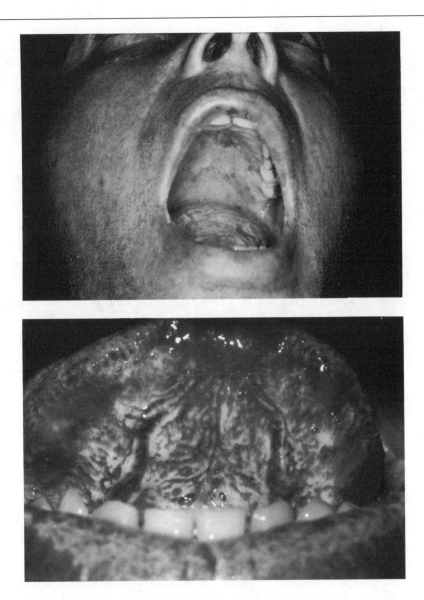

Figure 8.6 Lichen planus-type lesions are commonly found on the buccal (top) and labial mucosa (bottom), and frequently apear similar to oral candidiasis.

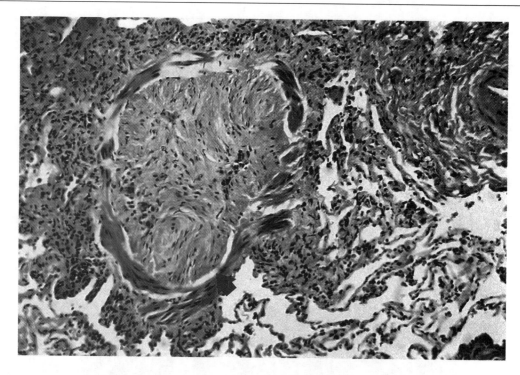

Figure 8.7   In approximately 5% to 10% of patients with chronic GVHD, lesions involving the bronchioles resulting from obliteration of the lumen occur and result in an obstructive small airway disease (Sullivan, 1986; Ralph, 1984)

plications of total body irradiation should be considered as causative factors (Klingemann, 1988).

Neuromuscular System

Clinical manifestations similar to those of myasthenia gravis have been observed in a small number of patients with chronic GVHD. These include muscular weakness, repetitive nerve stimulation, response to edrophonium, and elevated acetylcholine receptor antibodies. These symptoms were noted to occur after tapering of corticosteroid therapy and were thought to result from immune dysregulation and donor-host alloreactivity. Polymyositis, peripheral neuropathy (Klingemann, 1988), and recurrent acute inflammatory demyelinating polyradiculitis (Liedtke et al., 1994) have also been observed in chronic GVHD. Table 8.3 summarizes the late effects seen in chronic GVHD.

DIAGNOSIS, GRADING, AND PROGNOSIS

The diagnosis of GVHD is made by evaluating a combination of clinical manifestations and histologic findings. The safest and simplest

TABLE 8.3 Late effects of bone marrow transplantation: chronic graft-versus-host disease

Late effect	Incidence rate	Time post-BMT (days)	Signs and symptoms	Nursing management	Diagnostic tools	Medical treatment
Skin	95%	100–400	Rough, scaly skin Malar erythema Generalized rash Hypo- hyperpigmentation Dyspigmentation Premature graying Alopecia Joint contractures Scleroderma Loss of sweating	Use of nonabrasive soaps, lotions, sunscreen Cosmetic support, makeup, wigs Range-of-motion activities Patient/family education Monitor compliance to treatment protoocols Infection precautions until differential diagnosis is made Monitor LFTs Low-fat diet	Skin biopsy + for GVHD Karnofsky score	Lanolin-based creams Possible systemic immunosuppresive therapy with cyclosporin A, prednisone, azathioprine
Liver	30%	100–400	Jaundice	Infection precautions until differential diagnosis is made Monitor LFTs Low-fat diet	Alkaline phosphatase SGOT Bilirubin	Possible systemic immunosuppresive therapy with cyclosporin A, prednisone, azathioprine
Oral	80%	100–400	Pain, burning, dryness, irritation, soreness, loss of taste Lichenoic changes, atrophy, erythema in oral cavity Candida infection Stomatitis Dental caries Xerostomia	Encourage soft, bland diet Dental hygiene education Soft toothbrush, flossing Saline rinses Dental medicine referral/recommendation Salivary gland stimulants, sugarless mints, artifical saliva	Labial mucosa biopsy + for GVHD Secretory IgA levels Mouth culture + for bacterial and viral etiologies Radiographs	Possible systemic immunosuppresive therapy with cyclosporin A, prednisone, azathioprine Artificial saliva Clotrimazole troches or bystatin Swish and swallow Nystatin Appropriate topical medication Topical fluoride treatment Appropriate dental therapy
Ocular	80%	100–400	Grittiness, burning of eyes Dry eyes Sicca syndrome	Artifical tears Schirmer's tear test: If < 10 mm of wetting, refer to ophthalmologist	Kertoconjuntivitis Corneal ulceration Slit-lamp microscopy	Lacriset plugs Soft contact lenses Puntal ligation for obliteration of tear duct outflow Keratoplasty Tarsorrhaphies

Continued

191

TABLE 8.3 Late effects of bone marrow transplantation: chronic graft-versus-host disease *Continued*

Late effect	Incidence rate	Time post-BMT (days)	Signs and symptoms	Nursing management	Diagnostic tools	Medical treatment
GI tract, esophagus	36%	100–400	Anorexia Difficulty eating Painful swallowing Retrosternal pain Weight loss Vomiting	Serial weights High-calorie food supplements Recommend nutritional counseling	Barium swallow of esophagus and small bowel follow-through	Esophageal dilatation Possible systemic immunosuppressive therapy with cyclosporin A
Vagina	20%	100–400	Inflammation Stricture formation causing obstruction of menstrual flow Adhesions Dry vagina Painful intercourse Marital problems	Water-soluble lubricants Recommend sexual counseling and therapy	Papanicolaou smear	Vaginal stints Estrogen cream Surgical intervention

Source: Buchsel, P.C. 1986. Long-term complications of allogeneic bone marrow transplantation: nursing implications. Reprinted with permission from *Oncology Nursing Forum*, 13:67.

method is confirmation by skin biopsy. If the biopsy results are ambiguous, a repeat biopsy can be taken 3 to 7 days later. If liver or gastrointestinal manifestations occur in the absence of skin rash, a "blind" biopsy can be taken from the forearm. These biopsies can help to establish the diagnosis if biopsies of the other organs (i.e., gut or liver) are ambiguous or dangerous. Other sites helpful in establishing a diagnosis are the esophagus and muscle. If clinical manifestations exist in only one organ, multiple-site biopsies can be obtained. It is unusual for GVHD to be isolated to one site, except in chronic GVHD (Sullivan, 1983).

The clinical stage and grade of acute GVHD (see Table 8.1) is based on the severity of organ dysfunction of the skin, liver, or gut. The incidence of moderate to severe (II–IV) acute GVHD in patients that have HLA-matched donors and have sustained engraftment is between 30% to 50% (Weisdorf et al., 1990). Of these patients, 30% to 60% die from either GVHD or related infectious complications (Weisdorf et al., 1990).

The prognosis in GVHD depends on the overall severity of the disease. Additional factors that have been correlated with poor survival in patients developing acute GVHD include:

1. older age of the patient,
2. refractory to random donor platelets,
3. lack of LAF isolation (Storb et al., 1983), and
4. lack of complete response or resistance to GVHD treatment (Weisdorf et al., 1990).

In chronic GVHD, oral biopsies and lacrimal function studies facilitate staging the extent of the disease (Sullivan et al., 1981b). The Karnofsky performance scale has also been used to grade the severity of the disease (Sullivan, 1985). Table 8.4 shows a classification system for chronic GVHD.

TABLE 8.4 Clinicopathological classification of chronic graft-versus-host disease

Limited chronic graft-versus-host disease (either or both)	Extensive chronic graft-versus-host disease

Localized skin involvement	Either
	  Generalized skin
	  involvement
	Or
	  Localized skin in-
	  volvement or hepatic
	  dysfunction due to
	  chronic GVHD or both
	plus:

Hepatic dysfunction (due to chronic GVHD)	Liver histology showing
	  chronic aggressive
	  hepatitis, bridging
	  necrosis, or cirrhosis,
	  or
	Involvement of eye
	  (Schirmer's test with
	  > 5 mm of wetting), or
	Involvement of minor
	  salivary glands or oral
	  mucosa demonstrated
	  on labial biopsy, or
	Involvement of any
	  other target organ

SOURCE: Adapted from Shulman et al., 1980.

Several risk factors for the development of chronic GVHD have been identified. They include female donor/male recipient sex-match particularly if the female donors had been pregnant or transfused, no GVHD drug prophylaxis, an increased number of posttransplant transfusions, no pretransplant trimethoprim-sulfamethoxazole treatment, and lower Karnofsky performance scores (Gale et al., 1987). Prior acute GVHD is a risk factor that has been identified in the development of chronic GVHD. The risk appears to increase with the increasing severity or grade of the prior acute GVHD (Wingard et al., 1989). Other risk factors include persistent severe thrombocytopenia (Sullivan et al., 1982), lichenoid changes on skin histology, and serum bilirubin greater than 1.2 mg/dl (Wingard et al., 1989). One factor that has been found to adversely influence survival in patients with chronic GVHD is the type of onset. The progressive onset from acute to chronic, without resolution of acute GVHD, correlates with the highest mortality (Wingard et al., 1989; Sullivan, 1981a).

Factors that have not been found to correlate with the development of GVHD include diagnosis, disease status at the time of transplant, interval from diagnosis to transplant, year of transplant, ABO compatibility, source of radiation, dose of radiation, dose rate, fractionation versus no fractionation, prior splenectomy, presence of infection in the week before transplant, bone marrow cell dose, posttransplant transfusion of unirradiated blood products, pretransplant gut decontamination, and conventional versus LAF isolation (Gale et al., 1987). Factors that have no association in the development of chronic GVHD include patient and donor sex, donor-recipient sex mismatching, donor age, or transplantation during remission or relapse of leukemia (Sullivan, 1983).

MEDICAL MANAGEMENT

Prophylaxis

With the increase of unrelated donor transplantation and peripheral blood cell transplantation, improved GVHD prophylactic regimens are needed. Most of the GVHD prevention protocols attempt to interfere with pathophysiological mechanisms occurring in the afferent phase by either depleting donor T cells or blocking their activation. The most effective strategy to reduce the incidence of GVHD in-

volves depleting T cells from the donor marrow prior to transplantation. This can be accomplished either by physically separating out the T cells via a process called *lectin agglutination* or by using T-cell–specific monoclonal antibodies (moAbs) (Ferrara and Deeg, 1991). Two techniques can be used in the moAb approach. One technique involves eliminating the T cells by toxin-conjugated antibodies. The other technique uses an incubation process in which the moAbs are added to the donor bone marrow and incubated, followed by the addition of complement. The moAb-coated T cells are then lysed by complement. T-cell depletion techniques have yielded 90% to 99.9% reductions in T-cell counts and have significantly reduced the incidence and severity of GVHD. Unfortunately, these techniques are associated with higher rates of graft failure (Ferrara and Deeg, 1991).

Ultraviolet irradiation of donor marrow prior to transplantation has also been found beneficial in inactivating or depleting T cells and dendritic cells (a type of APC) in the marrow inoculum (Hudson, Lawler, Pamphilon, 1994; Oluwole, Engelstad, James, 1993). Both in vivo and in vitro studies show a positive correlation between stem cell damage and dose of ultraviolet light (Hudson et al., 1994). Kapoor and colleagues (1992) utilized methyloxypsoralen plus ultraviolet A therapy in the treatment of chronic GVHD. While continuing to receive CsA and methylprednisolone, 15 patients received eight methyloxypsoralen plus ultraviolet A treatments. Lichen planus formations on the skin and oral mucosa improved while no improvements were seen in the visceral disease.

Currently, the gold standard of prophylaxis involves posttransplantation immunosuppressive therapy (Deeg, 1994). Single-agent therapy includes MTX (Sullivan, 1985), CsA (Aschan et al., 1994), and corticosteroids. The protocol used in the largest number of institutions consists of MTX administered on days 1, 3, 6, and 11 (day 11 eliminated in some protocols) and CsA begun on the day prior to transplantation continuing up to 24 months. Combination agent protocols include MTX and CsA (Storb et al., 1992; Aschan et al., 1994; Ringden et al., 1993), MTX, CsA, and folinic acid (Russell et al., 1994), antithymocyte globulin (ATG), MTX, and corticosteroids (Ramsay et al., 1982), MTX and FK506, a macrolide antibiotic derived from *Streptomyces tsukubaensis* that has potent immunosuppressive activity (Cooper et al., 1994; Fay et al., 1995), and prednisone with three different cytotoxic agents: procarbazine, azathioprine, or cyclophosphamide (Sullivan, 1983).

Storb and colleagues have studied the effectiveness of CsA versus MTX in preventing acute and chronic GVHD and examined each of their effects on leukemia relapse and long-term survival. An earlier study showed that the drugs were equivalent in almost all of the parameters examined—long-term survival of patients who received CsA was 62% and of patients who received MTX was 66%. Patients who received CsA did not exhibit impairment of hematopoietic engraftment or an increase in infection-associated deaths (Storb et al., 1985). A more recent long-term follow-up of three randomized prospective trials provided further support that MTX and CsA are comparable in their ability to prevent acute and chronic GVHD and that the probabilities of leukemia relapse, interstitial pneumonia, and overall survival are similar (Storb et al., 1992).

Data from several centers have shown a reduced incidence of relapse in patients with hematological malignancies who received MTX compared with those who received CsA for GVHD prophylaxis (Backman et al., 1988; Atkinson et al., 1988; Horowitz et al., 1989). Increases in leukemia relapse have been observed when both MTX and CsA were used in combination rather than as single agents

(Aschan et al., 1991). Conversely, data from other studies have found no increases in relapse (Ringden et al., 1993; von Bueltzingsloewen et al., 1993). Weaver and colleagues (1994), through a multivariate analysis, examined risk factors for relapse after HLA-identical bone marrow transplantation in 184 patients with acute myelogenous leukemia in first remission. Patients received either MTX, CsA, or MTX and CsA. While no differences in relapse were found with single-agent prophylaxis, a 2.34 increased relative risk of relapse was discovered in patients receiving the combination regimen. However, by increasing the cumulative dose of total body irradiation (TBI) from 12.0 Gy to 15.75 Gy, relapse rates have been found to decrease (Clift et al., 1990). No associations were found among patient age, sex, FAB subtype, and marrow cell dose and the risk of post-BMT relapse (Weaver et al., 1994).

The majority of drugs in GVHD prophylaxis is aimed at blocking the synthesis of cells critical in the afferent phase of GVHD. CsA, for example, inhibits the synthesis of IL-2 mRNA (Ferrara, 1994). FK506, while not structurally related to CsA, has similar bioactivity. This agent inhibits the transcription of the interleukins (specifically IL-1, IL-2, IL-3, and IL-4), granulocyte/macrophage colony-stimulating factor (GM-CSF), TNFα, and IFNγ. FK504, however, has 10 to 100 times the potency of CsA in inhibiting the proliferation of alloantigen-activated T cells in vitro and is more effective in suppressing allo- and xenogeneic organ transplant rejection in animal models (Cooper et al., 1994).

Methotrexate prevents mitosis and clonal expansion of the activated T cells (Jolivet et al., 1983). Glucocorticoids repress the expression of specific genes in the nucleus and block the production of IL-1 by antigen-presenting cells, the cells necessary for antigen presentation to T cells (Ferrara and Deeg, 1991). The combination of MTX, ATG, and prednisone has been found to be superior to MTX alone in preventing GVHD. However, no improvement in long-term survival was observed because the number of fatal infections was not reduced (Ramsay et al., 1982).

Although drug prophylaxis is effective in reducing the incidence and severity of GVHD, it can produce side effects, some of which can be rather serious. CsA has been found to delay red blood cell recovery. In vitro studies using bone marrow derived from canine erythroid colonies show suppression of erythroid colony formation when CsA was exogenously added. It was thought that this was due either to a direct suppression of erythroid precursors or to inhibition of an accessory cell (Deeg et al., 1980; Kennedy et al., 1983; Haus et al., 1983; Atkinson et al., 1983). Additional reported toxicities of CsA include nephrotoxicity (Yee et al., 1988), hypertension (Loughran et al., 1985), hepatotoxicity (Keown et al., 1982), and neurological disturbances (Storb et al., 1988). No statistically significant differences have been observed between CsA and MTX in regard to toxicities (Storb et al., 1988; Biggs et al., 1986).

Treatment

Established acute GVHD is treated primarily with corticosteroids, although other immunosuppressive therapies have been used including CsA, anti–T-cell immunotoxins, ATG (Weisdorf et al., 1990), moAbs, and FK506 (Deeg, 1994). A prospective study examining the effectiveness of ATG and corticosteroids showed a decrease in GVHD although there was no improvement in survival (Doney et al., 1981). Patients have been found to improve with methylprednisolone (2 mg/kg) or ATG (10–15 mg/kg) (Sullivan, 1985). Diminished clinical manifestations of GVHD have also been observed in patients receiving higher doses of corticosteroids. However, long-term survival has

not improved in these patients because they continue to die from infections (Kendra et al., 1981).

Several centers are examining the efficacy of IL-2 in inhibiting GVHD in both mice and humans. Szebeni and colleagues (1994) administered a short course of high-dose IL-2 to lethally irradiated mice that received T-cell–depleted allogeneic bone marrow and splenic suspensions. Serum IFNγ levels of allogeneically transplanted controls (i.e., those not receiving IL-2) were monitored and found to increase significantly, peaking on days 4 or 5 when compared with the sera of syngeneic bone marrow recipients. Mice receiving IL-2 exhibited a marked reduction in IFNγ levels, particularly on day +4. However, they also demonstrated early GVHD mortality. This finding suggests that decreasing IFNγ levels early in GVHD pathogenesis may decrease host resistance to microbial pathogens, which may be a secondary stimulatory signal for GVHD.

Przepiorka and colleagues (1994) administered IL-2 (3 MIU/m2 per day IV by continuous infusion for 96 hours beginning 4 hours after transplant) in addition to CsA and MTX to 7 patients with leukemia in relapse undergoing allogeneic transplantation. Five donor/recipient pairs were matched at only 1 HLA locus and two were complete mismatches. The two completely mismatched patients developed steroid and ATG-resistant grade 4 GVHD and subsequently died from GVHD-related complications. Three others developed grade 3 or 4 GVHD. Of the five with two antigen mismatches, two died from veno-occlusive disease, one from leukemia, and one from GVHD. The investigators suggest that the severity of GVHD in patients with two antigen mismatches can be reduced with IL-2 prophylaxis, but it is not sufficient in incomplete mismatches.

Treatment of chronic GVHD often includes steroids, CsA, and azathioprine alone or in combination (Wingard et al., 1989). Thalidomide, initially used as a sedative, has recently been used to treat chronic GVHD (Cole et al., 1994; Vogelsang et al., 1992) and has been found to be effective with minimal immediate side effects. Its actions include impairment of neutrophil phagocytosis and chemotaxis, decreased in antibody production in response to antigenic stimulation, increased suppressor T cells, reduced helper T cells, and inhibited TNF production. Its immediate side effects are typically mild and reversible, and include somnolence, constipation, headache, nausea, and dryness of mouth or skin. The most critical long-term side effect is peripheral neuropathy characterized by parathesias of the hands and feet, coldness, and cramping of extremities. No peripheral neuropathy has been reported with its use in pediatric patients. It has also been found to be teratogenic (Cole et al., 1994).

Patients experiencing chronic GVHD also require skillful supportive care to manage infections, fluid and electrolyte imbalances, and nutritional deficits. Hyperalimentation, fluid replacement, transfusions, and antibiotic therapy are often necessary (Gauvreau et al., 1981; Parker and Cohen, 1983).

NURSING MANAGEMENT

The nursing management of patients experiencing GVHD is complex and requires expert skills, knowledge, and creativity. Careful assessment is required to identify its early clinical manifestations and to distinguish GVHD from other complications such as reactions to antibiotics or chemotherapy, irritated bowel, infections, and radiation toxicity. An awareness of high-risk factors that increase the likelihood of developing GVHD and the identification of patients in this high-risk category are important so that scrupulous monitoring of these patients can occur during the period when GVHD is most likely to occur.

Providing appropriate skin care is important for patient comfort and prevention of infection (McConn, 1987). Placing oil in the bathwater or applying it after showering helps to decrease the skin dryness and to soothe the discomfort caused by pruritis. Antipruretic and steroid creams have been found to have marginal benefit for pruritis.

In some instances of acute GVHD, the rash progresses to bullae with subsequent desquamation of the outer epidermal layers. If this occurs, preventing infection and bleeding is important. Silicon bead or low air-loss beds may decrease discomfort caused by pressure points and to facilitate exudate absorption. Covering the desquamated areas with gauze pads in Burrow's solution soaked for approximately 10 minutes serves as a means of debridement. Skin desquamation can be intensely painful and require narcotic drips for pain control. Application of hydrogel dressings that have been painted with an antibiotic ointment has several advantages. It

- is nonadherent;
- absorbs wound exudate, bacteria, and odor;
- provides a physiologically moist environment; and
- is conducive to wound healing and tissue granulation (Caudell and Schauer, 1989).

Acute GVHD can also affect the gastrointestinal system, causing several liters of diarrhea per day. Strict monitoring of intake and output, daily weights, and serum electrolytes such as sodium, chloride, and potassium, is essential. Loss of these electrolytes can cause metabolic alkalosis. Severe diarrhea combined with intestinal sloughing can lead to malabsorption and result in malnutrition. Therefore, hyperalimentation may be needed to provide the patient with adequate nutritional support. Placement on an NPO diet to further reduce gut activation may be necessary. Proteins such as prealbumin and albumin, anthropometric measurements, and the creatinine height index are parameters that can be used to measure somatic and visceral protein (Behnke, 1986).

If the patient has moderate to severe diarrhea, he or she should be instructed to clean the perineal area thoroughly after each bowel movement. Sitz baths further cleanse the perineal area and soothe irritated skin. The patient should be assessed regularly for rectal lesions.

Mucosal sloughing that occurs in severe gut GVHD can also produce gastrointestinal bleeding. All emesis and stool output should be tested regularly for occult blood. GVHD stools often appear mahogany colored and have a strong, foul odor. If gastrointestinal bleeding occurs, the hemoglobin and hematocrit should be monitored carefully and appropriate blood-product therapy should be administered.

In liver GVHD, the patient may experience right upper-quadrant pain, hepatomegaly, jaundice, and elevated liver function studies. The serum alkaline phosphatase and bilirubin levels should be monitored (Sullivan, 1983). Although the SGOT may rise, it usually does so at a slower rate. If a liver biopsy is performed to obtain an accurate diagnosis, careful assessment for bleeding is necessary. However, a liver biopsy may be contraindicated in the presence of thrombocytopenia.

Moderate to severe acute GVHD (grades II–IV) has been strongly correlated with the incidence of nonviral infection (Paulin, 1987). Also, chronic GVHD has been found to be a major factor predisposing patients to infection (Englehard, 1986). For these reasons, patients who have either acute or chronic GVHD should be thoroughly assessed for infection, and appropriately trained in measures to prevent infection following discharge.

Patients who experience ocular sicca with resultant insufficient tear production should be advised to use artificial tears to prevent corneal erosion, perforation, and scarring. Sicca syndrome can also affect the mouth, genital tract, and the mucosa of the tracheobronchial tree. If the patient exhibits these symptoms, moisture-enhancing measures to treat these various areas include frequent mouth care and adequate lubrication of the vagina prior to intercourse. Ophthalmic preparations of pilocarpine have been used orally (5 mg tid) to stimulate saliva production and relieve mucosal atrophy, erythema, and discomfort (Singhal et al., 1995). The use of an air humidifier also may be recommended.

Nursing management of patients receiving medications to prevent or treat GVHD is also important. For instance, many nurses are familiar with the complex management of patients receiving high-dose steroids, but less familiar with managing the side effects of CsA (Truog and Wozniak, 1990; Klemm, 1985).

Nursing management of the variety of complications common to patients with acute and/or chronic GVHD is challenging. Nursing management of the effects of acute and chronic GVHD often continues after the patient is discharged from the hospital. The long-term effects of chronic GVHD are primarily within the realm of the ambulatory, home health, and long-term follow-up nursing staff (Buchsel and Kelleher, 1989; Buchsel, 1986). Standardization of nursing care based on systematic study of effective nursing interventions for GVHD is continuing. Nursing interventions and research focused on appropriate nursing interventions to treat the effects of GVHD is necessary and needs to correspond to the different and varied degrees of the disease until consistent GVHD prevention is a reality.

FUTURE DIRECTIONS

Despite HLA-identical donor/recipient transplants and prophylactic immunosuppressive therapy, GVHD continues to be a significant problem in patients who receive allogeneic bone marrow transplants. In addition, although blood cell transplantation provides rapid hematologic recovery, it is too early to tell if the incidence and severity of GVHD will be worse in these types of transplants.

Tissue Typing

Research directed at improving tissue typing, improving drug prophylaxis, and identifying better ways in which to deplete T cells from marrow inoculum without increasing graft failure is ongoing. Tissue-typing technology now allows successful matching at the molecular level of unrelated individuals. Unfortunately, while this may decrease the incidence and severity of GVHD, it may significantly reduce the potential donor pool (Deeg, 1994).

Pharmacological Treatments

Currently research is examining the efficacy of drugs such as FK506 (Cooper et al., 1994; Fay et al., 1995), thalidomide (Cole et al., 1994), rapamycin (Chang et al., 1991), mycophenolic acid (Dayton et al., 1992), and 15-deoxyspergualin (Yuh and Morris, 1993) in reducing the incidence and severity of GVHD. IL-2 is getting considerable attention in regards to a "protective effect" it may provide. This lymphokine is being examined as a component of posttransplantation prophylaxis (Przepiorka et al., 1994; Szebeni et al., 1994). Other studies are investigating the effects of IL-2-receptor antibody therapy in GVHD prophylaxis (Blaise et al., 1989; Belanger et al., 1993) and chronic GVHD (Blaise et al., 1995). To date, data from the IL-2 receptor antibody studies are providing mixed results.

Selective Cellular Depletion

The depletion of T cells in bone marrow inoculum is the most effective strategy in reducing the incidence of GVHD. However, as mentioned previously, it is also associated with a high risk of graft failure. For this reason, a number of investigators are examining the depletion of selective subsets of lymphocytes (Champlin et al., 1990) as well as other types of putative effector cells (Oluwole et al., 1993).

Ultraviolet Phototherapy

Ultraviolet therapy has been used to modulate accessory cells and T cells in bone marrow inoculum prior to transplantation (Oluwole et al., 1993; Hudson et al., 1994) and as a posttransplantation treatment for cutaneous GVHD (Kapoor et al., 1992). Other studies involve extracorporeal photopheresis, a method by which peripheral leukocytes sensitized by the drug 8-MOP are exposed to ultraviolet A via an extracorporeal flow system (Owsianowski et al., 1994). This study provided encouraging results in the treatment of chronic sclerodermatous GVHD.

SUMMARY

Many research centers are investigating a variety of prophylactic and therapeutic regimens to find the most effective in reducing the incidence of, morbidity from, and mortality from GVHD. As the field of immunology continues to increase its knowledge regarding the effects of cytokines on the immunopathogenesis of GVHD, investigators and clinicians may begin to make significant improvements in immunopharmacological treatments.

Because the occurrence of GVHD continues to afflict approximately half of allogeneic BMT patients and because blood cell transplantation procedures are becoming more widespread, it is critical that nurses working in the area of transplantation understand the etiology and the physiological mechanisms of GVHD, and the temporal sequencing of these pathophysiological events. Furthermore, it is essential that transplant nurses balance their knowledge of the pathophysiology and treatment with a sensitivity to the negative effects that GVHD may have on their patient's body image, self-esteem, and sexuality.

REFERENCES

Abbas, A.K., Lichtman, A.H., Pober, J.S. (Eds.) 1994. Self tolerance and autoimmunity. In *Cellular and Molecular Immunology*, 2d ed. Philadelphia: Saunders, 377-391.

Anasetti, C., Martin, P.J., Storb, R., et al., 1991. Prophylaxis of graft-vs-host disease by administration of the murine anti-IL-2 receptor antibody 2A3. *BMT* 7: 375-381.

Anderson, K.C., Weinstein, H.J. 1990. Transfusion-associated graft-versus-host disease. *N Engl J Med 321:* 56.

Antin, J.H., Bierer, B.E., Smith B.R., et al., 1991. Selective depletion of bone marrow T lymphocyte with anti-CD5 monoclonal antibodies: effective prophylaxis for graft-versus-host disease in patients with hematologic malignancies. *Blood* 78:2139-2149.

Antin, J.H., Ferrara, J.L.M. 1992. Cytokine dysregulation and acute graft-versus-host disease. *Blood* 80(12): 2964-2968.

Aschan, J., Ringden, O., Andstrom, E., et al., 1994. Individualized prophylaxis against graft-versus-host disease in leukemic marrow transplant recipients. *BMT* 14:79-87.

Aschan, J., Ringden, O., Sundberg, B., et al., 1991. Methotrexate combined with cyclosporin A decreases graft-versus-host disease but increases leukemic relapse compared to monotherapy. *BMT* 7:113-119.

Ash, R.C., Horowitz, M.M., Gale, R.P., et al., 1991. Bone marrow transplantation from related donors other than HLA-identical siblings: effect of T cell depletion. *BMT* 7:443-452.

Atkinson, K., Biggs, J.C., Concannon, A., et al., 1988. A prospective randomised trial of cyclosporin versus methotrexate after HLA-identical sibling marrow transplantation for patients with acute leukemia in first remission: analysis 2.5 years after last patient entry. *Aust N Z J Med* 18:594-599.

Atkinson, K., Biggs, J.C., Hayes, J., et al., 1983. Cyclosporin A associated nephrotoxicity in the first 100 days after allogeneic bone marrow transplantation: Three distinct syndromes. *Br J Haematol 54:*59-67.

Backman, L., Ringden, O., Tollemar, J., et al., 1988. An increased risk of relapse in cyclosporin-treated compared with methotrexate-treated patients: long-term follow-up of a randomized trial. *BMT* 3:463-471.

Barrett, A.J., Kendra, J.R., Lucas, C.F., et al., 1982. Cyclosporine A as prophylaxis against graft-versus-host disease in 36 patients. *Br Med J 285:*162-166.

Beatty, P.G., Clift, R.A., Mickelson, E.M., et al., 1985. Marrow transplantation from related donors other than HLA-identical siblings. *N Engl J Med* 313(13):765-771.

Behnke, M.C. 1986. Anorexia. In Carrieri, V.K., Lindsey, A.M., West, C.M., (Eds.) *Pathophysiological Phenomena in Nursing: Human Responses to Illness.* Philadelphia: Saunders, 110-111.

Belanger, C., Esperou-Bourdeau, H., Bordigoni, P., et al., 1993. Use of an anti–interleukin-2 receptor monoclonal antibody for GVHD prophylaxis in unrelated donor BMT. *BMT* 11:293-297.

Biggs, J.C., Atkinson, K., Gillett, E., et al., 1986. A randomized prospective trial comparing cyclosporin and methotrexate given for prophylaxis of graft-versus-host disease after bone marrow transplantation. *Transplant Proc XVIII(2):*253-255.

Billingham, R.E. 1966. The biology of graft-versus-host reactions. In *The Harvey Lectures.* New York: Academic Press, 21-78

Blaise, D., Maraninchi, D., Mawas, C., et al., 1989. Prevention of acute graft-versus-host disease by monoclonal antibody to interleukin-2 receptor. *Lancet* 1: 1333-1334.

Blaise, D., Olive, D., Hirn, M., et al., 1991. Prevention of acute GVHD by in vivo use of anti-interleukin-2 receptor monoclonal antibody (33b3.1): a feasibility trial in 15 patients. *BMT* 8:105-111.

Blaise, D., Olive, D., Michallet, M., et al., 1995. Impairment of leukaemia-free survival by addition of interleukin-2-receptor antibody to standard graft-versus-host prophylaxis. *Lancet* 345:1144-1146.

Brkic, S., Twoi, M.S., Mori, T., et al., 1985. Cellular interactions in marrow-grafted patients: normal interleukin-1 and defective interleukin-2 production in short-term patients and in those with chronic graft-versus-host disease. *Transplantation* 39:30-35.

Buchsel, P.C. 1986. Long-term complications of allogeneic bone marrow transplantation: Nursing implications. *Oncol Nurs Forum* 13(6):61-70.

Buchsel, P.C., Kapustay, P.M. 1995. Peripheral stem cell transplantation. *Oncol Nurs* 2(2):1-14.

Buchsel, P.C., Kelleher, J. 1989. Bone marrow transplantation. *Nurs Clin N Am* 24(4):907-938.

Calissendorff, B., el Azazi, M., Lonnquist, B. 1989. Dry eye syndrome in long-term follow-up of bone marrow transplantation patients. *BMT* 4:675-678.

Caudell, K.A. and Schauer, V. 1989. A dressing used for GVHD skin desquamation. *Oncol Nurs Forum* 16(5): 726.

Champlin, R., Gale, R.P. 1984. The early complications of bone marrow transplantation. *Semin Hematol* 21(2): 101-108.

Champlin, R., Ho, W., Gajewski, J., et al., 1990. Selective depletion of CD8+ lymphocytes for prevention of graft-versus-host disease after allogeneic bone marrow transplantation. *Blood* 76(2):418-423.

Chang, J.Y., Sehgal, S.N., Bansbach, C.C. 1991. FK506 and rapamycin: novel pharmacological probes of the immune response. *Trends Pharmacol Sci* 12:218-223.

Clift, R.A., Buckner, C.D., Appelbaum, F.R., et al., 1990. Allogeneic marrow transplantation in patients with acute myeloid leukemia in first remission: a randomized trial of two irradiation regimens. *Blood* 76(9): 1867-1871.

Cole, C.H., Rogers, P.C.J., Pritchard, S., et al., 1994. Thalidomide in the management of chronic graft-versus-host disease in children following bone marrow transplantation. *BMT* 14:937-942.

Cooper, M.H., Patrene, K.D., Vecchini, F., et al., 1994. Short-term myeloid reconstitution following TBI is not adversely affected by doses of FK506 that abrogate lethal GVHD. *BMT* 14:355-362.

Corson, S.L., Sullivan, K., Batzer, F., et al., 1982. Gynecologic manifestations of chronic graft-versus-host disease. *Obstetr & Gynecol* 60(4):488-492.

Dayton, J.S., Turka, L.A., Thompson, C.B., et al., 1992. Comparison of the effects of mizoribine with those of azathioprine, 6-mercaptopurine and mycophenolic acid on T lymphocyte proliferation and purine ribonucleotide metabolism. *Molecular Pharmacol* 41:671-676.

Deeg, H.J. 1988. Acute graft-versus-host disease. In Deeg, H.J., et al. (Eds.) *A Guide to BMT.* Berlin, Heidelberg: Springer-Verlag, 86-98.

Deeg, H.J. 1994. Prophylaxis and treatment of acute graft-versus-host- disease: current state, implications of new immunopharmacologic compounds and future strategies to prevent and treat acute GVHD in high-risk patients. *BMT 14*(suppl 4):S56-S60.

Deeg, H.J., Storb, R. 1984. Graft-versus-host-disease: pathophysiological and clinical aspects. *Ann Rev Med* 35:11-24.

Deeg, H.J., Storb, R., Thomas, E.D. 1984. Bone marrow transplantation: a review of delayed complications. *Br J Haematol* 57:185-208.

Deeg, H.J., Torok-Storb, B. Storb, R., et al., 1980. Effect of cyclosporin A (CyA) on marrow engraftment in vivo and on hematopoiesis in vitro. *Exp Hematol* 8:78 (abstr 138).

Deisseroth, A.B., Andreeff, M., Champlin, R., et al., 1993. Chronic leukemias. In DeVita, V.T. , Hellman, S., Rosenberg, S.A. (Eds.) *Cancer: Principles and Practice of Oncology,* 4th ed. Philadelphia: Lippincott, 1977.

Doney, K.C., Weiden, P.L., Storb, R., et al., 1981. Treatment of graft-versus-host disease in human allogeneic marrow graft recipients: a randomized trial comparing antithymocyte globulin and corticosteroids. *Am J Hematol* 11:1-8.

Englehard, D., Marks, M.I., and Good, R.A. 1986. Infections in bone marrow transplant recipients. *J Pediatr* 108(3):335-346.

Fay, J.W., Nash, R.A., Wingard, J.R., et al., 1995. FK506-based immunosuppression for prevention of graft-versus-host disease after unrelated donor marrow transplantation. *Transplant Proc* 27(1):1374.

Ferrara, J.L.M., Deeg, H.J. 1991. Mechanisms of disease: graft-versus-host disease. *N Engl J Med* 324(10): 667-674.

Ferrara, J.L.M. 1994. Pardigm shift for graft-versus-host disease. *BMT* 14:183-184.

Fischer, A.C., Ruvolo, P.P., Burt, R., et al., 1995. Characterization of the autoreactive T cell repertoire in cyclosporin-induced syngeneic graft-versus-host disease: a highly conserved repertoire mediates autoaggression. *J Immunol* 154(8):3713-3725.

Ford, R., Ballard, B. 1988. Acute complications after bone marrow transplantation. *Semin Oncol Nurs* 4(10): 15-24.

Fowler, D.H., Kurasawa, K., Smith, R., et al., 1994. Donor CD4-enriched cells of Th2 cytokine phenotype regulate graft-versus-host disease without impairing allogeneic engraftment in sublethally irradiated mice. *Blood* 84(10):3540-3549.

Galati, J.S., Wisecarver, J.L., Quigley, E.M.M. 1993. Inflammatory polyps as a manifestation of intestinal graft versus host disease. *Gastrointestinal Endoscopy* 39(5):719-722.

Gale, R.P., Bortin, M.M., van Bekkum, D.W., et al., 1987. Risk factors for acute graft-versus-host disease. *Br J Haematol* 67:397-406.

Gao, E.K., Lo, D., Cheny, R., et al., 1989. Abnormal differentiation of thymocytes in mice treated with cyclosporin A. *Nature* 336:176-179.

Gauvreau, J.M., Lenssen, P., Cheney, C.L., et al., 1981. Nutritional management of patients with intestinal graft-versus-host disease. *J Am Dietetic Assoc* 79(6):673-677.

Gratwohl, A., Speck, B., Wenk, M., et al., 1983. Cyclosporine in human bone marrow transplantation: serum concentration, graft-versus-host disease, and nephrotoxicity. *Transplantation* 36:40-44.

Grishaber, J.E., Birney, S.M., Strauss, R.G. 1993. Potential for transfusion-associated graft-versus-host disease due to apheresis platelets matched for HLA class I antigens. *Transfusion* 33(11):910-914.

Hale, G., Waldmann, H. 1994. Control of graft-versus-host disease and graft rejection by T cell depletion of donor and recipient with Campath-1 antibodies: results of matched sibling transplants for malignant diseases. *BMT* 13:597-611.

Haus, J.M., Chipping, P.M., Fairhead, S., et al., 1983. Nephrotoxicity in bone marrow transplant recipients treated with cyclosporin A. *Br J Haematol* 54:69-78.

Haus, J., Harris, R., Palmer, S., et al., 1981. Immunosuppression with cyclosporin A in allogeneic bone marrow transplantation for severe aplastic anemia: preliminary studies. *Br J Haematol* 48:227-236.

Holler, E., Kolb, H.J., Hintermeier-Knabe, R., et al., 1993. The role of TNF-alpha in acute graft-versus-host disease and complications following allogeneic bone marrow transplantation. *Transplant Proc* 25:1234-1238.

Holler, E., Kolb, H.J., Moller, A., et al., 1990. Increased serum levels of tumor necrosis factor α precede major complications of bone marrow transplantation. *Blood* 75(4):1011-1016.

Hood, A.F., Vogelsang, G.B., Black, L.P., et al., 1987. Acute graft-vs-host disease: development following autologous and syngeneic bone marrow transplantation. *Arch Dermatol* 123(6):745-750.

Horowitz, M.M., Gale, R.P., Barrett, A.J., et al., 1989. Effect of methotrexate on relapse after bone-marrow transplantation for acute lymphoblastic leukaemia. *Lancet* 1:535-537.

Hudson, J.G., Lawler, M., Pamphilon, D.H. 1994. Ultraviolet irradiation for the prevention of graft-versus-host disease and graft rejection in bone marrow transplantation. *BMT* 14:511-516.

Jenkins, M.K., Schwartz, R.H., and Pardoll, D.M. 1988. Effects of cyclosporin A on T cell development and clonal deletion. *Science* 241:1655-1658.

Jolivet, J., Cowan, K.H., Curt G.A., et al., 1983. The pharmacology and clinical use of methotrexate. *N Engl J Med* 309:1094-1104.

Kapoor, N., Pelligrini, A.E., Copelan, E.A., et al., 1992. Psoralen plus ultraviolet A (PUVA) in the treatment of chronic graft-versus-host disease: preliminary experience in standard treatment-resistant patients. *Semin Hematol* 29(2):108-112.

Kendra, J., Barrett, A.J., Lucas, C., et al., 1981. Response of graft-versus-host disease to high doses of methylprednisolone. *Clin Lab Haematol* 3(1):19-26.

Kennedy, M.S., Yee, G.C., Deeg, H.J., et al., 1983. Pharmacokinetics and toxicity of cyclosporin in marrow transplant patients. *Transplant Proc* 15:2416-2418.

Keown, P.A., Stiller, C.R., Luapacis, A.L., et al., 1982. The effects and side effects of cyclosporin: relationship to drug pharmacokinetics. *Transplant Proc XIV*(4):659-661.

Klemm, P. 1985. Cyclosporin A: use in preventing graft-versus-host disease. *Oncol Nurs Forum* 12(5):25-32.

Klingemann, H.-G. 1988. Chronic graft-versus-host disease. In Deeg, H.G., Klingemann, H.G., Phillips, G.L. (Eds.). *A Guide to Bone Marrow Transplants*. Berlin, Heidelberg: Springer-Verlag, 156-169.

Liedtke, W., Quabeck, K., Beelen, D.W., et al., 1994. Recurrent acute inflammatory demyelinating polyradiculitis after allogeneic bone marrow transplantation. *J Neurol Sci* 125:110-111.

Loughran, T.P. Jr., Deeg, H.J., Dahlberg, S., et al., 1985. Incidence of hypertension after marrow transplantation among 112 patients randomized to either cyclosporin or methotrexate as graft-versus-host disease prophylaxis. *Bri J Haematol* 59:547-553.

Lucas, C.F., Barrett, A.J. 1982. Bone Marrow Transplantation. *Update*, 2403.

McConn, R. 1987. Skin changes following bone marrow transplantation. *Cancer Nurs* 10(2):82-84.

McDonald, G.B., Shulman, H.M., Sullivan, K.M., et al., 1986. Intestinal and hepatic complications of human bone marrow transplantation. *Gastroenterology* 90:460-477 (part I);770-784 (part II).

McDonald, G.B., Sullivan, K.M., Schuffler, M.D., et al., 1981. Esophageal abnormalities in chronic graft-versus-host disease in humans. *Gastroenterology* 80:914-921.

Meyers, J.D., Flournoy, N., Thomas, E.D. 1986. Risk factors for cytomegalovirus infection after human marrow transplantation. *J Infect Dis* 153(3):478-488.

Mitsuyasu, R.T., Champlin, R.E., Gale, R.P., et al. 1986. Treatment of donor bone marrow with monoclonal anti-T cell antibody and complement for the prevention of graft-versus-host disease. *Ann Intern Med* 105:20-26.

Oluwole S.F., Engelstad, K., James, T. 1993. Prevention of graft-versus-host disease and bone marrow rejection:

kinetics of induction of tolerance by UVB modulation of accessory cells and T cells in the bone marrow inoculum. *Blood* 81(6):1658-1665.

Owsianowski, M., Gollnick, H., Siegert, W., et al., 1994. Successful treatment of chronic graft-versus-host disease with extracorporeal photopheresis. *BMT* 14:845-848.

Parker, N., Cohen, T. 1983. Acute graft-versus-host disease in allogeneic marrow transplantation. A nursing perspective. *Nurs Clin N Am* 18(3):569-577.

Paulin T., et al. 1987. Variables predicting bacterial and fungal infections after allogeneic marrow engraftment. *Transplantation* 43(3):393-398.

Postmus, P.E. et al. 1988. Graft-versus-host disease after transfusions of non-irradiated blood cells in patients having received autologous bone marrow: a report of 4 cases following ablative chemotherapy for solid tumors. *Eur J Canc Clin Oncol* 24(5):889-894.

Powles, R.L., Clink, H.M., Spence, D., et al., 1980. Cyclosporin A to prevent graft-versus-host disease in man after allogeneic bone marrow transplntation. *Lancet* 1(8164):327-329.

Przepiorka, D., Ippoliti, C., Koberda, J., et al., 1994. Interleukin-2 for prevention of graft-versus-host disease after haploidentical marrow transplantation. *Transplantation* 58(7):858-860.

Quiquandon, I., Janin, A., Noel-Walter, M.P., et al., 1994. Cytomegalovirus expression in minor salivary glands and chronic graft-versus-host disease. *BMT* 14:31-35.

Ralph, d.D., et al. 1984. Rapidly progressive airflow obstruction in marrow transplant recipients. *Am Rev Resp Dis* 129:641-644.

Ramsay, N.K.C., Kersey, J.H., Robinson, L.L., et al., 1982. A randomized study of the prevention of acute graft-versus-host disease. *N Engl J Med,* 306:392-397.

Ringden, O., Horowitz, M.M., Sondel, P., et al., 1993. Methotrexate, cyclosporin or both to prevent graft-versus-host disease after HLA-identical sibling bone marrow transplants for early leukemia? *Blood* 81:1094-1101.

Russell, J.A., Woodman, R.C., Poon, M.-C., et al., 1994. Addition of low-dose folinic acid to a methotrexate/cyclosporin A regimen for prevention of acute graft-versus-host disease. *BMT* 14:397-401.

Sale, G.E., Shulman, H.M., Shubert, M.M., et al., 1981. Oral and ophthalmic pathology of graft-versus-host disease in man: predictive value of lip biopsy. *Hum Pathol* 12:1022-1030.

Schubert, M.M., Sullivan, K.M. 1990. Recognition, incidence, and management of oral graft-versus-host disease. *NCI Monogr* 9:135-143.

Shulman, H.M. Sullivan, K.M. 1988. Graft-versus-host disease: allo- and autoimmunity after bone marrow transplantation. *Concepts in Immunopathology* 6:141-165.

Shulman, H.M., Sullivan, K.M., Weiden, P.L., et al., 1980. Chronic graft-versus-host syndrome in man: a long-term clinicopathological study of 20 Seattle patients. *Am J Med* 69:204-217.

Singhal, S., Mehta, J., Rattenbury, H., et al., 1995. Oral pilocarpine hydrochloride for the treatment of refractory xerostomia assicated with chronic graft-versus-host disease. *Blood* 85(4):1147-1148.

Storb, R., Deeg, H.J., Fisher, L., et al., 1988. Cyclosporine vs. methotrexate for graft-versus-host disease prevention in patients given marrow grafts for leukemia: long-term follow-up of three controlled trials. *Blood* 71(2):293-298.

Storb, R., Deeg, H.J., Pepe, M., et al., 1992. Long-term follow-up of three controlled trials comparing cyclosporin versus methotrexate for graft-versus-host disease prevention in patients given marrow grafts for leukemia. *Blood* 79(11):3091-3098.

Storb, R., Deeg, H.J., Thomas, E.D., et al., 1985. Marrow transplantation for chronic myelocytic leukemia: a controlled trial of cyclosporin versus methotrexate for prophylaxis of graft-versus-host disease. *Blood* 66:698-702.

Storb, R., Deeg, H.J., Whitehead, J., et al., 1986. Methotrexate and cyclosporin compared with cyclosporin alone for prophylaxis of acute graft-versus-host disease after marrow transplantation for leukemia. *N Engl J Med* 314(12):729-735.

Storb, R., Prentice R.L., Buckner, C.D., et al., 1983. Graft-versus-host disease and survival in patients with aplastic anemia treated by marrow grafts from HLA-identical siblings: beneficial effects of a protective environment. *N Engl J Med* 308:302-307.

Sullivan, K.M. 1983. Graft-versus-host disease. In Blume, K.G., Petz, L.D. (Eds.) *Clinical Bone Marrow Transplantation.* New York: Churchill Livingstone, 98-101.

Sullivan, K.M. 1985. Special care of the bone marrow transplant patient. In Wiernik, P.H., et al. (Eds.) *Neoplastic Diseases of the Blood.* New York: Churchill Livingstone, 1124-1129.

Sullivan, K.M. 1986. Acute and chronic graft-versus-host disease in man. *Int J Cell Cloning* 4:42-93.

Sullivan K.M., Kopecky, K.J., Jocom, J., et al., 1990. Immunomodulatory and antimicrobial efficacy of intravenous immunoglobulin in bone marrow transplantation. *N Engl J Med* 323:705-712.

Sullivan, K.M., Shulman, H.M., Storb, R., et al., 1981a. Chronic graft-versus-host disease in 52 patients: adverse natural course and successful treatment with combination immunosuppression. *Blood* 57(2):267-276.

Sullivan, K.M., et al., 1981b. Day 100 screening studies predict development of chronic graft-versus-host disease. *Blood* 58:176a (abstr).

Sullivan, K.M., et al., 1982. Preliminary analysis of a randomized trial of immunosuppressive therapy of chronic graft-versus-host disease. *Blood* 60:173a (abstr).

Szebeni, J., Wang, M.G., Pearson, D.A., et al., 1994. IL-2 inhibits early increases in serum gamma interferon levels associated with graft-versus-host disease. *Transplantation* 58(12):1385-1393.

Thomas, E.D. 1988. The future of marrow transplantations. *Sem Oncol Nurs* 4(1):74-78.

Truog, A.W., Wozniak, S.P. 1990. Cyclosporin A as prevention for graft-versus-host disease in pediatric patients undergoing bone marrow transplants. *Oncol Nurs Forum* 17(1):39-44.

Tsoi, M.S. 1982. Immunological mechanisms of graft-versus-host disease in man. *Transplantation* 13:459.

Vogelsang, G.B., Farmer, E.R., Hess, A.D., et al., 1992. Thalidomide for the treatment of chronic graft-versus-host disease. *N Engl J Med* 326:1055-1058.

von Bueltzingsloewen, A., Belanger, R., Perreault, C., et al., 1993. Acute graft-versus-host disease prophylaxis with methotrexate and cyclosporin after busulfan and cyclophosphamide in patients with hematologic malignancies. *Blood* 81:849-855.

Weaver, C.H., Clift, R.A., Deeg, H.J., et al., 1994. Effect of graft-versus-host disease prophylaxis on relapse in patients transplanted for acute myeloid leukemia. *BMT* 14:885-893.

Weiden, P.L., Flournoy, N, Thomas, E.D., et al., 1979. Antileukemic effect of chronic graft-versus-host disease in human recipients of allogeneic marrow grafts. *N Engl J Med* 300(19):1068-1073.

Weisdorf, D., Haake, R., Blazar, B., et al., 1990. Treatment of moderate/severe acute graft-versus-host disease after allogeneic bone marrow transplantation: an analysis of clinical risk features and outcome. *Blood* 75(4):1024-1030.

Wingard, J.R., Piantadosi, S., Vogelsang, G.B., et al., 1989. Predictors of death from chronic graft-versus-host disease after bone marrow transplantation. *Blood* 74(4):1428-1435.

Yee, G.C., Self, S.G., McGuire, T.R., et al., 1988. Serum cyclosporin concentration and risk of acute graft-versus-host disease after allogeneic marrow transplantation. *N Engl J Med* 319(2):65-70.

Yuh, D.D., Morris, R.E. 1993. The immunopharmacology of immunosuppression by 15-deoxyspergualin. *Transplantation* 55:578-591.

9

Hematologic Effects of Transplantation

Frances Walker, Shelley Burcat

Hematopoietic dysfunction is a major complication of bone marrow and blood cell transplantation. Patients undergoing a transplantation receive radiotherapy and/or chemotherapy as part of the conditioning regimen. These treatments eradicate hematopoietic functioning, resulting in profound pancytopenia and immune dysfunction (Schuening et al., 1994).

During the time of pancytopenia, patients are at risk for complications such as infection and bleeding. The greater the degree and the longer the duration of pancytopenia, the greater the associated morbidity and mortality. Neutropenia may last for 2 or 3 weeks after bone marrow and blood cell transplant (Hiemenz and Greene, 1993). Neutrophil defects persist for months after engraftment (Lazarus and Rowe, 1994).

Nurses must be knowledgeable about hematologic side effects of transplantation. Assessments should be done for anticipated as well as unexpected reactions (Ford and Eisenberg, 1990). Appropriate nursing interventions can minimize or eliminate complications. This chapter provides an overview of common hematologic complications associated with bone marrow transplantation (BMT) and blood cell transplantation (BCT).

HEMATOLOGIC EFFECTS

Leukopenia and Neutropenia

In patients who receive transplants, treatment-related factors produce profound leukopenia, or a decrease in the number of circulating white blood cells to fewer than 100 cells per microliter (μl) (Lin, 1993). High-dose chemotherapy causes both neutropenia and lymphopenia. Severe neutropenia, defined as fewer than 500 neutrophils/μl, usually lasts for 2 to 4 weeks after the conditioning (Caudell and Whedon, 1991). Lymphopenia, which is a decrease in the number of lymphocytes in the blood, also results from the high-dose regimen. Stem cells and immature neutrophils and lymphocytes in the process of differentiation are the most sensitive to the effects of chemotherapy.

Total body irradiation is also used to ablate marrow function in BMT patients. Radiation causes bone marrow supression due to the inclusion in the radiation field of active sites of bone marrow (skull, sternum, ribs, vertebrae, pelvis, and long bones). Radiation therapy destroys stem cells, therefore the duration of neutropenia is prolonged. The patterns of neutropenia seen with chemotherapy may be exaggerated or prolonged when radiation therapy is administered prior to or during chemotherapy. In addition, certain marrow-purging techniques interfere with hematopoietic function, resulting in prolongation of the neutropenic recovery period (Schafer, 1993). Graft failure or graft rejection also decreases the chance of bone marrow recovery and increases the risk of graft-versus-host disease and superinfections with antibiotic-resistant pathogens (Schafer, 1993).

Other factors also complicate neutropenia in some transplant patients. Protein-calorie malnutrition is associated with the gastrointestinal side effects of chemotherapy and radiation therapy; the effects include anorexia, taste alterations, stomatitis, esophagitis, nausea, vomiting, and diarrhea. Disruption of the integrity of the skin or mucous membranes as well as failure to provide an adequate protective environment may also complicate the neutropenic period by predisposing the patient to infection (Caudell and Whedon, 1991). The immunosuppressive effects of steroids can also predispose a patient to complications during the neutropenic period by inhibiting the inflammatory response and by causing impaired cell-mediated immunity and protein-calorie malnutrition through increased catabolism (Schafer, 1993).

Infection occurs when the body or a specific anatomical site is invaded by pathogenic microbes (bacteria, viruses, protozoa, fungi, or yeast) that have the ability to multiply under favorable conditions and cause cellular injury or destruction (Schafer, 1993). Infections related to marrow aplasia, immunosuppressive therapy, and delay or failure of immune reconstitution following transplantation are a major cause of morbidity and mortality. The risk of infection in transplant patients is divided into three phases: (1) the pre-engraftment phase, (2) the early postengraftment phase, and (3) the late postengraftment phase. The predominant host problem during the pre-engraftment phase (within 30 days after transplantation) is neutropenia (Wujcik et al., 1994). The infections most commonly seen at this time are bacterial and fungal, similar to those seen in neutropenic patients with leukemia (Shaffer and Wilson, 1993).

Bacterial Infections

The combination of neutropenia and altered mucosal barriers allows easy entry of gram-negative bacteria into the systemic circulation (Wingard, 1990a; Caudell and Whedon, 1991). Sites frequently infected include the lungs, urinary tract, skin wounds, intravenous or indwelling catheter sites, the perianal and rectal area, the pharynx, and the mouth (Rostad, 1991). The standard treatment of infections is to initiate at the first sign of fever empirical broad-spectrum antibiotic therapy with a cephalosporin and a penicillin (Wade, 1992). The third-generation cephalosporins protect against gram-negative aerobic organisms and provide some gram-positive coverage (Allan, 1987). Infection prophylaxis with a fluoroquinolone such as ciprofloxacin or ofloxacin is now standard therapy. This provides coverage against gram-positive and gram-negative organisms and preserves normal gastrointestinal flora (Feld, 1989). The fluoroquinolones can be administered orally or intravenously and have broad-spectrum activity against aerobic gram-negative organisms. Fluoroquinolones are usually well tolerated and when given prophylactically have demonstrated reduced gram-negative infections (Feld, 1989; Maiche, 1991).

Gram-positive infections are prevalent with the use of indwelling central venous catheters. The most common organism is *Staphylococcus epidermitis* (Wingard, 1990b; Caudell and Whedon, 1991). Because many are resistant to methicillin, vancomycin is administered both prophylactically and for treatment (Armstrong, 1991).

Fungal Infections

Fungal infections occur as a result of broad-spectrum antibiotic use. Overgrowth of fungi leads to penetration of damaged mucosa and systemic infection. Infection with the candida species is common (Wujcik et al., 1994). Infection with *Candida albicans* occurs more frequently but is less virulent than *candida tropicalis*. The latter occurs less frequently but is associated with a more serious infection. Amphotericin B is administered intravenously (IV) for persistent fever after 5 to 7 days of broad-spectrum antibiotic coverage. Amphotericin B is very toxic, causing fever, rigors, and nephrotoxicity. Clinical trials of a liposomal formulation are in progress in the hope of finding a less toxic formulation that is equally efficacious (Tollemar et al., 1993; de Marie, 1996).

More recently, imidazoles are being used for prophylaxis of fungal infections. Imidazoles are antifungal agents that block enzymes required for synthesis of the cell membrane. Fluconizole is used for prophylaxis of the candida organism (Wingard, 1990a). Oral nystatin and ketoconazole are useful in treating oral candida but have not proved useful against systemic infection (Armstrong, 1991).

The risk of infection with *Aspergillus* increases with the duration of neutropenia (Wingard et al., 1988). The portal of entry is the repiratory tract and pulmonary invasion is the most life-threatening infection. *Aspergillus* infections require confirmation with tissue culture. In the past this was accomplished with open lung biopsy or bronchoscopy. Rapid diagnosis can now be achieved with bronchial lavage (Wujcik et al., 1994). Amphotericin B in dosages of 1 mg/kg per day IV is the only effective treatment (Wingard et al., 1988).

Viral Infections

If viral infection does occur, reactivation of latent virus is the most common cause. Herpes viruses include herpes simplex virus (HSV) types I and II, cytomegalovirus (CMV), and varicella-zoster (VZ). Without therapy with acyclovir, 70% to 80% of seropositive patients experience infection (Wingard, 1990; Sugar, 1990; Klastersky, 1992). In the pre-engraftment period, infections of HSV type I are manifested by oral ulcerative mucositis, and type II reactivation appears as genital or extragenital vesicles. Because oral ulceration is a common side effect of chemotherapy and irradiation, a viral culture is necessary to distinguish viral etiology. Although acyclovir is highly effective when given as prophylaxis and treatment, there is evidence of an increasing frequency of acyclovir-resistant herpes viruses (McLauren et al., 1985; Englund et al., 1990). Therefore, other antiviral agents may be indicated (Safrin et al., 1991; Verdonck, 1993).

At 30 to 100 days posttransplant (the early postengraftment phase), patients are at risk for infection from viruses, principally cytomegalovirus and herpes simplex, and intracellular organisms such as mycobacteria, fungi, and protozoa (Wingard, 1990b; Winston and Gale, 1991). Illness may be the result of a new infection in seronegative patients or represent reactivation in a seropositive patient. These infections are related to deficient cell-mediated immunity. Neutrophil recovery has usually occurred by this time. Immunologic recovery is related to delayed recovery of the immune system or to immunosuppressive therapy, and/or to acute graft-versus-host disease (GVHD) in allogeneic patients (Atkinson, 1990; Wingard, 1990b).

Patients are also at risk for interstitial pneumonia (IP) during this time (McFadden, 1992). Interstitial pneumonia is the most common cause of death in the first 100 days after

BMT, and the most common cause of IP is CMV. CMV infection can be transmitted from the donated marrow in the allogeneic setting or from infected blood products. Factors that increase risk include prior infection, GVHD, increasing age, and histoincompatibility. Although CMV infection can be asymptomatic, clinical manifestations include fever, hepatitis, pancytopenia, retinitis, enteritis, and pneumonitis (Wujcik et al., 1994).

The use of CMV-negative blood products is indicated in patients who are CMV negative. To prevent reactivation of viral infection, high-dose acyclovir (500 mg/m^2 every 8 hours) is given to patients who are HSV and or CMV positive before transplant (Schimpff, 1992). Gancyclovir is more active than acyclovir when treating CMV. Prophylactic gancyclovir is indicated in patients who are shedding CMV (Wingard, 1990a). The combination of gancyclovir and IV immunoglobulin has been shown to resolve CMV pneumonitis (Reed et al., 1988).

Parasitic Infections

In the past, patients were at risk for *Pneumocystis carinii* pneumonia. This has been virtually eliminated with prophylactic trimethoprim-sulfamethoxazole, which is initiated at the time of engraftment and continues until recovery of the immune system. Because the drug has some myelosuppressive activity, it cannot be administered any sooner in the BMT process (Wingard, 1990).

In the late postengraftment phase, infections in bone marrow transplant patients are associated with a prolonged defect in humoral immunity, most frequently seen in patients with chronic graft-versus-host disease and increasing immunosuppressive drug therapy. Infecting organisms include pyrogenic bacteria such as *Pneumococcus* (Wujcik et al., 1994), *Streptococcus pneumoniae*, and *Haemophilus influenzae* (Deeg and Storb, 1986). There is also reac-

tivation of varicella zoster in up to 50% of patients. Patients are maintained on an oral antibiotic and acyclovir to reduce the risk of these infections (Wujcik et al., 1994).

Anemia

The intense antineoplastic regimens used in BMT create a deficiency in circulating red blood cells (anemia). Chemotherapy creates a hypoproliferative anemia because of its effects on the bone marrow. In addition, radiation therapy results in a decrease in production of red blood cells (RBCs) when certain treatment fields (pelvis, sternum, proximal ends of long bones) are included (Clark, Landis, McGee, 1987). Anemia is indicated by a reduction in the hemoglobin level and hematocrit value. The effects of anemia include fatigue and dyspnea during exertion, as well as headaches, dizziness, and irritability. As the anemia becomes more severe, tachycardia, tachypnea, hypotension, and tissue hypoxia can occur (Maxwell, 1984; Goodman, 1989).

Most transplant programs suggest maintaining hematocrit levels of 25% to 30%. The majority of the RBCs transfused are required in the first 4 weeks following BMT. Most increases in RBC transfusion requirements are due to ABO-incompatible transplants, which often result in delayed engraftment (Slichter, 1994). The only other factor that has been shown to increase transfusion requirements in the bone marrow transplant population is increased age (Wulff et al., 1983).

A variety of techniques, including RBC antigen phenotyping and cytogenetic analysis, have been used to distinguish between a host or donor source forerythrocyte repopulation following allogeneic BMT (Bar et al., 1989). This information can be useful when attempting to distinquish engraftment of donor marrow and regeneration of host marrow. If the RBCs are of host origin, it may be due to an inadequate conditioning regimen and may result in disease relapse (Caudell and Whedon, 1991). Return of normal hematopoiesis is generally first evidenced by the appearance of reticulocytes in the circulation (Griffin, 1986).

The reticulocyte maturation index (RMI), which has been used to study erythropoiesis, is another measurement of engraftment in autologous transplants and has been shown to detect engraftment sooner than the reticulocyte or the erythrocyte count. The RMI is a proportional measurement of reticulocyte maturity determined by the content of reticulocyte RNA using flow cytometric reticulocyte quantification with thiazole orange (Caudell and Whedon, 1991).

Thrombocytopenia

Thrombocytopenia is an abnormal decrease in the number of circulating platelets and usually results in bleeding or hemorrhage. Platelets are critical to the process of hemostasis. They ensure the continued maintenance of vascular integrity, the initial arrest of bleeding by platelet plug formation, and the stabilization of clot formation (Bennett and Shattil, 1990). When thrombocytopenia is present, the most frequent sites of bleeding are the mucous membranes, skin, gastrointestinal system, respiratory system, genitourinary system, and the intracranial area. Thrombocytopenia results when there is a decrease in the production of megakaryocytes, which are precursors of platelets. This can occur in transplant patients as a result of the toxic effects of chemotherapy on stem cells. Radiation therapy to the active sites of bone marrow function (skull, ribs, sternum, vertebrae, pelvis, and ends of long bones) can also result in a decreased platelet count (Petursson, 1993).

When the platelet count falls below $20,000/mm^3$, spontaneous hemorrhaging is a major clinical concern and bruising, petechiae, and mucosal bleeding may be detectable. There is a strong association between intracranial bleeding and a platelet count of less than $5000/mm^3$ (Rostad, 1991).

Megakaryocyte colony-stimulating activity (Meg-CSA) or growth-promoting activity (Meg-GPA) after BMT have been measured to determine their relationships to megakaryocyte engraftment and platelet count after BMT (Adams et al., 1990; de Alarcon et al., 1988; Fauser et al., 1988). There is a biphasic increase in Meg-CSA after BMT, starting with an initial peak following the marrow conditioning program, a gradual decline, and then a second peak approximately 2 weeks after BMT (de Alarcon et al., 1988). The initial peak was seen in all 23 study patients and was postulated to be due to tissue injury from the conditioning program with release of stored Meg-CSA. However, the second peak was seen only in patients who engrafted (Fauser et al., 1988). These factors remain under investigation for clinical usefulness. Persistent and prolonged thrombocytopenia can indicate a worse overall prognosis (First et al., 1988; de Alarcon et al., 1988).

IMMUNOHEMATOLOGIC COMPLICATIONS

Considerable evidence supports the hypothesis that normal hematopoiesis depends on the interaction of the immune system and the hematopoietic system (Mangan, 1987a, 1987b). In addition to intrinsic failure of the hematopoietic system to function, normal hematopoiesis following transplantation may be adversely affected by (1) failure of the immune system to provide the normal physiologic stimuli for hematopoiesis and (2) active suppression of hematopoiesis by the immune system (Klumpp, 1991).

Several hypotheses have been proposed to explain the development of adverse interactions between an immune system and a hematopoietic system that were previously interacting normally. The first applies only to allogeneic transplantation. It is well established that in most patients, the engrafted immune and hematopoietic systems are of donor origin following BMT (Roy et al., 1990; Sparkes et al., 1979; Ginsburg et al., 1985). However, unlike the situation in solid organ transplant, the recipient immune and/or hematopoietic systems may linger for weeks or months following transplantation of the donor marrow (Bensinger et al., 1982; Barge et al., 1989). Therefore two separate immune systems and two separate hematopoietic systems can coexist in a single host. It is therefore not surprising that mismatches in the ABO and other alloantigen systems can lead to adverse interactions (Klumpp, 1991).

A second hypothesis that applies to both allogeneic and autologous transplantation is that regulatory elements of the immune system are damaged during the transplant process itself. There is evidence that the pretransplant regimen may predispose the development of autoimmunity directed against hematopoietic elements (Minchinton et al., 1984; Chapman et al., 1986).

There is a third hypothesis for which a paucity of supporting data exists. This hypothesis states that certain immunologically relevant surface antigens on hematopoietic cells may be transiently or permanently altered as a result of the transplant process itself (Minchinton et al., 1984).

It is important to clarify the terms *alloimmune* and *autoimmune* when discussing immunohematologic complications of bone marrow transplantation. Both host-versus-donor and donor-versus-host interactions are described as alloimmune. Autoimmune applies to host-versus-host and donor-versus-donor reactions (Klumpp, 1991).

Graft Failure

Graft failure is the lack of functional hematopoiesis after marrow transplantation. Primary graft failure is the failure to establish hematopoiesis, and the causes may be multifactorial. In autologous transplants, this may be due to inadequate volume or quality of stem cells, which is possibly related to prior treatment, damage during collection or cryopreservation. In allogeneic transplants, graft failure is especially common with the use of HLA-mismatched donor marrow or with transplantation of T-cell–depleted marrow. The latter suggests that the donor immune system may be capable of reducing host-derived host-versus-graft immunity (Klumpp, 1991). In the absence of myelosuppressive drug therapy or infectious complications, primary graft failure should be attributed to rejection of the marrow allograft by residual immunocompetent cells in the patient (Filipovich, 1990; Anasetti et al., 1989; Kernan et al., 1987).

Secondary graft failure or graft rejection is the failure of functional hematopoiesis after the occurrence of transient hematopoiesis. This can be due to myelosuppression from medications or infections, but is often rejection mediated by immunological factors (Kernan, 1988). Classically, the transient hematopoiesis that characterizes graft rejection is of donor-derived marrow. This is followed by an increase in the number of lymphocytes from the cells of host origin, and either failure of all hematopoietic activity or the return of host hematopoiesis (Quinones, 1993).

In the past, there was 30% incidence of graft failure in genotypically matched patients with aplastic anemia who had been transfused multiple times (Champlin et al., 1989). The problem of graft rejection in this population has been overcome by the development of improved strategies of increased immunosuppression including radiation (total body irradiation or total lymphoid irradiation), infusion of donor immunocompetent cells, and in vivo anti–T-cell therapy (Storb et al., 1987).

It is often not possible to distinguish true graft rejection from intrinsic graft failure since the two are so closely related. Another clinically similar syndrome is post-BMT autoimmune pancytopenia. Although rare, the latter syndrome is important to recognize because it may respond well to treatment with corticosteroids (Klumpp et al., 1990).

Therapy for graft rejection is limited by difficulty in recognizing the complication in its early stages because delayed engraftment can also be caused by infection and drug toxicity. The fragility of the new marrow, and the lack of effective agents to prevent rejection also complicate treatment (Quinones, 1993). At present, therapy for graft rejection is based on the use of corticosteroids and ATG (antithymocyte globulin) or other in vivo anti–T-cell serotherapy (Kernan et al., 1989). Hematopoietic growth factors are also employed for this purpose. Attempts to reconstitute hematopoiesis in patients after graft rejection are of limited success and require additional cytoreduction with chemotherapy and radiation (Kernan et al., 1989).

MANAGEMENT OF THE BMT PATIENT WITH MYELOSUPPRESSION

Neutropenia

Prevention, early detection, and prompt management of infections in patients with neutropenia are essential if sepsis and septic shock are to be avoided. An absolute granulocyte count greater than 500 is generally achieved within 2 weeks after a bone marrow transplant (Whedon, 1991). It is important to be aware of some of the factors that place bone marrow transplant patients at a particularly high risk for infection. These risk factors include:

1. hematologic or lymphoid malignancy
2. previous treatment with high dose chemotherapy and/or radiation
3. type of preparative treatment
4. prolonged neutropenia and immune deficiency
5. graft-versus-host disease (GVHD) and immunosuppressive therapy to prevent and/or treat acute or chronic GVHD
6. altered mucosal barriers
7. microorganism colonization
8. prolonged use of antibiotics (Paulin et al., 1987; Buchsel, 1990).

A thorough assessment is vital when patients are at risk for infection. A comprehensive physical assessment is performed at least every 4 to 8 hours, with special attention to catheter sites, lungs, integument, oral mucosa, and the rectal area. Special attention is given to signs and symptoms of infection at common sites of occurrence. Temperature and vital signs are assessed for trends and deviations from normal at least every 4 hours during the immediate post-BMT phase. A complete blood count and absolute neutrophil count is obtained daily (Caudell and Whedon, 1991). Finally, immunoglobulin (IG) levels are evaluated before IV administration of IG (Mangan et al., 1991).

Infection can be prevented or at least minimized if the nurse implements various protective interventions. People who have or might have a communicable infection should be screened from contact with a neutropenic patient. The patient with neutropenia should avoid crowds and should wear an isolation mask when out of the protective environment (Rostad, 1991).

Protective Isolation

A variety of techniques may be employed to protect patients from nosocomial microbial flora. These techniques range from simple protective precautions to total protective environments (Rostad, 1991). The type of protective isolation depends on the philosophy of the transplant center.

A *total protective environment* is achieved by several means, including laminar air flow rooms, with sterilization of the entire room and its contents and of every item brought into the room, and low-microbial diets. Oral nonabsorbable antibiotics can be used to decontaminate the patient, as can skin antiseptics, antibiotic sprays, and ointments (Hawthorne and Pizzo, 1989). A private room that includes a sterile patient zone separated from an anteroom by a transparent curtain is necessary. Air and water cultures are usually done weekly. Indirect patient care (e.g., infusion of IV solutions and blood, oral medication, diet) is performed through the curtain. Direct patient care such as physical assessment, treatments, and vital signs are performed inside the sterile patient zone. The required attire by the caraegiver may include masks, head covers, gowns, gloves, and shoe covers. There is also high efficiency particle air (HEPA) filtration with continuous horizontal or positive-pressure air flow (Caudell and Whedon, 1991; ONS, 1994).

Strict protective isolation also requires a private room, routine air and water cultures, and HEPA and/or positive air pressure. Meticulous hand washing is required prior to entering the unit, upon entering the patient's room, and after leaving the patient's room. Direct and indirect nursing care is provided at the bedside. The required attire varies among centers and may include masks, gloves, head covers, gowns, and shoe covers (Caudell and Whedon, 1991; ONS, 1994).

Simple protective isolation is generally the same protocol as strict protective isolation. The only variation is that masks, gowns and/or gloves may not be worn (Caudell and Whedon, 1991; ONS, 1994). It is important to promote meticulous personal hygiene as part of infection

control. Skin decontamination with antimicrobial soap is helpful. It is also essential to promote meticulous oral and perineal hygiene, although solutions and protocols vary among centers (ONS, 1994).

Oral cavity assessment should be performed a minimum of once per shift. An assessment tool that measures the appearance as well as the level of function of the oral cavity should be used (Beck, 1993; Eilers, Berger, Peterson, 1988; Kolbinson et al., 1988; Western Consortium for Cancer Nursing Research, 1991). The frequency of oral care is based on the grade of stomatitis. When the goal is to prevent stomatitis, after meals and at bedtime is the recommended frequency for oral care. For mild to moderate stomatitis, every 2 hours while awake and every 6 hours during the night is the usual frequency. If severe stomatitis should develop, oral care needs to be done every 2 hours during the day and every 4 hours at night (Goodman and Stoner, 1991). Topical analgesics/antifungals/cryoprotective agents are used for mild to moderate stomatitis (Epstein, 1990). Systemic analgesics are used for severe stomatitis (ONS, 1994).

The care of the BMT patient also involves administering and monitoring the patient's response to antifungal, antiviral, and antibacterial prophylaxis and treatment. Important areas of assessment include

- vital signs
- intake and output
- BUN and creatinine
- liver function tests
- complete blood count
- electrolytes
- hearing
- respiratory status (ONS, 1994).

Nurses caring for patients with absent or very low white blood cell counts play a vital role in their outcomes. Nursing interventions aimed at decreasing or eliminating the likelihood of infection must be an essential part of the daily care of the BMT patient.

Since it is common for pathogens to invade the respiratory tract, the use of the respiratory incentive spirometer should be encouraged and breath sounds should be assessed at least every 4 hours. Central venous catheters and any other externally placed tubes need meticulous care on a daily basis. It is also essential to avoid unnecessary invasive procedures such as enemas, rectal temperatures, bladder catheterizations, and finger sticks for blood sampling. Viral, fungal, and bacterial cultures are to be obtained in a timely fashion according to the protocol of the transplant center. Nursing assistance in obtaining other diagnostic tests is helpful in ensuring their completion as well as in adhering to precautions against infections. CMV-negative blood products should be administered to seronegative BMT recipients. A low bacterial or sterile diet must be maintained according to institutional protocol. Vaccines such as pneumovax, flu, tetanus, DPT, and MMR should be admininstered at appropriate times; however, it is essential that BMT patients avoid individuals who have received live virus vaccines during the first year post transplant (Lum, 1990). Fresh flowers and uncooked fruits and vegetables are to be avoided in patients' rooms. Patients and families need education about signs and symptoms of infection as well as prophylaxis and treatment (ONS, 1994).

Bleeding

Bleeding and anemia also require prompt attention and skill in order to prevent life-threatening emergencies. The preparative regimens used in transplantation often result in profound thrombocytopenia and anemia. Platelet engraftment is delayed in patients who develop GVHD (First et al., 1985), those on cy-

closporin (Bensinger, 1989), and those whose marrow has been purged (Ball et al., 1990; Korbling et al., 1989). The administration of myelosuppressive medications such as methotrexate, trimethoprim-sulfamethoxazone, gancyclovir, and interferon also contributes to poor graft function and the resulting thrombocytopenia and anemia (Storb, 1989). Coagulation abnormalities resulting from hepatotoxicity, GVHD, disseminated intravascular coagulation (DIC), and/or sepsis may also contribute to abnormal bleeding (ONS, 1994). Other risk factors include veno-occlusive disease with impaired production of coagulation factors (Ballard, 1991), altered mucosal barriers (Vanacek, 1991), viral infections (Cahn, 1989), and ABO incompatible allogeneic BMT (Petz, 1989).

The nursing management of patients at risk for bleeding begins with a thorough assessment for signs or symptoms of bleeding. Laboratory data including red blood cell count, hemoglobin, hematocrit, platelet count, and coagulation studies are closely monitored at least daily. Bleeding episodes can be minimized by the avoidance of unnecessary invasive procedures such as enemas, rectal temperatures, suppositories, bladder catheterizations, venipunctures, finger sticks, nasogastric tubes, and intramuscular or subcutaneous injections. Medications that inhibit platelet function such as aspirin-containing products are also to be avoided (ONS, 1994).

Blood Product Support

The administration of blood products to transplant recipients is another essential component of their daily care during the first few weeks after transplant. It is imperative that nurses possess a thorough understanding of the rationale behind the administration of each specific blood product as well as the special considerations required for administration.

Because viable lymphocytes, which are thought to be capable of triggering GVHD, are present in all cellular transfusion products, irradiation is recommended in order to inactivate T lymphocytes (Petz and Scott, 1983). The usual dose of gamma radiation is between 1.5 and 3.0 Gy (1500–3000 cGy) (Petz, 1989). Although transfusion-induced GVHD can occur in both allogeneic (Petz, 1989) and autologous patients (Postmus et al., 1988), it does occur more frequently with lesser degrees of match. Leukocyte-reduction filters are used for PRBCs and platelets to reduce exposure to HLA antigens (Sniecinski et al., 1988) and prevent adverse reactions as a result of the transfusions (Caudell and Whedon, 1991). CMV serologically tested negative blood products are given to patients who are CMV serologically negative. Because the virus is carried on the granulocyte, the risk of CMV infection may increase if CMV-postive products are used (Bowden et al., 1991; Petz and Scott, 1983).

Red blood cells (RBCs) are administered over 2 to 4 hours to patients with symptomatic anemia due to blood loss. It is expected that one unit of packed RBCs will increase the patient's hemoglobin to 1 gm/dl above the pretransfusion hemoglobin. It is important for RBCs to be ABO compatible. Leucocyte-poor or filtered RBCs are given to patients at risk for febrile transfusion reactions.

Platelets from random donors are given over 5 to 10 minutes per unit for bleeding due to thrombocytopenia. ABO compatibility is not required for platelet transfusions. It is worth noting that random donor platelets are not usually effective for BMT recipients who have received many prior platelet transfusions.

Platelets from a single donor are given over 20 to 60 minutes in order to increase the platelet count to 40,000 per unit. Single-donor platelets are given to patients who are bleeding due to thrombocytopenia and who possess antiplatelet antibodies. Single-donor platelets may be random or HLA matched. HLA-matched platelet products are indicated if a patient's platelet count failed to increase after multiple transfusions. Patients who receive multiple transfusions may develop lymphocytotoxic anti-HLA antibodies and platelet refractoriness (Fuller, 1990).

Fresh frozen plasma, which contains plasma, all coagulation factors, and complement, is given over 10 to 15 minutes. Coagulation factors are increased by 5% to 10% per unit. It is given for a coagulation factor deficiency or for disseminated intravascular coagulation (DIC). ABO compatibility is necessary when transfusing fresh frozen plasma.

Cryoprecipitate contains plasma and stable clotting factors. It is given over 15 to 30 minutes and increases factor VIII, factor XIII, and fibrinogen levels. It is given to treat deficiencies of stable clotting factors (II, VII, IX, X, XI) and disseminated intravascular coagulation. ABO compatibility is preferred (Hardaway and Adams, 1989; Jassak and Godwin, 1991; Snyder, 1987; ONS, 1994).

It is important to monitor ABO titers in patients who received ABO-incompatible marrow. The recipient's ABO type will change to that of the donor approximately 3 to 4 months after transplant. The titers are followed to determine when the ABO type of the transfusion is changed from the recipient's to the donor's type.

Nursing interventions are aimed at closely monitoring patient symptomatology regarding the need for blood products. Essential nursing care also includes assessing for signs and symptoms of bleeding and intervening to stop or minimize bleeding when and if it does occur as well as educating patients and families regarding bleeding precautions. Other specific interventions are

- testing urine, stool, and emesis for occult blood

- encouraging the use of a soft toothbrush and discouraging flossing
- administering topical agents such as thrombin, adrenalin, and cocaine to stop bleeding
- administering H2 antagonists to prevent ulcers and estrogen to prevent menstruation
- administering bladder irrigations and IV hydration for prevention and management of hemorrhagic cystitis
- applying pressure to sites of invasive procedures when possible (ONS, 1994).

The actual transfusion of blood products necessitates careful monitoring for adverse reactions. Premedications with an antipyretic, an antihistamine, and possibly a steroid are usually a routine part of the transfusion administration. Close monitoring of vital signs and patient symptoms is essential especially during the first hour of transfusion (ONS, 1994).

SUMMARY

Bone marrow and blood cell transplantation continues to grow as a challenging and rewarding subspecialty of nursing. The hematologic system is the system that first indicates the success of the transplant. Most of the care provided to patients during transplant is necessitated by the hematologic effects. As a broader range of diseases continue to be treated with transplantation, and as the techniques continue to evolve and be refined, the nursing care needs to progress in the same way and at the same pace.

During the last 10 years, the use of blood stem cells as well as growth factors such as G-CSF (granulocyte colony-stimulating factor) which affects granulocytes, GM-CSF (granulocyte-macrophage colony-stimulating factor) which affects both granulocytes and macrophages, and erythropoietin which affects red blood cells have revolutionized bone marrow transplantation. These agents have the capacity

to minimize the severity and duration of myelosuppression, which then decreases recovery time and shortens the hospitalization period for the BMT patient (Moore, 1991).

Other growth factors that stimulate even more of the cell line continue to be investigated. Among them are M-CSF (macrophage colony-stimulating factor), IL-3 (interleukin-3), SCF (stem cell factor), and PIXY 321 (GM-CSF and IL-3) (Abernathy, 1995). As these growth factors are developed, as more patients become candidates for bone marrow transplantation to treat more diseases, and as more donor-recipient combinations become possible, the hematologic system will be affected in new ways. The time line for a BMT is likely to change as techniques to allow ex vivo expansion of small numbers of stem cells become a reality (Broxmeyer, 1994). Nurses will continue to play key roles in the outcomes of patients' treatments through precision in assessing and caring for patients and through intensive education of patients in a variety of settings.

REFERENCES

Abernathy, E. 1995. Role of hematopoietic growth factors in post-induction treatment. In Wujcik, D. (Ed.) *Nursing Care Issues in Adult Leukemia,* vol 2. Huntington, NY: PRR INC., 20-27.

Adams, J.A., Gordon, A.A., Jiang, Y.Z., et al. 1990. Thrombocytopenia after bone marrow transplantation for leukaemia: changes in megakaryocyte growth and growth-promoting activity. *Br J Haematol* 75:195-201.

Alkire, K., Collingwood, J. 1990. Physiology of blood and bone marrow. *Semin Oncol Nurs* 6(2):99-108.

Allan, J.D. 1987. Antibiotic combinations. *Med Clin North Am* 71:1079-1091.

Anasetti, C., Amos, D., Beatty, P.G., et al. 1989. Effect of HLA compatibility on engraftment of bone marrow transplants in patients with leukemia or lymphoma. *N Engl J Med* 320:197.

Armstong, D. 1991. Empiric therapy for the immuno-compromised host. *Rev Infect Dis* 13:s763-s769.

Ball, E.D., Mills, L.E., Cornwell, G.G., et al. 1990. Autologous bone marrow transplantation for acute myeloid leukemia using monoclonal antibody-purged bone marrow. *Blood* 75:1199-1206.

Ballard, B. 1991. Renal and hepatic complications. In Whedon, M.B. (Ed.) *Bone Marrow Transplantation: Principles, Practices, and Nursing Insights.* Boston: Jones & Bartlett, 240-261.

Bar, B.M., Schattenberg, A., Van Oijk, B.A., et al. 1989. Host and donor erythrocyte repopulation patterns after allogeneic bone marrow transplantation analyzed with antibody-coated fluorescent microspheres. *Br J Hematol* 72:239-245.

Barge, A.J., Johnson, G., Witherspoon, R., Torok-Storb, B. 1989. Antibody-mediated marrow failure after allogeneic bone marrow transplantation. *Blood* 74: 1477-1480.

Beck, S. 1993. Prevention and management of oral complications in the cancer patient. In Hubbard, S.M., Greene, P.E., Knobf, M.T. (Eds.) *Current Issues in Cancer Nursing Practice Updates.* Philadelphia: Lippincott, 1-12.

Bennett, J.S., Shattil, S.J. 1990. Platelet function. In Williams, W.J., et al. *Hematology.* New York: McGraw-Hill, 1233-1242.

Bensinger, W.I., Buckner, C.D., Thomas, E.D., Clift, R.A. 1982. ABO-incompatible marrow transplants. *Transplantation* 33:427-429.

Bensinger, W., Peterson, F.B., Banaji, M., et al. 1989. Engraftment and transfusion requirements after allogeneic marrow transplantation for patients with acute nonlymphocytic leukemia in first complete remission. *BMT* 4(4):409-414.

Bowden, R.A., Slichter, S.J., Sayers, et al. 1991. Use of leukocyte-depleted platelets and cytomegalic-seronegative red blood cells for prevention of primary cytomegalovirus infection after marrow transplant. *Blood* 78 (1):246-250.

Broxmeyer, H.E. 1994. Stem cell expansion. *Blood Cells* 20(2,3):223-629.

Buchsel, P.C. 1990. Bone marrow transplantation. In Groenwald, S.L., Frogge, M.H., Goodman, M. Yarboro, C.H. (Eds.) *Cancer Nursing: Principles and Practice* 2d ed. Boston: Jones & Bartlett, 307-337.

Cahn, J.Y. 1989. Autoimmune-like thrombocytopenia after bone marrow transplantation. *Blood* 74:2771.

Caudell, K.A., Whedon, M.B. 1991. Hematopoietic complications. In Whedon, M.B. (Ed.) *Bone Marrow Transplantation: Principles, Practice, and Nursing Insights.* Boston: Jones & Bartlett, 135-159.

Champlin, R.E., Horowitz, M.M., von Bekkum, D.W., et al. 1989. Graft failure following bone marrow trans-

plantation for severe aplastic anemia: risk factors and treatment results. *Blood* 73(2):606-613.

Chapman, J.F., Murphy, M.F., Minchinton, et al. 1986. Autoimmune thrombocytopenia and neutropenia after remission induction therapy for acute leukemia. *Br J Haematol* 63:693-702.

Clark, J., Landis, L., McGee, R. 1987. Nursing management of outcomes of disease, psychological response, treatment and complications. In Ziegfield, C.R. (Ed.) *Core Curriculum for Oncology Nursing.* Philadelphia: Saunders, 272-274.

Dale, D. 1994. Physiology, function, and role of the neutrophil in host defense (monogr). Thousand Oaks, CA: Amgen Inc.

de Alarcon, P.A., Schmieder, J.A., Gingrich, R., Klugman, M.P. 1988. Pattern of response of megakaryocyte colony-stimulating activity in the serum of patients undergoing bone marrow transplantation. *Exper Hematol* 16:316-319.

Deeg, H.J., Storb, R. 1986. Acute and chronic graft versus host disease: Clinical manifestations, prophylaxis and treatment. *J Nat Canc Inst* 76:1325.

de Marie, S. 1996. Liposomal and lipid based formulations of amphotericin B. *Leukemia* 10(2):93-96.

DiJulio, J. 1991. Hematopoiesis: an overview. *Oncol Nurs Forum* 18(2 suppl):3-6.

Eilers, J., Berger, A.M., Petersen, M.C. 1988. Development, testing and application of the oral assessment guide. *Oncol Nurs Forum* 15:325-330.

Englund, J.A., Zimmerman, M.E., Swierkosz, E.M. 1990. Herpes simplex virus resistant to acyclovir: a study in a tertiary care center. *Ann Intern Med* 112:416-422.

Epstein, J.B. 1990. Infection prevention in bone marrow transplantation and radiation patients. (NCI monogr). *Oral Complications of Cancer Therapy,* 9:73-85.

Fauser, A.A., et al. 1988. Megakaryocytic colony-stimulating activity in patients receiving a bone marrow transplant during hematopoietic reconstitution. *Transplantation* 46(4):43-548.

Feld, R. 1989. The compromised host. *Eur J Canc Clin Oncol* 25:s1-s7.

Fidler, I., Meltzer, M. 1991. Mononuclear phagocytes host defense master series (monogr). East Hanover, NJ: Sandoz Pharmaceuticals Corp. and Schering-Plough Corp.

Filipovich, A.H., Vallera, D., McGlave, P., et al. 1990. T cell depletion with anti-CD5 immunotoxin in histocompatible bone marrow transplantation: the correlation between residual CD5 negative cells and subsequent graft-vs-host disease. *Transplantation* 50:410.

First, L.R., Smith, B.R., Lipton, J., Nathan, D.G., Parkman, R., Rappaport, J.M. 1985. Isolated thrombocytopenia after allogeneic bone marrow transplantation: Existence of transient and chronic thrombocytopenic syndromes. *Blood* 65:368-374.

Ford, R., Eisenberg, S. 1990. Bone marrow transplant: recent advances and nursing implications. *Nurs Clin North Am* 25(2):405-422.

Fuller, A.K. 1990. Platelet transfusion therapy for thrombocytopenia. *Semin Oncol Nurs* 6:123-128.

Ginsburg, D., Antin, J.H., Smith, B.R., Orkin, S.H., Rappeport, J.M. 1985. Origin of cell populations after bone marrow transplantation: analysis using DNA sequence polymorphisms. *J Clin Investig* 75:596-603.

Glaspy, J., et al. 1992. The cells of the hematopoietic cascade (mongr). Seattle, WA: Immunex Corp.

Goodman, M. 1989. Managing the side effects of chemotherapy. *Semin Oncol Nurs* 5(21 suppl):29-52.

Goodman, M., Stoner, C. 1991. Mucous membrane integrity, impairmant of, related to stomatitis. In McNally, J.C., Somerville, E.T., Miaskowski, C., Rostad, M. (Eds.) *Guidelines for Oncology Nursing Practice*. Philadelphia: Saunders, 241-247.

Griffin, J.P. 1986. Physiology of the hematopoietic system. In Griffin, J.P. (Ed.) *Hematology and Immunology: Concepts for Nursing*. Norwalk, CT: Appleton-Century-Crofts, 19-40.

Hardaway, R.M., Adams, W.H. 1989. Transfusions. *Prob Crit Care* 3(2):249-270.

Hawthorne, J.W., Pizzo, P.A. 1989. Infectious complications in the pediatric cancer patient. In Pizzo, P.A., Poplack, D.G. (Eds.) *Principles and Practice of Pediatric Oncology*. Philadelphia: Lippincott, 837-868.

Hays, K. 1990. Physiology of normal bone marrow. *Semin Oncol Nurs* 6(1):3-8.

Herberman, R.B. 1987. Elements of the immune system: cetus immune primer series (monogr). Pittsburgh, PA: Cetus Corp.

Hiemenz, J.W., Greene, J.N. 1993. Special considerations for the patient undergoing allogeneic or autologous bone marrow transplantation. *Hematol Oncol Clin North Am* 7(5):961-1002.

Jassak, P.F., Godwin, J. 1991. Blood component therapy. In Baird, S.B., McCorkle, R., Grant, M. (Eds.) *Cancer Nursing: A Comprehensive Textbook*. Philadelphia: Saunders, 370-384.

Kernan, N.A. 1988. Graft failure following transplantation of T-cell–depleted marrow. In Burakoff, S.J., Deeg, H.J., Ferrara, J.L.M., Atkinson, M.K. (Eds.) *Graft-vs-*

Host Disease: Immunology, Pathophysiology, and Treatment. New York: Marcel Dekker, 57.

Kernan, N.A., Bordignon, C., Heller, G., et al. 1989. Graft failure after T-cell–depleted human leukocyte antigen identical marrow transplants for leukemia. I. Analysis of risk factors and results of secondary transplants. *Blood* 74:2227.

Kernan, N.A., Flomenberg, N., Dupont, B., O'Reilly, R.J. 1987. Graft rejection in recipients of T-cell–depleted HLA-nonidentical marrow transplants for leukemia. *Transplantation* 43:842.

King, C.R. 1995. Outpatient management of myelosuppression. *Clin Perspect Oncol Nurs* 1(4):1-12.

Klastersky, J. 1992. Infections in patients with cancer: prevention. In Moose, A.R., Schimpff, S.C., Robson, M.C. (Eds.) *Comprehensive Textbook of Oncology*, vol 2(2). Baltimore: Williams & Wilkins, 1749-1753.

Klumpp, T.R. 1991. Immunohematologic complications of bone marrow transplantation. *BMT* 8:159-170.

Klumpp, T.R. 1995. Complications of peripheral blood stem cell transplantation. *Semin Oncol* 22(3):263-270.

Klumpp, T.R., Caligiuri, M.A., Rabinowe, S.N., et al. 1990. Autoimmune pancytopenia following allogeneic bone marrow transplantation. *BMT* 6:445-447.

Kolbinson, D.T., Schubert, M.M., Flourney, N., Truelove, E.L. 1988. Early changes following bone marrow transplantation. *Oral Surg Oral Med Oral Pathol* 66: 130-138.

Korbling, M., Hunstein, W., Fliedner, T.M., et al. 1989. Disease-free survival after autologous bone marrow transplantation in patients with acute myelogenous leukemia. *Blood* 74:1898-1904.

Lazarus, H.M., Rowe, J.M. 1994. Clinical use of hematopoietic growth factors in allogeneic bone marrow transplantation. *Blood Rev* 8:169-178.

Lin, E.M., Tierny, D.K., Stadtmauer, E.A. 1993. Autologous bone marrow transplantation: a review of the principles and complications. *Canc Nurs* 16(3):204-213.

Lum, L.G. 1991. Immune recovery after bone marrow transplantation. *Hematol Oncol Clin North Am* 4(3): 659-675.

Mangan, K.F. 1987a. Immune disregulation of hematopoiesis. *Ann Rev Med* 38:61-70.

Mangan, K.F. 1987b. Immunologic control of hematopoiesis: implications for quality of the graft after allogeneic bone marrow transplantation. *Transplant Proc* 19:23-28.

Mangan, K., Klumpp, T., Rosenfeld, C., Shadduck, R.K. 1991. Bone marrow transplantation. In Makowka, L.

(Ed.) *The Handbook of Transplantation Management.* Austin: Landis, 374-376.

Maiche, A.G. 1991. Use of quinolones in the immunocompromised host. *Eur J Clin Microbiol Infect Dis 13:* 361-367.

Maxwell, M.B. 1984. When the cancer patient becomes anemic. *Canc Nurs* 7(4):321-326.

McFadden, M.E., Sartorius, S.E. 1992. Multiple systems organ failure in the patient with cancer. Part 1. *Oncol Nurs Forum* 19:719.

McFadden, M.E., Sartorius, S.E. 1992. Multiple systems organ failure in the patient with cancer. Part 2. *Oncol Nurs Forum* 19:727.

McLauren, C., Chen, M.S., Ghazzouli, I., et al. 1985. Drug resistance patterns of herpes simplex virus isolated from patients treated with acyclovir. *Antimicrob Agents Chemother* 28:740-744.

Minchinton, R.M., Waters, A.H., Malpas, J.S., et al. 1984. Platelet and granulocyte-specific antibodies after allogeneic and autologous bone marrow grafts. *Vox Sang* 46:125-135.

Moore, M.A.S. 1991. The clinical use of colony stimulating factors. *Ann Rev Immunol* 9:159-191.

Oncology Nursing Society, 1994. *Manual for Bone Marrow Transplant Nursing.* Pittsburgh: Oncology Nursing Press.

Paulin, R., Ringden, O., Nilsson, et al. 1987. Variables predicting bacterial and fungal infections after allogeneic marrow engraftment. *Transplantation* 43:393-398.

Petursson, C. 1993. Bleeding due to thrombocytopenia. In Yasko, J.M. (Ed.) *Nursing Management of Symptoms Associated with Chemotherapy,* 3d ed. Philadelphia: Meniscus Health Care Communications, 135-141.

Petz, L. D. 1989. Bone marrow transplantation. In Petz, L.D., Svisher, S. (Eds.) *Clinical Practice of Transfusion Medicine.* New York: Churchill Livingstone, 485-508.

Petz, L.D., Scott, E.P. 1983. Supportive care. In Blume, K.G., Petz, L.D. (Eds.) *Clinical Bone Marrow Transplant.* New York: Churchill Livingstone, 177-213.

Quinones, R.R. 1993. Hematopoietic engraftment and graft failure after bone marrow transplantation. *Am J Pediatr Hematol Oncol* 15(1):3-17.

Reed, E.C., Bowden, R.A., Dandliker, P.S., et al. 1988. Treatment of cytomegalovirus pneumonia with gancyclovir and intravenous immunoglobulin in patients with bone marrow transplant. *Ann Intern Med* 15:783-788.

Rostad, M.E. 1991. Current strategies for managing myelosuppression in patients with cancer. *Oncol Nurs Forum* 18 (2 suppl):7-15.

Roy, D.C., Tantravahi, R., Murray, C., et al. 1990. Natural history of mixed chimerism after bone marrow transplantation with cd-6 depleted allogeneic marrow: a stable equilibrium. *Blood* 75:296-304.

Safrin, S., Crumpacker, C., Chatis, P., et al. 1991. A controlled trial comparing foscarnet with vidarabine for acyclovir-resistant mucocutaneous herpes simplex in the acquired immunodeficiency syndrome. *N Engl J Med 325:*551-555.

Schafer, S.L. 1993. Infection due to leukopenia. In Yasko, J.M. (Ed.) *Nursing Management of Symptoms Associated with Chemotherapy,* 3d ed. Philadelphia: Meniscus Health Care Communications, 143-168.

Schimpff, S.C. 1992. Infections in patients with cancer: overview and epidemiology. In Moosa, A.R., Schimpft, S.C., Robson, M.C. (Eds.) *Comprehensive Textbook of Oncology.* Philadelphia: Williams & Wilkins, 1720-1732.

Schuening, F.G., Nemunaitis, J., Appelbaum, F.R., Storb, R. 1994. Hematopoietic growth factors after allogeneic marrow transplantation in animal studies and clinical trials. *BMT 14*(suppl 4):574-577.

Shaffer, S., Wilson, J.N. 1993. Bone marrow transplantation: critical care implications. *Crit Care Nurs Clin North Am* 5(3):531-542.

Slichter, S.J. 1994. Principles of transfusion support before and after bone marrow transplantation. In Forman, S.J., Blume, K.G., Thomas, E.D. (Eds.) *Bone Marrow Transplantation* Boston: Blackwell Scientific.

Sniecinski, L., O'Donnell, M.R., Nowicki, B., Hill, L.R. 1988. Prevention of refractoriness and HLA alloimmunization using filtered blood products. *Blood* 71:1402-1407.

Snyder, E.L. (Ed.) 1987. *Blood Transfusion Therapy: A Physician's Handbook.* Arlington, VA: American Association of Blood Banks.

Sparkes, R.S., Sparkes, M.C., Gale, R.P. 1979. Immunoglobulin synthesis following bone marrow transplantation in man: conversion to donor allotype. *Transplantation* 27:212-213.

Storb, R. 1989. Bone marrow transplantation. In DeVita, V.T., Hellman, S., Rosenberg, S. (Eds.) *Cancer Principles and Practice of Oncology.* Philadelphia: Lippincott, 2474-2489.

Storb, R., Weiden, P.L., Sullivan, K.M., et al. 1987. Second marrow transplants in patients with aplastic anemia rejecting the first graft: use of a conditioning regimen including cyclophosphamide and antithymocyte globulin. *Blood* 70:116-121.

Sugar, A.M. 1990. Empiric treatment of fungal infections in the neutropenic host: Review of the literature and guidelines for use. *Arch Intern Med 150*: 2258-2264

Taylor, D.L. !984. Immune response physiology, signs, and symptoms. *Nursing 5*:52-54.

Tollemar, J., Ringden, O., Anderson, S., et al. 1993. Prophylactic use of liposomal amphotericin B (ambisome) against fungal infections: a randomized trial in bone marrow transplant recipients. *Transplant Proc 25*:1495-1497.

Vanacek, K. S. 1991. Gastrointestinal complications of bone marrow transplantation. In Whedon, M.B. (Ed.) *Bone Marrow Transplantation: Principles, Practice, and Nursing Insights.* Boston: Jones & Bartlett, 206-239.

Verdonck, L. F., Cornelissen, J.J., Smit, J., et al. 1993. Successful foscarnet therapy for acyclovir-resistant mucocutaneous infection with herpes simplex virus in a recipient of allogeneic BMT. *BMT 11*:177-179.

Wade, J.C. 1992. Infections in patients with cancer: treatment. In Moosa, A.R., Schimpff, S.C., Robson, M.C. (Eds.) *Comprehensive Textbook of Oncology,* vol. 2, 2d ed. Baltimore: Williams & Wilkins, 1740-1748.

Western Consortium for Cancer Nursing Research. 1991. Development of a staging system for chemotherapy-induced stomatitis. *Canc Nurs 14*:6-12.

Whedon, M.B. 1991. Allogeneic bone marrow transplantation: clinical indications, treatment process, and outcomes. In Whedon, M.B. (Ed.) *Bone Marrow Transplantation: Principles, Practice and Nursing Insights.* Boston: Jones & Bartlett, 20-48.

Wingard, J.R. 1990a. Advances in the management of infectious complications after bone marrow transplantation. *BMT 6*:371-383.

Wingard, J.R. 1990b. Management of infectious complications of bone marrow transplantation. *Oncology 4*(2): 69-75.

Wingard, J.R., Mellits, E.D., Sostrin, M.B., et al. 1988. Interstitial pneumonia after allogeneic bone marrow transplantation: nine years experience at a single institution. *Medicine 67*:175-186.

Winston, D.J., Gale, R.P. 1991. Prevention and treatment of cytomegalovirus infection and disease after bone marrow transplantation in the 1990s. *BMT 8*:7-11

Wujcik, D., Ballard, B., Camp-Sorrell, D. 1994. Selected complications of allogeneic bone marrow transplantation. *Semin Oncol Nurs 10*(1):28-41.

Wulff, J.C., Santner, T.J., Storb, R., et al. 1983. Transfusion requirements after HLA-identical marrow transplantation in 82 patients with aplastic anemia. *Vox Sang 44*:366-374.

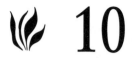

10

Gastrointestinal Effects

Constance Engelking, Deborah Rust

Complications of the gastrointestinal (GI) system are the first clinical problems experienced by patients undergoing all types of bone marrow (BMT) and blood cell transplantation (BCT) procedures (Ford and Ballard, 1988). An array of GI sequelae pose dramatic physical challenges to these patients. Despite advances in ameliorating certain causative factors during the past two decades, transplant-related GI morbidity continues to be a significant problem. The introduction of effective GVHD prophylaxis and antiviral agents targeted at eliminating infections of herpes simplex (HSV) and cytomegalovirus (CMV) has reduced the incidence of associated hepatic and intestinal complications experienced by transplant patients (Einsele et al., 1988; Erice et al., 1987; Laskin et al., 1987; Schmeiser et al., 1988; Shuhart and McDonald, 1994). Similarly, the arrival of the serotonin antagonists on the antiemetic scene has helped to diminish the acute emetogenicity of dose-intensive chemotherapy (Dilly, 1994; Egan, Taggart, Bender, 1992). However, GI-associated morbidity and mortality remains high as a result of three factors: (1) veno-occlusive disease (VOD) of the liver in response to increasingly aggressive cytoreductive therapies, (2) a rise in GVHD as the number of allogeneic transplants using matched but unrelated donors grows (Shuhart and McDonald, 1994), and (3) delayed nausea, vomiting, and anorexia, which are not well controlled with currently available antiemetic strategies.

Gastrointestinal sequelae associated with marrow and stem cell transplantation are generally attributable to one or more of the following causes (Wolford and McDonald, 1988):

- the effects of dose-intensive conditioning regimens (i.e., chemotherapy ± total body or total nodal radiation);
- side effects of supportive pharmaceuticals or treatments administered during the transplant process;
- acute or chronic graft-versus-host disease (primarily allogeneic setting); and
- infection involving any segment of the GI tract or liver.

Dose-intensive cytoreductive regimens are especially implicated in the causation of acute GI toxicities that occur early in the transplant process. In contrast to standard-dose antineoplastic regimens, high-dose (HD) regimens typically cause GI complications that are more severe in nature and of longer duration. Only preliminary quantitative and qualitative data is available to describe clearly the character of the complications produced by the etiologic factors associated with the transplant experience (Chapko et al., 1989). However, several facts remain. First, both the occurrence and intensity of GI sequelae are contingent upon the intrinsic toxic properties of the particular treatment regimen employed and the individual host's response. Second, the combined effects of dose-intensive antineoplastic drug therapy and total body irradiation (TBI) produce more extensive tissue and organ damage than either therapy alone. Finally, prior exposure to cytotoxic agents and radiation therapy may alter the incidence and severity of GI effects experienced by patients who undergo transplantation.

Transplant-related GI pathophysiology ranges in character from complications that are mild, temporary disturbances to protracted, life-threatening clinical events. Though many present early patient-care challenges for nurses, certain complications produce continuing long-term problems, requiring specialized nursing management. The most common toxic effects of transplant conditioning regimens include:

- severe emetic responses with persistent nausea and anorexia;
- mucositis extending the length of the alimentary tract with accompanying dysphagia, xerostomia, and esophagitis;
- diarrhea with abdominal cramping and pain;
- GI bleeding and, in some instances, major gastric or intestinal hemorrhage; and
- elevated LFTs, cholestasis, hepatitis, and VOD of the liver.

The impact of major etiologic factors on incidence and severity of secondary GI dysfunction varies among patients; yet GI related transplant sequelae continue to be perceived as the most uncomfortable and distressing aspects of the entire process for both patients and providers. In fact, one recent study identified loss of appetite, diarrhea, and mucositis among eight symptoms ranked as most distressing by BMT patients and nurses (Larson et al., 1993). Further, GI complications can actually threaten survival. Possbile life-threatening outcomes include a heightened risk of sepsis produced in the presence of widespread mucosal disruption, significant nutritional deficiencies resulting in profound electrolyte and biochemical disturbances, and irreversible organ damage induced by conditioning therapies or GVHD.

Nurses play a vital role in the early detection, monitoring, and delivery of therapeutic interventions aimed at managing GI problems and minimizing discomfort during the entire transplant process.

PATHOPHYSIOLOGIC GI RESPONSES

Primary GI responses to both allogeneic and autologous transplantation can be categorized according to target sites in the GI system and include emetic, mucosal, glandular, and hepatic sequelae. The particular target site affected dictates the specific clinical manifestations, though there is considerable overlap in sites affected and in the subsequent symptom profile.

The incidence, duration, severity, and reversibility of GI complications vary greatly depending on individual host factors, source of stem cells, prescribed conditioning regimen, and supportive therapies. Whether they occur independently, concomitantly, or sequentially, GI problems invariably have the potential to undermine protective functions, jeopardize biochemical homeostasis, impair nutritional status, and produce discomfort. Early and effective management is critical to preventing evolution from what may initially appear to be minor problems to those that are life threatening. However, the multicausal and dynamic etiologies associated with transplant-related GI problems create significant challenges to symptom management.

The Emetic Response

Nausea, vomiting, and anorexia comprise a symptom complex that is experienced almost universally by patients at some point during the transplant process (Shuhart and McDonald,

1994). Generally, the emetic response is the first significant GI problem to occur in patients undergoing BMT/BCT. The physiologic mechanisms associated with the emetic response involve stimulation of the true vomiting center (TVC) in the fourth ventricle of the brain via central (e.g., cerebral cortex, chemoreceptor trigger zone) or peripheral (e.g., vagal and sympathetic afferent nerves) pathways. Emetic messages are thought to be mediated by certain neurotransmitters (e.g., dopamine, serotonin, histamine, acetylcholine). These mechanisms are described in depth elsewhere (Blower, 1994; Hogan, 1990; Wickham, 1989).

Anorexia often accompanies nausea and vomiting. The mechanisms underlying anorexia and its relationship to nausea and vomiting are not well understood. There is speculation, however, that the occurrence of anorexia may be related to elevated serum levels of circulating lipids, peptides, and certain cytokines such as tumor necrosis factor and interleukin-1 (Bruera and MacDonald, 1989; Holler et al., 1990). A spectrum of persistent taste alterations secondary to TBI, selected chemotherapeutic agents, oral infection, and antibiotic therapy are commonly experienced by BMT patients and can contribute to the problem of anorexia (Barale et al., 1982; Cunningham et al., 1983; Huldij et al., 1986).

The pattern and duration of emetic symptoms are quite variable. Though not well described in the literature, it is likely that acute emetic patterns associated with transplant conditioning differ from those produced by standard-dose chemotherapy (Gilbert et al., 1995). The character of delayed nausea, vomiting, and anorexia also is poorly described. Typically, nausea and vomiting occur in concert and early in the process during the period beginning within 24 hours of initiating the conditioning regimen and extending through the infusion of marrow and/or stem cells. These symptoms are generally followed within a short period by the onset of anorexia. Often nausea with or without vomiting persists, overlapping the patient's loss of appetite and lasting 3 to 6 weeks (Chapko, 1989). Not all patients fit this classic picture, though, since the particular symptoms and the pattern of occurrence are directly linked to specific causative factors that differ somewhat from patient to patient. In studies of long-term survivors of allogeneic transplant, it has been noted that at 1 year after transplant, up to 28% continue to experience weight loss and 6% to 8% are still coping with anorexia (Lenssen et al., 1990; Schmidt et al., 1993).

Outcomes of unremitting acute nausea and vomiting include life-threatening electrolyte disturbances, Mallory-Weiss tears, aspiration resulting in pneumonia, severe nutritional disturbances, protracted hospital stays and, ultimately, diminished quality of life (Lazlo, 1983). Uncontrolled emetic responses also result in significant emotional distress for patients, families, and caregivers (Jenns, 1994). In conjunction with removal of the causative factor(s) and appropriate antiemetic therapy, timely and consistent nursing intervention can minimize the intensity of the emetic response, resulting possibly in a reduction of patients risk of life-threatening secondary outcomes, lower levels of anxiety in patients and families and enhanced quality of life.

Causation and Character

The emetic response may be acute or chronic and is initiated by a variety of causative factors including host response to emetogenic antineoplastic therapies, supportive pharmaceuticals, infectious processes, and graft-versus-host disease (GVHD). Psychoneurologic factors can also play a role in the causation and/or intensity of the emetic response (Jenns, 1994). Knowledge of the primary etiologies prepares the nurse to anticipate, characterize, and plan for each patient's emetic response during transplantation.

Conditioning Regimens. Certain antineoplastic agents and radiation therapy to abdominal, whole brain, and sacral or lumbar fields are noxious stimuli known to initiate the emetic response by direct or indirect stimulation of midbrain vomiting centers. The drug and radiation configuration of the conditioning regimen dictate the risk for nausea and vomiting. Regimens that are platinum based and/or involve TBI are considered more highly emetogenic than other conditioning regimens, resulting frequently in a more severe emetic response of earlier onset and longer duration. With regard to individual drugs, carmustine, carboplatin, cyclophosphamide, and busulfan in high dosages have all been noted to produce moderate to severe emetic responses in both allogeneic and autologous transplant conditioning (Dorr and Von Hoff, 1994; Fetting et al., 1983; Gilbert et al., 1995; Owen, Clove, Cotanch, 1981). In contrast, the emetogenicity associated with single-agent high-dose (HD) melphalan is described as only moderately severe (Samuels and Bitran, 1995) and short lived (Dorr and Von Hoff, 1994). Similarly, emetic responses produced by HD etoposide and mitoxantrone are characterized as falling within the mild to moderate range of intensity (Dorr and Von Hoff, 1994). Projecting severity of the emetic response, however, becomes more difficult in the setting of multiagent regimens.

In addition to particular drugs at HD levels and the inclusion of TBI in the conditioning regimen, emetogenic intensity appears to be directly proportionate to the precise dosages of drugs and radiation. In one comparative trial of two conditioning regimens for allogeneic transplant, for example, Chapko and colleagues (1989) noted differences in both severity and duration of nausea depending on specific doses administered. Though both populations were receiving cyclosphosphamide in high doses, patients with aplastic anemia who received higher doses of cyclophosphamide (200 mg/kg) experi-

enced more nausea than did patients with hematologic malignancies being conditioned with lower cyclophosphamide doses (120 mg/kg) and TBI. Higher dose fractions of TBI (1575 cGy versus 1200 cGy) were also associated with more nausea.

Most current guidelines for projecting emetogenicity are general and emphasize responsible agents without attention to dose-related variations in symptomatology. Building on an expanded classification of the emetogenic potential of the antineoplastic agents, which incorporates dosage levels recently developed by Hesketh and colleagues (1995), may enhance the accuracy of projections of emetogenicity produced by transplant conditioning regimens (Table 10.1).

Route of administration plays a role as well. For example, the intrathecal instillation of methotrexate to eradicate disease in the central nervous system is known to produce nausea and vomiting in some patients though relatively low doses are employed (Dorr and Von Hoff, 1994).

Supportive Pharmaceuticals. A spectrum of pharmaceuticals are employed to manage transplant-associated complications and generally support patients through the engraftment phase of the transplant process when they are most vulnerable to life-threatening infectious and nutritional sequelae. Many of these agents affect appetite and have the capacity to cause nausea with or without vomiting. Oral nonabsorbable antibiotics (e.g., nystatin, trimethoprim-sulfamethoxazole, pentoxifylline), parenteral antifungals (e.g., cyclosporin, amphotericin), and opioids to control pain associated with mucositis are among the primary offenders (Shuhart and McDonald, 1994; Wolford and McDonald, 1988). Total parenteral nutrition (TPN), lipid infusions, and steroid therapy, which can all produce high serum glucose and amino acid levels, are other pharmaceuticals

TABLE 10.1 Emetogenic potential of antineoplastic agents

Moderate	Moderate to high	High
Cisplatin ≥ 70 mg/m²	Carboplatin 200–400 mg/m²	Methotrexate 100–250 mg/m²
Cytarabine > 1 g/m²	Cisplatin 20–69 mg/m²	Milomycin ≥ 8 mg/m²
Cyclophosphamide ≥ 1,000 mg/m²	Dacarbazine < 500 mg/m²	Cyclophosphamide < 600 mg/m²
Dacarbazine ≥ 500 mg/m²	Cyclophosphamide 600–999 mg/m²	Doxorubicin 20–75 mg/m²
Carmustine ≥ 200 mg/m²	Cytarabine 250–1,000 mg/m²	
Streptozocin	Carmustine < 200 mg/m²	
Mechlorethamine	Doxorubicin ≥ 75 mg/m²	
Dactinomycin	Methotrexate ≥ 250 mg/m²	
	Cyclophosphamide 400–599 mg/m² and Doxorubicin ≥ 40 mg/m²	Cyclophosphamide 100 mg/m² orally and Methotrexate 40–60 mg/m² and Fluorouracil 600–700 mg/m²

NOTE: IV administration unless otherwise indicated.
SOURCE: Hesketh et al., 1995.

associated with nausea and anorexia. Surprisingly, the impact of TPN on appetite may extend up to 3 weeks after its discontinuation, which creates implications for the post-hospital phase of the transplant process (Martyn, Hansen, Jen, 1984)

Infection. Infectious processes also contribute to the problem of nausea, vomiting, and anorexia. Infections of viral origin are most commonly associated with the emetic response, though the onset of symptoms is much later in the transplant process (i.e., up to 54 days) than with other etiologies. In the absence of prophylactic antiviral therapy, the incidence of viral infection is as high as 70% to 80% (Wujcik et al., 1994), though not all affected patients present with emetic symptoms. The organisms most often associated with emetic symptoms prior to the development of gancyclovir and acyclovir were CMV and HSV (Shuhart and McDonald, 1994). In one prospective study,

esophageal and intestinal CMV were documented in 38% of 50 BMT patients who presented with unexplained persistent vomiting (Spencer et al., 1986). HSV esophagitis also has been associated with incessant vomiting (McDonald et al., 1985). Protracted nausea is attributed to tenacious active viral infection, acid-peptic reflux, and gastric and intestinal ulceration. Viral infections are less common today, currently occurring most often as a result of reactivated pretransplant viral infection or after premature discontinuation of gancyclovir necessitated by patient toxicity. In contrast to the protracted nausea produced by viral infections, fungal and bacterial infections are noted to cause anorexia (Shuhart and McDonald, 1994).

Graft-versus-Host Disease. Emetic responses may be early indicators of acute intestinal GVHD. The average onset of GVHD-induced nausea and vomiting is at day 34 (Wolford and

McDonald, 1988). Anorexia soon followed by nausea and vomiting or retching are among the earliest manifestations of this complication (Wujcik, Ballard and Camp-Sorrell, 1994; Shuhart and McDonald, 1994). Uncontrolled retching of early onset, however, generally subsides despite continuation of nausea, vomiting, and anorexia (McDonald et al., 1986). In a prospective trial, Spencer and colleagues (1986) found that 42% of 50 BMT patients who developed unexplained vomiting during the period extending from day 20 to day 100 actually had GVHD. Weisdorf and colleagues (1990) determined that nausea and vomiting were the primary clinical indicators of gut GVHD in 60% of patients with biopsy-proven GVHD of the stomach and small intestine.

Psychoneurologic Factors. Unknown physiologic reasons for vomiting have been reported in BMT patients (Spencer et al., 1986). In many instances, psychological causes are implicated. Nausea and vomiting also may be anticipatory or conditioned responses by certain patients to perceived noxious stimuli in the environment (Duigon, 1986). Though there is no scientific proof, there is speculation that a significant number of BMT/BCT patients experience conditioned emetic responses based on previous negative exposure to highly emetogenic chemotherapy regimens. Other psychological symptomatology common to transplant patients such as anxiety, depression, powerlessness, and exaggerated responses to pain may set the emotional stage for protracted nausea, vomiting, and anorexia. Despite the large role that psychoneurologic factors may play in producing emetic responses, this area remains largely unexplored.

Prevention and Management
Effective control of the emetic response in BMT/BCT populations requires a plan that in-

corporates comprehensive assessment in conjunction with both preventive and management strategies. Prophylaxis of acute emetic responses entails baseline assessment focused on factors that might predispose the patient to nausea, vomiting, and anorexia. These include host factors (e.g., previous emetic patterns, response to antiemetic approaches, history of dystonic reactions or other side effects), currently prescribed emetogenic agents or therapies, and anticipated clinical problems (e.g., GVHD, infection, GI ulceration).

For emetic responses that persist or occur later in the transplant process, it is critical to perform meticulous ongoing assessment that characterizes the patient's particular emetic pattern (e.g., onset, timing, duration, intensity, associated symptomatology) and tracks specific trends in the patient's emetic experience (e.g., response to current antiemetic strategies, occurrence of other symptoms, impact on nutrition, etc.). A standardized grading scale is essential to accurate evaluation of the patient. Table 10.2 provides examples of existing scales.

Both pharmacologic and nonpharmacologic interventions are employed to prevent, minimize, or eliminate emetic responses during all phases of the transplant process. Many of the approaches are empiric, however, because few substantial clinical trials evaluating antiemetic approaches in the BMT population have been conducted. The focus of the antiemetic plan differs according to the specific etiology.

Control of acute conditioning-induced emesis is primarily preventive; control of nausea and vomiting associated with other etiologies relies on eradication of the underlying cause(s).

Conditioning-Induced Emetic Responses. Pharmacologic approaches are the key to controlling conditioning-induced emetic responses. Unfortunately, no one antiemetic agent or multidrug regimen demonstrates the capacity to

TABLE 10.2 Grading scales to evaluate transplant-related GI complications

	0	1	2	3	4
(A) Nausea and/or vomiting	None	Able to eat, reasonable intake, one episode vomiting in 24 h	Intake significantly decreased but able to eat, 2–4 episodes of vomiting in 24 h	No significant intake, 5–10 episodes of vomiting in 24 h	> 10 Episodes of vomiting in 24 h, requires parenteral nutrition
(B) Stomatitis	Pink, moist intact mucosa	Gingival erythema, buccal/glossal ridging or blanching, ± oral sensitivity	Gingival erythema, isolated ulceration, ± pain and white plaques	Confluent ulceration or denuding > 25–50% oral mucosa, mod pain, ± white plaques	Confluent ulceration > 50% oral mucosa, marked pain, ± white plaques oozing or active bleeding
(C) Perianal skin integrity	No redness	Mild erythema without inflammation	Moderate erythema, inflammation, pruritis or burning	Severe erythema, inflammation with bullae and/or vesicles	Ulceration, open area of skin > 0.5 × 0.5 cm, necrotic tissue, eschar, or drainage
(D) Diarrhea	Normal number of stools, asymptomatic	2–3 Loose stools/day, asymptomatic	4–6 Loose stools/day and/or nocturnal stools, abdominal cramping	7–9 Loose stools/day and/or incontinence, severe cramping	> 10 Loose stools/day and/or grossly bloody diarrhea, requires parenteral support

Sources: Data from (A) Schubert and Sullivan, 1990; (B) Westchester County Medical Center; (C) Yeomans et al., 1991 (Perirectal Skin Assessment Tool); (D) Schubert and Sullivan, 1990.

prevent or ablate the nausea and vomiting produced by transplant conditioning therapies. With the exception of a few small clinical trials, little research has been conducted to identify definitive antiemetic therapy in the transplant setting. The paucity of research is likely due to the difficulties imposed by multiple variables such as the wide disparity in conditioning regimens and individual host factors. As a result, therapeutic strategies to prevent and manage conditioning-induced emetogenicity are drawn from clinical observation and anecdotal reports of successful interventions. The approaches chosen typically are based on the principles that govern antiemetic therapy for standard-dose chemotherapy; that is, liberal and regular use of combination antiemetic regimens that incorporate drugs with different mechanisms of action, nonoverlapping toxicities, demonstrated efficacy as single agents, and ideal administration routes and schedules (Gralla et al., 1987).

Generally, prophylactic multiagent antiemetic therapy beginning prior to the initiation of conditioning and extending 24 to 48 hours post conditioning is critical to controlling the acute emetic response to HD therapy. As with standard-dose chemotherapy, it is the practice to select antiemetic agents from a spectrum of drug classes for combination in multidrug regimens. Key antiemetic agents traditionally used in the transplant setting include metoclopramide, lorazepam, dexamethasone, diphenhydramine, prochlorperazine, thiethylperazine, and haloperidol.

More recently, the serotonin antagonists, ondansetron and granisetron, have been added to the antiemetic armamentarium. The success of these agents in controlling chemotherapy-induced emetic responses is based on their novel receptor binding mechanism of action (Blower, 1994; Egan, Taggart, Bender, 1992). Though scientific proof of efficacy in the management of emetic responses to HD alkylator-based transplant conditioning therapy is limited, the results of three small studies have been reported. In these trials of single-agent ondansetron in standard dosages, subject accrual ranged from 12 to 33 patients. The size of the population limits generalization; however, ondansetron was found to be efficacious in controlling acute nausea and vomiting that accompanied conditioning for transplantation with a HD multiagent conditioning regimen consisting of cisplatinum, carmustine, and etoposide (Lazarus et al., 1990), with HD melphalan (Viner et al., 1990), and with HD cyclosphophamide with TBI (Croockewit, 1990).

One major advantage of these newer agents is that they produce fewer side effects than traditional antiemetic drugs, especially with regard to sedation, anticholinergic and extrapyramidal effects. Cost is a concern. However recent observations are that the oral route of administration may provide equal or superior control of emesis at lower cost than intravenously administered antiemetics. Conclusions based on clinical observation, extrapolation from studies of antiemetic efficacy with standard chemotherapy regimens, and the few small studies targeting BMT populations are that the serotonin antagonists seem to offer better control of emetic responses to certain conditioning regimens while at the same time paring down the number of antiemetic agents required for effective prophylaxis of acute conditioning-induced nausea and vomiting. These observations have prompted many centers to develop antiemetic strategies that use these agents often in combination with one or two other drugs. Both ondansetron and granisetron frequently are combined with dexamethasone since the combination of a serotonin antagonist with a steroid has been demonstrated to produce better antiemetic overall outcomes (Roila et al., 1991).

It also is becoming clear that the phenomena of acute (i.e., occurring within 24 to 48 hrs of therapy) and delayed (i.e., occurring later than 48 hrs post therapy) onset nausea and vomiting are mediated by different physiologic mechanisms, and therefore, require different pharmacologic approaches. Though highly effective in managing acute emetic responses, neither of the serotonin antagonists has demonstrated efficacy in controlling delayed nausea and vomiting. Consequently, in some centers the antiemetic plan for BMT/BCT patients is progressive, beginning with a serotonin antagonist in conjunction with a steroid and followed after 48 hours with a dopamine antagonist plus the steroid and an antihistamine. This approach not only appears to be highly effective in minimizing emetogenic responses but also may reduce cost.

Considerable research is still needed to identify superior antiemetic strategies for this population that also are cost effective. Selected prophylactic antiemetic regimens currently used in conjunction with transplant conditioning appear in Table 10.3.

Though the combination of antiemetic agents can result in diminished emetic responses, the use of multidrug regimens also can be problematic. For example, Gilbert and colleagues (1995) concluded from their placebo-controlled double-blind randomized trial of selected four drug regimens (i.e., metoclopramide plus dronabinol or placebo versus prochlorperazine plus dronabinol or placebo in conjunction with an anxiolytic and an antihistamine) in 126 patients undergoing HD cisplatinum, cyclophosphamide, carmustine conditioning with autologous rescue that both metoclopramide

TABLE 10.3 Selected antiemetric regimens used in BMT conditioning

Medications	Dosing schedule	Comments
SCHEDULE I		
Diphenhydramine	30 mg/m^2 intravenously 30 min before each metoclopramide dose × 6 doses for each chemotherapy infusion; continued every 4 h × 6 doses after last dose of chemotherapy	Antihistamine: not a potent antiemetic, but prevents extrapyramidal side effects of dopamine recpetor antagonists and has sedative properities; can be used alone in some infants and children at 0.5–1.0 mg/kg per dose every 4–6 h
Metoclopramide	40 mg/m^2 intravenously every 4 h × 6 doses for each chemotherapy infusion	Dopamine and serotonin receptor antagonist: extra-pyramidal side effects, use cautiously in children
Droperidol	3 mg/m^2 intravenously every 2 h × 12 doses for each chemotherapy infusion	Dopamine receptor antagonist: extrapyramidal side effects; use cautiously in children
SCHEDULE II		
Ondansetron by Bolus Dosing	0.15 mg/kg intravenously before chemo-therapy, then at 4 and 8 h after chemotherapy	Serotonin receptor antagonist: doses may become less effective over time
Lorazepam	0.25–2.0 mg intravenously every 4–6 h	Benzodiazepine: often a useful adjunct to ondansetron, especially for anticipatory vomiting, because of its sedative and anxiolytic effects
SCHEDULE III		
Ondansetron by Bolus Dosing	0.15 mg/kg intravenously before chemo-therapy, then at 4 and 8 h after chemotherapy	Serotonin receptor antagonist: doses may become less effective over time
Dexamethasone	10–20 mg intravenously 30–45 min before chemotherapy or with first dose of ondansetron	Corticosteroid: useful as an ad-junct to ondansetron for regi-mens that contain cisplatin; side effects include hyper-glycemia and mental status changes

NOTE: The medications in schedules I and II are effective during cyclophosphamide and etoposide infusions. Nausea from busulfan is usually less problematic: preventive therapy with diphenhydramine and lorazepam may suffice. The medications in schedule III are effective for regimens that contain cisplatin.

and prochlorperazine in combination with lorazepam and diphenhydramine offer good control of nausea and vomiting. However, because of the CNS-depressant effects of these regimens and risk for cardiotoxicity, the use of these regimens is limited to the inpatient setting where patients can be monitored closely.

As the penetration of managed care increases and transplant technology continues to move from acute care to ambulatory settings, it is clear that antiemetic regimens that are both cost effective and feasible for use in outpatient situations must be identified.

Nonpharmacologic approaches such as dietary modification, relaxation strategies (e.g., rhythmic breathing exercises, progressive muscle relaxation), and distraction by a variety of methods (visual imagery, biofeedback, hypnosis) can serve as valuable adjuncts to preventive antiemetic drug regimens. Evaluating the appropriateness of patients for relaxation and distraction interventions is critical to their ultimate effectiveness. These strategies are especially useful for patients capable of participating fully, motivated to pursue them as part of the antiemetic plan, and previously successful with such alternatives (Cotanch, 1983; Morrow and Morrell, 1982; Redd and Andrykowski, 1982).

Other Etiologies. Little information regarding management of emetic responses due to etiologies other than conditioning therapies is available. Nausea, vomiting, and anorexia secondary to supportive pharmaceuticals can partially be alleviated through the use of antiemetic agents (Cunningham et al., 1983). Discontinuing responsible medications is seldom an option because many of the drugs employed during the engraftment period are necessary for prevention or treatment of life-threatening complications and without them full recovery would not be possible. However, a full review of the patient's drug profile to identify agents that could be

discontinued or replaced with less emetogenic agents is warranted. In some cases, switching from the oral to parenteral route of administration can be helpful, especially with agents such as cyclosporin.

The management of protracted emetic responses caused by infectious processes or GVHD involves successful treatment of the underlying etiology. For more specific information on preventive and therapeutic approaches to managing these complications, see Chapter 8.

The Salivary Gland Response

Pairs of sublingual, submandibular, parotid, and numerous minute buccal glands comprise the network of salivary glands responsible for producing saliva, the watery secretion that serves the important functions of cleansing the oral cavity and facilitating the passage of the food bolus along the alimentary canal. The salivary glands are highly sensitive to radiation. The acinar cells of the parotid glands, the largest pair of salivary glands, are affected to a greater extent than the mucinous acinar cells in other areas of the mouth (Carl, 1983). As a result, the 1 to 1.5 liters of saliva normally discharged into the oral cavity every 24 hours diminishes significantly after radiation therapy to the head and neck, rendering the saliva scant, tenacious, and ropy. In addition, the saliva produced becomes more acidic, thus altering normal patterns of microbial flora, increasing the risk for oral superinfection, and aggravating existing therapy-induced mucositis (Carl, 1983).

Bilateral parotitis (inflammation of the parotid glands) and partial xerostomia are frequently reported problems in allogeneic transplant patients following TBI (Carl and Higby, 1985). The parotitis associated with TBI is characterized as tender transient "mumpslike" neck swelling that occurs shortly after the initiation of TBI and resolves spontaneously in 24 to 48 hours of completing therapy. Xerostomia generally begins later and is of longer duration. Evaluating early oral changes in BMT patients, Kolbinson and colleagues (1988) reported salivary viscosity, xerostomia, and patient complaints of oral dryness as the most frequent changes during the first 2 weeks post conditioning. Xerostomia persisted for the entire 5-week study period. TBI was cited as the probable major causative factor for oral changes. Salivary gland dysfunction also is attributable to causes other other than TBI in the transplant population. The fibrotic effects of chronic GVHD (Sale et al., 1981), certain antineoplastic agents such as combination alkylating agent therapy and methotrexate (Barrett, 1986), and anticholinergic drugs have all been implicated in the causation of salivary gland damage and/or dysfunction.

The primary goals in the management of salivary gland dysfunction and resulting xerostomia overlap those in the mucositis management plan and include

1. stimulation of existing salivary gland function
2. lubrication and hydration of oral mucosa
3. infection prevention
4. control of pain or discomfort
5. prevention of resulting nutritional deficits

A regimen of meticulous oral hygiene during the conditioning and engraftment phases of the transplant process followed by regular dental care that incorporates a long-term plan for prevention and management of xerostomia-induced oral complications (e.g., the development of dental caries and periodontal disease) is critical to patients experiencing salivary gland dysfunction.

The acute neck and shoulder pain associated with parotitis that occurs during TBI conditioning is managed symptomatically with analgesics and topical cold applications (e.g., an ice collar). The management of xerostomia entails lubricants, frequent oral intake of fluids or hydrating sprays, and artificial saliva products as tolerated and according to the patient's preference (e.g., Salivart, Xerolube, Oralube, Moistir). Avoidance of mechanical (e.g., hard bristle brushing, rough foods) and thermo-chemical (e.g., hot or spicy foods, alcohol, or cigarette smoke) trauma to the oral mucosa is critical to maintaining mucosal integrity. Foods accompanied by sauces or gravies or otherwise high in water content facilitate swallowing and keep the mucosa moist. Family consultation with a dietician prior to discharge can be helpful in defining necessary dietary modifications. Regular dental follow-up is necessary post discharge, especially for patients experiencing salivary gland effects of chronic GVHD.

The Mucosal Response

The mucosal lining of the entire alimentary tract undergoes dramatic change in response to the effects of dose-intensive conditioning therapies, infectious processes, and the occurrence of GVHD. Manifestations of the damaging effects of these causative factors include oral and esophageal mucositis severe enough to impair comfort, speech, swallowing, and nutrition and gastric and intestinal ulceration with clinically significant diarrhea and subsequent hemorrhage or perforation (Armstrong, 1994; Cox et al., 1994; Peterson, 1990; Raybould et al., 1994; Schubert et al., 1984). With the exception of the mucosal damage associated with chronic GVHD, these alterations are characteristically temporary and self-limiting. Nevertheless, they set the stage for life-threatening events during the period that they are experienced.

Causation and Character

Stomatitis. Alterations in the oropharyngeal mucosa are clinically evident at various points in the transplant process, depending on etiology. The incidence of stomatitis in transplant patients is quite high, occurring in 36% to 89% of patients after transplant conditioning regimens (Carl and Higby, 1985; McGuire et al., 1993; Schubert et al., 1983; Woo et al., 1993; Zerbe et al., 1992) and in up to 80% of patients with extensive GVHD (Nims and Strom, 1988; Schubert and Sullivan, 1990). Mucosal lesions also occur commonly in this population as a result of bacterial, fungal, and viral infections (Peterson, 1990). Incidence rates, character, and severity vary according to specific conditioning regimens, types of transplant, infecting organisms, and occurrence of GVHD.

Oral complications affect patients following allogeneic BMT more often than after autologous or syngeneic BMT and with greater frequency in chronic than acute GVHD. The risk for significant oral and esophageal effects is higher for patients undergoing conditioning that incorporates TBI and GVHD prophylaxis with methotrexate (Ford and Ballard, 1988; Zerbe et al., 1992) and in those who are seropositive for HSV infection pretransplant (Montgomery et al., 1986; Peterson, 1990).

Certain antineoplastic agents used in chemotherapy conditioning regimens are known to be more stomatotoxic than others. Mucositis is the dose-limiting toxicity associated with HD busulfan, etoposide, melphalan, and thiotepa (Dorr and Von Hoff, 1994). Cytarabine, cyclophosphamide, and methotrexate also can produce mucositis in a significant number of patients (Carl and Higby, 1985; Dorr and Von Hoff, 1994).

Stomatitis develops initially in response to dose-intensive conditioning therapies. Occurring within 1 to 2 weeks of the administration of stomatotoxic therapies and peaking between 7 and 11 days post conditioning, the course of mucositis generally parallels closely that of neutropenia (Gordon et al., 1994; Lockhardt and Sonis, 1979). The clinical presentation is rapidly progressive, beginning with some combination of gingival edema and erythema. These mucosal changes often are accompanied by patient complaint of oral dryness, tingling or burning sensations. Within days these changes progress to bilateral buccal "scalloping" (i.e., blanching along the teeth line), isolated ulcerative lesions with or without pseudomembrane formation. As the mucosal effects evolve, there is sloughing of pseudomembranous plaques and ulceration becomes confluent, often encompassing more than 50% of the oral cavity at its peak.

The most common sites of ulceration are the nonkeratinized mucosa of the floor of the mouth, tongue, cheek, and soft palate (Barasch et al., 1995; Kolbinson et al., 1988; Peterson, 1990; Seto et al., 1985), though lesions may appear anywhere from the lips up to and including the esophagus. At its worst, therapy-related oropharyngeal mucositis is complicated by bleeding caused by thrombocytopenia and superinfection.

Oral infection is often difficult to distinguish from drug- and radiation-induced effects because infectious complications generally do not occur as isolated events. Rather, they are superimposed on existing therapy-related changes in the oropharyngeal mucosa. Further, the clinical presentation of oral infectious processes depends on the responsible organism. Gram-negative bacterial infections usually present as creamy but nonpurulent, raised, shiny erosions on an erythematous foundation. In contrast, gram-positive staphylococcal and streptococcal infections appear as dry, raised, wartlike, yellowish-brown, round plaques (Brager and Yasko, 1984).

HSV infections occur either because of primary exposure or more commonly as a result of reactivation of the latent virus between 8 and 12 days in allogeneic BMT patients (Kolbinson et al., 1988; Strohl, 1989) and somewhat less frequently in autologous BMT patients. HSV is manifest as discrete vesicular lesions on the lips or anywhere in the oral cavity and can take on the appearance of other oral infections or lesions secondary to therapy. Oral candidiasis presents as pinpoint lesions under yellowish or whitish curdlike plaques on the tongue and buccal mucosa (Brager and Yasko, 1984). In addition, patients with oropharyngeal candidal infections often complain of burning, pain, and/ or dysgeusia. Because the oropharyngeal area is rife with normal flora as well as pathogens, differential diagnosis relies on oral cultures or biopsy (McDonald et al., 1985).

The oral manifestations of acute GVHD are not yet well documented. Existing descriptions are general and cite clinical elements of the clinical presentation similar to those associated with other etiologies such as painful desquamation, mucosal ulceration, erythema, plaques, and lichenoid keratoses (Barrett and Bilous, 1984; Kolbinson et al., 1988). These findings mimic those observed with conditioning-induced stomatitis and, therefore, may be misdiagnosed as an exacerbation of that problem rather than the onset of this new clinical situation.

In contrast, the presenting signs reported with chronic GVHD differ significantly from those related to other etiologies and include gingival atrophy and patchy erythema or lichenoid lesions of the buccal and labial mucosa, salivary gland fibrosis, and oral pain. Ulcerative lesions are not typical except in patients with severe chronic GVHD. Persistent dryness of the oral cavity also has been reported (Rodu and Glockerman, 1983; Schubert et al., 1984). Another distinguishing factor is the onset, which does not occur until at least 3 months and as long as 12 months post transplant.

Seven major descriptive studies further detail the onset, duration, and character of stomatitis in the BMT population (see Table 10.4). More research evaluating the phenomenon of stomatitis is necessary to fully document its presentation and natural course in BMT/BCT subpopulations (e.g., predisposing factors, effects associated with unstudied conditioning regimens, source of stem cells, use of cytokines, relationship to infectious etiologies, etc.).

Esophagitis. Mucosal changes also occur in the eophagus, though they are more difficult to characterize because of the inability to directly visualize the area except by invasive means (e.g., endoscopy). Consequently, for routine evaluation clinicians rely on patients' subjective complaints of dysphagia, epigastric pain, or burning in conjunction with observations of trends in the evolution of oropharyngeal mucosal alterations and the appearance of indicators of oral infection, which may extend into the esophagus. As with alterations of oropharyngeal mucosa, mucosal impairments of the esophagus are due primarily to the damaging effects of conditioning therapies, infectious processes, and GVHD. Mucosal tears resulting from the trauma of intense retching and gastroesophageal acid reflux also may impair esophageal mucosa (Shuhart and McDonald, 1994).

Bacterial, viral, and fungal infections of the esophagus all occur with relative frequency in BMT/BCT patients. Bacteria, along with viral and fungal pathogens derived from the oral flora, can infect the esophagus early in the engraftment period. The result is a polymicrobial infectious process (Walsh, Belitsos, Hamilton, 1986). This condition necessitates endoscopic biopsy to confirm the diagnosis and distinguish the process from GVHD (McDonald et al., 1985; Shuhart and McDonald, 1994).

Viral esophagitis due primarily to HSV and CMV is another serious complication occurring in BMT patients (Apperly and Goldman, 1988; Shuhart and McDonald, 1994). In patients who have allogeneic BMTs, it may appear between 30 and 75 days (Wolford and McDonald, 1988). CMV is less common in patients undergoing autologous transplantation (Wingard et al., 1988), but HSV occurs in both populations, especially patients who were seropositive prior to transplant.

TABLE 10.4 Key studies of stomatitis in patients undergoing BMT

Investigators	Population	Key findings
Barrett, 1986	15 allogeneic BMT patients	60%–90% experienced ulceration, bleeding, infection 2 HSV, candida, bacteria
Eilers et al., 1988	18 autologous BMT patients 2 allogeneic BMT patients	Stomatitis severity peaked from day +5 to day +12
Kolbinson et al., 1988	21 allogeneic BMT (2 syngeneic) patients	Incidence rates not reported; onset of oral changes prior to marrow infusion with worsening over 2-week post-BMT period; actual ulceration between day +7 and day +11; followed by progressive resolution; pain onset between day +4 and day +14 with 70% pts. requiring IV narcotics
McGuire et al., 1993	28 autologous BMT patients 19 allogeneic BMT patients	42 pts. (89%) developed stomatitis; average onset at day +3; average duration day +9.5; resolution at day +12.6 36 pts. (86%) reported pain; average onset at day +4; average duration day +6.5; resolution at day +11
Weisdorf et al., 1989	100 BMT patients	Stomatitis average onset between day +4 and day +8; peak at day +10 to day +15; gradual resolution around day +24
Wingard et al., 1991	47 BMT patients	17 pts. (36%) developed ulcerative stomatitis; average onset between day –2 and day +18 with median at day +4; incidence 19 × higher in pts. receiving bucy or bucy + VP –16 than CY along or CY +TBI (P < 0.001)
Zerbe et al., 1992	12 allogeneic BMT patients 8 autologous BMT patients	Onset of mucosal changes at day –2, peaked at day +8 and returned to baseline between day +20 and day +25; 15 pts. required continuous infusion narcotic to control oral pain

SOURCE: Adapted from Armstrong, 1994.

Mucosal alterations differ according to the infecting virus. Changes associated with HSV include the development of small vesicles in the squamous epithelium of the mid and distal regions of the esophagus. Sloughing of infected epithelial tissue produces ulcers with raised erythematous borders, which may coalesce and result in large denuded areas. When thrombocytopenia precludes endoscopic biopsy, diagnosis of HSV can be made with brushings alone (Shuhart and McDonald, 1994).

Unlike HSV, CMV infects endothelial cells and fibroblasts in the esophageal submucosa. Endoscopically, CMV infection appears as shallow ulcers with erythematous edges. Though ulcers can be as large as 10 to 12 cm, some normal epithelium is visible. Biopsy is the most reliable diagnostic method, though it requires the patient have adequate platelet counts to avoid hemorrhagic complications (Shuhart and McDonald, 1994). Definitive diagnosis of CMV esophagitis by biopsy and culture is very important because visceral dissemination can occur if the patient is receiving immunosuppressants to prevent GVHD (McDonald et al., 1986).

Clinically, nausea and vomiting are prominent features. Other clinical symptoms include fever, dysphagia, severe retrosternal pain, and esophageal ulceration. With HSV infections, vomiting may be incessant and strictures may be a late complication (Wolford and McDonald, 1988; Shuhart and McDonald, 1994). Fortunately, viral esophagitis is rare today since the advent of prophylactic antiviral therapy with gancyclovir and acyclovir (Reed et al., 1988; Shuhart and McDonald, 1994).

Fungal esophagitis is due primarily to various species of candida and aspergillus and occur usually during the neutropenic period immediately following conditioning. Anorexia is pronounced. Other clinical manifestations include dysphagia, epigastric pain expressed as "heartburn," GI bleeding, and fever. Esophagitis may occur with or without oral candidiasis. Because the classic creamy adherent plaques are absent during granulocytopenia and cultures do not distinguish between colonization and tissue infection, definitive diagnosis relies on brushings and esophageal biopsy. As with viral esophagitis, prophylactic antifungal therapies appear to be decreasing the incidence of esophagitis of fungal origin (Shuhart and McDonald, 1994).

Approximately 10% of patients with extensive chronic GVHD have esophageal involvement characterized by dysphagia, pain, weight loss, and aspiration (Wolford and McDonald, 1988). Radiographically, esophageal webbing, ring formation, and strictures are seen (Deeg and Storb, 1986).

Ulceration and GI Bleeding. Patients undergoing BMT/BCT are at risk for gross or occult bleeding from various sites in the GI tract where the mucosal wall has been damaged. Approximately 5% to 15% of patients develop severe bleeding during the first 100 days as evidenced by hematemesis, melena, or gross rectal bleeding (Shuhart and McDonald, 1994). A significantly larger population experience spontaneous occult or minor bleeding during periods of severe thrombocytopenia, especially when thrombocytopenia is refractory to platelet transfusion therapy. Though not necessarily life-threatening, oropharyngeal and nasal bleeding are particularly problematic and anxiety provoking for patients.

The most common sites associated with severe GI hemorrhage in the transplant population are the esophageal and intestinal regions of the alimentary tract. The specific causes of severe bleeding from those sites include traumatic injury to the mucosa due to uncontrollable retching and ulceration secondary to acid-peptic reflux or viral and fungal infection (Shuhart and McDonald, 1994). Mallory-Weiss tears at the gastroesophageal junction and intramural hematomas generally pose hemorrhagic problems only until platelet counts rise above 60,000/mm^3. Resolution of hematomas occurs without surgical intervention at about 10 to 14 days (Wolford and McDonald, 1988).

Similarly, esophageal bleeding due to reflux ulceration responds to keeping platelet counts adequate and controlling the acid-peptic reflux. Surgical intervention might be necessary when ulcers become chronic and expose submucosal vessels that bleed persistently (Wolford and McDonald, 1987). Ulceration secondary to infectious agents has been all but eliminated by antiviral and antifungal prophylaxis, though it was previously a primary cause of GI hemorrhage (Goodrich et al., 1991; Goodman et al., 1992; Perfect et al., 1992).

Enteritis and Diarrhea. Mucosal damage resulting in inflammation, significant diarrhea, hemorrhage, and occasional perforation of the gastric and intestinal regions of the alimentary tract occur in the BMT/BCT population secondary to many of the same causative factors responsible for upper-tract mucosal impairment. Acute diarrheal illness is a particularly complex problem that, if not adequately controlled, can be life threatening in this population. Multiple etiologies for intestinal dysfunction can give rise to diarrhea. The toxic effects of chemoradiation conditioning therapy on the intestinal mucosa and of certain supportive pharmaceuticals (e.g., antibiotics, metoclopramide, oral magnesium, antacids) produce diarrhea early in the transplant process. Viral, bacterial, and parasitic infections and the effects of GVHD are primary causative factors during later phases (e.g., days 20 through 100). (Cascinu, 1995; Cox et al., 1994; Shuhart and McDonald, 1994).

The diarrhea associated with BMT/BCT procedures are classified as chemotherapy-induced, secretory, exudative, osmotic, or dismotility types depending on the likely etiology, onset, and clinical features. Each type of diarrhea is associated with specific effects on the intestinal mucosa. The clinical manifestations of diarrheal illness vary according to etiopathologic category.

Chemotherapy-induced mucosal alterations are generally not well understood, but morphologic changes associated with diarrhea include mucosal crypt aberrations, decreased villus height, and distortion of surface epithelium and villous architecture. These changes cause secretion of intestinal fluid to peak 7 to 10 days after the initiation of conditioning therapy and normalize between 12 and 15 days (Cascinu, 1995; Fegan, Poynton, Whittaker, 1990). By day 20 mucosal regeneration is complete (Shuhart and McDonald, 1994).

Chemotherapy-related diarrhea is characterized as watery stools with crampy abdominal pain and anorexia. Intestinal bleeding also may be observed if mucosal damage is extensive (Champlin and Gale, 1984). The pattern of symptom resolution parallels the time period for regeneration of the normal marrow elements, generally a few weeks (Fegan, Poynton, Whittaker, 1990). Diarrhea is a particularly notable effect of certain antineoplastic agents used in HD transplant conditioning regimens including busulfan, cytarabine, paclitaxel, melphalan, and methotrexate. The uroprotectant, mesna, is also implicated (Dorr and Von Hoff, 1994).

The principal mucosal alterations in the gut produced in *secretory syndrome* are

- an increased intestinal secretion of fluid and electrolytes initiated by morphologic changes in the crypt cells and mediated by a spectrum of secretagogues (e.g., hormones, inflammatory substances; enterotoxins), in conjunction with
- a reduced absorptive capacity of the enterocytes lining the villi due to architectural changes in and the loss of brush border enzymes from the intestinal villi.

Secretory-type diarrhea presents as large volume (>1000 ml/day) watery stools (stool osmolality approaching that of plasma) that persist even in the absence of oral intake, and begins later in the transplant process.

Primary etiologies associated with secretory diarrhea include noninvasive infectious organisms known to produce enterotoxin (e.g., *Clostridium difficile*) and intestinal GVHD. In BMT/BCT patients secretory-type diarrhea due to infection is most often associated with *C. difficile,* astrovirus, and adenovirus.

Secretory syndrome is the prominent feature of acute GVHD of the gut in allogeneic BMT patients. Stool volume in this setting is proportionate to the extent of mucosal damage. Severe damage can produce losses of up to 10 to 15 liters per day accompanied by severe dehydration, protein and electrolyte disturbances

(Cascinu, 1995; Shuhart and McDonald, 1994). The dramatic stool volume lost as a result of GVHD occurs because the intestinal regions most often affected by GVHD, the ileum and cecum, are primarily responsible for fluid absorption (Shuhart and McDonald, 1994). The abrupt onset of diarrhea is related to a cascade of events beginning with local cytokine release (e.g., tumor necrosis factor), which produces mucosal edema, increases vascular permeability, and enhances the movement of fluid across the intestinal wall (Holler et al., 1990). Stools appear watery and greenish with ropy mucoid strands indicative of protein loss (Weisdorf et al., 1990). In severe cases of GVHD, intestinal bleeding or hemorrhage often accompany diarrhea, making stools melanotic or frankly bloody (Wolford and McDonald, 1987).

Exudative diarrhea results when the mucosal integrity of the intestinal wall is disrupted by inflammation and ulceration. Subsequently, mucus, blood, and serum proteins are discharged through the damaged wall into the bowel lumen. Unlike the clinical picture presented with secretory syndrome, exudative-type diarrhea presents with high frequency stools (> 6 stools per day) of variable volume but generally less than 1000 ml per day. Hypoalbuminemia and anemia also are part of the exudative picture. Exudative diarrhea is associated with radiation injury and infection with invasive pathogens (Shigella, Salmonella, Strongyloides, Giardia lamblia, rotavirus) (Cascinu, 1995; Wadler, 1994).

Osmotic and *dismotility-type diarrheas* are not associated with mucosal changes but rather with mechanical disturbances that affect the bowel wall. In the former, osmotic forces are disrupted by luminal exposure to hyperosmolar stimuli (e.g., magnesium-based antacids, intraluminal blood); in the latter, peristaltic enhancement secondary to alterations in a variety of mechanical stretch or neural receptors (e.g., due to peristatic stimulants) is the responsible mechanism. These intestinal disturbances often are triggered by mucosal aberrations responsible for the other types of diarrhea described (Cascinu, 1995; Fruto, 1994). Osmotic diarrhea is characterized by a large volume of watery stools that resolve when the causative agent is withdrawn. The stools associated with bowel hypermotility are frequent, small, semisolid to liquid.

The multicausal nature of transplant-related diarrhea makes diagnosis of underlying etiologies, which often overlap, difficult and subsequently delays the implementation of effective management strategies. It is especially difficult to distinguish infectious and noninfectious etiologies. In one recent study of 126 patients undergoing autologous and allogeneic transplant, for example, the incidence of acute diarrhea after day 20 was 43%. Biopsy-proven intestinal GVHD was responsible for 48% of cases and intestinal infection was documented in 13%, but the investigators were unable to identify with certainty the cause of diarrhea in 39% of patients (Cox et al., 1994). The low incidence of infection and the high number of cases in which etiology could not be specifically identified are especially notable. Clearly, more research is necessary to further describe diarrheal illness in the transplant population.

Perirectal Lesions. The effects of conditioning regimens and diarrheal illness also can impair mucosal integrity in the perirectal area. This is particularly problematic in highly immunosuppressed patients since the rectum and perianal area provide an ideal environment for the numerous preexisting skin flora and fecal organisms to flourish while impaired mucosa permits invasion of tissues and ultimately sepsis and death. Organisms predominantly associated with rectal infection include *Pseudomonas aeruginosa*, *E. coli*, and *Klebsiella* species. Other organisms identified as causative for rectal infection are group-D *Streptococcus*, *Staphylococcus aureas*, *Hemophilus influenzae*, *Enterobacter cloacae*, *Candida albicans*, and

Bacteroides fragilis (Yeomans, 1986; Yeomans et al., 1991). Vancomycin-resistant enterococci are a newer group of resistant bacteria that pose more difficult challenges to infection control in this highly immunosuppressed population (CDC, 1994; Montecalvo et al., 1994).

Fever, a sign often difficult to distinguish from other febrile causes, and perirectal pain, which patients typically attribute to hemorrhoidal problems, comprise the prodromal symptom profile. Fever generally precedes diagnosis of perirectal infection by 3 to 6 days, the onset of pain having been about 2 to 3 days prior. Though rectal infections can take on various clinical presentations and can progress to expansive necrotic lesions, the development of point tenderness and poorly demarcated induration are among the earliest consistent findings associated with rectal abscess (Barnes et al., 1984; Yeomans, 1986; Yeomans et al., 1991). Knowing that early indicators can easily be confused with other etiologies, clinicians must maintain a high degree of suspicion regarding perirectal infection as a cause when patients complain of "hemorrhoidal" pain in the presence of unexplained fever.

Assessment and Management

Effective management of mucosal responses to the sequelae of BMT/BCT depends largely on accurate identification of the underlying causative factor(s). Sorting through etiologies for alimentary mucosal wall impairment and its manifestations is an especially challenging task in this population because of the multicausal nature of the mucosal aberrations and the inability to visualize large regions of the alimentary tract without invasive means. Routine visual inspection is an option for assessment only of the oropharyngeal and perianal areas of the tract. Consequently, since they are visible and readily accessed, the tendency has been to focus attention and research on those regions. Assessment of esophageal and intestinal impairments is considerably more difficult, which re-

sults in less comprehensive assessment and more empiric managerial approaches. Another important consideration when planning therapeutic approaches is that strategies used to manage certain causative factors can at the same time be responsible for mucosal impairment. Consequently, the risk of new or enhanced mucosal injury must be balanced against the potential benefits of the intervention to resolve the manifestations at specific points along the alimentary tract.

Stomatitis. Considerable attention has been focused on characterizing and treating stomatitis in the patient undergoing transplant procedures, yet no concrete standards addressing this complication in the transplant setting exist. A recent national survey of oral care practices in 92 BMT centers in the United States conducted by Ezzone and colleagues (1993) revealed a wide spectrum of assessment strategies and intervention plans for stomatitis. A majority of responding centers reported assessment strategies that incorporate pretransplant dental consultations, and routine assessment by nurses (i.e., every shift) and physicians (i.e., daily). Though 42% reported using an oral evaluation instrument to cue assessment and document findings, there was no consistency among centers as to the particular tool. The variety of tools reportedly in use ranged from comprehensive detailed documents such as the Oral Assessment Guide developed by Eilers, Berger, and Peterson (1988) to more simple grading scales as depicted in Table 10.2.

Parameters employed by more than 85% of the respondents to guide assessment include observations for the presence of oral ulceration, discoloration of the oral mucosa, tissue sloughing, indicators of infection, indicators of bleeding such as petechiae or bruising, and xerostomia. The condition of the lips also was high on the list. Patients' perceptions of pain or discomfort and functional ability have also been cited as important data when evaluating oral mucosal impairment (Beck, 1979; Western Consortium for Nursing Research, 1991).

Despite a plethora of recommendations for oral care of patients undergoing cancer therapies in the medical, nursing, and dental literature, there are no proven methods of preventing therapy-induced oropharyngeal lesions. Consequently, realistic management goals include preventing the incidence of secondary infection and minimizing the intensity of subsequent pain. Though some themes are identifiable, there is wide institution-based variation in the specific solutions, techniques, and devices reportedly used in core cleansing regimens for patients who undergo BMT/BCT. Infection-control and pain-management components of the regimens described also vary significantly. Table 10.5 illustrates the spectrum of interven-

TABLE 10.5 Findings of survey of interventions to manage stomatitis in the BMT population (N = 92 BMT centers)

Interventions	Responses	Interventions	Responses
Frequency of Oral Assessment		**Oral-Cavity Lubricants**	
Every 2–4 hours	7%	Oral fluids	76%
Every 4 hours	17%	Artifical saliva	57%
Every 8 hours	44%	Hard candy	54%
Every 12 hours	14%	Chewing gum	25%
Daily	17%	Glycerine swabs	7%
Oral-Care Techniques/Tools		Normal swabs	5%
Toothettes	68%	**Infection-Control Strategies**	
Mouthwash only	28%	Fungal prophylaxis	78%
Soft toothbrush	14%	Chlortrimazole troches	73%
Gauze	5%	Nystatin swish, swallow	82%
Swabs	5%	**Oral-Pain Management**	
Jet spray	3%	Viscous lidocaine	65%
Oral-Care Solutions		Lidocaine/Benadryl/antacid mixture	45%
Peridex	36%	Systemic analgesics	36%
Normal saline	33%	**Indications for Modification**	
Sodium bicarbonate	17%	**of Regimen**	
Water only	14%	Change in oral care	
Peroxide	10%	Trigger point: WBC	47%
Commercial mouthwash	3%	Trigger point: platelet count	72%
Betadine	1%	Change in toothbrushing techniques	
Lip Lubricants		Trigger point: WBC < 500 mm^3	23%
Petroleum	82%	Trigger point: platelet count	41%
Water-based lubricant	11%	< 50,000 mm^3	
Ointments with vitamins A, D	8%	Change in flossing techniques	
Lanolin	7%	Trigger point: WBT < 1000 mm^3	16%
Glycerin	5%	Trigger point: platelet count	22%
Other	9%	< 50,000 mm^3	

SOURCE: Ezzone et al., 1993.

tions employed in protocols to manage stomatitis in the transplant population.

Most regimens include vigorous, frequent oral cleansing to avoid the development of a debris-laden environment conducive to microbial growth, to reduce the residing pathogen load, and to enhance the patient's comfort. Routine brushing with a soft-bristled toothbrush and flossing are recommended until marrow function is suppressed, though standard cytopenic trigger points at which this practice should be discontinued have not yet been defined. Simple tools such as toothettes or gauze-covered tongue blades are the suggested non-traumatic replacements for the toothbrush despite the finding that they are not effective in removing debris or stimulating gingival tissue (Miaskowski, 1990; Ezzone et al., 1993). More complex devices (e.g., water jet sprays) are cited but there is little information about effectiveness or attendant risks.

Patients are routinely encouraged to remove dentures or other oral appliances because they can be a source of mucosal irritation and prevent adequate cleansing. Commercial mouthwashes are generally discouraged because many contain isopropyl alcohol, which can have a drying effect on the oral mucosa (Brager and Yasko, 1984). Instead, saline and sterile water alone or in solution with sodium bicarbonate or hydrogen peroxide (Daeffler, 1980; Tombes and Gallucci, 1993) and broad-spectrum antimicrobial mouthrinses with chlorhexidine gluconate (Ferretti et al., 1988; Raybould et al., 1994; Weisdorf et al., 1989), amikacin (Brown et al., 1990), or amphotericin (Viele, C., personal communication, 1994) in varying frequency schemes have all been proposed.

Prophylaxis of oral infection is further accomplished empirically by initiating antiviral and antifungal agents at some point pretransplant for a predetermined duration during the transplant process. Because the HSV reactivation rate is high in transplant patients (i.e., approximately 75%), prophylactic oral or parenteral acyclovir is administered to HSV-seropositive patients in a majority of surveyed centers (Ezzone et al., 1993; Poland, 1989; Saral, 1989). To prevent fungal infections, especially *Candidiasis,* topical antifungal agents are used. Sequenced immediately after the cleansing procedure, antifungal troches (i.e., clotrimazole 10 mg p.o. 5x daily) slowly dissolved in the mouth or suspensions (i.e., nystatin 30 ml of 100,000 U/ml solution 3x daily) using a swish-and-swallow approach have been incorporated as standard practice into the routine oral-care regimen in BMT centers (Ezzone et al., 1993). However, the introduction of fluconazole (100 mg–200 mg p.o. daily) raises questions about the need to also use topical antifungals in transplant and leukemia populations.

Pain control in patients who develop mild to moderate stomatitis involves dietary modification to eliminate irritating food and fluids in conjunction with topical anesthetics (e.g., Dyclone 0.5%; lidocaine viscous 2%; cetacaine spray). Though a swish-and-expectorate technique often is recommended with these agents, in the case of isolated lesions, local application with a cotton-tipped swab or directed spray results in targeted pain control without numbing the entire oral cavity. Admixtures of varying combinations of antacid, antihistamine, and topical anesthetic also have been described. However, the use of such solutions can produce thick tenacious secretions, obscure visualization of the oral mucosa and, impairment of the patient's gag reflex (Engelking, 1988).

In cases of severe stomatitis, the pain often reaches an intensity that precludes mastication, swallowing, and speaking. Parenteral nutrition usually is initiated and systemic narcotic analgesia is delivered parenterally by continuous infusions, by intermittent bolusing, or by patient-controlled devices. An oral-suction device that has a nontraumatic tip and that is easily used by patients to suction secretions also should be made available.

Some innovative approaches recently investigated involve prostaglandin E_2 prophylaxis (Labar et al., 1993), novel uses of existing agents such as allopurinol rinses (Elzawawy, 1991; Loprinzi et al., 1990), and propantheline to minimize mucosal contact with antineoplastics (Ahmed et al., 1993), pain reduction strategies using benzocaine in a mucoadhesive base (LeVeque et al., 1992), and vitamin E (Wadleigh et al., 1992), cryotherapy (Rocke et al., 1993), and low energy helium-neon laser therapy (Barasch et al., 1995).

Currently, there are no consistent scientific findings to indicate the superiority of one cleansing regimen over another, support the efficacy of prophylactic antimicrobial interventions, or identify the best strategies for pain control. Key controversies with regard to the core cleansing regimen include the timing and frequency of interventions, the appropriateness of incorporating routine prophylactic antimicrobial swish solutions, and oral cleansing devices (e.g., toothettes, power sprays). In the infection-control component, unanswered questions concern the risks and benefits of repetitive use of prophylactic systemic antiviral therapy and topical antifungal agents in the presence of systemic therapy, and the most efficacious and cost-effective length of therapy.

Issues relevant to the management of oral pain revolve around the use of multiagent mixtures to produce topical analgesia and the risk/benefit ratio of systemic opioid infusions to control severe pain. The need to modify regimens based on identified etiology and the setting (inpatient versus outpatient) also is yet to be defined. However, the fact remains that establishment and implementation of a systematic approach to assess and treat stomatitis, regardless of the specific intervention, is more beneficial than random management strategies (Beck, 1979; Peterson, 1990).

Esophagitis and Dysphagia. The management of esophagitis is an extension of the stomatitis management plan with overlapping goals and interventions. Primary medical mangement of esophagitis is directly linked to the identified etiology. The goals for controlling infectious complications resulting in esophagitis are similar to the infection-control objectives of the oral-care regimen—prevention in patients at risk (e.g., HSV seropositive) and targeted antimicrobial intervention for documented infection. As in the prevention of oral HSV reactivation, current antiviral prophylaxis for HSV esophagitis involves acyclovir (e.g., 5 mg/kg every 8 hours). When HSV is documented, those isolates resistant to acyclovir generally respond to a course of foscarnet (Shuhart and McDonald, 1994).

CMV prophylaxis entails the use of immune globulin and CMV-seronegative blood products to patients who were seronegative pretransplant (Bowden et al., 1986). When esophageal CMV infection is diagnosed, gancyclovir administered in high doses for the first 2 weeks followed by lower doses for 2 weeks or more has demonstrated efficacy in eliminating the infection. However, resolution of esophageal ulceration and concomitant symptoms is slow (Reed et al., 1990).

Foscarnet may be an alternative though little conclusive data is available with regard to its efficacy in the BMT population (Ringden et al., 1987; Shuhart and McDonald, 1994). Antifungal prophylaxis is accomplished with oral fluconazole (100 mg–200 mg daily). IV amphotericin is indicated by the presence of documented fungal infection or when granulocytopenia is coupled with suspicious systemic symptoms. Newer liposomal formulations may reduce amphotericin-induced hypersensitivity that makes the agent difficult for patients to tolerate, though it is a costly drug and studies to determine its efficacy in controlling untoward effects in the transplant population are complete.

Esophageal reflux and ulceration are managed symptomatically. Strategies recommended for reducing gastric acid production and reflux include head-of-bed elevation, omeprazole, and intraesophageal antacid drips to alkalinize the esophagus (Shuhart and McDonald, 1994). H_2-receptor antagonists are avoided in the transplant population since they are known to produce granulocytopenia (Agura et al., 1988).

Ulceration and GI Bleeding. The approach to management of GI bleeding depends on the site and the severity. Patients are observed closely for overt and occult bleeding. All stools and emesis should be tested for occult blood. Laboratory indices reflective of risk for or actual bleeding (e.g., platelet counts, hematocrit, coagulation studies) are routinely monitored. For minor oral and nasal bleeding, topical strategies include applications of cold and topical coagulants as targeted applications, rinses, or packings (e.g., thrombin, aminocaproic acid, absorbable gelatin film). Not only should patients be discouraged from dislodging clot formations, but also the vigor of oral care must be attenuated to prevent the abrupt disturbance of clots. Close monitoring for obstructive symptoms and breathing difficulties is paramount and oral suction should be readily available. Involving the patient and family in the management plan whenever possible and reassurance that breathing will be maintained helps to minimize anxiety.

In cases of severe GI bleeding, medical interventions are aimed at maintaining hemodynamic stability, and determining and eradicating the specific hemorrhagic source. Maintaining platelet counts at or above established trigger points (e.g., 20,000/mm^3) is accomplished with more frequent platelet transfusions. Single-donor platelets are employed in refractory patients. Continuous infusions of platelets and aminocaproic acid are given to patients unresponsive to less aggressive inter-

ventions. Endoscopic procedures, angiography, and surgical resection of ulcerated intestines depend on the risk-benefit analysis conducted by the medical team (Wolford and McDonald, 1988).

Enteritis and Diarrhea. The management of diarrhea in the transplant population is dictated by its type and severity. Comprehensive assessment is necessary to pinpoint the precise cause and to accurately characterize the patient's diarrhea and its overall impact. Assessment should include stool character and pattern, abdominal evaluation, hydration and electrolyte status, perianal skin integrity, and associated signs and symptoms such as fever and pain. Stool analyses and blood cultures are required to distinguish infectious and noninfectious etiologies (Jones et al., 1988). Endoscopic evaluations and enteric biopsy may be necessary to establish GVHD as a definitive diagnosis, especially in the case of risk for CMV enteritis. The criteria for rating severity of diarrhea (Table 10.2) are useful in monitoring the diarrhea pattern over time. Actual volume of diarrhea is a key in the grading and staging of intestinal GVHD (Atkinson et al., 1989). Once the patient's diarrhea has been characterized and the underlying cause identified, diarrhea management goals include

1. reestablishment of the normal bowel pattern,
2. restoration and maintenance of fluid and electolyte balance,
3. protection of skin integrity, and
4. maintenance of the patient's comfort and dignity.

Reestablishment of the normal bowel pattern in the setting of enteric infections entails administration of appropriate antimicrobial therapy (e.g., vancomycin or metronidazole for *C. difficile;* acyclovir for HSV; gancyclovir or foscarnet for CMV). Immunosuppressive therapy is dramatically effective in controlling the diarrhea associated with intestinal GVHD. Half the patients in one retrospective study responded immediately to initial therapy with prednisone, cyclosporin, or antithymocyte globulin (Martin et al., 1990). Dietary modification to eliminate bowel stimulants or irritants also can help to normalize bowel pattern. A bland, low-residue diet is most appropriate. In severe cases, intake is restricted to parenteral nutrition in an attempt to rest the bowel.

In the absence of infectious etiologies, a variety of pharmaceutical agents are used to further restore the normal bowel pattern and provide symptomatic relief. They include absorbents (e.g., aluminum hydroxide, pectin), adsorbents (e.g., kaolin), anticholinergics (e.g., belladonna, atropine sulfate), opiate derivatives (e.g., loperamide, codeine, paregoric), and antisecretory agents (e.g., clonidine, octreotide acetate). The antiperistaltic, loperamide, has been the most used antidiarrheal agent. More recently, interest has been generated in determining the usefulness of the synthetic somatostatin analogue, octreotide acetate, in controlling transplant-related diarrhea.

Efficacy has been demonstrated in managing diarrhea due to GVHD in several small pilot studies (Bianco et al., 1990; Ely et al., 1991). One recent trial comparing the two agents in the control of chemotherapy-induced diarrhea in 36 BMT and leukemia patients suggested that oral loperamide had greater efficacy than continuous infusion of octreotide, but noted that results may differ at higher doses and in the population of BMT patients receiving TBI as a component of the conditioning regimen. Since loperamide is available only as an oral preparation, octreotide was suggested as an alternative for patients with severe mucositis and/or dysphagia (Geller et al., 1995). More research is needed to identify superior antidiarrheal agents and establish the most effective doses.

The management plan for diarrhea also must attend to the integrity of the patients' hydration, perianal skin, and comfort. Fluids and electrolytes are monitored closely and replaced or supplemented as needed. Strict intake and output, daily or twice-daily weights, and cardiovascular parameters provide the data necessary for assessing the adequacy of volume. Perianal skin requires meticulous attention after each diarrheal episode. Nondetergent soaps or plain water are preferable for cleansing and friction should be avoided when drying the area. To further protect the skin, a moisture barrier that is easily cleansed should be applied after careful cleansing and drying.

In severe cases of diarrhea, an external collection device is necessary to minimize skin exposure to the corrosive effects of stool. There is little information specific to the transplant population, however, additional interventions for maintaining integrity of perianal skin can be found in the literature dealing with wounds, ostomy, and continence (Basch and Jensen, 1991).

Perirectal Abscess. The ability to directly examine the perianal area is advantageous to the clinician in detecting early skin and mucosal changes that may be harbingers of serious rectal infection or abscesses that can lead to septicemia and death in the transplant population. The Perirectal Skin Assessment Tool (PSAT) developed by Yeomans and colleagues (1991) is an excellent guide for visual inspection of the perianal area of patients who complain of rectal pain (Table 10.2).

In addition to routine hygiene after each bowel movement, anecdotally reported preventive measures involve perianal skin decontamination with daily antimicrobial scrubs or sitz baths and the application of antiinfective ointments (Crane, Emmer Grguras, 1989). The particular products vary considerably from institution to institution, ranging from simple soap and water to chlorhexidine or providone-iodine scrubs (Yeomans et al., 1991). Though a number of studies have demonstrated that routine chlohexidine can reduce microbial count in the perianal region (Davis et al., 1977), there is no evidence that a prophylactic scrub or bath protects against infection. One small comparative study revealed no difference in the incidence of perirectal infections or skin impairments between chlorhexidine or nonmedicated soap among patients using prophylactic perianal scrub protocols (Yeomans et al., 1991). Though warm-water sitz bathing has been suggested in the past, concerns have arisen about the risk of infection associated with this procedure. Until that issue has been resolved, regular showering with a handheld shower head or the use of a peri bottle to direct the flow of warm water can help to keep the perianal area scrupulously clean in patients with preexisting hemorrhoids, fissures, and/or perianal breakdown due to frequent diarrhea.

Patients can be taught self-care of the rectal area but should be monitored to ensure that their technique is effective and to address factors (e.g., weakness, fatigue, use of CNS depressants, lack of understanding) that might interfere with compliance. Normalizing bowel elimination patterns altered by constipation or diarrhea and avoiding rectal manipulations such as digital examinations, rectal suppositories, thermometers, and enemas also are common precautions to minimize risk for perirectal infection.

Acute perirectal inflammation and abscess are managed with antiinfective therapy, which includes broad-spectrum antibiotics, and antifungal and antiviral agents depending on the organism(s) isolated and possibly even surgical incision or drainage (Barnes et al., 1984; Shaked, Shinar, Freund, 1986). Wound care to prevent the development of superinfection and to enhance healing must be implemented once perianal lesions become obvious.

The complexity of the wound-care plan is dictated by the severity of the perianal skin impairment. Consultation with a wound-care specialist or enterostomal therapist is recommended to devise a wound-care protocol that is feasible and appropriate to the patient's specific situation, and that can be consistently followed by the patient's caregivers. Because an array of wound-care products are available, the specialist can assist in selection and proper usage of the products chosen. At a minimum, the wound-care protocol should define (1) solutions, techniques, and frequency of wound cleansing; (2) antimicrobial ointments or creams, skin barrier products, or wound-dressing materials to be applied after cleansing; and (3) pain control. Procedures for managing perianal lesions in the BMT/BCT population are not specifically described. However, the guiding principles and specific wound-care procedures from which to extrapolate protocol are detailed elsewhere (Bryant, 1992; Fowler, 1987; Sieggren, 1987).

The Hepatic Response

The liver is affected by various events in the transplant process. The causes of liver toxicity in transplant patients can be predicted from the time the transplant process begins to their presentation. Treatment-related toxicity caused by conditioning with HD chemotherapy with or without TBI, drug-induced toxicity associated with support medications, veno-occlusive disease (VOD), GVHD, infection, and recurrent disease are all possible factors (Shuhart and McDonald, 1994; Ayash, 1992). Resulting damage to the hepatocytes leads, ultimately, to loss of liver function. The loss in function can range from a transient elevation in liver function studies to the serious disorder of VOD. Because the pathogenesis and management of VOD and the hepatic effects of GVHD are detailed elsewhere, only the nutritional implications of these complications are addressed in this chapter. Other etiologies associated with liver complications in the transplant population are summarized briefly.

Causation and Character

Liver Infection. Pretransplant hepatitis can be as threatening to patients undergoing transplant procedures as infections that occur later in the process. The presence of hepatitis prior to transplantation carries three risks for BMT patients: (1) an increased risk of fatal VOD following conditioning therapy, (2) viral hepatitis post transplant, and (3) progressive liver disease after the recovery from BMT (Shuhart and McDonald, 1994). Consequently, a routine pretransplant evaluation includes the recognition and evaluation of risk factors before initiation of the conditioning regimen and proceeding to transplantation.

Bacterial and fungal infections generally are seen early in the postconditioning granulocytopenic period, whereas viral liver infections are seen later due to the delay in viral replication (Shuhart and McDonald, 1994). Bacterial and fungal infections can result in liver abscesses, causing pain and fever. Bacterial infections are most commonly associated with empiric prophylactic antibiotic therapy. In contrast, fungal liver infection often is a component of widespread fungal disease and is manifested by fever and hepatomegaly.

Associated liver function abnormalities vary widely in clinical significance. Asymptomatic elevations in alkaline phosphatase and bilirubin may reflect intrahepatic cholestasis (Wingard, 1990). Diagnostic techniques include computerized tomography (CT scan), magnetic resonance imaging (MRI), ultrasound, fine-needle aspiration, and liver biopsy.

All transplant patients are at risk for hepatitis C virus (HCV, formerly non-A, non-B hepatitis) due to the high number of blood transfusions used for supportive therapy.

HCV is considered the causative agent for the chronic hepatitis that develops 6 to 12 months after BMT. Until 1990, the prevalence of viral hepatitis among BMT patients was 15% to 20%, due primarily to HCV-contaminated blood products. The recent implementation of methods for screening blood products has resulted in a decreased incidence of HCV (Aach et al., 1991).

Chronic hepatitis B (HBV) infection pretransplant has been reported to result in active replication during the postconditioning period of immunosuppression, resulting in fulminant hepatitis when the immune system recovers after day 70 (Chen et al., 1990). However, based on reports of more than 50 HBV-positive patients who did not go on to develop HBV, the risk of HBV after transplantation has been estimated at less than 6 in 100 (Shuhart and McDonald, 1994).

Other viral etiologies that can cause liver dysfunction specifically in the allogeneic transplant patient include CMV, HSV, varicella zoster virus (VZV), adenovirus, and Epstein-Barr virus (Ayash, 1992). Liver biopsy is necessary to establish a definitive diagnosis of viral infections of the liver. Liver function tests may reflect variably elevated serum transaminase levels. CMV infection can arise from a seropositive donor via a blood transfusion, by reactivation of latent virus, or by reinfection with a new viral strain. Approximately 50% of patients undergoing allogeneic BMT develop active CMV; 15% to 20% of them die from the disease. The onset of symptomatic infection usually occurs between day +30 and day +110 (Ayash, 1992). HSV serology is performed pretransplant to identify patients at risk for reactivation of the latent virus. The use of prophylactic acyclovir can decrease the risk of active infection. When liver infection does occur, it is usually an indication of systemic infection. (Ayash, 1992). VZV also occurs in a reactivated form in a seropositive recipient , usually 5 months after transplant. Reported incidence varies form 16% to 40%. It is more common in patients who receive allogeneic BMTs, especially in the presence of GVHD (Wingard, 1990).

Drug-Induced Liver Injury. In addition to the hepatotoxic effects of the conditioning regimens, certain medications administered to patients undergoing transplant have the potential to cause liver dysfunction. Some responsible medications include cyclosporin and methotrexate, given as GVHD prophylaxis, antithymocyte globulin, and antimicrobial agents (e.g., trimethoprim-sulfa-methaxazole) used for the *Pneumocystis carinii* prophylaxis, and mezlocillin (Shuhart and McDonald, 1994). This list is not all inclusive, however, because of the evolution of new drugs and therapeutic approaches used in BMT patients. Total parenteral nutrition (TPN) may also negatively affect the liver, causing hepatitis and cholestatis (Sax and Bowser, 1988). Careful monitoring of liver function studies, specifically an increase serum transaminase and alkaline phosphatase levels, can be the clinical indices to detect and prevent complications. The increase in liver function studies usually resolve after TPN is discontinued (Balistreri and Bove, 1990).

Veno-occlusive Disease. VOD is a transplant-related liver toxicity clinically characterized by right upper quadrant pain, rising serum bilirubin, jaundice, sudden weight gain, ascites, hepatomegaly, and hepatic encephalopathy. This disorder can occur 1 to 3 weeks post transplant and may be associated with significant morbidity and mortality for the BMT patient.

Assessment and Management
Antimicrobial therapy for treating bacterial, fungal, and viral infections has been addressed earlier. Drugs suspected to be hepatotoxic may be withheld, administered every other day, or undergo some other form of dosage modification, depending on the severity of liver dysfunction. Nursing management of BMT/BCT pa-

tients experiencing liver dysfunction involves close monitoring of trends in liver function tests (i.e., serum bilirubin, SGOT and SGPT, alkaline phosphatase), serum ammonia coagulation studies and cultures. Deviations from normal values or progressively worsening trends should be reported immediately. Because encephalopathy occurs with progressive liver dysfunction, the patient's level of consciousness and potential for aspiration should be evaluated regularly and the appropriate safety precautions initiated. Because abnormal fluid shifts and renal dysfunction from poor renal perfusion may occur concomitantly with a failing liver, the patient's BUN and creatinine, volume status, and electrolytes also need to be monitored.

Management of abdominal pain from liver injury in transplant patients is difficult. It requires great care and caution in selecting medications for treatment. The metabolism of many narcotics, anxiolytics, and sedatives is prolonged in the setting of liver dysfunction. The ideal narcotics for pain management in this situation should be short-acting and given in small doses (e.g., morphine and hydromorphone); sedatives and anxiolytics that are renally cleared are preferred to those that are metabolized by the liver (Cherney and Portenoy, 1994).

NUTRITION FOR THE BMT/BCT PATIENT

The nutritional support of patients experiencing the complex series of events typical during the transplant process is an exceedingly important element of medical and nursing care. A variety of the nutritional strategies that can be employed to manage specific GI complications have been addressed earlier in this chapter. The remaining nutritional concerns for transplant population are related to metabolic alterations, nutritional assessment, low-microbial diets, and the role of parenteral and enteral nutrition.

Metabolic and Nutritional Alterations

Patients undergoing transplant can have an alteration in their metabolic functioning related to the current or previous treatment they received or their diseases. A thorough understanding of the metabolic alterations is essential in order to provide adequate nutritional support for these patients. BMT can be divided into three phases, each presenting distinct metabolic challenges: (1) conditioning period with therapies causing tissue damage, (2) neutropenic period and tissue repair, and (3) engraftment, which can be complicated by GVHD, graft failure, or sepsis.

The acute effects of dose-intensive conditioning regimens and longer term treatment-related complications can all decrease the intake of nutrients, putting the patient on the path to malnutrition. The effect on the central nervous system which causes severe vomiting is the first barrier to oral nutrition. Intestinal dysmotility due to narcotic analgesics can exacerbate vomiting. The conditioning regimen also causes painful mucositis. Taste alteration has also been reported. Many of the gastrointestinal complications, such as mucositis, GVHD, fever, infection, enteritis, diarrhea, and nausea make the nutritional requirements of a transplant patient paramount. The normal growth and repair of the gastrointestinal mucosa is disrupted (Weisdorf and Schwarzenberg, 1994). The loss of functioning intestinal epithelium results in malabsorption, which results in diarrhea and leads to protein loss in the feces.

Following the conditioning regimen, the BMT patient is profoundly neutropenic. This places the patient at risk for bacterial infections. The damaged intestine serves a portal of entry for the invasion of pathogens. Narcotic analgesia can cause intestinal stasis, predisposing the mucosa to bacterial overgrowth, which in turn leads to further intestinal damage. Systemic effects of infection, such as fever, have a significant appetite-suppressant effect. Tissue damage and nitrogen mobilization from protein breakdown also are exacerbated by infection. During the neutropenic period, tissue repair is also occurring, thus increasing nutrient requirements.

After engraftment, mucosal lesions heal and patients are often able to resume some oral intake. With the absence of enteral nutrients, which stimulate the intestine, absorption can be affected, delaying epithelial cell repair and regeneration. Diarrhea can occur during this time, caused either by GVHD or infection. This can once again lead to mucosal cell breakdown or tissue necrosis. Clinically, GVHD diarrhea is similar to that during the conditioning regimen, but is more severe and prolonged. It can cause massive protein loss and a profound decrease in nitrogen balance (Weisdorf and Schwarzenberg, 1994).

Several nutritional effects result from GVHD prophylaxis and treatment with high-dose corticosteroids. Corticosteroids promote muscle breakdown increasing the urea cycle and causing a loss of nitrogen. With this loss of protein, fluid overload can result from the IV fluids and nephrotoxic agents, including cyclosporin and antibiotics.

In spite of interventions aimed at improving oral intake, changes in oral metabolism may further contribute to weight loss and malnutrition. A thorough understanding of both the generalized and specific metabolic alterations is essential in providing effective nutritional support.

Protein

The transplant procedure has been associated with prolonged negative nitrogen balance. Nitrogen balance is a measure of protein metabolism and is largely influenced by calorie and protein intake. An increase in calories and protein may improve both total body weight and nitrogen balance (referred to as anabolism). Protein catabolism or the destruction of body protein such as muscle leads to negative nitrogen balance, even with the provision of adequate calories. Despite adequate caloric and protein intake, protein catabolism may not be preventable. If protein needs of the BMT patient are not met, skeletal and visceral muscle mass may be depleted. What is observed clinically includes loss of respiratory muscle mass, which increases the potential for complications such as pneumonia or loss of skeletal muscle, which leads to decreased mobility. Last, without adequate protein, lymphocyte production is decreased, causing prolonged immunosuppression.

Measurement of protein loss must be quantified (i.e., via diarrhea, urine, pleural effusion). This will allow for replacement of exogenous protein. To meet nitrogen needs, dietary protein must be provided in adequate daily amounts (Rust and Schuster, 1993). The protein requirements of a BMT patient range from 1.2 to 1.5 g/kg per day, which is double the requirement of a healthy adult. Protein needs increase in BMT patients with severe stress such as GVHD, sepsis, and diarrhea (Keenan, 1989; Kaproth et al., 1990).

Carbohydrates

Treatments associated with BMT may have a significant effect on metabolism of carbohydrates. Human metabolism depends on carbohydrates or glucose. Carbohydrates, a primary energy source, provide 50% to 60% of required daily calories. When carbohydrate intake is inadequate, gluconeogenesis occurs and glucose is obtained from protein and fat. Anaerobic metabolism is the breakdown of glucose without oxygen. It yields less energy, produces lactic acid, and leads to poor tissue perfusion. In the BMT patient, steroids, often used in conjunction with immunosuppressive therapy, can precipitate hyperglycemia. Specific antineoplastic agents used in conditioning regimens also can cause alterations in carbohydrate metabolism. For example, L-asparaginase can precipitate

insulin-dependent diabetes whereas bulsulfan can cause direct damage to the pancreatic beta cells (Herrmann and Petruska, 1993).

Glucose intolerance causing insulin-dependent diabetes has been assessed in patients undergoing autologous BMT. Glucose intolerance was noted in this group of patients by a decrease in peak insulin concentration, suggesting that there is impairment in pancreatic cell function (Smedyr et al., 1990). In a review of nine patients with glucose intolerance, Scholten and colleagues (1990) found organ failure, suggesting that these alterations in carbohydrate metabolism may predispose patients to significant toxicity and morbidity.

Lipids

The normal response to the ingestion of food allows carbohydrates to be used immediately for energy. Dietary protein is incorporated into enzymes, collagen, and serum proteins. Ingested fat in the presence of insulin is stored. Fat is used for energy if inadequate amounts of carbohydrates are ingested. If the amount and type of food eaten are more than the body's current needs, the food will be stored as fat in the adipose tissue. This normal process does not occur in the patient with cancer. The cancer patient's ability to store fat is limited. Therefore, wasting of stored body fat and increased levels of serum lipids in transplant patients may occur (Kern and Norton, 1988). Desai and Kinze (1990) observed that certain lipids can inhibit the immune system. This can further compromise a neutropenic transplant patient, especially since many of the interventions employed to increase caloric intake use fats in the diet. Immunosuppressive therapy, specifically cyclosporin, also has been associated with altered lipid metabolism. Elevated serum cholesterol and triglyceride concentrations have been reported (Neumunaitis, Deeg, Yel, 1986).

Energy needs in the initial 30 to 50 days post transplant have been estimated to be

170% of the basal energy expenditure and approximately 130% to 150% at the time of discharge. Protein requirements at the recommended daily allowance (Aker, 1983) for the BMT patient can be estimated by the Harris Benedict equation. Many investigators have proved that 30 to 35 kcal/kg per day are needed for the adult BMT patient; however, Szeluga and colleagues (1985) found that up to 50 kcal/kg per day are needed by most adult patients with acute GVHD. Others have demonstrated the energy requirements of BMT patients to be 130% to 150% times their predicted basal energy expenditure (Kaproth et al., 1990).

Nutritional Assessment

The primary goals of nutritional assessment of the BMT patient are to (1) identify risk factors, (2) determine nutritional requirements, and (3) evaluate the effectiveness of the nutritional support in maintaining a patient's nutritional status (Aker, 1990). Nutritional assessment begins prior to transplant and continues until the patient is no longer taking medications and/or is without signs of GVHD.

The majority of BMT patients have an acceptable nutritional status prior to treatment. It is best to evaluate the patient prior to the initiation of therapy, however nutritional assessment is an ongoing process. During the pretransplant phase, an initial nutritional assessment and screening should be performed. Accurate measurements of height and weight are recorded for baseline information and for the calculation of chemotherapy drug dosages. Body weight may not be an accurate indicator of a patient's nutritional status. Changes in body weight can be influenced by aggressive hydration, fluid shifts, TPN, vomiting, or diarrhea, however body composition or body mass may not change (Keenan, 1989).

Key components of baseline assessment include the patient's nutritional practices: current nutritional intake, food allergies, factors that influence oral intake, activity level, special dietary likes and dislikes, identification of the food preparer, and medications.

Pretransplant assessment and counseling includes an introduction to the nutrition-related problems associated with transplantation and the concept of parenteral and/or enteral supplementation. Baseline nutritional assessment of the BMT patient is of critical importance to determine the nature and extent of nutritional deficiencies in order to rapidly prepare for and intervene with nutritional strategies to prevent further deterioration during very stressful treatment. If the patient is well nourished prior to transplantation, then the goal of nutritional support is maintenance.

The nurse and dietitian should collaborate with the transplant team on a continual basis to promote optimum nutrition. Elements the nurse can use to evaluate nutrition of the BMT patient are outlined in Table 10.6.

Anthropometric measurements have been used to assess changes in the BMT patient's body composition, however the fluid and electrolyte abnormalities leading to overhydration or dehydration limit their usefulness.

A number of serum markers are traditionally used for nutritional assessment. The total lymphocyte count is affected by treatment-induced neutropenia and immunosuppression, which can limit its usefulness for nutritional assessment. Plasma proteins such as albumin, transferrin, and prealbumin have been regarded as parameters of nutritional assessment and repletion. Factors that can alter serum albumin concentration are hydration and blood component therapy. Overhydration will cause a falsely low reading with the value decreased in the event of hepatic dysfunction.

Low-Microbial Diets

Low-microbial, reduced-bacteria, and sterile diets are common for the immunocompromised

TABLE 10.6 **Nutritional assessment of the BMT patient**

History and Physical Assessment
Height and weight
  Usual and current
  Percentage deviation from ideal body weight
Age and sex
Educational level
Relevant medical history
Hydration status
Oral cavity and dental status
Energy/activity level and exercise tolerance
Gastrointestinal symptoms
  anorexia, dysgeusia (altered taste), mucositis, dysphagia, xerostomia, reflux esophagitis, nausea, diarrhea, constipation
Current medications
Insurance coverage

Dietary History
Current appetite
Previous treatment and their nutritional side effects
Food allergies
Food aversions/preferences
Dietary practices at home
  meal patterns
  timing of meals
  person responsible for food preparation and shopping
Unproven dietary practices such as vitamin therapy
Religious or cultural preferences

Laboratory Data
CBC (WBC, hematocrit, hemoglobin, platelet)
PT, PTT
Magnesium, calcium, phosphorus
Electrolytes
  sodium, chloride, potassium, carbon dioxide, glucose
BUN, creatinine
Total bilirubin, SGOT, SGPT, alkaline phosphatase, LDH
Plasma proteins
  albumin, serum transferrin

BMT/BCT patient. The theoretical purpose of such diets is to minimize the transmission of foodborne pathogens from foodstuffs to the immunocompromised patient and to determine how best to prevent infection (Aker and Cheney, 1983). The gastrointestinal tract serves as an important barrier to infection by preventing the migration of pathogenic microorganisms into the systemic circulation. The most important stimulus for mucosal cell proliferation is the presence of nutrients in the gut (Johnson, 1988). The absence of nutrients in the gut results in atrophy of the mucosal villi, which leads to decreased activity of the gut enzymes and affects gut-associated lymphoid tissue, which are essential to maintaining the integrity of the intestinal barrier (Rombeau and Cauldwell, 1990).

Other factors that reduce the efficiency of the gut barrier include decreased gastric motility secondary to narcotics analgesia, increased gastric pH, and disrupted gastrointestinal flora (Smith, 1990). Therefore, malnutrition, ileus, acid-sequestering drugs, and antibiotic therapy, all common in BMT patients, can interfere with the protective mechanism of the gut. This interference can allow transmission of bacteria to the accessory intestinal organs and into the systemic circulation, resulting in sepsis.

Food Vehicles of Infections
Many organisms can infect the immunocompromised BMT patient. The following discussion details organisms that can be transmitted by food, lists the microorganisms, their food sources, and the best methods of preventing infection or intoxication.

Camphylobacter jejuni is a leading cause of gastroenteritis. Its incidence is greater than *Salmonella,* with the ingestion of a few hundred cells leading to an infection in the immunocompetent host. This suggests that even a smaller dose could cause infection in an immunocompromised host (Notermans and Hoogenboom-Verdegaal, 1992). As with any infectious organism, there is a potential for dissemination that results in sepsis. Fresh fruits and vegetables are the potential sources of *Camphylobacter*. One study reported a higher incidence in fruits and vegetables purchased at a farmer's market than in those purchased at a grocery store (Park and Saunders, 1991). Patients must be taught the importance of cleaning fruits and vegetables and the need to peel away outer skins before eating.

Clostridium perfringens is a notable organism in foods. Spores of *Clostridium* can survive the cooking process and resume cell growth once the food reaches a suitable temperature (Weil and Rovelli, 1986). The prevention of clostridium is accomplished during food preparation and storage. The BMT patient must be taught how to cool foods effectively and rapidly by using small, shallow containers and by putting hot and warm foods immediately into the refrigerator or freezer. A common misconception about food preparation is that food should be brought to room temperature before refrigeration. This not necessary.

Escherichia coli is common intestinal flora, yet it is not usually associated with foodborne disease. The primary concern about *E. coli* arises from inadequately cooked beef or untreated water. However, *E. coli* has recently been associated with food dissemination from the gastrointestinal tract to other organs. In patients undergoing BMT, infection with *E. coli* can cause hemorrhagic colitis and can result in hemolytic uremic syndrome (HUS) that progresses to acute renal failure and death (Doyle, 1990).

Staphylococcus aureus produces an enterotoxin that results in staphylococcus aureus intoxication when ingested. Normally, when a staph aureus infection occurs, enteric symptoms occur, though these symptoms resolve uneventfully within 1 to 2 days. Intoxication results in ineffective absorption of immunosuppressive therapy, which can alter the therapeutic effect and result in GVHD. Although raw foods are not a source of *Staph. aureus,* cooked foods may be. Cooking food eliminates other organisms but allows *Staph. aureus* to flourish. Inadequately cooled and refrigerated foods can lead to a *Staph. aureus* infection.

Salmonella is the most notable cause of foodborne disease. When *Salmonella* is disseminated through the GI barrier into the systemic circulation, mortality is high (Fang, Araujo, Guerrant, 1991). *Salmonella* infection can occur from exposure to as few as 10 organisms (Notermans and Hoogenboom-Vererdegaal, 1992), which makes strict adherence to the prevention guidelines essential.

Fungal infections are difficult to treat and can be life threatening. The primary method of fungi transmission is via decaying fruits and vegetables or from the soil. Cryptococcus is a fungus that is an encapsulated yeast, found in the soil. The concern for patients is associated with fruit and vegetables. It is necessary that careful inspection of fruits and vegetables, washing and peeling of the skin be done.

An array of dietary interventions are used to maintain nutritional status of patients undergoing transplantation. In general, three types of transplant diet include a sterile diet, the low-microbial diet, and the modified house diet. Sterile diets include germ-free foods that are tested for microbes. Sterility is achieved by autoclaving, canning, prolonged oven baking, or irradiation (Dezenhall et al., 1987). Low-microbial diets include well-cooked foods or foods containing a minimum number of pathogens, specifically bacteria or fungus. Modified house diets are the most liberal and are essentially regular diets without fresh fruits or vegetables. Over the last several years, the need for and efficacy of the low-microbial diet in reducing infections in neutropenic BMT patients have been questioned.

There has been no study comparing low-microbial diet with a regular diet reported in the literature. One unpublished Dutch study indicated that profoundly neutropenic patients undergoing gut decontamination and protective isolation did not appear to benefit from a low-microbial diet (Pinner et al., 1992).

A recent survey of 54 transplant centers revealed some notable findings and trends in BMT dietary practices (Fierini, 1995). Data indicate that the trend continues to move away from strict sterile diets and toward more permissive diets such as the low-microbial or modified house diets (Fierini, 1995; Dezenhall et al., 1987). Of 50 transplant centers in the Fierini study that use a low-microbial diet, three centers serve a house diet with the omission of raw fruits and vegetables. Only one center exclusively serves a sterile diet. Of the remaining 33 transplant centers, some serve a form of a low-microbial diet. The researcher noted the significant controversy among transplant centers relating to timing of the initiation and discontinuation of a low-microbial diet. The most common standard for starting the low-microbial diet was at the start of the conditioning regimen or when a patient's neutrophil count was $1.0 \times 10^9/l$; however, discontinuing the diet ranged from day 10 to 1 year after transplantation. The researcher also noted that the frequently reported criteria to discontinue the low-microbial diet were related to a variety of factors. The criteria include infectious disease concerns, food-service limitations pertaining to cost and space, nursing and physician concerns, review of the literature that indicates no conclusive evidence, information from other transplant centers, and the microbiological testing of the food done within the center.

High-Risk Foods. A variety of methods can prevent cross-contamination of high-risk foods, specifically raw meats, poultry, and seafood. One method is to designate separate cutting boards for meats and other foods. Cutting boards should be washed and sanitized. Plastic boards with knife grooves provide an environ-

ment for the transmission of organisms. Separate utensils should be used when preparing meats. Food preparers should thoroughly wash their hands, lathering for at least 20 seconds. Marinades, gravies, and sauces should be brought to boiling if they contain meat juices or if they have been in contact with raw meat. Meats should be thawed on the bottom shelf of the refrigerator, in a dish with sides to prevent the meat juices from coming in contact with other foods. At the grocery store, meats should be wrapped and packaged separately from non-meat foods (Cabelof, 1994).

Water. Patients with private water supplies such as wells should be instructed to have their water checked when a change in taste, odor, or color is noted. Water should be checked quarterly thereafter. In the event of substantial rainfall or flooding, water should be checked for bacteria. Patients with a public water supply do not need to have their water checked for bacteria, because the Safe Drinking Water Act of 1974 regulates strict community standards established by the EPA and/or state (Cabelof, 1994).

Methods of preventing transmission of foodborne pathogens are summarized in Table 10.7. These guidelines are strict and are intended for BMT patients at high risk for developing foodborne infections. Further detail and teaching by the nurse is necessary, as well as assessment of the patient's risk for infection. Clinical judgment should determine which guidelines will be most beneficial for each patient based on risk of infection, lifestyle, and level of malnutrition.

Additional research is needed to define the optimal low-microbial dietary practices for BMT patients. Cost in relationship to the therapeutic outcome should also be examined. The collaborative relationship of the nurses and dieticians is critical for effective implementation of any strategies. Patients and family members re-

TABLE 10.7 Guidelines for foods for the immunocompromised host

Meats and Proteins
Avoid raw animal foods.
Adequately cook meats.
    Beef: Cooking temperature should reach 160°F (71°C).
                No pink meat should be visible or eaten.
                Avoid cooked meats that have been in contact with raw meats or juice.
    Eggs: Yolks and whites should be firm.
                Consider egg substitutes.
                Avoid dishes made with uncooked eggs (i.e., Caesar salad, custard).
    Poultry: Cooking temperature should be 180°F (82°C).
    Seafood: Cook until flesh is firm.
                Harvest seafood from clean waters.
    Leftovers: Warm at uniform temperature to 165°F (74°C).

Dairy Products
Drink only pasteurized milk.
Avoid chocolate milk.

Fruits and Vegetables
Wash fruits and vegetables well by using a scrub brush and chlorinated water; even when the outer skin will not be consumed.
Peeling is necessary if the food will be consumed raw.

Water
Have private water supplies checked regularly for bacterial contamination.

Food Preparation and Handling
Avoid cross-contamination.
Thaw foods properly.
Maintain adequate storage temperatures.
    Use 40°F (4°C for refrigeration).
    Use 0°F (−17°C for freezing).
Maintain proper hygiene prior to and during food preparation (i.e., scrubbing hands for at least 20 seconds).
Properly and quickly cool and refrigerate foods after preparation.
Discard decaying or outdated foods.
Discard foods that may be contaminated by insects or rodents.

quire education in the rationale and importance of the selected dietary practice, both during and after hospitalization.

Oral Intake. Oral intake can resume when mucositis subsides, and narcotic therapy is reduced. Narcotic weaning as mucositis improves and pain subsides allows for reintroduction of oral intake. Oral intake is often severely decreased during the first month after transplant. During the times of acute GI distress, however, oral intake should be neither forced nor over emphasized (Moe et al., 1985). It could severely discourage the patient who has a fear of eating and create a negative atmosphere, thus preventing successful refeeding. During this period, many patients consume only water or ice chips.

When the patient becomes clinically stable, teaching can be initiated to suggest foods and fluids that are appealing and easily tolerated. In one of two published studies of food-intake patterns in one BMT center (Gauvreau-Stern et al., 1989), researchers reported that beverages were the most frequently requested item, followed by bread products, and cooked fruits and vegetables. Another group of investigators (Mattsson et al., 1992) reported that the initial food desired by BMT patients is usually cold or very sweet. Taste is altered after BMT, with a decreased threshold for sweet and salt that can last for more than 1 year. As appetite improves, previously rejected foods may become more acceptable; the patient should be encouraged to retry foods (Gauvreau-Stern et al., 1989).

Oral intake can become a major nursing effort, particularly when the patient is approaching discharge. Patients usually consume 60% of their oral intake on the day prior to discharge. Food plans must be designed to provide a variety of foods at frequent intervals to meet patients' needs and therefore reduce dependence on TPN (Gauvreau-Stern et al., 1989). It is critical that the patient be able to maintain an adequate oral intake, and especially crucial for patients receiving cyclosporin. This will prevent dehydration, thereby minimizing the need for hospital readmission or intravenous fluid hydration in the home setting.

The role of the nurse in enhancing oral intake is critical throughout the treatment process. Nurses can identify barriers to eating such as refractory nausea, food aversions, depression, medications causing GI disturbances, and other GI complications that plague the BMT patient. They can coordinate a plan of care that includes monitoring of daily oral food and fluid intake, nutritional strategies to manage GI symptoms (Strohl, 1983), and patient/family education and support. Families frequently find support from hearing that patients other than their family member have difficulty eating.

Nutrition classes and support groups may be helpful, not only for education but also for motivation. It has been noted that oral intake frequently improves when patients are able to eat food they are more familiar with: home cooked or ethnic foods rather than hospital food (Weisdorf and Schwarzenberg, 1994). Nurses, physicians, and dieticians should collaborate to mobilize all resources available to enhance oral intake by the BMT patient.

Parenteral and Enteral Nutrition

Poor oral intake with a poor performance and a debilitated nutritional status is a central concern in the BMT patients. All of the gastrointestinal complications such as mucositis, GVHD, fever, infection, enteritis diarrhea, xerostomia, dysgeusia, nausea with or without vomiting, and organ damage predispose the transplant patient to severe metabolic disorders, catabolism, and almost certainly the inability to meet nutritional requirements both during and frequently after discharge. Nutritional consequences are compounded by the fact that many transplant candidates were nutritionally compromised pretransplant from their disease, previous treatment, psychological stress, or underlying gastrointestinal complaints.

Enteral Nutrition

Prior to the acceptance of total parenteral nutrition (TPN) to support BMT patients, enteral nutrition was the mainstay of nutritional support at many centers (Weisdorf and Schwarzenberg, 1994). Currently enteral nutrition is not typically used in BMT patients for several reasons. Gastrointestinal side effects associated with BMT result in poor tolerance of enteral feedings. Evidence indicates that the intestinal tract may be a significant portal of entry for bacteria into the blood stream and visceral organs in the immunocompromised patient

(Bodey, 1984). There is also a concern about thrombocytopenia and the risk of infection.

The need for central venous access for infusion of chemotherapy, blood products, and support medications has made it convenient to provide nutritional support via TPN. Recent research, however, showing benefits of feeding via the gastrointestinal tract and the focus on cost in health care, has caused many BMT centers to be interested in the enteral feedings of BMT patients (Katz, Kwetan, Askawazi, 1990). There have been two studies comparing enteral and parenteral nutrition support in BMT patients. Both the Szeluga (1987) and Mulder (1989) groups demonstrated that enteral feedings were an acceptable alternative to TPN. Enteral nutrition has been clearly demonstrated to help maintain intestinal mucosal integrity and support the barrier function of the gut; this protective effect of enteral feeding is not realized with TPN.

Enteral feeding alone, however, can be difficult for patients because of the severe nausea and vomiting. A common conditioning regimen for patients undergoing autologous transplant for metastatic breast cancer is cyclophosphamide, etoposide, and cisplatin. This regimen can cause severe nausea and vomiting in most patients. Parenteral nutrition supplemented with at least some enteral intake may be a reasonable form of nutritional support for these patients.

Factors to be considered when initiating enteral feedings are disease status, marrow function, control of GI symptoms, estimated duration of enteral feedings, availability of caregivers, and insurance. Allogeneic BMT patients who fail to thrive may benefit from placement of a percutaneous endoscopic gastrostomy (PEG) tube for long-term nutritional support.

Parenteral Nutrition

Total parenteral nutrition is frequently a supportive care strategy for the BMT patient. The severe gastrointestinal side effects of HD cytoreductive conditioning regimens in conjunction with fever, infection, organ dysfunction, and GVHD often preclude oral diets or enteral feedings. The transplant procedure has been associated with prolonged negative nitrogen balance and loss of muscle mass in the BMT patient. Literature indicates that if parenteral nutrition is delayed in the BMT patients, it is difficult to "catch up," particularly as organ failure develops after treatment, impeding the tolerance of fluids and high concentrations of proteins, carbohydrates, and fats (Herrmann and Petruska, 1993; Cunningham et al., 1983).

Energy requirements and TPN for the BMT patient have been the focus of numerous studies (Michallet et al., 1989; Cheney et al., 1987; Weisdorf et al., 1987; Szeluga et al., 1987; Hutchinson et al., 1984; Weisdorf et al., 1984).

Prophylactic TPN. One early study demonstrated the advantages of prophylactic TPN in well-nourished BMT patients, including rapid hematologic recovery (Weisdorf et al., 1984). However, the investigators noted that overall improvement in survival, relapse, GVHD, sepsis, and length of hospital stay were not found to be influenced or statistically significant. A larger randomized trial in well-nourished BMT patients (N = 137; allogeneic, syngeneic, autologous patients) to evaluate prophylactic TPN (starting 1 week prior to transplant) has shown significant improvements in overall survival, time to relapse, and disease-free survival in the experimental TPN group (Weisdorf et al., 1987). The control group received dextrose maintenance fluids, electrolytes, minerals, trace elements, and vitamins; 61% of these patients required intravenous nutritional support prior to discharge.

Further multivariant analysis of the data suggested that TPN has a significant influence on survival and relapse, independent of the type of transplant, risk category for relapse, and incidence of GVHD (in allogeneic patients). Variables not found to be significant between the two groups included engraftment, duration of hospitalization, incidence of GVHD, and bacteremia.

Enteral Nutrition versus TPN. Though parenteral nutritional support of the immunocompromised patient undergoing transplant is a standard treatment modality, it can be associated with profound toxicity. Some investigators have attempted to compare TPN to enteral nutrition in the BMT patient with conflicting results. A small prospective randomized study of 57 evaluable patients compared the efficacy of nutritional support in the BMT patient receiving TPN and the patient receiving enteral feeding. (Szeluga et al., 1987). The two areas of the study had comparable numbers of allogeneic patients, and fewer autologous patients. The enteral feeding program was individualized to the patient, involving strategies such as counseling, positive reinforcement, menu selection, snacks, commercial supplements, and tube feedings. Enteral patients also received a daily vitamin-mineral supplement. Enteral feeding patients who had inadequate oral protein intake received supplements until their oral protein intakes met the study's standard or treatment failed.

Findings indicated no differences in the rate of hematologic recovery, length of hospital stay, or survival. The TPN group did experience an increase in fluid overload requiring diuretics, hyperglycemia, and catheter-related complications; the enteral nutrition group experienced a greater incidence of hypomagnesemia and tube occlusion. The costs of nutrition support were 2.3 times higher in the TPN group. Investigators concluded that TPN was not clearly superior to an individualized enteric feeding program and recommend that TPN be reserved for those patients failing enteral feeding interventions.

Other investigators have performed prospective randomized studies that compared TPN with enterally supported regimens and confirmed the feasibility of enteral support in BMT patients. Mulder and colleagues (1989) reported a lower incidence of diarrhea in patients supported with enteral nutrition than in those given TPN alone. In another prospective study there was no difference in recovery from myelosuppression, rate to engraftment, length of hospitalization, and survival (Szeluga et al., 1987).

TPN Administration. The primary clinical goals of TPN administration include the prevention of nitrogen imbalance and loss of lean body mass while not overloading patients with excessive fluids and nutrients. The availability of different concentrations of amino acids, dextrose, and lipid solutions allows the dietician, TPN pharmacist, and physician to specify a TPN regimen to the nutritional needs of the transplant patient (Herrmann and Petruska, 1993; Cunningham et al., 1983). The role of the nurse in caring for the transplant patient receiving TPN includes the administration of the solution, monitoring the patient for tolerance of the TPN solution, and monitoring for adverse complications.

Central venous catheters facilitate administration of TPN in the transplant patient. The number of lumens depends on the alternative care needs of the patient. Several studies have examined the rate of catheter-related sepsis in patients who had triple-lumen central venous catheters inserted. It is well documented that the incidence of infection is directly proportionate to the number of catheter lumens (Baranowski, 1993; Freedman and Boserman, 1993; Eastridge and LeFor, 1995). In a recent prospective study of 143 Hickman catheters in 111 BMT patients, 44% had positive blood cultures during the lifetime of the catheter. Of these infections, 40 of 63 cultures were positive for Staphylococcus, suggesting line sepsis rather than catheter contamination from a bloodborne enteric source. The majority of such infections are treated with antibiotics without catheter removal (Ulz et al., 1990). Another researcher found a significant incidence of systemic sepsis and infections at entry sites; it was recommended that percutaneously inserted catheters not be used in patients requiring long-term TPN (McCarthy et al., 1987).

Meticulous care must be exercised to maintain asepctic technique when caring for a patient receiving TPN via central venous catheter. Institutional policies and procedures should reflect current literature related to infection control in TPN administration including the changing of TPN tubing every 24 to 48 hours, maintaining a closed system, and avoiding collection of blood specimens through the TPN tubing except in an emergency or when changing or discontinuation of tubing is planned (Baranowski, 1993; Williams, 1985). When parenteral nutrition lumens are used for multiple purposes in the transplant patient, careful maintenance and care should be used to minimize risk of infection.

Other complications of TPN administration to BMT patients are varied because of the possible impact of concomitant metabolic disturbances from organ system dysfunction and other medications. Hyperglycemia, for example, may result because of the TPN and concurrent steroid therapy and/or sepsis. Hypoglycemia may result from abruptly stopping the solution or from excess insulin administration. Hypokalemia and hypomagnesemia may result despite supplementation of these electrolytes, because of the effects of parenteral antibiotics, amphotericin B, and diarrhea. Hypermagnesemia, hyperkalemia, and hyperphosphatemia may result from renal failure. Sudden weight gain may reflect impending veno-occlusive disease or volume overload, whereas significant volume depletion may occur because of prolonged vomiting or diarrhea. Fluid overload is also a frequent complication of intensive nutritional therapy in chronically undernourished patients (Apovian, McMahon, Bistrian, 1990).

The nurse must be aware of all possible etiologies for the metabolic disturbances in BMT patients on TPN. Routine chemistries, careful assessment of fluid volume status, and electrolyte supplementation are all necessary interventions when caring for these patients. Certain laboratory studies are indicated to anticipate and correct potential metabolic problems that can be caused by parenteral nutrition as well as metabolic problems of other causes being treated with parenteral nutrition. Hyperglycemia may require management of frequent serum-glucose testing with the addition of insulin to the TPN or sliding-scale insulin coverage. There is an association between hyperglycemia and candida sepsis (Weisdorf and Schwarzenberg, 1994); therefore, awareness of glucose levels can be helpful in anticipating infectious complications as well as metabolic complications. Hypoglycemia can be avoided by properly tapering solutions as ordered.

Management of fluids overload may require diuresis and concentration of medications (antibiotics) to the minimum permissible volume of the drug. Some researchers (Herrmann and Petruska, 1993; Cheney et al., 1987) indicate that a shift of fluid from the intracellular compartment occurs during the first 4 weeks after marrow engraftment; TPN can result in such fluid shifts. Strict intake and output and daily weights need to be monitored. Weight is assessed primarily to judge hydration status, which is reflected by electrolytes, BUN, creatinine, and albumin levels. Constant weight fluctuations often reflect difficulty in managing fluids, rather than actual gains and losses in body mass (Weisdorf and Schwarzenberg, 1994).

Cycling of TPN (i.e., administration over 10 to 18 hours) can be successful in the BMT patient in order to create a daily infusion-free period (Reed et al., 1983). In this way the catheter is available for administering other medications and blood products. The nurse may encounter difficulty with the timely administration of drugs and blood products when TPN is infusing continuously into one lumen. Cycling may allow the patient some freedom by temporarily being disconnected from intravenous infusion lines.

Home TPN. The inability to sustain caloric and protein intake sufficient to meet energy demands is not unusual at the time of discharge from the hospital (primarily in allogeneic patients). Anorexia is often an ongoing issue due to protracted gastrointestinal complications such as GVHD and/or medications to manage these complications. Outpatient TPN is a therapeutic option that has been used in the BMT setting, specifically for allogeneic BMT patients (Aker, 1990; Lenssen et al., 1983).

In a retrospective study of 246 BMT patients, researchers noted that parenteral nutrition (PN) after discharge was used in 65% of patients (Lenssen et al., 1983). Indications for PN included stomatitis, esophagitis, nausea and vomiting not associated with fever or GI lesions, anorexia, and malaise associated with fever or viral syndrome, or failure to thrive not associated with GI or clinical symptoms. Continuing stomatitis was the central reason for PN among adults, and failure to thrive the central reason among the adolescents and children in this study. GVHD was another frequently cited etiology. PN provided most of the nutrition during the weeks of acute GVHD. Patients with leukemia required outpatient PN more frequently than those with aplastic anemia. Patients in this study required outpatient PN for a median of 10 to 15 days, however some patients were on PN much longer.

Cost/benefit analysis of outpatient PN has been addressed in several studies. Although the costs of outpatient PN are considerable, some authors (Gouttebel et al., 1987) reported that

this strategy still reduces annual costs by 50% to 70%; other benefits cited include medical efficiency, prevention of prolonged hospitalization, and psychosocial benefits for patients who regain a more normal life at home. Others (Lenssen et al., 1983) noted that the cost of outpatient therapy is only a fraction of the cost of intensive care for a BMT patient; the daily cost of maintaining an outpatient on PN at their center was approximately one sixth the cost of maintaining a patient in the hospital.

Experimental Nutritional Therapies

A variety of experimental nutritonal support therapies may improve the ability to nourish the transplant patient effectively The trend in nutritional support is toward specific modifications during the critical neutropenic period (Wilmore, 1991). Four novel therapies being investigated for the BMT patient are the use of glutamine, branched-chain amino acids, growth hormone, and early initiation of enteral alimentation.

Glutamine

Supplemental glutamine has been studied recently to determine its effects on sepsis and immunologic response. The mechanism of action through which glutamine may improve nutrition of BMT patients is unclear. Investigators in two recent randomized trials suggest a number of possible mechanisms including altering immune system functioning, promoting repair of the mucosal barrier integrity, maintaining antioxidant levels in tissues, and reducing catabolic stress (Ziegler, 1992; Schloerb and Amare, 1993). Ziegler and colleagues (1992) demonstrated that glutamine-supplemented parenteral nutrition in allogeneic BMT patients clearly improves nitrogen balance, reduces the incidence of sepsis, and shortens the duration of hospitalization. In spite of the benefits, no difference was seen in the incidence of fever or time to engraftment in the glutamine-supplemented group. Schloerb and Amare (1993) used glutamine in both autologous and allogeneic BMT patients, reporting shorter hospitalization and less fluid retention.

It is important to determine the optimal route of administration for glutamine. Several centers are attempting to provide glutamine orally to patients. The powdered form is usually diluted in liquid such as juice and given three times per day. There have been reports of patients having difficulty tolerating glutamine due to nausea and the taste. There is a need for additional research to study the supplementation as well as the optimal route of administration.

Branched-Chain Amino Acids

Amino acid solutions enriched by the branched-chain amino acids (BCAA; isoleucine, leucine, and valine) have been shown to improve nitrogen balance in some critical-care situations. The improvement in nitrogen balance is small in most studies, and the BCAA parenteral solution costs considerably more than the standard TPN solution. It is unclear as to which metabolic pathway is altered; however, it is theorized that BCAA oxidation has a protein-sparing effect on somatic protein stores (Weisdorf and Schwarzenberg, 1994).

Parenteral support enriched by BCAA was studied in a group of BMT patients, randomly selected to receive TPN containing 23% or 45% BCAA. It was noted that nitrogen balance was maintained during the first month after BMT, though the number in the study is small (N = 19). Of note, the patients who received 45% BCAA were treated with more frequent and higher dose steroids than those who received 23% BCAA (Lenssen et al., 1987). This study has not settled the controversy associated with BCAA use in BMT patients.

Growth Hormone

Growth hormone, a polypeptide produced in the pituitary gland, is an anabolic hormone.

Clinical trials in several centers have demonstrated its use in promoting nitrogen balance in sepsis, as well as in other settings (i.e., severe burns, trauma, after surgery) (Piccolboni et al., 1991; Ziegler et al., 1990). In a group of patients receiving prednisone, it was noted that growth hormones decreased the catabolism associated with prednisone therapy, therefore preventing protein loss (Bennet and Haymond, 1992). Though published studies have small numbers of patients, they hold promise for BMT patients. Additional studies are needed before this therapy can be used clinically.

Early Enteral Alimentation

Several groups have challenged the assumption that TPN is superior to enteral nutrition during the acute phase of critical illness (i.e., sepsis). It has been demonstrated that an aggressive protocol for early enteral nutrition may decrease infection rates (Moore et al., 1989). Patients undergoing transplant procedures are generally not good candidates for enteral nutrition by feeding tube because of mucositis, neutropenia, nausea, and vomiting associated with the conditioning regimen and GVHD. However, the results of one comparative study addressing the predominant use of enteral feeding over TPN suggest that BMT patients could be supported by aggressive enteral feeding.

Szeluga and colleagues (1987) randomly assigned patients to two nutritional support modalities during BMT—30 to an enteral program and 27 to parenteral nutrition. Of the 30 receiving enteral nutrition 73% patients required supplemental intravenous feedings for adequate nutritional support; 23% were crossed over to TPN because of the inability to achieve adequate intake via the enteral system. The study showed that patients who received parenteral nutrition had more days of diuretic use, hyperglycemia, and more catheter-related complications, but fewer episodes of hypomagnesemia. No difference was noted in length of hospital stay, engraftment, or survival. The researchers indicated that due to the high cost of parenteral nutrition, TPN should be used only for patients who fail on enteral nutrition. This study introduces the importance of this treatment option, which can provide mucosal-preserving advantages; however, this method would be challenging to use in the critically ill BMT patient.

SUMMARY

Numerous GI complications can plague the patient undergoing transplant procedures, both during and after the actual transplant process. A spectrum of etiologies are responsible for these complications and involve the combined impact of various therapeutic interventions and their sequelae. Nurses caring for this population of patients are faced with formidable challenges because the management of these complications is labor intensive, difficult, and costly. All of these complications profoundly affect the patient's nutritional status. It is likely that consensus regarding assessment of GI complications will emerge as transplant technology continues to evolve; the current lack of uniformity in assessment approaches limits multicenter trials describing the character and efficacy of managing stomatitis, esophagitis, enteritis, and ulcerative pathologies. However, additional nursing research is necessary to provide information on the most efficacious ways to manage GI difficulties and to enhance nutritional intake throughout the process.

Acknowledgment

We would like to acknowledge with appreciation the contribution of our colleague, Karen Ohly Vanacek, MSN, RN, who laid the groundwork for this chapter in the first edition of this book.

REFERENCES

Aach, R.D., et al. 1991. Hepatitis C virus infection in post transfusion hepatitis: an analysis with first and second generation assays. *N Engl J Med* 325:1325-1329.

Agura, E.D., et al. 1988. The use of ranitidine in bone marrow transplantation. *Transplantation* 46:53-56.

Ahmed, T., et al. 1993. Propantheline prevention of mucositis from etoposide. *BMT* 12:131-132.

Aker S.N. 1983. Nutritional assessment in the marrow transplant patient. *Nutr Supp Serv* 3:22-37.

Aker, S.N., Cheney, C.L. 1983. The use of sterile and low microbial diets in ultraisolation environments. *J Parenteral & Enteral Nutr* 7:390-397.

Aker, S.N. 1990. Bone marrow transplantion: nutritional support and monitoring. In Block, A. (Ed.) *Nutritional Care of the Cancer Patient*. Rockville: Aspen, 199-224.

Apovian, C.M., McMahon, M.M., Bistrian B.R. 1990. Guidelines for refeeding the marasmic patient. *Crit Care Med* 18:1030-1033.

Apperly, J.F., Goldman, J.M. 1988. Cytomegalovirus: biology, clinical features, and methods for diagnosis. *BMT* 3:253-264.

Armstrong, T. 1994. Stomatitis in the bone marrow transplant patient: an overview and proposed oral care protocol. *Canc Nurs* 17(5):403-410.

Atkinson, K., et al. 1989. Consensus among bone marrow transplanters for diagnosis, grading, and treatment of chronic graft-versus-host disease. *BMT* 4:247-254.

Ayash, L.J. 1992. Hepatic complications of bone marrow tranplantation. In Armitage, J.O., Antman, K. (Eds.) *High Dose Cancer Therapy: Pharmacology, Hematopoietins, Stem Cells*. Baltimore: Williams & Wilkins, 487-554.

Balistreri, W.F., Bove, K.E. 1990. Hepatobiliary consequences of parenteral hyperalimentation. In Popper, H., Schaffner, F. (Eds.) *Progress in Liver Disease*. Philadelphia: Saunders, 567-602.

Barale, K.V., et al. 1982. Primary taste thresholds in children with leukemia undergoing marrow transplantation. *J Parenteral and Enteral Nutr* 6:287-290.

Baranowski, L. 1993. Central venous access devices: current technologies, uses, and management strategies. *J Intrav Therapy* 16(3):167-194.

Barasch, A., et al. 1995. Helium-neon laser effects on conditioning-induced oral mucositis in bone marrow transplantation patients. *Cancer* 76(12):2550-2556.

Barnes, S.G., et al. 1984. Perirectal infections in acute leukemia: improved survival after incision and debridement. *Ann Intern Med* 100:515-518.

Barrett, A.P. 1986. Oral complications of bone marrow transplantation. *Aust NZ J Med* 16:239-240.

Barrett, A.P., Bilous, A.M. 1984. Oral patterns of acute and chronic graft-versus-host disease. *Arch Dermatol* 120:1461-1465.

Basch, A., Jensen, L. 1991. Management of fecal incontinence. In Doughty, D. (Ed.) *Urinary and Fecal Incontinence: Nursing Management.* Philadelphia: Mosby Year Book, 235-268.

Beck, S. 1979. Impact of systematic oral care protocol on stomatitis after chemotherapy. *Canc Nurs* 2:185-199.

Bennett, W.H., Haymond, M.W. 1992. Growth hormone and lean tissue catabolism during long term glucocorticoid treatment. *Clin Endocrinol* 36:161-164.

Bianco, J.A., et al. 1990. The somatostatin analogue octreotide in the management of the secretory diarrhea of the acute intestinal graft-versus-host disease in a patient after bone marrow transplantation. *Transplantation* 49:1194-1195.

Blower, P.R. 1994. Comparative pharmacology of 5-HT3-receptor antagonists. *Hosp Formul* 29(suppl 5): S4-S9.

Bodey, G. 1984. Current status of prophylaxis of infection with protected environments. *Am J Med* 76: 678-684.

Bowden, R.A., et al. 1986. Cytomegalovirus immune globulin and seronegative blood products to prevent primary cytomegalovirus infection after marrow transplant. *N Engl J Med* 314:1006-1010.

Brager, B.L., Yasko, J. 1984. *Care of the Client Receiving Chemotherapy.* Reston, VA: Reston Publishing.

Brown, A.T., et al. 1990. In vitro effect of chlorhexidine and amikacin on oral gram-negative bacilli from bone marrow transplant recipients. *Oral Surg Oral Med Oral Pathol* 70:715-719.

Bruera, E., MacDonald R. 1988. Nutrition in cancer patients: an update and review of our experience. *J Pain Sympt Manag* 3:133-140.

Bryant, R.A. (Ed.). 1992. *Acute and Chronic Wounds: Nursing Management.* Philadelphia: Mosby Year Book.

Cabelof, D.C. 1994. Preventing infection from food borne pathogens in liver transplant patients. *J Am Diet Assoc* 94(10):1140-1144.

Carl, W. 1983. Oral complications in cancer patients. *Am Fam Physician* 27:161-170.

Carl, W., Higby, D. 1985. Oral manifestations of bone marrow transplantation. *Am J Clin Oncol* 8:81-87.

Cascinu, S. 1995. Drug therapy in diarrheal diseases in oncology/hematology patients. *Crit Rev Oncol/Hematol* 18:37-50.

Centers for Disease Control and Prevention. 1994. Preventing the spread of vancomycin resistance—report from the Hospital Infection Control Practices Advisory Committee, Atlanta, GA. *Fed Regist* 59:25758-25763.

Champlin, R.E., Gale, R.P. 1984. The early complications of bone marrow transplantation. *Semin Hematol* 21(2):101-108.

Chapko, M.K., et al. 1989. Chemoradiotherapy toxicity during bone marrow transplantation: time course and variation in pain and nausea. *BMT* 4:184-186.

Chastanger, P., et al. 1989. Role of parenteral antibiotic therapy in gastrointestinal tract flora suppression: a study in children with high-dose chemotherapy and autologous bone marrow transplantation. *BMT* 4:393-398.

Chen, P.M., et al. 1990. Changing of hepatitis B viral markers in patients with BMT. *Transplantation* 49: 708-713.

Cheney, C.L., et al. 1987. Body composition changes in marrow transplant recipients receiving total parenteral nutrition. *Cancer* 59:1515-1519.

Cherney, N.I., Portenoy, R.K. 1994. Practical issues in management of cancer pain. In Wall, P.D., Melzack, R. (Eds.) *Textbook of Pain.* Edinburgh: Churchhill Livingstone.

Cotanch, P.H. 1983. Relaxation training for control of nausea and vomiting in cancer patients. *Canc Nurs* 6: 277-283.

Cox, G. J., et al., 1994. Etiology and outcome of diarrhea after marrow transplantation: a prospective study. *Gastroenterol* 107:1398-1407.

Crane, L.R., Emmer, D.R., Grguras, A. 1989. Prevention of infection in an oncology unit. *Nurs Clin North Am* 15:843-846.

Croockewit, S. 1990. The efficacy of ondansetron in emesis induced by total body irradiation. *Proceedings of Symposium at the European Society of Medical Oncology Meeting.* Copenhagen, December 2, 15-17.

Cunninghham, B.A., et al. 1983. Nutritional considerations during marrow transplanation. *Nurs Clin North Am* 18:585-595.

Daeffler, R. 1980. Oral hygeine measures for patients with cancer, II. *Canc Nurs* 3:427-432.

Davis, J., Babb. J.R., Ayliff, G., et al. 1977. The effect on the skin flora of bathing with antiseptic solutions. *J Antimicrobial Chemother* 3:473-481.

Deeg, H.J., Storb, R. 1986. Acute and chronic graft-versus-host disease: clinical manifestations, prophylaxis and treatment. *J Natl Canc Inst* 76:1325-1328.

Desai, T.K., Kinze, J. 1990. Meta analysis of 12 prospective randomized controlled trials of parenteral nutrition during cancer chemotherapy: association between parenteral lipid infusion and infection. *J Parenteral & Enteral Nutr* 14:7S.

Dezenhal, A., et al. 1987. Food and nutrition services in bone marrow transplant centers. *J Am Diet Assoc* 87: 1351-1353.

Dilly, S. 1994. Overview of clinical experience with new 5-HT3-receptor antagonists. *Hosp Formul* 29(suppl 5): S10-S17.

Dorr, R.T., Von Hoff, D.D. 1994. *Cancer Chemotherapy Handboook.* Norwalk: Appleton and Lange.

Doyle, M.P. 1990. Food borne illness: pathogenic E. Coli and Vibro parahaemoyticus. *Lancet* 336:1111-1115.

Duigon, A. 1986. Anticipatory nausea and vomiting associated with cancer chemotherapy. *Oncol Nurs Forum* 13(1):35-40.

Egan, A.P., Taggart, J.R., Bender, C.M. 1992. Management of chemotherapy-related nausea and vomiting using a serotonin antagonist. *Oncol Nurs Forum* 19(5): 791-795.

Eastridge, B., Lefor, A. 1995. Complications of indwelling venous access devices in cancer patients. *J Clin Onc* 13(10):233-238.

Eilers, J., Berger, A., Petersen, M. 1988. Development, testing and application of the oral assessment guide. *Oncol Nurs Forum* 15(3):325-330.

Ely, P., et al. 1991. Use of a somatostatin analogue octreotide acetate in the management of acute gastrointestinal graft-versus-host disease. *Am J Med* 90:707-710.

Elzaway, A. 1991. Treatment of 5-fluorouracil-induced stomatitis by allopurinol mouthwashes. *Oncology* 48: 282-284.

Engelking, C. 1988. Managing stomatitis: a nursing process approach. In Moore, P (Ed.) *Supportive Care for the Patient with Cancer.* Valley Cottage, NY: Medical Marketing Interaction, 20-38.

Einsele, H., et al. 1988. Significant reduction of cytomegalovirus (CMV) disease by prophylaxis with CMV hyperimmune globulin plus oral acyclovir. *BMT* 3:607-617.

Erice, A., et al. 1987. Ganciclovir treatment of cytomegalovirus disease in transplant recipients and other immunocompromised hosts. *JAMA* 257:3082-3087.

Ezzone, S., et al. 1993. Survey of oral hygiene regimens among bone marrow transplant centers. *Oncol Nurs Forum* 20(9):1375-1381.

Fang, G., Araujo, V., Guerrant, R. 1991. Enteric infections associated with exposure to animals or animal products. *Infect Dis Clin North Am* 5:681-701.

Fegan, C., Poynton, C.H., Whittaker, J.A. 1990. The gut mucosal barrier in bone marrow transplantation. *BMT* 5:373-377.

Ferreti, G.A., et al. 1988. Control of oral mucositis and candidiasis in marrow transplantation: a prospective, double-blind trial of chlorhexidine digluconate oral rinse. *BMT* 3:283-493.

Fetting, J.H., et al. 1983. The course of nausea and vomiting after high-dose cyclophosphamide. *Canc Treat Rep* 66:1487-1493.

Fierini, D. 1995. Is the low microbial diet effective? Can this question be answered? *Marrow Transplant Nutrition Network* 3(1):1.

Ford, R., Ballard, B. 1988. Acute complications after bone marrow transplantation. *Semin Oncol Nurs* 4(1): 15-24.

Fowler, E. M. 1987. Equipment and products used in the managment and treatment of pressure ulcers. *Nurs Clin North Am* 22:449-461.

Freedman, S., Boserman, G. 1993. Tunnelled catheters: technologic advances and nursing care issues. *Nurs Clin North Am* 28(4):851-858.

Fruto, L.V. 1994. Current concepts: management of diarrhea in acute care. *J WOCN* 21:199-205.

Gauvreau-Stern, J.M., et al. 1989. Food intake patterns and food service requirements on a marrow transplant unit. *J Am Diet Assoc* 89:367-372.

Geller, R.B., et al. 1995. Randomized trial of loperamide versus dose escalation of octreotide acetate for chemotherapy-induced diarrhea in bone marrow transplant and leukemia patients. *Am J Hematol* 50:167-172.

Gilbert, C. J., et al. 1995. Randomized, double-blind comparison of a prochlorperazine-based versus a metoclopramide-based antiemetic regimen in patients undergoing autologous bone marrow transplantation. *Cancer* 76:2330-2337.

Goodman, J.L., et al. 1992. A controlled trial of fluconazole to prevent fungal infections in patients undergoing bone marrow transplantation. *N Engl J Med* 326:845-851.

Goodrich, J.M., et al. 1991. Early treatment with ganciclovir to prevent cytomegalovirus disease after allogeneic bone marrow transplantation. *N Engl J Med* 325: 1601-1607.

Gordon, B., et al. 1994. Effect of granulocyte-macrophage colony-stimulating factor on oral mucositis after hematopoietic stem-cell transplantation. *J Clin Oncol* 12:1917-1922.

Gouttebel, M.C., et al. 1987. Ambulatory home total parenteral nutrition. *J Parenteral & Enteral Nutr* 11: 475-479.

Gralla, R., et al. 1987. The management of chemotherapy-induced nausea and vomiting. *Med Clin North Am* 71(2):289-301.

Herrmann, V.M., Petruska, P.J. 1993. Nutrition support in bone marrow transplant recipients. *Nutr Clin Pract* 8:19-27.

Hesketh, P.J., et al. 1995. Adjusting the dose of intravenous ondansetron plus dexamethasone to the emetogenic potential of the chemotherapy regimen. *J Clin Oncol* 13:2117-2122.

Hogan, C. 1990. Advances in the management of nausea and vomiting. *Nurs Clin North Am* 25:475-497.

Holler, E., et al. 1990. Increased serum levels of tumor necrosis factor-*a* precede major complications of bone marrow transplantation. *Blood* 75:1011-1016.

Huldij, A., et al. 1986. Alterations in taste appreciation in cancer patients during treatment. *Canc Nurs* 9:38-42.

Hutchinson, M.L., et al. 1984. Energy expenditure estimation in recipients of marrow transplants. *Cancer* 54:1734-1738.

Jenns, K. 1994. Importance of nausea. *Canc Nurs* 17 (6):488-493.

Johnson, L.R. 1988. Regulation of gastrointestinal mucosal growth. *Physiol Rev* 68:456-502.

Jones, B., et al. 1988. Gastrointestinal inflammation after bone marrow transplantation: graft-versus-host disease or opportunistic infection? *AJR* 150:277-281.

Kaproth, P.L., et al. 1990. Parenteral nutrition in a bone marrow transplant patients with hepatic complications. *Nutr Clin Pract* 5:18-22.

Katz, D.P., Kwetan, V., Askanazi, J. 1990. Enteral nutrition: potential role in regulating immune function. *Curr Opin Gastroenterol* 6:199-203.

Keenan, A.M. 1989. Nutritional support of the bone marrow transplant patient. *Nurs Clin North Am* 24 (2):383-393.

Kern, K.A., Norton, J.A. 1988. Cancer cachexia. *J Parenteral & Enteral Nutr* 12:286-298.

Kolbinson, D.A., et al. 1988. Early oral changes following bone marrow transplantation. *Oral Surg Oral Med Oral Pathol* 66:130-138.

Labar, B., et al., 1993. Prostaglandin E2 for prophylaxis of oral mucositis following BMT. *BMT* 11:379-82.

Larson, P.J., et al. 1993. Comparison of perceived symptoms of patients undergoing bone marrow transplant and the nurses caring for them. *Oncol Nurs Forum* 20(1):81-88.

Laskin, R.L., et al. 1987. Gancyclovir for the treatment and suppression of various infections caused by cytomegalovirus. *Am J Med* 83:201-208.

Lazlo, J. 1983. Nausea and vomiting as major complications of cancer chemotherapy. In Lazlo, J. (Ed.) *Drugs, Chemotherapy-Induced Emesis: Focus on Metaclopromide 25* (suppl 1). Balgowah, NSW, Australia: ADIS Press Australasia 1-7.

Lazarus, H.M., et al. 1990. Antiemetic efficacy and pharmacokinetic analyses of the serotonin antagonist ondansetron (GR38032F) during multiple-day chemotherapy with cisplatin prior to autologous bone marrow tranplantation. *J Natl Canc Inst* 82:1776-1778.

Lenssen, P., et al. 1983. Parenteral nutrition in marrow transplant recipients after discharge from the hospital. *Exp Hematol* 11:974-981.

Lenssen, P., et al. 1987. Intravenous branched chain amino acid in marrow transplant recipients. *J Parenteral & Enteral Nutr* 11:112-118.

Lenssen, P., et al. 1990. Prevalence of nutrition-related problems among long-term survivors of allogeneic marrow transplantation. *J Am Diet Assoc* 90:835-842.

Lenssen, P., Bruemmer, B., Aker, S. 1994. Relationship between IV lipid dose and incidence of bacteremias and fungemias in 492 marrow transplant patients. *J Parenteral and Enteral Nutr* 18(suppl):22S.

LeVeque, F.G., et al. 1992. Clinical evaluation of MGUI 209, an anesthetic, film-forming agent for relief from painful oral ulcers associated with chemotherapy. *J Clin Oncol* 10:1963-1968.

Lockhardt, P.B., Sonis, S.T. 1979. Relationship of oral complications to peripheral blood leukocyte and platelet counts in patients receiving cancer chemotherapy. *Oral Surg Oral Med Oral Pathol* 48:210-218.

Loprinzi, C.L., et al. 1990. A controlled evaluation of an allopurinol mouthwash as prophylaxis against 5-flourouracil–induced stomatitis. *Cancer* 65:1879-1882.

Martin, P.J., et al. 1990. A retrospective analysis of therapy for acute graft-versus-host disease: Initial treatment. *Blood* 76:1464-1472.

Martyn, P.A., Hansen, B.C., Jen, K. 1984. The effects of enteral and parenteral nutrition on appetitite in monkeys. *Nurs Res* 33:336-342.

Mattsson, T., et al. 1992. Alterations in taste acuity associated with allogeneic bone marrow transplantaion. *J Oral Pathol Med* 21:31-37.

McCarthy, M.C., et al. 1987. Prospective evaluation of single and triple lumen catheters in total parenteral nutrition. *J Parenteral & Enteral Nutr* 11:259-262.

McDonald, G.B., et al. 1985. Esophageal infections in immunocompromised patients after marrow transplantation. *Gastroenterol* 88:1111-1117.

McDonald, G.B., et al. 1986. Intestinal and hepatic complications of human bone marrow transplantation, parts I, II. *Gastroenterol* 90:460-477, 770-784.

McGuire, D.B., et al. 1993. Patterns of mucositis and pain in patients receiving preparative chemotherapy and bone marrow transplantation. *Oncol Nurs Forum* 20 (10):1493-1502.

Miaskowski, C. 1990. Management of mucositis during therapy. *NCI Monogr* 9:95-97.

Michallet, M., et al. 1989. Nutritional assessment of allogeneic BMT patients: role of parenteral nutrition and protein intake *BMT* 3(suppl 1):309 (abstr).

Moe, G., et al. 1985. Enteral managment. In Lensenn, P., Aker, S.N. (Eds.) *Nutritional Assessment and Management during Marrow Transplantation: A Resource Manual.* Seattle: Fred Hutchinson Cancer Ctr, 31-44.

Moller, J., et al. 1982. Protection against graft-versus-host disease by gut sterilization? Clinical experience with bone marrow transplantation in protective isolation. *Exp Hematol* 10:101-102.

Montecalvo, M.A. et al. 1994. Outbreak of vancomycin-, ampicillin-, and aminoglycoside-resistant enterococcus faecium bacteremia in an adult oncology unit. *Antimicrob Agents Chemother* 38:1363-1367.

Montgomery, M.T., et al. 1986. The incidence of oral herpes simplex virus infection in patients undergoing cancer chemotherapy. *Oral Surg Oral Med Oral Pathol* 61:238-242.

Moore, F.A., et al. 1989. TEN vs TPN following major trauma-induced septic morbidity. *J Trauma* 29:916-923.

Morrow, G.R., Morrell, C. 1982. Behavioral treatment for the anticipatory nausea and vomiting induced by cancer chemotherapy. *N Engl J Med* 307 (24): 1476-1480.

Mulder, P.O., et al. 1989. Hyperalimentation in autologous bone marrow transplantation for solid tumors: comparison of total parenteral versus partial parenteral plus enteral nutrition. *Cancer* 64:2045-2052.

National Institutes of Health Consensus Development Conference Statement. 1989. *Oral Complications of Cancer Therapies: Diagnosis, Prevention and Treatment.* 7:1-32.

Nemunaitis, J., Deeg, H.J., Yel, G.C. 1986. High cyclosporin concentration after bone marrow transplantation associated with hypertriglyceridemia. *Lancet* 2: 744-745.

Nims, J., Strom, S. 1988. Late complications of bone marrow transplant recipients: nursing care issues. *Semin Oncol Nurs* 4(1):47-54.

Nimer, S.D., et al. 1990. Successful treatment of hepatic veno-occlusive disease in bone marrow transplant patients. *Transplantation* 49:819-821.

Notermans, S., Hoogenboom-Verdegaal, A. 1992. Existing and emerging food borne disease. *Int J Food Microbiol* 15:197-205.

Owen, H., Klove, C., Cotanch, P.H. 1981. Bone marrow harvesting and high-dose BCNU therapy: nursing implications. *Canc Nurs* Jun:199-205.

Park, C.E., Saunders, G.W. 1991. Occurrence of thermtolerant camphylobacters in fresh vegetables sold at farmers' outdoor markets and supermarkets. *Can J Microbiol* 38:313-316.

Perfect J.R., et al. 1992. Prophylactic intravenous amphotericin B in neutropenic autologous bone marrow transplant recipients. *J Infect Dis* 165:891-897.

Peterson, D.E. 1990. Pretreatment strategies for infection prevention in chemotherapy patients. *Nat Canc Inst Monogr* 9:61-71.

Petz, L.D., Scott, E.P. 1983. Supportive care. In Blume, K.G., Petz, L.D. (Eds.) *Clinical Bone Marrow Transplantation.* New York: Churchill Livingstone, 177-213.

Piccolboni, D., et al. 1991. Nutritional and hormonal effects of biosynthetic human growth hormone in surgical patients on TPN. *Nutrition* 7:177-184.

Pinner, R.W., et al. 1992. Role of foods in sporadic listeriosis: microbiologic and epidemiologic investigation. *JAMA* 267(15):2046-2050.

Poland, J. 1989. Differential diagnosis of oral HSV infection. *Nurs Acumen* 1:3.

Raybould, T.P., et al. 1994. Emergence of gram-negative bacilli in the mouths of bone marrow transplant recipients using chlorhexidine mouth rinse. *Oncol Nurs Forum* 2(4):691-698.

Redd, W.H., Andrykowski, M.A. 1982. Behavioral interventions in cancer treatment: controlling aversion reactions to chemotherapy. *J Consult Clin Psychol* 50: 1018-1029.

Reed, E.C., et al. 1988. Ganciclovir treatment of cytomegalovirus infection of the gastrointestinal tract after marrow transplantation. *BMT* 3:199-206.

Reed, E.C., et al. 1990. Ganciclovir for the treatment of cytomegalovirus gastroenteritis in bone marrow transplant patients: a randomized, placebo-controlled trial. *Ann Intern Med* 112:505-510.

Reed, M., et al. 1983. Cyclic parenteral nutrition during bone marrow transplantation in children. *Cancer* 51: 1563-1570.

Ringden, O., et al. 1987. A pilot trial using foscarnet for cytomegalovirus infections in marrow transplant recipients. In Gale, R.P., Champlin, R. (Eds.) *Progress in*

Bone Marrow Transplantation. New York: A.R. Liss, 589-593.

Rocke, L.K., et al. 1993. A randomized clinical trial of two different durations of oral cryotherapy for prevention of 5-fluorouracil–related stomatitis. *Cancer* 72: 2234-2238.

Rodu, B., Gockerman, J.P. 1983. Oral manifestations of the chronic graft-v.-host reaction. *JAMA* 249:504-507.

Roila, F., et al. 1991. Prevention of cisplatin-induced emesis: a double-blind multicenter randomized crossover study comparing ondansetron and ondansetron plus desamethasone. *J Clin Oncol* 9:675-678.

Rombeau, J.L., Caldwell, M.D. 1990. Critical illness and sepsis. In Rombeau, J.L., Caldwell, M.D. (Eds.) *Clinical Nutrition: Enteral and Tube Feeding.* Philadelphia: Saunders, 294-299.

Rust, D.M., Schuster M.H. 1993. Anorexia and protein calorie malnutrition associated with chemotherapy. In Yasko, J.M. (Ed.) *Nursing Management of Symptoms Associated with Chemotherapy.* Columbus: Adria Labs, 47-66.

Sale, G.E., et al. 1981. Oral and ophthalmic pathology of graft-versus-host disease in man: predictive values of lip biopsy. *Hum Pathol* 12:1022-1030.

Samuels, B.L., Bitran, J.D. 1995. High dose intravenous melphalan: a review. *J Clin Oncol* 13:1786-1799.

Saral, R. 1989. Morbidity from HSV infection: yesterday, today and tomorrow. *Nursing Acumen* 1:2.

Saral, R., et al. 1983. Acyclovir prophylaxis against herpes simplex infection in patients with leukemia. *Ann Intern Med* 99:773-776.

Sax, H.C., Bowser, R.H. 1988. Hepatic complations of total parenteral nutrition. *J Parenteral & Enteral Nutr* 12: 615-618.

Schloerb, P.R., Amare, M. 1993. Total parenteral nutrition with glutamine in bone marrow tranplantation and other clinical applications. *J Parenteral & Enteral Nutr* 17:407-413.

Schmeiser, T., et al. 1988. Antimicrobial prophylaxis in neutropenic patients after bone marrow transplantation. *Infection* 16:19-24.

Schmidt, G.M., et al. 1993. Extended follow-up in 212 long-term allogeneic bone marrow transplant survivors: addressing issues of quality of life. *Tranplantation* 55: 551-557.

Scholten, H.C., et al. 1990. Diabetes mellitus or an impaired glucose intolerance as a potential complicating factor in patients treated with high dose therapy and autologous bone marrow tranplantation. *BMT* 6: 333-335.

Schubert, M.M., et al. 1983. Oral complications of bone marrow transplantation. In Peterson, D.E., and Sonis, S.T. (Eds.) *Oral Complications of Cancer Chemotherapy.* Boston: Martinus Nijhoff, 93-112.

Schubert, M.M., et al. 1984. Oral manifestations of chronic graft-v-host disease. *Arch Intern Med* 144: 1591-1595.

Schubert, M.M., Sullivan. 1990. Recognition, incidence, and management of oral graft-versus-host-disease. *NCI Monogr* 9:135-143.

Seto, B.G., et al. 1985. Oral mucositis in patients undergoing bone marrow transplantation. *Oral Surg Oral Med Oral Path* 60:493-497.

Shaked, A.A., Shinar, E., Freund, H. 1986. Managing the granulocytopenic patients with acute perianal inflammatory disease. *Am J Surg* 152:510-512.

Shuhart, M.C., McDonald, G.B. 1994. Gastrointestinal and hepatic complications. In Forman, S.J., Blume, K.G., Thomas, E.D. (Eds.) *Bone Marrow Transplantation.* Boston: Blackwell Scientific, 454-481.

Sieggren, M.Y. 1987. Healing physical wounds. *Nurs Clin North Am* 22:439-447.

Smedmyr, B., et al. 1990. Impaired glucose tolerance after bone marrow tranplantation. *BMT* 6:89-92.

Smith, S.L. 1990. *Tissue and Organ Transplantation: Implications for Professional Nursing Practice.* St. Louis: Mosby.

Spencer, G.D., et al. 1986. A prospective study of unexplained nausea and vomiting after marrow tranplantation. *Transplantation* 42:602-607.

Strohl, R.A. 1983. Nursing management of the patient experiencing taste changes. *Canc Nurs* 6:353-359.

Strohl, R. 1989. Herpes simplex virus infections in the bone marrow transplant patient: nursing considerations. *Nursing Acumen* 1:1, 5.

Szeluga, D.J., et al. 1985. Energy requirements of parenterally fed bone marrow transplant recipients. *J Parenteral & Enteral Nutr* 9:139-143.

Szeluga, D. J., et al. 1987. Nutritional support of the bone marrow transplant recipients: a prospective, randomized clinical trial comparing total parenteral nutrition to an enteral feeding program. *Canc Res* 47: 3309-3316.

Tombes, M.B., Gallucci, B. 1993. The effects of hydrogen peroxide rinses on the normal oral mucosa. *Nurs Res* 42:332-337.

Ulz, L., et al. 1990. A prospective study of complications in Hickman right atrial catheters in marrow transplant patients. *J Parenteral & Enteral Nutr* 14:27-30.

Viner, C.V., et al. 1990. Ondansetron: a new and safe antiemetic in patients receiving high-dose melphalan. *Canc Chemother Pharmacol* 25:449-453.

Wadleigh, R.C., et al. 1992. Vitamin E in the treatment of chemotherapy-induced mucositis. *Am J Med* 92: 481-484.

Wadler, S. 1994. Secretory diarrhea: induction by chemotherapy. East Hanover, NJ: Sandoz Pharmaceuticals, 1-12 (monogr).

Walsh, T. J., Belitsos, N.J., Hamilton, S.R. 1986. Bacterial esophagitis in immunocompromised patients. *Arch Intern Med* 146:1345-1349.

Weil, M., Rovelli, M. 1986. Infectious disease and transplantation. In Sigardson-Poor, F.M., Haggerty, L.M. (Eds.) *Nursing Care of the Transplant Recipient*. Philadelphia: Saunders.

Weisdorf, D. J., et al. 1989. Oropharyngeal mucositis complicating bone marrow transplantation: prognostic factors and the effect of chlorhexidine mouth rinse. *BMT* 4:89-95.

Weisdorf, D.J., et al. 1990. Acute upper gastrointestinal graft-versus-host disease: clinical significance and response to immunosuppressive therapy. *Blood* 76: 624-629.

Weisdorf, S. A., et al. 1984. Total parenteral nutrition in bone marrow transplantation: a clinical evaluation. *J Pediatr Gastro Nutr* 3:95-100.

Weisdorf, S. A., et al. 1987. Positive effect of prophylactic total parenteral nutrition on long-term outcome of bone marrow transplantation. *Transplantation* 43: 833-838.

Weisdorf, S.A., Schwarzenberg, S.J. 1994. Nutritional support of bone marrow transplantation recipients. In Forman, S.J., Blume, K.G., Thomas, E.D. (Eds.) *Bone Marrow Transplantation*. Boston: Blackwell Scientific, 327-336.

Western Consortium for Cancer Nursing Research. 1991. Development of a staging system for chemotherapy-induced stomatitis. *Canc Nurs* 14:6-12.

Wickham, R. 1989. Managing chemotherapy-related nausea and vomiting: the state of the art. *Oncol Nurs Forum* 16:563-574.

Williams, W. 1985. Infection control during parenteral nutrition therapy. *J Parenteral & Enteral Nutr* 9: 735-745.

Wilmore, D.W. 1991. Catabolic illness: strategies for enhancing recovery. *N Engl J Med* 325:695-702.

Wingard, J.R. 1990. Advances in the management of infectious complications after bone marrow transplantation. *BMT* 6:371-383.

Wingard, J.R., et al. 1988. Cytomegalovirus infection after autologous bone marrow transplantation with comparison to infection after allogeneic bone marrow transplantation. *Blood* 71:1432-1437.

Wolford, J.L., McDonald, G.B. 1987. Gastrointestinal bleeding after marrow transplantation: a prospective study of risk factors, etiology, and outcome. *Gastroenterol* 92:1697.

Wolford, J.L., McDonald, G.B. 1988. A problem-oriented approach to intestinal and liver disease after marrow transplantation. *J Clin Gastroenterol* 10(4): 419-433.

Woo, S.B., et al. 1993. A longitudinal study of oral ulcerative mucositis in bone marrow transplant recipients. *Cancer* 72:1612-1617.

Wujcik, D., Ballard, B., Camp-Sorrell, D. 1994. Selected complications of allogeneic bone marrow transplantation. *Semin Oncol Nurs* 10(1):28-41.

Yeomans, A.C. 1986. Rectal infections acute leukemia. *Canc Nurs* 9(6):295-300.

Yeomans, A., et al. 1991. Efficacy of chlorhexidine gluconate use in the prevention of perirectal infections in patients with acute leukemia. *Oncol Nurs Forum* 18 (7):1207-1213.

Zerbe, M.B., et al. 1992. Relationships between oral mucositis and treatment variables in bone marrow transplant patients. *Cancer Nurs* 15(3):196-205.

Ziegler, T.R., et al. 1990. Use of human growth hormone combined with nutritional support in a critical care unit. *J Parenteral & Enteral Nutr* 14:574-581.

Ziegler, T.R., et al. 1992. Clinical and metabolic effects of glutamine supplemented parenteral nutrition after bone marrow transplantation. *Ann Intern Med* 116: 821-828.

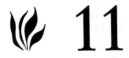

11

Pulmonary and Cardiac Effects

Teresa Wikle Shapiro

Pulmonary complications continue to be a major source of morbidity and mortality for people who undergo bone marrow transplantation (BMT) or blood cell transplantation (BCT). Irrespective of underlying disease, type of transplant, or transplant center, pulmonary disease continues to be the main cause of death in the majority of reports on overall allogeneic BMT results over the past two decades (Quabeck, 1994). A lesser but significant number of autologous recipients are plagued by pulmonary problems as well (Fort and Graham-Pole, 1989). Interstitial pneumonitis accounts for about 40% of transplant-related deaths (Weiner et al., 1986). In a meta-analysis of 1345 allogeneic and autologous BMT patients from 1973 to 1993 patients, 43% died from therapy-related complications (Quabeck, 1994). Pneumonia was noted as the primary cause of death in 39% of these patients.

All patients who undergo BCT and BMT are routinely screened pretransplant for underlying pulmonary disease with baseline pulmonary function tests, including a measurement of diffusion capacity. Poor pulmonary function often indicates underlying pulmonary disease. These patients may not be considered viable candidates for transplant because underlying pulmonary disease places the patient at an extremely high risk for the development of lethal pulmonary complications.

Cardiac complications occur in about 25% of patients who undergo allogeneic and autologous BMT and BCT, with a higher incidence in the autologous population. Cardiac complications, however, are rarely the cause of death of a BMT patient (Bearman et al., 1988; Pihkala et al., 1994). Baseline cardiac function should also be assessed in all patients. Such an evaluation is accomplished through echocardiography or radionuclide ventriculography. Patients with poor left ventricular function (diminished shortening fraction or ejection fraction) are generally at too high a risk to undergo the process, and are therefore usually denied a BMT or BCT as a therapeutic option.

Nursing plays a vital role in the prevention, detection, and intervention of cardiopulmonary complications of blood cell and marrow transplantations. This necessitates that nurses caring for these patients have a strong base of knowledge in the medical, scientific, and nursing interventions for dealing with these often grave complications.

PULMONARY COMPLICATIONS

Pathogenesis

Pulmonary interstitial pneumonitis (IPn) is a general term referring to an inflammatory process involving the intra-alveolar linings of the lung. Many complex interacting factors contribute to the development of IPn (Figure 11.1) (Bortin, 1983; Wikle, 1991). The three major predisposing factors are (1) an immunosuppressed host, (2) lung damage, and (3) the presence of opportunistic microorganisms (Bortin, 1983). Any of these alone or in combination can lead to the development of IPn. IPn usually occurs from day 30 to day 100 post BMT, and approximately 50% of these cases are fatal. Other common risk factors predispose the BMT patient to the development of IPn (see Table 11.1).

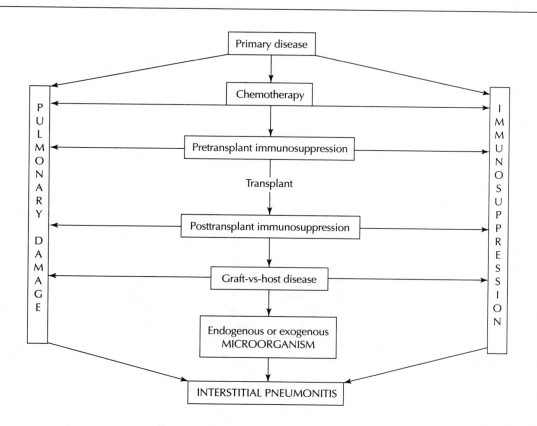

Figure 11.1 Possible pathways for the pathogenesis of interstitial pneumonitis

SOURCE: Bortin, 1983. Used with permission.

TABLE 11.1 Risk factors for the development of interstitial pneumonitis

1. Immunosuppressive agents (corticosteroids, MTX, cyclosporin, ATG)
2. High-dose cyclophosphamide prior to BMT
3. Graft-versus-host disease
4. High-dose rate of radiation therapy
5. High total lung dose rate
6. Single fraction radiation therapy
7. Total body irradiation
8. Increased age at time of transplant
9. Seropositivity to CMV pretransplant
10. Matched unrelated or haploidentical bone marrow donor

TABLE 11.2 Agents associated with interstitial pneumonitis that are immuno-suppressive and/or cause lung damage

Actinomycin	Irradiation[a]
BCNU	Melphalan
Bleomycin[a]	Methotrexate
Busulfan	Mitomycin
Chlorambucil	Procarbazine
Cyclophosphamide[a]	Vincristine

[a]Frequent association

SOURCE: Bortin, 1983. Used with permission.

Immunosuppression

A sequence of pre- and post-transplant events contribute to the severe immunosuppressed state and leave the patient vulnerable to infection. For example, a significant number of patients with malignancies receive chemotherapy for remission induction and consolidation for weeks or months prior to transplant. This therapy has significant immunosuppressive activity. In addition, some cancers such as leukemia or lymphoma affect immune function. The patient's pretransplant conditioning regimen has profound immunosuppressive effects as well. Many of the immunosuppressive agents that are administered pretransplant have also been found to cause lung damage (see Table 11.2).

Posttransplant immunosuppression with methotrexate, cyclosporin A, antithymocyte globulin, and other immunosuppressive agents administered to prevent or treat graft-versus-host disease (GVHD) adds to and prolongs the patient's immunosuppressed state. In addition, GVHD has been found to have immunosuppressive effects.

Patients who undergo BMTs have multiple interacting factors that result in virtual destruc-

tion of the defense against infection. Opportunistic pathogens are often found in the lungs of patients with IPn, suggesting that the severe and prolonged injury to the immune system may allow the growth of these microorganisms. This may especially be true of lung tissue that is already damaged.

Lung Damage

The same sequence of events that leads to immunosuppression in the transplant patient also leads to lung damage. For example, at the time of diagnosis, patients with a history of leukemic infiltrates have already suffered a pulmonary insult even if the infiltrates resolve by the time of transplant. Patients may receive at some time many of the chemotherapeutic agents listed in Table 11.2 for either induction or consolidation therapy. Perhaps of greater importance is the fact that many of these drugs have been reported to interact with radiation by increasing the amount of damage to normal lung tissue (Bortin, 1983). At the present time, many patients who undergo transplant are treated with cyclophosphamide and/or methotrexate along with total body irradiation (TBI); lung damage is magnified when either of these drugs is administered in close proximity to radiation to the lung (Bortin, 1983).

Although it is well known and documented that irradiation injures the lungs, the precise role of TBI in the pathogenesis of IPn has yet to be identified. Dose rates, the use of fractionated TBI, and the total dose received by the lung affects the patient's risk for the development of IPn.

Finally, although the lung is not considered a primary target organ for GVHD, chronic lung damage and decreased pulmonary function can occur with both acute and chronic GVHD.

Opportunistic Microorganisms

Opportunistic microorganisms such as cytomegalovirus (CMV) and *Pneumocystis carinii* are often found in the lungs of BMT patients with IPn. Damaged lungs in immunosuppressed patients with IPn provide a suitable environment for the overgrowth of opportunistic pathogens. BMT patients are exposed to many endogenous or exogenous sources of CMV and other dangerous microorganisms. The presence of lung damage in an immunosuppressed host strengthens the hypothesis that these microorganisms are the causative agents, and therefore infection is responsible for many cases of IPn.

However, approximately 30% to 50% of IPn cases are categorized as "idiopathic," meaning no causative organism was isolated either through lung biopsy or, all too often, tissue obtained post-mortem (Meyers, Flourney, Thomas, 1982).

Diagnosis of Pulmonary Interstitial Pneumonitis and Pneumonia

The differential diagnosis of pulmonary disease includes various infectious and noninfectious processes including congestive heart failure; septic and aseptic emboli; adult respiratory distress syndrome; hemorrhage; radiation injury; hypersensitivity disorders; toxic reactions; and

an expanding list of bacterial, fungal, viral, and protozoan infections (Shelhamer et al., 1992). Table 11.3 outlines the altered host defenses common to BMT patients and their associated pulmonary processes.

Interstitial pneumonitis has been defined as a clinical syndrome characterized by dry cough, dyspnea, fever, hypoxemia (arterial $Po_2 < 70$ mmHg at room air) and interstitial or reticulonodal pulmonary infiltrates on chest X ray (Granena et al., 1993). IPn may be associated with an infection, most commonly CMV, or may be idiopathic. Pneumonia is most commonly associated with bacterial and fungal pathogens. Apart from a thorough physical exam, relevant diagnostic tests of the transplant patient with acute or chronic lung disease include PFTs, venous or arterial blood gas (ABG) analysis, chest radiographs (CXRs) or computerized tomography (CT) scan, sputum specimens, bronchial alveolar lavage (BAL) with transbronchial biopsy (TBB), and open lung biopsy (OLB).

The basic principles by which infections should be diagnosed and treated are the same for BMT and BCT patients as for other high-risk patients. Intensive evaluation, including appropriate biopsies, should be performed in an attempt to identify specific pathogens responsible for the pulmonary process. If a specific pathogen or pathologic process is identified, tailored drug therapy can be instituted. The rapidity with which a specific diagnosis is made and effective therapy is instituted is the most important variable in determining the patient's outcome (Wingard et al., 1988).

Radiological Studies

Because prompt diagnosis and treatment of pulmonary disease is essential if the patient is to survive, weekly screening CXRs are commonly performed throughout the acute post-

TABLE 11.3 **Altered host defenses and assciated pulmonary processes in BCT and BMT patients**

INFECTIOUS CAUSES OF PULMONARY INFILTRATES

Granulocytopenia

Gram-negative bacilli: *P. aeruginosa, E. coli, Enterobacter* species

Gram-positive cocci: *S. aureus, S. epidermis,* group D *Streptococci,* alpha-hemolytic streptococci

Gram-positive bacilli: *Bacillus* species, *Clostridium* species

Fungi: *Aspergillus* species, *Fusarium* species, *Candida* species, *Torulopsis glabrata*

Celluar (T Lymphocyte) Immune Defects (due to CyA, steroids, GVHD)

Bacteria: *Mycobacterium* species, *Legionella* species, *Listeria, Salmonella* species

Viruses: CMV, varicella zoster, herpes simplex, Epstein-Barr virus

Protozoan: *P. carinii, Toxoplasma gondii*

Fungi: *Cryptococcus neoformans, Histoplasma capsulatum*

Coccidioides Humoral (B Lymphocyte) Immune Deficiency (due to low levels of IgG)

Bacteria: *Streptococcus pneumoniae, Haemophilus influenzae*

Impaired tracheobonchial clearance (due to mucositis, sedation, altered neurologic status)

Bacteria and fungi colonizing lower respiratory tract

NONINFECTIOUS CAUSES OF PULMONARY INFILTRATES

Congestive heart failure

Drug-induced pneumonia

Pulmonary infarction (septic emboli, embolism)

Adult respiratory distress syndrome

Alveolar hemorrhage

Hypersensitivity pneumonitis

Radiation pneumonitis

KEY: CyA = cyclosporin, GVHD = graft-versus-host disease, IgG = immunoglobulin G, CMV = cytomegalovirus

transplant period. The CXR remains the major signpost of pneumonitis. Although no radiographic pattern of pneumonitis is specific either for a particular disease process in the lungs or for a particular infectious agent, some radiologic findings are more characteristic of some diseases than of others. This does little to simplify the process of differential diagnosis, however, because since a multitude of causative organisms are possible (Shelhamer et al., 1992).

In patients who have tachypnea, dyspnea, cough, or abnormal physical findings, ABGs and a CXR should be performed without delay. It is recommended that for the patient with significant clinical signs and symptoms, the CXR should be two views, both anteroposterior and left-lateral, while the patient is in the standing position. The CXR may not reveal pathologic changes, especially during aplasia, because potential lesions lack granulocytic infiltration, thus making them less dense and therefore more difficult to detect on a plain CXR (Quabek, 1994).

High-resolution CT scan with contrast may allow detailed imaging not only of the extent and localization of pulmonary disease, but also of the possible nature of the lesions (i.e., isolated fungal lesions, diffuse viral process). In addition, CT scan can facilitate further diagnostic measure such as BAL or OLB.

The performance of a two-view CXR and a CT scan often requires that the patient temporarily leave protective isolation. This should not be viewed as a major obstacle in view of the need for an exact diagnosis (Quabek, 1994).

Conventional Sputum Examination

Examination of expectorated sputum for gram stain and culture can sometimes be helpful in the diagnosis of pulmonary infections, especially if the patient has not expectorated secretions in the past. The gram stain and culture are helpful in the compromised host even if only to determine that the sputum contains the patient's own normal flora. Unfortunately in the immunocompromised BMT patient, particularly those who are also granulocytopenic, sputum samples provide confusing information.

Diagnostic limitations of sputum analysis include the inability to diagnose some viral (CMV) or fungal (aspergillosis, candida, torulopsis) pneumonias. The distinction between colonization and actual infection by some fungi and bacteria frequently is not feasible and requires further evaluation with other procedures to assess the clinical significance of these isolates. Further, there is often an inability to diagnose noninfectious processes such as pulmonary hemorrhage, diffuse alveolar damage, and drug toxicities (Shelhamer et al., 1992). Because of such limitations, other diagnostic techniques usually must be employed to determine the etiology of pulmonary disease.

Bronchoalveolar Lavage and Transbronchial Biopsy

Bronchoalveolar lavage (BAL) has become an established approach to the diagnosis of pulmonary disease in the BMT patient. This procedure entails lavaging the diseased sections of the lung via the bronchoscope, and then submitting the lavaged fluid for analysis. BAL is particularly useful in the diagnosis of opportunistic infection and confirming pulmonary hemorrhage. It is also useful in the identification of cellular elements, such as lymphocytes and macrophages, seen in noninfectious and inflammatory conditions of the lung. Special stains and cultures of the lavaged material result in a diagnosis in 30% to 55% of cases (Shelhamer et al., 1992). BAL is valuable in BMT patients who have low platelet counts or bleeding disorders, or who are being treated with positive pressure ventilation and are therefore at increased risk for bleeding with open lung biopsy or transbronchial biopsy.

Transbronchial biopsy (TBB) in conjunction with BAL is considered a "middle-level" diagnostic technique that is employed in the less emergent situations in which the diagnosis cannot be made by noninvasive approaches. TBB provides an actual biopsy of lung tissue during fiberoptic bronchoscopy. TBB and BAL together increase the diagnostic yield.

The patient must be closely monitored following TBB for signs of bleeding, infection of the pulmonary tree, and pneumothorax. The nurse should also send the first sputum expectorated post TBB for culture because it may also increase the diagnostic yield of the procedure.

Open Lung Biopsy

Open lung biopsy is often instituted if the above-mentioned procedures fail to establish a diagnosis or if the patient continues to deteriorate despite tailored therapeutic measures. These transplant patients should be considered diagnostic emergencies, especially if the patient's hypoxemia is intensifying and the pulmonary infiltrates are spreading rapidly. Transplant patients tolerate OLB poorly due to the need for general anesthesia, thoracotomy, and postoperative chest tube. Because many patients with IPn require mechanical ventilation following the procedure, thoracic surgery teams hesitate to operate on these patients.

Open lung biopsy has been an important diagnostic procedure in this patient population because a specific pathogen is found in 50% to 90% of them (Bortin, 1983). Brown and colleagues (1990), in a randomized trial of 24 patients with pulmonary infiltrates, examined the use of OLB versus empiric antimicrobial therapy in non-neutropenic BMT patients. The findings from this study suggest (1) establishment of a diagnosis by OLB did not result in changes in antibiotic therapy and (2) empiric antibiotic therapy appears to be as successful as and potentially less toxic than an OLB. Due to the overall morbidity of the OLB procedure, its use is becoming less commonplace in BMT centers (Wingard et al., 1988)

Whatever diagnostic procedure is employed, a detailed analysis of the lung material is carried out. The lung sample is gram stained and cultured for aerobic and anaerobic bacterial pathogens, as well as mycobacteria, fungi, viruses, mycoplasmas, and the *Legionella* species. In addition, materials are processed with methenanine silver staining for *Pneumocystis* and with immunofluorescent staining for *Legionella*, CMV, and other organisms that are difficult to culture. Polymerase chain reaction (PCR) studies are now used to test for a number of microbes. Improved PCR techniques have resulted in increased rapidity with which a diagnosis of infection can be confirmed or excluded since the turnaround time for most PCRs is less than 3 days.

In summary, the diagnosis of pulmonary disease is essential if appropriate therapeutic measures are to be successful for the BMT patient. Diagnosis is based on symptomatology, chest X ray, sometimes sputum examination, and tissue culture. The transplant nurse plays an active role in early detection and treatment of IPn by frequently assessing the patient's pulmonary status during activity and at rest, and by reporting changes as they occur.

Pulmonary Edema

Pulmonary toxicity developing early after BMT is usually due to the individual or collective effects of the pretransplant conditioning chemotherapy, radiation therapy, and marrow infusion. These early effects are seen in the form of pulmonary edema 7 to 28 days after transplant (Fort and Graham-Pole, 1989). This syndrome is presumed to be due primarily to leaky pulmonary vasculature. High-dose cytosine arabinoside (Ara-C), which is used in several pretransplant conditioning regimens, has been shown to cause capillary leakage of proteinlike serous fluid into the aveolar spaces (Cardozo et al., 1985). Total body irradiation causes similar capillary leakage. Radiation doses in excess of 1000 cGy to the lung are associated with increased vascular permeability, alveolar wall edema, alveolar protein leakage, loss of pulmonary surfactant, and formation of an alveolar hyaline membrane. High-dose cyclophosphamide can cause myocardial damage with resultant pulmonary edema. In addition, patients with marginal cardiac status pretransplant are also at greater risk for pulmonary edema during the early posttransplant period due to cardiac failure.

Although the occurrence of pulmonary edema in the early posttransplant phase is well documented, detailed information on its incidence and risk factors are lacking (Quabek, 1994). Symptoms of pulmonary edema include tachypnea, rales, orthopnea, lethargy, restlessness, weight gain, and cardiac enlargement on CXR. Lung changes on CXR may mimic those induced by infection. Resolution of the above findings by fluid restriction and diuretic therapy usually confirms a diagnosis. For severe cases in patients who experience true congestive heart failure, management includes fluid restriction, diuretics, nitroglycerine, and dobutamine. Digitalis may be indicated if prolonged medication is required. Nursing management of the BMT patient with pulmonary edema includes assisting the patient to maintain oxygenation, maintenance of strict intake and output, and assisting the medical team with precise fluid management along with the judicious use of diuretics. With astute management, the patient can be assisted through this initial phase of BMT with complete resolution of the process.

Acute hemorrhagic pulmonary edema may also develop early in the transplant process. This is much less common than the edema caused by increased vascular permeability, and seems to affect patients receiving HLA-mismatched transplants (Hamilton et al., 1986). It is associated with hemorrhage into the alveolar sacs, low central venous pressure, fluid retention, hypotension, and renal failure. Once this complication develops, it is fatal 90% of the time.

Pulmonary Infections Associated with BMT

Infections are a major cause of pulmonary pathology following BMT. Among the numerous causes, about two thirds of them have a documented infectious agent causing pneumonitis (viral, bacterial, fungal, or protozoal); other cases are attributable to the effects of drugs, radiation therapy, or GVHD. The infections may take the form of intra-alveolar lobar consolidation (pneumonia) or involve the interalveolar linings (interstitial pneumonitis). The symptoms associated with infectious pulmonary infiltrates include dyspnea, tachypnea, cyanosis, dry rales, and a cough. These symptoms are a result of inadequate gas exchange, which results from the abnormal alveolar structure producing an alveolar/capillary block.

Intensive evaluation, including appropriate biopsies, should be performed to identify the specific organisms responsible for the pulmonary infection (see Table 11.4). If a specific pathogen is identified, then the appropriate antibiotic/drug therapy should be instituted as soon as possible. If a specific pathogen cannot be found (idiopathic) or is not found because the patient cannot undergo the required diagnostic procedures, then empiric, broad-spectrum antibiotics should be administered to cover any or all microorganisms that could be causing the infection. The patient is usually receives medications to treat all possible bacterial, fungal, protozoal, viral, and chlamydial infections. Caring for a patient being treated for all likely infectious sources can be one of the

TABLE 11.4 Microorganisms frequently associated with interstital pneumonitis

Aspergillus	*Mycoplasma*
Candida	*Pneumococcus*
Cryptococcus	*Pneumocystis*
Cytomegalovirus	*Pseudomonas*
Herpes simplex	*Toxoplasma*
Histoplasma	Varicella zoster
Klebsiellsa	

SOURCE: Wikle, 1991. Used with permission.

greatest challenges a transplant nurse can experience. Venous access, renal compromise, and fluid overload may complicate the patient's management overall because of the large number of medications that must administered.

The objectives of therapy to treat infectious IPn are twofold: (1) treatment and or reversal of the causative factor(s) and (2) adequate ventilation/oxygenation. Unfortunately, the treatment of established IPn has been unsuccessful for the most part. This negative experience may partly reflect the irreparable pulmonary damage produced by the large quantities of pathologic organisms that are likely present in established pneumonia. For this reason, the effectiveness of any therapeutic modality is severely limited. Efforts at prevention of the pneumonia(s) appear to be more successful.

Bacterial Pneumonia

Bacterial pneumonia commonly occurs within the first 6 months post BMT and is most frequently seen in patients with chronic GVHD and those with incomplete HLA donor matching. Risk factors include prolonged neutropenia, B-cell immune deficiency, impaired splenic function, and IgA deficiency. In normal individuals, the flora of the upper respiratory tract are primarily gram-positive organisms, which are relatively nonvirulent and sensitive to antibiotics. Because of a special interaction between these bacteria and the specialized receptors on the surface of the upper respiratory tract, colonization with gram-negative bacilli is prevented. In the immunocompromised BMT patient, this ecological system is disturbed, resulting in a high rate of colonization of the respiratory tract by gram-negative organisms (Rubin, 1988).

Bacterial infections usually take the form of consolidation of the alveolar sacs in the lungs. Both gram-positive organisms such as *Staphylococcus aureus, Staph. epidermidis,* and *Streptococcus pneumoniae,* and gram-negative organisms like *Klebsiella,* and the *Pseudomonas* species are the common causative pathogens. In addition, patients with chronic GVHD have a higher incidence of pneumococcal pneumonia. *Legionella, Chlamydia, Mycobacteria,* and *Mycoplasma* are also being more frequently isolated in these patients. Several resistant strains of gram-positive organisms are more frequently seen late into the BMT patient's treatment, and many of these organisms are sensitive only to vancomycin.

The approach to therapy for pulmonary bacterial infections is as mentioned earlier: if a specific pathogen is identified, then antibiotic therapy should be tailored according to the culture and sensitivity reports. Frequently, if the patient is neutropenic, he or she will require other antibiotic coverage as well so that superinfection will not occur. Double or triple antibiotic coverage is standard in these patients because a vast number of other bacteria may pose a threat. Prophylactic use of trimethoprim-sulfamethoxazole (TMP-SMZ) may lower the frequency of streptococcal pneumonia and certain gram-negative infections, but further study in this area is required. The present pneumococcal vaccine seems to offer no protection for the post-BMT patient with chronic GVHD. However, patients who are being treated for chronic GVHD should receive prophylactic antibiotic coverage against encapsulated bacteria such as *Streptococcus pneumonia* and *Haemophilus influenzae,* for the duration of their immunosuppressive therapy.

Although sometimes fatal, bacterial pneumonias are generally more sensitive to drug therapy than the viral, fungal, and protozoal infections. This is most likely due to the fact that the alveolar wall becomes increasingly thickened in the nonbacterial IPns, thus rendering the lung more resistant to penetration with drug therapy and repair.

Viral Pneumonia

Viral infections are the most common documented cause of IPn in the BMT patient population. Very little success has been achieved in the treatment of IPn associated with viral pathogens. Most attempts to treat viral IPn have focused on CMV infections since the mortality rate of CMV pneumonia following BMT is so high. CMV is the most common viral pathogen isolated in these patients and is responsible for about 50% of cases of IPn post BMT (Granena et al., 1993).

Cytomegalovirus infection usually presents 6 to 8 weeks after BMT, either as multiifocal disease suggestive of hematologic dissemination, or strictly localized to the lungs suggestive of airway dissemination. CMV pneumonitis may represent (1) reactivation of latent CMV virus in the BMT recipient, (2) acquisition of the virus from an infected marrow donor, or (3) acquisition of the virus through a transfusion that is infected with the CMV virus.

Prolonged immunosuppression is the single most important factor in the development of CMV pneumonitis. This is supported by the increased incidence of CMV pneumonitis in patients who have received antithymocyte globulin for GVHD prophylaxis, and in patients being treated with high doses of steroids for acute GVHD. The patient's resistance to CMV infection is mediated by cellular immunity. Although the total number of WBCs and phagocytes may be normal in patients after transplant, T- and B-cell–mediated immune function may be reduced for up to 2 years after transplant. This is especially true of the allogeneic BMT population (Lum, 1987).

However, the question has remained unanswered: Why do some patients infected with CMV develop CMV disease while others do not? It has been speculated that, in addition to the presence of virus in the lung, an immunopathological reaction mediated by lymphocytes, especially cytotoxic T cells which are elevated in GVHD, is essential for the establishment of disease (Quabeck, 1994). This may explain why there is an extremely low incidence of CMV pneumonitis in BCT and autologous marrow transplant patients.

The most promising current management for post-BMT CMV infection is prophylaxis with immune globulin containing a high titer of CMV antibody, along with intravenous ganciclovir. Intravenous immunoglobulin administered 1 week prior to, and for the first 3 to 4 months after BMT probably reduces the incidence of pneumonitis, although the data is conflicting. The use of CMV-seronegative blood products in recipients who are seronegative and who also have a seronegative donor has assisted in decreasing the incidence of CMV infection. At some transplant centers, these prophylactic measures against CMV are generally isolated to allogeneic BMT patients since the incidence of CMV in autologous transplant patients ranges from only 0% to 8.6% (Ljungman et al., 1994). However, in spite of the limited availability of CMV seronegative blood products, transplant centers are now able to provide "CMV-safe" blood products to all BCT, autologous, and allogeneic BMT patients by the use of an in-line blood filter, which has been shown to be 90% effective in removing the virus from contaminated blood products (Bacigalupo et al., 1992).

Various antiviral agents have shown increasing efficacy in prevention of CMV pneumonitis (Bacigalupo et al., 1992). Ganciclovir (DHPG) has shown some promise in the prevention of CMV disease (Goodrich et al., 1993). Although some patients who receive ganciclovir prophylaxis develop CMV disease, studies have shown that prophylactic use of ganciclovir may decrease the severity of the CMV infection (Bacigalupo et al., 1994). However, ganciclovir has marked myelosuppressive activity and is therefore difficult to use early after BMT. Forcarnet, which has no myelosuppressive effects, has also been used prophylactically against CMV, but with slightly less success than ganciclovir (Reusser et al., 1991). As is seen in all therapies for established CMV pneumonitis, both ganciclovir and foscarnet have limited effect on overall survival of patients with active CMV pulmonary infection (Emanuel et al., 1988; Ljungman et al., 1992; Quabeck, 1994). Some trials have shown an improved disease response when ganciclovir is used in conjunction with CMV immune globulin.

Adenine arabinoside, an antiviral agent used in the treatment of herpes simplex viral encephalitis, has been used in the treatment of proven CMV pneumonitis with poor results. Human leukocyte interferon is another antiviral agent that has been effective against herpes-zoster infections and hepatitis B infections, but has been ineffective against CMV.

In summary, all regimens to treat established CMV pneumonia after BMT have so far been unsuccessful. Due to the devastating effects of CMV pneumonitis, nurses can expect many new clinical trials in both the treatment and prevention of this grave complication of BMT.

Although CMV is the most common viral etiology of IPn, other viruses account for 7% to 10% of the infectious cases of IPn (Fort and Graham-Pole, 1989). These include adenovirus, herpes simplex virus (HSV), and varicella zoster

(VZ). Acyclovir prophylaxis has decreased the incidence of IPn caused by the herpes viruses and has also reduced the severity of established infections. Epstein-Barr virus (EBV), respiratory syncytial virus (RSV), influenza, and parainfluenza infections are rare, and often fatal, causes of IPn in BMT patients (Englund et al., 1988; Wendt et al., 1992).

Fungal Pneumonia

The pulmonary fungal infections that occur in the BMT patient can be divided into three categories: (1) opportunistic infections caused by organisms that primarily invade the lung (e.g., *Aspergillus* species and *Cryptococcus neoformans*), (2) opportunistic infections that reach the lung either by way of the circulating blood from another site, or as organisms superinfecting a lung that was previously injured by a viral or bacterial process (e.g., the *Candida* species and the *Aspergillus* species), and (3) systemic mycoses that resemble tuberculosis by lying dormant for many years after the initial infection but subsequently undergo reactivation during the patient's immunosuppressed state (e.g., blastomycosis, coccidioidomycosis, histoplasmosis, and mucormycosis). This type of infection is rare in the transplant setting (Morrison and McGlave, 1993; Rubin, 1988).

Invasive aspergillosis is the most important fungal infection in terms of both incidence and severity. *Aspergillus* accounts for about 10% of the cases of posttransplant pulmonary disease and has an overall incidence of 5.6% (Paulin et al., 1987; Saugier-Verber et al., 1993). Invasive pulmonary Aspergillus carries an 82% mortality rate (Saugier-Verber et al., 1993). The *Aspergillus* species most commonly associated with invasive infections are *A. fumigatus* and *A. flavum*. A typical clinical setting for the development of invasive aspergillosis is the patient with severe granulocytopenia or the patient with GVHD receiving high-dose corticosteroids who has received broad-spectrum antibiotics within the previous month.

The presenting clinical symptoms of invasive pulmonary aspergillosis are usually subtle, with persistent fever often being the sole manifestation. In time, a mild productive cough may develop, which may cause pleuritic-type chest pain. As the disease progresses, fever worsens, rales develop, and pulmonary infiltrates appear. Invasive pulmonary aspergillosis causes a necrotizing bronchopneumonia with or without a hemmorhagic infarction. It is not unusual to aspirate lung tissue while suctioning the intubated patient who has an invasive aspergillosis infection due to the necrotizing process.

The most characteristic CXR of invasive aspergillosis reveals a rapidly progressing nodular infiltrate, often cavitating, and that frequently crosses lung fissures (Rubin, 1988). Figure 11.2 shows these cavitating lesions in a patient with invasive aspergillosis.

One of the most challenging aspects of an *Aspergillus* infection is that it rapidly spreads to the central nervous system (CNS). CNS symptoms may be the nurse's first indication that *Aspergillus* is a threat, even while the primary pulmonary site of infection is relatively asymptomatic. Therefore, major emphasis is placed on early diagnosis via bronchial alveolar lavage or open lung biopsy in the patient with this type of infiltrate, even if the patient displays no signs of pulmonary compromise. Surgical wedge resection is sometimes performed in patients who have isolated, cavitating lesions in hope of removing the primary site of infection.

Several transplant centers have suffered devastating epidemics of invasive pulmonary aspergillosis secondary to contamination of the hospital air conditioning system with *Aspergillus* spores. Protective environments, particularly laminar air flow, seem to decrease the incidence of *Aspergillus* pneumonitis. Fungal prophylaxis with fluconazole early after transplant and in patients on immunosuppressive therapy after transplant for GVHD can be effective in preventing *Aspergillus* as well as other types of fungal infections. At present, the most reasonable approach to early intervention is the empiric use of amphotericin B for the treatment of the neutropenic BMT patient who develops a fever that is unresponsive to broad-spectrum antibiotics after approximately 7 days. This alone may prevent pulmonary seeding of organisms such as the *Candida* and *Aspergillus* species via the circulating blood.

Presumptive therapy should be initiated in the BMT patient who has a clinically compatible syndrome and CXR and has either *A. fumigatus* or *A. flavus* isolated from their respiratory secretions (Rubin, 1988). The treatment of choice for pulmonary fungal infections is amphotericin B. However, successful treatment using amphotericin B is limited by the toxicity of the drug and the organism's intrinsic resistance to its antifungal activity. Maintenance doses of 0.6 to 0.7 mg/kg per day are often used, but higher doses of up to 1.5 mg/kg per day may be implemented. Neither miconazole, 5-fluorocytosine, nor ketoconazole are an acceptable substitute for amphotericin B. However, some data do support the use of 5-FC, rifampin, or tetracycline in combination with amphotericin B (Shelhamer et al., 1992). Because of the excessively high mortality rate associated with pulmonary aspergillosis, further study in the prevention and treatment of this lethal infection is warranted.

Parasitic Pneumonia

Two different opportunistic parasites are capable of producing pneumonia in the immunosuppressed patient—*Pneumocystis carinii* and *Toxoplasma gondii*. The most important is *P. carinii*. The typical CXR appearance of *Pneu-*

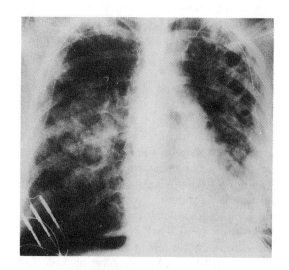

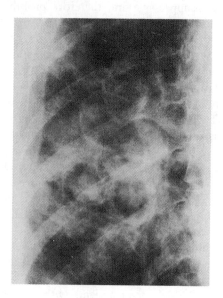

Figure 11.2 **X ray of cavitations caused by** *Aspergillus*

SOURCE: Rubin, 1988. Used with permission.

mocystis infection in the lungs is that of a diffuse interstitial alveolar pneumonia that often becomes confluent as the disease progresses. Usually, the disease affects the lower lobes and is bilateral and symmetric. The patient presents with a nonproductive cough, tachypnea, hypoxemia, and a restrictive defect on pulmonary function testing. These symptoms may be present despite a normal CXR. In such patients, a gallium scan can be useful in suggesting the presence of a *Pneumocystis* infection.

Prior to prophylaxis with TMP-SMZ, *P. carinii* was a common cause of severe pneumonia in all immunocompromised patients. Since the institution of TMP-SMZ prophylaxis, *P. carinii* accounts for less than 5% of pulmonary disease post BMT. TMP-SMZ prophylaxis can be myelosuppressive and therefore prohibitive in a number of patients. TMP-SMZ prophylaxis is administered two times per day, three times weekly. After successful prevention of *Pneumocystis* pneumonia in the HIV-infected population, dapsone-pyrimethamine is now commonly used in BMT patients who cannot take TMP-SMZ (Girard et al., 1993). Prophylaxis is administered once daily. Dapsone is also effective prophylaxis against *Toxoplasma gondii* (Girard et al., 1993). Dapsone should be used with caution in patients who are allergic to TMP-SMZ since there are reports of allergic cross-reactivity between TMP-SMZ and dapsone.

Pentamidine administered intravenously or by inhalation is also effective prophylaxis for patients who have poor compliance in taking oral TMP-SMZ, or in patients with an allergy to TMP-SMZ or dapsone. The advantage of inhaled pentamidine is that it only requires monthly administration.

Although *P. carinii* rarely develops in patients who are receiving prophylaxis, there is a 30% mortality rate. This is presumably due to the emergence of resistant strains of the organism. In this unusual patient, intravenous TMP-SMZ is the drug of choice for initial treatment because it is less toxic than pentamidine. The dosages are 20 mg/kg of trimethoprim per day and 100 mg/kg of sulfamethoxazole per day in four equal doses (Winston et al., 1983). Therapy is given for approximately 14 days. Using this approach, a therapeutic response is expected in about 70% of patients. Deaths are frequently associated with concomitant viral or fungal infections.

Such therapy, however, can have profound adverse effects in BMT patients. A new agent with activity against *P. carinii*, atovaquone, has been used in clinical trials for patients who cannot tolerate therapeutic doses of TMP-SMZ due to myelosuppression. These studies, however, demonstrated that atovaquone is not so effective in treating *P. carinii* as TMP-SMZ (Hughes et al., 1993).

Recently, several series have suggested that systemic corticosteroid therapy can decrease mortality, hasten defervescence, improve symptoms, and improve gas exchange in patients with *P. carinii* infection. In a prospective, double-blind, randomized, placebo-controlled trial of 37 HIV-infected patients with *P. carinii*, Montaner and colleagues (1990) found that corticosteroids, if used early, can prevent deterioration and increase tolerance of exercise. Clearly, further investigation into the use of corticosteroids in BMT patients infected with *P. carinii* is warranted.

Toxoplasmosis is an uncommon cause of pneumonia in BMT patients. Prophylaxis against *Toxoplasmosis gondii* with weekly administration of pyrimethamine was evaluated for efficacy and toxicity by Foot and colleagues (1994). They found pyrimethamine to be an effective prophylactic agent against toxoplasmosis. In addition, the 69 patients who received pyrimethamine were on no PCP prophylaxis; however, no patients in the trial experienced PCP pneumonia. Pyrimethamine may be included in the increasing list of prophylactic agents that can be given safely to BMT patients. As a rule, if *Toxoplasmosis gondii* does infect the lung, almost invariably other pathogens, particularly one or more of the herpes group of viruses or *Pneumocystis carinii,* are also present.

Drug-Induced Pulmonary Damage

Certain drugs used in the pretransplant conditioning regimens are known pulmonary toxins, and may be implicated in some cases of idiopathic IPn. As mentioned, Table 11.2 lists chemotherapeutic agents most commonly associated with IPn. This toxicity may be an acute single-dose effect or a cumulative effect from the combination of drugs the patient received prior to transplant. Such toxicity becomes compounded when these drugs are used in conjunction with radiation therapy and other treatments such as oxygen therapy and positive pressure ventilation (Weiss et al., 1980; Bortin, 1983). This additional lung damage may account for the difficulty in weaning the mechanically ventilated BMT patient.

Two clinical syndromes of drug-induced pneumonitis are recognized. The first is a subacute, progressive IPn characterized by fever, nonproductive cough, and dyspnea. This form is usually seen weeks to months following BMT, and resembles a viral or *P. carinii* infection both clinically and on CXR. The second is a chronic interstitial fibrosis that occurs insidiously. Diagnosis is generally made by use of a gallium scan that is usually positive in the inflammatory form of the disease. Pulmonary function tests reveal progressive pulmonary restriction and a decreased diffusing capacity. Transbronchial or open lung biopsy is usually required for a diagnosis (Rubin, 1988).

Bleomycin is one of the most pulmonary-toxic chemotherapeutic agents currently in use. Although not commonly used in BMT conditioning regimens, many patients, especially those with lymphoma, have received bleomycin sometime in the past. Bleomycin is distributed in the skin and the lungs (Bortin, 1983); therefore, when additional toxins such as radiation are given to patients who have received bleomycin, additional pulmonary insults ensue. Patients suffering from such toxicity present with a dry, hacky cough and exertional dyspnea that can progress to resting dyspnea, tachypnea, and cyanosis. The physical exam and CXR findings are often preceded by abnormal pulmonary functions tests. Bleomycin causes pulmonary fibrosis, which appears to be dose related. This fibrosis can develop in up to 40% of patients who are receiving doses of greater than 150 units. This type of fibrosis is usually irreversible and often fatal (Weiss et al., 1980). The route of bleomycin administration may play a role in toxicity, with continuous infusion being less toxic than IV bolus or intramuscular therapy. The dose at which pulmonary toxicity occurs is much lower when combined with other pulmonary toxins such as alkylating agents, radiation therapy, and high oxygen tensions to the lung (Ginsberg et al., 1982; Jules-Elysee and White, 1990).

One study of patients undergoing operative procedures necessitating elevated oxygen tensions during the procedure, showed 100% mortality of patients who had received cumulative doses of bleomycin between 200 and 400 units/m^2 (Weiss et al., 1980). All of those patients died of IPn and progressive pulmonary fibrosis. Synergy also exists between bleomycin and radiation therapy. The frequency of severe pulmonary toxicity when radiation is used with bleomycin is 35% to 50%, with 50% of those cases being fatal (Ginsberg et al., 1982; Elysee and White, 1990). Currently there is no effective treatment for the pulmonary fibrosis caused by bleomycin.

Occasionally hypersensitivity to bleomycin is seen as fever, eosinophilia, and diffuse pulmonary infiltrates. These patients, however, often respond to corticosteroid therapy (Ginsberg et al., 1982).

The nitrosureas (BCNU, CCNU, semustine, and chlorotocin) are pulmonary toxins with a reported incidence of pulmonary complications in about 20% to 30% of patients. BCNU is commonly used in BMT conditioning of patients who have Hodgkin's and non-Hodgkin's lymphoma. Such patients have often received previous pulmonary toxins such as bleomycin and mantel irradiation prior to transplant conditioning.

The doses at which symptoms develop with BCNU are unknown, but there is usually a 6-month or greater delay from the time of drug exposure to the development of symptoms. Symptoms normally seen are progressive dyspnea, tachypnea, and a nonproductive cough. The patient's CXR shows a reticulonodular pattern, pulmonary edema, and often pleural effusions. Pulmonary function tests (PFTs) reveal a restrictive lung defect with hypoxemia and a decreased carbon monoxide diffusion capacity (DLCO). Tissue evaluated from open lung biopsy or upon autopsy show interstitial fibrosis, alveolar septal thickening, and protein-filled alveoli. Although the outcome varies, and is probably dose dependent, mortality secondary to nitrosurea pulmonary toxicity ranges from 24% to 60%. Corticosteroids are of little benefit in the treatment of pulmonary toxicity from nitrosureas.

Methotrexate produces a variable pulmonary toxicity, which is independent of the dose the patient receives. Pulmonary damage can also result from any route of administration. PFTs usually show hypoxemia, a decreased DLCO, and a restrictive defect. A hypersensitivity drug reaction is the most common pulmonary toxic effect seen with methotrexate. Leucovorin does not seem to protect against the pulmonary toxicity. Fortunately, recovery usually occurs after the methotrexate is stopped. Corticosteroids appear to be of some benefit in the treatment of methotrexate-induced pulmonary toxicity, but do not induce a complete reversal of the pulmonary changes.

The alkylating agents, cyclophosphamide, busulfan, chlorambucil, and melphalan, probably have additive toxicity when used in combination with bleomycin or BCNU (Weiss et al., 1980; Ginsberg et al., 1982). Cyclophosphamide can cause intra-alveolar inflammation and edema leading to fibrosis, with similar PFT changes to those seen with the nitroureas. Infiltration can lead to a complete "whiting out" of the entire lung. Fortunately, early drug cessation can lead to a complete clinical and radiological resolution (Weiss et al., 1980). Like methotrexate, route of administration and total drug dose do not appear to determine how much toxicity the patient will suffer. Symptoms can begin while the patient is receiving cyclophosphamide, and can occur as late as 8 years following therapy.

Busulfan and cyclophosphamide can produce similar symptoms such as hypoxemia and a restrictive ventilatory defect. Many transplant protocols require the combination of these two antineoplastic agents. These patients are especially at high risk for pulmonary toxicity, and should be monitored closely for pulmonary compromise. However, in one study (Hartsell et al., 1995), fatal IPn was more commonly associated with cyclophosphamide and TBI conditioning regimens than those with busulphan and cyclophosphamide. Onset of symptoms with busulfan pulmonary toxicity are insidious, and are usually seen as cough, tachypnea, fever, and crepitant rales. Symptoms usually arise while the patient is on therapy, and often progress over weeks or months, unfortunately leading to a fatal outcome. Clinical improvement has been reported after discontinuing the busulfan, along with treating the patient with high-dose steroids.

Melphalan rarely causes pulmonary toxicity, but may occasionally damage the alveolar epithelium by causing dysplasia that can progress to fibrosis. This is caused by the proliferation of epithelial cells in the bronchi and the alveoli, which then results in the infiltration of these areas with plasma. Such a reaction is rarely seen in the BMT setting.

Cytosine arabinoside (Ara-C), as mentioned earlier in this chapter, can increase pulmonary vascular permeability, leading to non-cardiogenic pulmonary edema. Lung tissue in such patients reveals extensive fibrinous exudate suggestive of capillary leakage. This seems to correlate with the time course of drug administration, and not with the dose of the drug. In other words, the pulmonary toxic effects of Ara-C are increased if the drug is given in close proximity to other pulmonary toxins prior to the patient's transplant-conditioning regimen. The noncardiogenic pulmonary edema secondary to high-dose Ara-C is usually reversible with vigorous supportive care, including the administration of massive doses of corticosteroids (Andersson et al., 1990).

Although most drugs can cause toxicity through pulmonary parenchymal inflammation and fibrosis, procarbizine, like methotrexate causes pneumonitis through a hypersensitivity reaction. Permanent fibrosis can result if the hypersensitivty reaction is prolonged. Fortunately, symptoms usually resolve if the procarbazine is stopped.

The chemotherapy that patients receive prior to transplant is administered in large doses over a short period of time. Despite the development of symptoms, the patient is usually committed to receive the full conditioning regimen because the transplant is the patient's most likely chance for cure. Therefore, with the exception of methotrexate for GVHD prophylaxis, chemotherapeutic agents are rarely stopped due to the development of pulmonary or other serious symptomatology.

Radiation-Induced Pulmonary Damage

In addition to infections and chemotherapy-induced pulmonary toxicity, radiation therapy is a major cause of BMT-related pulmonary damage. The damage associated with total body irradiation (TBI) usually develops 2 to 3 months after treatment (Barrett et al., 1983; Bortin, 1983; Gross, 1977; Tait, 1990). Shielding the lungs, reducing the total exposure of TBI to 600 cGy or less, fractionating the TBI over several days, and decreasing the dose delivery rate all seem to decrease the incidence of IPn. Unfortunately many of these solutions are impractical. Shielding the lungs may increase risk of relapse for the patient since hidden tumor cells may be present in the shielded area. Many patients require greater than 600 cGy to achieve the required immunosuppression and antineoplastic effects that TBI offers. Much research is presently focused on the elimination of TBI, and thus its toxicities, so that most patients would be conditioned pretransplant with chemotherapy only. However, this may significantly increase the patient's risk of cardiac and other serious complications (Hartsell et al., 1995).

Signs and symptoms of radiation-induced pneumonitis are progressive dyspnea, high spiking fevers, a nonproductive cough with occasional hemoptysis, and chest pain secondary to pleural inflammation. Radiation-induced pulmonary damage usually resolves slowly, but may progress to fibrosis. Late symptoms include cyanosis, clubbing of the nails, orthopnea, and chronic cor pulmonale. Scoliosis with a midline shift may result from loss of pulmonary volume in the irradiated field in patients who receive local irradiation as part of their pretransplant conditioning. On CXR progressive fibrosis has a "ground glass" appearance with hazy pulmonary markings. As fibrosis develops, linear streaked consolidation with an occasional midline shift occurs. Bronchiolectatic cysts may also develop in the fibrosed lung. Corticosteroids offer some benefit in chronic radiation fibrosis. Unfortunately, symptoms usually reappear with tapering of the steroids. The time course for resolution or progression of the radiation damage is related to the severity of the pulmonary insult (Gross, 1977; Hartsell et al., 1995).

Graft-versus-Host Disease and Pulmonary Damage

Thirty to seventy percent of allogeneic BMT patients develop GVHD as a complication. These patients are predisposed to lung infections because of the immunosuppression that accompanies GVHD and its treatment. Additionally, GVHD appears to have a direct effect on the pulmonary epithelium. The sicca syndrome of chronic GVHD, which is recognized to have other target organs, can also exert its effect on the lungs. This is demonstrated as a decrease in the production of IgA and reduced local humoral immunity. Because of the death of epithelial cells, ciliary function is decreased, as are bronchial secretions. The bronchial mucosa is thus exposed. This results in a loss of its normal protective action, thus predisposing the patient to bronchopneumonia (Bortin, 1982).

A lymphocytic bronchitis can also occur concurrently with the development of acute GVHD. Studies in animals have found that small numbers of donor T cells in the transplanted marrow may not aid engraftment, but significantly increase the risk for pulmonary toxicity (Down et al., 1992). Such findings suggest that immunologically, the lungs of allogeneic BMT patients are different from those of BCT or autologous transplant patients.

Signs and symptoms of lymphocytic bronchitis secondary to acute GVHD include dyspnea, tachypnea, and a nonproductive cough due to bronchospasm with occasional progressive airway obstruction. With this syndrome there is lymphocytic infiltration of the mucosa, submucosa, and mucularis, with necrosis of epithelial cells, loss of cilia, and decreased goblet cells. This decreased ciliary function predisposes the patient to bronchopneumonia.

Bronchiolitis obliterans affects about 10% of patients with chronic GVHD. It is characterized by granulation tissue plugs in the small airways, often extending into the alveolar ducts (Holland, 1988). The tissue in the upper airways remain normal. Granulomas can also plug the alveolar spaces secondary to the sicca syndrome seen in chronic GVHD (Ostrow et al., 1985). Clinically the patient rapidly develops shortness of breath, inspiratory rales, a nonproductive cough, and airway obstruction. The patient's CXR is usually normal except for mild hyperinflation. Unfortunately, the obstruction is irreversible, unresponsive to bronchodilators, mucolytic agents, or steroids, and it usually progresses to recurrent pneumothoraces and hypoxia and leads to death.

Bronchiolitis Obliterans Organizing Pneumonia

A new pulmonary syndrome, bronchiolitis obliterans organizing pneumonia (BOOP), has been reported in a number of BMT patients in the past few years. The term *BOOP* (also known as cryptogenic organizing pneumonia) has led to confusion because its first two words are identical to bronchiolitis obliterans, a completely different disease in terms of histopathology, clinical picture, and prognosis (Quabek, 1994). An increased incidence of BOOP has been identified in patients with chronic GVHD and those receiving matched, unrelated donor transplants or haploidentical transplants (Mathew et al., 1994). Additionally, several cases of BOOP have also been reported with the use of FK506 for GVHD prophylaxis (Fay et al., 1995)

Various immunological, toxic, or inflammatory insults to the lung may lead to the characteristic histopathological lesions associated with BOOP. These lesions consist of exudates with plugs of granulation and connective tissue in the distal airways extending into the alveoli

(Costabel and Guzman, 1991). Lymphocytes, plasma cells, and granulocytes can be identified in the center of the plugs. A small amount of interstitial inflammation and fibrosis are also present.

Bronchiolitis obliterans organizing pneumonia usually occurs 2 to 4 months post transplant. Patients with BOOP usually present with progressive dyspnea preceded by a flulike illness. PFTs show a restrictive defect. CXR or CT scan reveal patchy, predominantly peripheral infiltrates. In the majority of patients, this radiological pattern is clearly distinguishable from bronchopneumonia.

Treatment with high doses of corticosteroids and additional antimicrobial therapy according to BAL findings usually leads to rapid resolution of BOOP (Quabek, 1994).

Malignant Infiltration

With the increasing use of autologous BMT for malignancies involving the bone marrow, another theoretical source of pulmonary disease associated with transplantation is infiltration with malignant cells. Although bone marrow purging is frequent, the procedure may not be adequate to remove all malignant cells from the marrow. Although infrequent, this must be a part of the differential diagnosis in patients with diffuse pulmonary infiltrates after autologous BMT (Glorieux et al., 1986). Leukemic infiltration can also be associated with pulmonary compromise associated with fever.

Diffuse Alveolar and Pulmonary Hemorrhage

A syndrome of diffuse alveolar hemorrhage (DAH) has been reported in up to 21% of autologous BMT patients (Robbins et al., 1989). Robbins and colleagues inaugurated a BAL surveillance program in autologous BMT patients and reported DAH within the first few weeks post transplant. In contrast to secondary hemorrhage from infectious agents (such as *Aspergillus*), infectious agents could not be identified in these patients. The onset of DAH is frequently associated with severe oral mucositis, renal insufficiency, and bone marrow engraftment. Symptoms include progressive dyspnea, cough, hypoxemia, and diffuse consolidation on CXR. While hemoptysis is not observed, the BAL fluid in these patients is extremely bloody. Corticosteroids have shown some efficacy against DAL, however the mortality rate continues to be about 80% (Chao et al., 1991; Robbins et al., 1989).

The poor prognosis of DAH resembles findings of idiopathic pneumonia syndrome seen in the allogeneic setting. In a BAL surveillance program with allogeneic patients, DAH was an extremely rare finding (Quabek, 1994). On the basis of these findings, it can be assumed that conditioning toxicity is the main cause of DAH (Chao et al., 1991; Quabek, 1994; Robbins et al., 1989).

Occult pulmonary hemorrhage may evolve as a primary or secondary event in thrombocytopenic patients. Pulmonary hemorrhage can be a result of trauma or secondary to an underlying pulmonary process such as aspergillosis infection. It is important to note that any of these causes can be complicated by an underlying infection in this group of patients, particularly if the patient has undergone endotracheal intubation as part of overall pulmonary management (Rubin, 1988).

Miscellaneous Pulmonary Complications

A less common cause of lung disease associated with BMT is pulmonary embolism due to infusing fat particles and bone spicules from unfiltered bone marrow. This finding has been been detected at autopsy from patients who died from other causes, and their significance is uncertain.

An unusual cause of febrile pneumonitis syndrome is a leukoagglutinin reaction. This syndrome is characterized by the abrupt onset of fever, rigors, tachypnea, nonproductive cough, and respiratory distress within the first 24 hours following the transfusion of a blood product. The clinical picture stems from the interaction of preformed antibodies and antigen in the blood. These antibodies may be directed against the patient's leukocytes. These reactions are most commonly seen following granulocyte transfusions, and can best be avoided by using transfusions that are washed, packed, or frozen if possible.

Pulmonary veno-occlusive disease has also been documented (Hamilton et al., 1986; Shulman and Hinterberger, 1992; Wingard et al., 1989). This is probably an unusual response to high-dose chemotherapy and TBI. In addition, lung disease on the basis of preexisting liver disease is a reported phenomenon referred to as *hepatopulmonary syndrome* (Quabek, 1994). Some relationship between hepatic veno-occlusive disease (VOD) and the subsequent development of pulmonary complications has been described by several authors (Shulman and Hinterberger, 1992; Wingard et al., 1989). Although the nature of such pulmonary complications remain ill defined, it is obvious that an idiopathic pneumonia syndrome was one of the major causes.

Pulmonary thromboembolism is a rare event in BMT patients, but is most often related to thrombosis associated with central venous catheter (CVC). Air embolism is also very rare, but might also occur with improper handling of the CVC.

Pleural effusions may also develop secondary to infection, CHF, VOD, or pulmonary thromboembolism (Quabek, 1994). In patients with malignancies, pleural effusions as well as focal or multifocal alveolar infiltrates may mean pulmonary metastasis. If present pre-transplant, such effusions may resolve with the conditioning regimen.

Late effects of BMT on pulmonary function have been described in long-term survivors. Chronic conditions such as small airway disease, pulmonary fibrosis, and obstructive lung disease have been reported (Carlson et al., 1994; Chan et al., 1987; Clark et al., 1987; Clark et al., 1989; Kaplan et al., 1994). Frequently these alterations are associated with a history of GVHD and multiple pulmonary toxins.

NURSING DIAGNOSIS, PLANNING, AND INTERVENTION

It is obvious that all patients who undergo BMT or BCT are at risk for lethal pulmonary complications. The transplant nurse plays a key role in the prevention, detection, and treatment of patients who develop acute pulmonary complications. Pulmonary diseases are perhaps the most devastating of any that we deal with in this clinical setting.

Preventive Nursing Measures

An important preventive measure performed by the nurse is encouraging patients to exercise, despite their obvious decrease in activity level. This poses a great nursing challenge, especially for patients who are isolated in a laminar air flow (LAF) environment. Many transplant centers use a variety of exercise equipment such as exercise bikes and treadmills. Consultation with the physical therapist may also be of some benefit. These types of activities may also improve the patients' state of mind, and may increase their motivation to participate in their own care.

Good pulmonary toilet should also be encouraged. This can be accomplished in the form of coughing and deep breathing every 2 to 4 hours, as well as the use of incentive spirometry. These two techniques can aid in the prevention of atelectasis, and thus facilitate gas exchange as each alveolus is filled (Ellis and Nowlis, 1989). Caution should be taken with percussion and postural drainage; pulmonary trauma can occur secondary to thrombocytopenia in these patients.

Maintaining appropriate isolation to avoid infections from exogenous sources is vital to the well-being of the BMT patient. Isolation of the BMT patient from possible infection involves either minimal protection such as wearing masks, thorough washing of hands, and minimal contact with people, to very strict isolation through the use of laminar air flow isolation rooms. Successful transplants are performed in both settings (Hutchison and King, 1983). No one quite knows which isolation technique is optimal, and there is great disparity in isolation procedures among transplant centers (Wikle, 1991). The use of laminar air flow does decrease colonization of aspergillosis while the patient is hospitalized.

Finally, the nurse will be involved in the prophylactic use of many of the agents already mentioned. The nurse will continue to be involved in a variety of research protocols aimed at the prevention and treatment of IPn.

Nursing Assessment and Diagnosis of the BMT Patient with IPn

Continuous and astute nursing observation of the patient for alterations in respiratory function is an essential component of the patient's nursing care. The transplant patient should have his or her lungs auscultated at least every 8 hours because expeditious intervention is key to the patient's survival. Once impaired gas exchange develops, the patient's respiratory status should be assessed a minimum of every 4 hours.

Care of the Intubated BMT Patient with Adult Respiratory Distress Syndrome

There are several causes of adult respiratory distress syndrome (ARDS) in the BMT patient population including (1) septic shock, (2) infection of the lung and/or IPn, (3) exposure to toxins (i.e. chemotherapy/radiation therapy), and (4) immunologic reactions. ARDS is usually the terminal demise of the BMT patient with IPn, and is manifested by increased permeability of pulmonary capillaries to water and plasma proteins. Management of the patient with ARDS involves finding and treating the "cause" of the process, maintaining a Po_2 above 55 mmHg, and avoiding potentially fatal complications.

These patients frequently require endotracheal intubation and mechanical ventilation in order to maintain oxygenation. Maintenance of an adequate arterial Po_2 is accomplished by careful management of fluids and ventilator. A number of complicated ventilators are used in BMT/intensive care units to aid in sustaining respirations for the BMT patient with IPn. Most of these ventilators work on the principle of positive pressure to inflate the lungs, but can be set to meet the individual needs of a particular patient with regards to the rate and depth of respirations, as well as the concentration of oxygen needed to maintain the Po_2. Close assessment of the arterial blood gases allows constant assessment and readjustment of the ventilator. Frequently these patients require an invasive arterial pressure line, so that frequent blood gas measurements can be made.

Positive end-expiratory pressure (PEEP) has been demonstrated to improve the Po_2 in the patient with ARDS (Faber-Langendon, Caplan, McGlave, 1993; Spragg, 1980). Applied during continuous mechanical ventilation, or during intermittent mandatory ventilation with positive airway pressures (IMV/CPAP), PEEP may help decrease cardiac output by decreasing the venous return to the chest, thus leading to an increase in the pulmonary vascular resistance. BMT patients often require large amounts of PEEP and CPAP to maintain adequate oxygenation.

Because careful fluid management is so important if the treatment is to be a success, frequent measurement of the patient's cardiac output is required. This can be accomplished through the use a of a Swan-Ganz thermodilutional catheter. Because a physiologic consequence of IPn is a shunting of venous blood through the nonventilated areas of the lungs, the Swan-Ganz catheter allows measurement of the extent of this shunting. Measurement of the pulmonary artery wedge pressures and cardiac output is mandatory in many of these patients. An adequate cardiac output, along with a low pulmonary artery wedge pressure helps minimize the extravascular lung "water" that plagues these patients.

Unfortunately, despite all of the above-described efforts, mortality approaches 70% of BMT patients with IPn who are intubated and receive more than 50% oxygen for 24 hours or longer. Very often the patient quickly experiences multisystem organ failure. As more complications arise, so does the rate of mortality.

Faber-Langendon, Caplan, and McGlave (1993) of the University of Minnesota BMT group retrospectively evaluated all of their adult patients (N = 191) in a 13-year period who required mechanical ventilation. Of these, 84% died on the ventilator within hours of intubation; 10% survived 1 week after extubation, and 3% survived 6 months. Survival was not predicted by type of transplant, use of TBI in the conditioning regimen, or reason for intubation. The patient's age and timing of intubation were predictive of survival. Of patients older than 40 years, 98% died within 30 days. Similarly, of those intubated within the first 90 days of transplant, 94% died within 1 week of intubation. These authors conclude that mechanical ventilation is rarely effective in achieving long-term survival in adult BMT recipients. They go on to imply that, based on cost/benefit consideration and medical futility, an argument can be made to withhold mechanical ventilation in certain patient subsets apart from a clinical research trial (Faber-Langendon, Caplan, McGlave, 1993).

Regardless of such findings, clinicians caring for BMT patients often pursue mechanical ventilation for patients with respiratory compromise. Despite often heroic measures, ventilatory efforts are often futile. If a pneumonia develops, the patient and family need emotional support. Most transplant patients and families fear pneumonia and may express fears of impending death. Additionally, the family, patient, and transplant team may have to face the possibility of life-support mechanisms if the pneumonia progresses (Hutchison and King, 1983). At times patients are given the choice of less aggressive medical interventions if the causative agent(s) of the pulmonary compromise is found to carry a poor prognosis. The nurse plays a large role in working with the medical team to inform and support the patient and family in making this kind of decision. Living wills are sometimes used in this setting so that the patient can choose from the outset whether he or she wishes to be placed on mechanical life support.

This chapter would be remiss without mentioning the emotional impact that caring for the intubated BMT patient with ARDS has not only on the nurse caring for the patient, but on the entire nursing staff. The human resources required to manage one of these patients are tremendous and rarely successful. Support groups for the transplant staff are often warranted following the death of one of their patients.

CARDIAC COMPLICATIONS

Cardiac complications of BMT and BCT are not uncommon, but are rarely the cause of death in this patient population.

The overall incidence of cardiac complications with BMT and BCT is 25%. However, cardiac complications have been reported to occur in about 40% of autologous BMT patients, and account for about 10% of the deaths associated with autologous BMT (Baello et al., 1986; von Herbay et al., 1988). This incidence is most likely attributable to regimen-related toxicity, and the large amount of antineoplastic drugs these patients receive prior to transplantation. Therefore, all patients, especially those who have been heavily treated with anthracyclines or cyclophosphamide and/or radiation to the chest, must be carefully screened prior to their acceptance for transplantation (Cazin et al., 1986; Pihkala et al., 1994).

In high-risk cancers, bone marrow toxicity has been the most important factor that limits the use of adequate doses of chemotherapy and/or radiation therapy for curative treatment. The use of BMT in cancer therapy permits dose escalation with the promise of a cure in the treatment of leukemia, lymphomas, and a variety of solid tumors. However, toxic effects on other organs are now becoming manifest and may account for many of the cardiac complications seen in these patients (von Herbay et al., 1988). Table 11.5 lists factors that place the BMT patient at risk for cardiac complications.

Chemotherapy-Induced Cardiac Damage

The cardiotoxicity of adriamycin is known to occur at doses greater than 450 mg/m². Although infrequently used in pretransplant conditioning regimens, a large number of patients with solid tumors may have received a significant amount of adriamycin for induction and/or consolidation therapy. Another an-

TABLE 11.5 Risk factors for cardiac complications after BMT

1. History of previous anthracyclines
2. History of radiation to the chest
3. Total dose of cyclophosphamide > 150 mg/kg
4. Cyclophosphamide as pretransplant conditioning, especially if patient has had previous Ara-C or 6-TG
5. Cyclophosphamide and TBI as pretransplant conditioning
6. Sepsis
7. History of mitral valve disease
8. Pretransplant ejection fraction of < 50%
9. Diagnosis of Hurler syndrome or thalassemia

SOURCE: Wikle, 1991. Used with permission.

thracycline, daunorubicin, also can contribute to cardiac damage. Both of these agents have been correlated with cardiac failure in the BMT patient (von Herbay et al., 1988). Even if these drugs are not used in pretransplant conditioning regimens, history of their use may significantly increase the patient's risk of cardiac toxicity after BMT.

The heart damage caused by anthracyclines is from a loss of myocardial fibrils, mitochondrial changes, and cellular degeneration. Necrosis of the cardiac fibers is often seen on autopsy of these patients, along with necrosis of the contraction bands in the heart. Chronic changes such as fibrosis are also common. The cardiac damage associated with anthracyclines is, for the most part, irreversible. Cells termed *adria cells* are often seen in patients who receive large doses of adriamycin, and are characterized by a "clumping" of myocardial cell nuclei. These cells are often associated with severe cardiomyopathy.

Cardiac toxicity induced by anthracyclines may occur very early in the posttransplant period. This is most likely due to the pretransplant conditioning regimen, adding to the cardiac insult. The period of marrow aplasia also places the patient under extreme physical stress. Pulmonary edema may arise secondary to myocardial damage. Symptoms for which the nurse should observe are weight gain, peripheral edema, tachycardia, dyspnea with exertion, orthopnea, rales, and rhonchi. At the first indication of cardiac difficulty, the patient should have a cardiac ejection fraction measured to compare with the preadmission baseline study.

Unfortunately, if the chronic and progressive damage associated with anthracyclines has occurred, supportive measures are rarely successful. Precise fluid management, and the judicious use of diuretics, digitalis, and preload reduction agents, along with lowering the stress to the heart, presently seem to be the best approach.

Cardiac complications associated with cyclophosphamide have been well documented at the doses used in the transplant setting. Cyclophosphamide is an alklyating agent that has been shown to have both potent immunosuppressive properties and antineoplastic activity and is a mainstay in most pretransplant conditioning regimens. Most transplant centers use 50 to 60 mg/kg per day, with total pretransplant doses in the range of 120 mg to 200 mg. Cardiac complications rarely occur at doses below this. Cardiac damage may be worsened if the patient has received cardiotoxic drugs, TBI, high-dose Ara-C, or 6-thioguanine in the past.

Cyclophosphamide causes hemorrhagic myocardial necrosis, thickening of the left ventricular wall, sero-sanguinous pericardial effusions, and a fibrinous pericarditis. Autopsy results on these patients have shown many areas of myocardial necrosis along with fibrin microthrombi near the areas of capillary damage (Goldberg et al., 1986). These type of changes are usually seen at doses greater than 150 mg/kg, although damage has been reported at doses as low as 120 mg/kg (Levine, 1982).

Clinical signs of cyclophosphamide-induced cardiac damage are severe and occur 1 to 10 days following cyclophosphamide administration (Goldberg et al., 1986). Symptoms are those associated with pulmonary edema, cardiomegaly, poor peripheral perfusion, and systemic edema. Decreased voltage is noted on the patient's electrocardiograph (ECG). The presence of sepsis may worsen the patient's cardiac dysfunction (Goldberg et al., 1986). Symptoms may progress to hemorrhagic myocarditis, cardiac tamponade, and death. If symptoms occur prior to completion of the patient's course of cyclophosphamide, the drug may be stopped and replaced with some other chemotherapeutic agent, usually nitrogen mustard.

Like the toxicity suffered with anthracyclines, little can be done to treat cyclophosphamide-induced cardiac damage. Supportive care also involves astute fluid management and diuretics and digitalis. Pericardiocentesis and placement of a pericardioperitoneal window are sometimes performed on patients who suffer from pericardial effusions since cardiac tamponade is a threat with cyclophosphamide-induced cardiac damage.

Long-term follow-up of patients who received cyclophosphamide and TBI as conditioning agents has shown that about 23% of patients suffer a decrease in their resting ejection fraction (Baello et al., 1986). Thus, long-term cardiac surveillance of such patients is indicated post transplant because treatment is more effective if the patient has yet to become symptomatic.

It is important to note that children seem to have a lower incidence of cyclophosphamide induced cardiac damage. Because children have a relatively smaller ratio of weight to body surface area than do adults, children may actually receive less cyclophosphamide than adult patients. Also, obese patients are more likely to be overdosed when treated based on milligrams per kilograms. It is recommended that dosage for these patients be calculated on an ideal body weight.

Radiation-Induced Cardiac Damage

Cardiac complications of radiation therapy are well known. Lowered dose rates and fractionation of total body and/or total lymphoid irradiation (TLI) appear to lessen the cardiac toxicity in transplant patients. Thus, pure radiation-induced cardiotoxicity is unlikely (von Herbay et al., 1988). However, there does seem to be a synergistic effect between chemotherapy and radiation (Baello, 1986).

Transplant patients at highest risk for radiation-induced cardiac damage are those patients who have received radiation to the chest prior to the transplant conditioning regimen. Patients who have borderline cardiac function prior to transplant may have their hearts shielded for TBI in order to decrease their chances of suffering a fatal cardiac complication.

Cardiac irradiation has been associated with the development of pericardial effusions and constrictive pericarditis, which predisposes the patient to pulmonary edema. This toxicity may be triggered by the microvascular damage that is noted with cyclophosphamide (von Herbay et al., 1988). It is also possible that radiation therapy may have a synergistic effect with the hyperlipidemia that is caused by long-term corticosteroid therapy for GVHD (Chan et al., 1989). Supportive measures for radiation induced cardiac damage are the same as those for cyclophosphamide toxicity.

In conclusion, the cardiac damage seen with regimen-related toxicity has similar results, regardless of the causative factors. Although only fatal in about 10% of cases, little can be done to reverse the cardiac damage that results from high-dose chemotherapy and radiation therapy. Many patients suffer from mild and often undetected cardiac toxicity. If the toxicity progresses, the patient will suffer from oliguria and fluid retention refractory to diuretics, cardiomegaly with persistent pericardial effusions, a fall in blood pressure, worsening pulmonary edema, cardiac collapse, and death. Research directed at decreasing the toxicity of and improving conditioning regimens is currently being conducted so that cardiac and other serious complications will lessen the threat of morbidity and mortality in patients who undergo BMT.

Cardiac Infections

Despite patient's severe immunocompromised states, cardiac infections in BMT and BCT patients are rare, and therefore little is published regarding such infections. If they do occur, infections can affect the pericardium, endocardium, and myocardium. Among the most common causative organisms are *Candida albicans, Aspergillus, Pseudomonas, Clostridia, Streptococcus, Staphylococcus toxoplasmosis,* coxsackie virus, and adenovirus (Sale and Shulman, 1984). Noninfectious endocarditis rarely occurs in these patients, and is usually secondary to subclavian central venous lines.

Bacterial Infections

Rarely do bacterial infections disseminating from the gut of the BMT patient seed the heart (Sale and Schulman, 1984). These infections can cause microabscesses containing organisms such as *Pseudomonas* and *Clostridium. Streptococcus viridans,* an organism commonly found in the oral cavity can also cause endocarditis if the patient's heart valves are already damaged (Guzzetta, 1984). This makes the pretransplant dental exam very important. *Staphylococcus aureus* is a more virulent organism, and can attack normal heart valves.

The pathogenesis of acute infectious endocarditis is related to the presence of a bacteremia caused by a highly virulent organism.

Because 50% to 60% of acute infections occur in patients without previous cardiac valvular deformities, several theories have been formulated to explain why some types of bacteria affect normal heart valves. One explanation is that *S. aureus* and other gram-positive bacteria exhibit a unique property that permit them to adhere to the endothelial surface of the heart valve. It appears that only a few highly virulent organisms are necessary to establish the infection (Guzzetta, 1984). Infections forming on the heart valves produce endothelial lesions, referred to as *vegetations*. The organisms lie deep in the layers of these vegetations. This explains why patients who receive adequate intravenous

antimicrobial therapy can still experience progressive valvular infection (Wikle, 1990). Figure 11.3 shows infective endocarditis vegetations of the mitral valve.

Infective endocarditis often goes unnoticed in these patients. Clinical signs are fever, chills, cough, malaise, and headache. The patients temperature will normally range from 39.4°C to 40°C. The patient may already experience many of these symptoms soon after transplant. More specific symptoms include a new murmur, a pericardial friction rub, and symptoms of congestive heart failure. Positive blood cultures may also be present. The ECG may show conduction or rhythm disturbances or even myocardial ischemic changes. An echocardiogram may reveal vegetations on the patient's heart valves. The patient should also be monitored closely for symptoms of an embolus because these vegetations can break away from the valves into the circulating blood.

Empiric, broad-spectrum antibiotic therapy is especially important for prevention and early treatment of this complication since sepsis is most common the cause. Pulling of the central venous catheter may be necessary if bacterial seeding from the line is suspected. Intracardiac infections secondary to central venous catheters are rare, but should not be ruled out if the patient is symptomatic. Precise management of fluids is also essential. Patients who survive this complication may require a heart valve replacement sometime in the future.

Fungal Infections

The deep-seated and disseminated fungal infections that produce multiple fungal emboli to other organs often involve the heart as well, with *Candida albicans* and *Aspergillus* the most common organisms.

The predominant form of cardiac involvement with *Aspergillus* is pericarditis. Pathogenesis of the infection appears to include

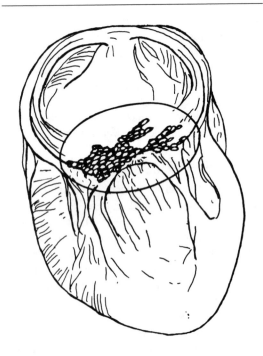

Figure 11.3 Infective endocarditis vegetations (*circle*) of the mitral valve

initial myocardial involvement with eventual spread to the pericardium. Spread to the heart appears to be by direct invasion from infected lung tissue adjacent to the heart, or by fungus in the circulating blood from involved pulmonary veins (Laszewski et al., 1988). Involvement of the endocardium is common in patients who have widespread aspergillosis since thromboemboli disseminate from the primary source. It is these fungal microemboli that can cause a myocardial infarction if they become lodged in the coronary arteries. Death from myocardial infarction secondary to *Aspergillus* embolization to the coronary arteries has also been reported in patients following BMT (Laszewski et al., 1988).

Symptoms of fungal endocarditis closely resemble those of bacterial endocarditis. In most cases of aspergillosis, there is some radiographic or clinical sign or symptom of a respiratory infection or pleuritis, even when the patient's blood cultures are negative. Spread to the heart by embolization may occur even if the patient has no signs of a primary pulmonary infection. The patient may simply complain of substernal chest pain that is refractory to pain medications. Further cardiac workup may a reveal an ECG with ischemic changes, an abnormal echocardiogram, and elevated cardiac isoenzymes. If the ischemia continues, the patient will most likely suffer from congestive heart failure and/or cardiac arrest, and die.

Fortunately, aspergillosis of the heart remains a rare complication of BMT. The difficulty in diagnosing aspergillosis prior to the patient's death is well recognized, as well as the importance of early detection so that appropriate treatment and possible cure can occur. For these reasons, the empiric use of antifungal therapy (i.e., amphotericin B) has been widely advocated for the immunosuppressed BMT patient who remains febrile and symptomatic despite antibacterial therapy. Supportive measures also include precise fluid management,

digitalis if needed, judicious use of diuretics, and nitroglycerin for relief of chest pain.

There are increasing numbers of case reports of fungal infections affecting the endocardium, myocardium, and pericardium of patients post BMT. This suggests that disseminated aspergillosis or candidiasis needs to be included in the differential diagnosis of chest pain and ECG changes in the immunocompromised BMT patient for early detection and successful treatment to be possible.

Viral Infections

Viral infections of the heart are rare and not well documented in the literature. The viruses most frequently documented are the coxsackie virus and adenovirus. Although CMV infections frequently occur in allogeneic patients, rarely does this virus affect the heart. Viruses, when they do occur, generally attack the myocardium, sometimes causing irreversible myocardial damage. Because viral infections are difficult to detect, they are often mistaken for drug and/or radiation toxicity (Sale and Schulman, 1984). Symptoms are due to decreased myocardial contractibility, diminished cardiac output, and secondary pulmonary edema. Supportive measures are the same as described previously. Little can be offered in the way of antiviral therapy, especially since most viral infections of the heart go undetected.

Graft-versus-Host Disease and Cardiac Damage

Evidence for GVHD affecting the heart is conflicting. Several case reports describe an acute inflammatory endocarditis strongly associated with the occurrence of severe, acute GVHD (Kupari et al., 1990). Animal studies have shown chronic inflammation involving the valves and, in rare instances, the myocardium and the coronary arteries. Most recent autopsy studies of GVHD have shown that myocardial abnormalities were present in about half of the animals, but consisted only of interstitial edema and sparse lymphocyte infiltration (Sale and Schulman, 1984). The relationship of cardiac problems and GVHD in humans remains controversial. Concentric intimal sclerosis of the major coronary arteries has been seen in some BMT patients with chronic GVHD. These changes are most likely due to the same processes that cause scleroderma and other connective-tissue changes in patients with chronic GVHD. However, it is unclear whether these changes are due to a viral infection or to late, toxic effects of the pretransplant conditioning regimen. However, there is anecdotal evidence that chronic GVHD may be associated with coronary atherosclerosis. Whether this is due to the GVHD itself or to the hyperlipidemia caused by high-dose corticosteroid therapy is unclear (Chan et al., 1989).

Cardiac Toxicity Associated with Infusion of Cryopreserved Cells

Several studies have reported cardiac toxicity associated with the infusion of cryopreserved bone marrow and peripheral blood stem cells (Davis et al., 1990; Keung et al., 1994; Lopez-Jimenez et al., 1994). There are several possible causes for the development of such toxicity. These include acute volume expansion leading to reflex slowing of the heart rate, electrolyte imbalance, vagal responses to the coldness of freshly thawed infusate, reaction to the DMSO, and cell lysis products.

Lopez-Jimenez and colleagues (1994) found that 82% of 17 patients who received autologous bone marrow infusion developed cardiac arrhythmia, of which 65% (11) developed sinus bradycardia, 24% (4) second-degree heart block, and 1 patient experienced a complete heart block. The onset of bradycardia occurred 15 to 513 (median 56) minutes following the start of the infusion. Heart block was seen 30 to 680 (median 234) minutes after starting the infusion. Hypertension was also noted in 41% of patients and usually occurred 2 hours after the infusion. Of note however, is the fact that none of these clinical findings were associated with clinical symptoms or mortality. However, death following autologous marrow infusion has been reported (Davis et al., 1990; Rapoport et al., 1991).

Lopez-Jimenez and colleagues (1994) prospectively evaluated 29 patients receiving stem cell infusion. Fifteen allogeneic BMT patients were used as a control for their study. Patients were evaluated, using a Holter monitor, 2 hours prior to infusion and 24 hours following completion. They found no significant differences in cardiovascular parameters between the two groups; however, the patients who had blood cell infusion were found to have an increased number of ventricular and atrial ectopic beats as well as a higher rate of hypertension post infusion.

Cardiac Tamponade

Acute cardiac tamponade without concurrent cardiac disease has been noted in about 2% of patients undergoing allogeneic BMT for thalasssemia (Angelucci et al., 1994; Saunders et al., 1993). In such cases patients experience tachycardia and pleuritic-type chest pain or may go on to develop sudden cardiac decompensation with hypotension. Treatment includes removal of the pericardial fluid and hemodynamic support.

Late Effects on Cardiac Function

Little is reported in the BMT literature regarding the long-term effects of BMT on cardiac function. However several reports have emerged describing asymptomatic cardiac abnormalities in 15% to 25% of long-term pediatric and adult BMT survivors (Carlson et al., 1994; Pihkala et al., 1994). Such effects include subclinical disturbances in cardiac function at rest and with exercise, diminished left ventricular function, and QRS voltage changes. Although late cardiotoxicity seems to be subclinical, long-term cardiac follow-up may be warranted.

NURSING THE TRANSPLANT PATIENT WITH CARDIAC COMPLICATIONS

Keen assessment and identification of BMT candidates at risk for cardiac complications should be included in the patient's nursing history prior to initiating the patient's pretransplant conditioning regimen. Close attention is given to risk factors. It is essential for the transplant team to know what chemotherapy and radiation therapy the patient has received. Pretransplant baseline studies should include a cardiac ejection fraction and a 12-lead ECG. Auscultation of the patient's heart and lungs should be performed upon admission, and at least every 8 hours throughout the patient's transplant hospitalization.

Twelve-lead electrocardiograms are suggested prior to the administration of cyclophosphamide and anthracyclines if these drugs are a part of the patient's pretransplant conditioning. Some centers monitor the patient via bedside cardiac monitors throughout the patient's course of cyclophosphamide and for 24 hours following its completion. A follow-up 12-lead ECG should also be done 7 days after cyclophosphamide administration (Hutchison and King, 1983). If ECG changes occur, the physician should be notified. Weighing the patient twice a day on the days the patient receives cyclophosphamide is also a frequent practice.

Nursing assessment for murmurs, friction rubs, and breath sounds are key in the early detection of infective endocarditis. Comfort measure for fever management, appropriate antibiotic administration, and balancing rest with activity are also important. Frequent assessment for signs of cardiac tamponade include tachycardia, pleuritic-type chest pain, and distended neck veins; a positive pulsus paradoxus should also be included in the BMT nurse's assessment. Detection of these symptoms should result in prompt medical intervention. The nurse should prepare the patient to undergo pericardiocentesis if cardiac tamponade should occur.

For the patient with cardiac-induced pulmonary edema and or congestive heart failure, the primary nursing focus should be on maintaining oxygenation and resolution or reduction of edema. These patients may require endotracheal intubation and the use of CPAP/PEEP, or may simply need a small amount of oxygen delivered by nasal cannula. It is important to stress the patient's heart as little as possible. Rest periods between procedures can be helpful. Strict intake and output, close monitoring of the patient's electrolytes, administering diuretics as ordered, and weighing the patient at least daily are essential in managing the patient's fluid balance. Transplant patients have a tendency to become overloaded with fluids due to the excessive amounts of blood products and medications they receive. It is important to administer the patient's fluid medications in as small a volume as possible.

For patients in congestive heart failure, frequent skin care and evaluation is needed, especially if the patients have excessive peripheral edema. If a patient is on digitalis therapy, the nurse should monitor the patient's drug levels and watch for signs of digitalis toxicity. These symptoms include, nausea, anorexia, headache, bigeminy and ectopic beats, confusion, and a pulse deficit. These symptoms should be reported as soon as possible to the physician.

It is important to note that cardiac complications are infrequently seen in the BMT patient population, thus cardiology consultants can be extremely helpful in the overall management of these patients. Currently, potential cardiac toxicity is one of the most limiting factors for BMT. It has therefore been suggested that transplantation be done as early as possible so that patients will not have to receive pretransplant excessive doses of cardiotoxic drugs that further increase their risk of serious cardiac complications.

REFERENCES

Andersson, B.S., Luna, M.A., Yee, C., et al. 1989. Fatal pulmonary failure complicating high-dose cytosine arabinoside therapy in acute leukemia. *Cancer 65:* 1079-1084.

Angelucci, E., Mariotti, E., Lucarelli, G. 1994. Cardiac tamponade in thalassemia. *BMT 13:827-829.*

Atkinson, J.B., Connor, D.H., Robinowitz, M., et al. 1984. Cardiac fungal infections: review of autopsy findings in 60 patients. *Hum Pathol 15:935-942.*

Bacigalupo, A., van Lint, M.T., Tedone, E., et al. 1994. Early treatment of CMV infection in allogeneic bone marrow transplant recipients with foscarnet or ganciclovir. *BMT 13:753-758.*

Baello, E.B., Ensberg, M.E., Ferguson, O.W., et al. 1986. Effect of high-dose cyclophosphamide and total body irradiation on left ventricular function in adult patients with leukemia undergoing allogeneic bone marrow transplantation. *Canc Treat Rep 70(10):1187-1193.*

Barrett, A., Depledge, M.H., Powles, R.L. 1983. Interstitial pneumonitis following bone marrow transplantation after low dose rate total body irradiation. *Intern J Radiat Oncol 9:1029-1033.*

Bearman, S.I., et al. 1988. Regimen-related toxicity in patients undergoing bone marrow transplantation. *J Clin Oncol 6(10):1562-1568.*

Bortin, M.M. 1983. Pathogenesis of interstitial pneumonitis following allogeneic bone marrow transplantation for acute leukemia. In Gale, R.P. (Ed.) *Recent Advances in Bone Marrow Transplantation.* New York: A.R. Liss, 445-460.

Bortin, M.M., et al. 1982. Factors associated with interstitial pneumonitis after bone marrow transplantation. *Lancet 1:437.*

Brown, N.J., Potter, D., Gress, J., et al. 1990. A randomized trial of open lung biopsy versus empiric antimicrobial therapy in cancer patients with diffuse pulmonary infiltrates. *J Clin Oncol 8(2):222-229.*

Buja, L.M., Ferrans, V.J., Graw, R.G., Blitt, C.D. 1976. Cardiac pathologic findings in patients treated with bone marrow transplantation. *Hum Pathol 7:15-45.*

Cardozo, B.L. 1985. Interstitial pneumonitis following bone marrow transplantation: pathogenesis and therapeutic considerations. *Eur J Canc Clin Oncol 21:43-47.*

Carlson, K., Smedmyr, B., Backlund, L., Simonsson, B. 1994. Subclinical disturbances in cardiac function at rest and in gas exchange during exercise are common findings after autologous bone marrow transplantation. *BMT 14:949-954.*

Carlson, K., Backlund, L., Smedmyr, G., Simonsson, B. 1994. Pulmonary function and complication subsequent to autologous bone marrow transplantation. *BMT 14:* 805-811.

Cazin, B., Gorin, N.C., Laporte, J.P., et al. 1986. Cardiac complications after bone marrow transplantation. *Cancer 57:2061-2069.*

Chan, C.K., Hyland, R.H., Hutchenon, M.A., et al. 1987. Small-airways disease in recipients of allogeneic bone marrow transplants. *N Engl J Med 66(5):327-340.*

Chan, K.W., Taylor, G.P., Shephard, J.D., Shephard, W.E. 1989. Coronary artery disease following bone marrow transplantation. *BMT 4:327-330.*

Chao, N.J., Duncan S.R., Long, G.D., Horning, S.J., Blume, K.G. 1991. Corticosteroid therapy for diffuse alveolar hemorrhage in autologous bone marrow transplant recipients. *Ann Intern Med 114(2):145-146.*

Chien, J., Chan, C.K., Chamberlain, D., et al. 1990. Cytomegalovirus pneumonia in bone marrow transplantation: an immunopathological process? *Chest 98:* 1034-1037.

Clark, J.G., Crawford, S.W., Madtes, D.K., et al. 1989. Obstructive lung disease after allogeneic marrow transplantation. *Ann Intern Med 111:368-376.*

Clark, J.G., Schwartz, D.A., Flourney, N., et al. 1987. Risk factors for airflow obstruction in recipients of bone marrow transplants. *Ann Intern Med 107:648-656.*

Corso, S., Vukelja, S.J., Wiener, D., Baker, W.J. 1993. Diffuse alveolar hemorrhage following autologous bone marrow infusion. *BMT 12:301-303.*

Costabel, U., Guzman, J. 1991. BOOP: what is old, what is new? *Eur J Resp Dis 4:771-773.*

Davis, J.M., Rowley, S.D., Braine, H.G., et al. 1990. Clinical toxicity of cryopreserved bone marrow graft infusion. *Blood 75:781-786.*

Daniele, R.P., Elias, J.A., Rossman, M.D. 1985. Bronchoalveolar lavage: role in the pathogenesis, diagnosis, and management of interstitial lung disease. *Ann Intern Med 102(1):93-108.*

Down, J.D., Mauch, P., Warhol, M., et al. 1992. The effects of donor T lymphocytes and total body irradiation on hemopoietic engraftment and pulmonary toxicity following experimental allogeneic bone marrow transplantation. *Transplantation* 54(5):802-808.

Ellis, J.R., Nowlis, E.A. (Eds.) 1989. Supporting oxygenation. *Nursing: A Human Needs Approach*. Boston: Houghton Mifflin, 788-797.

Emanuel, D., Cunningham, I., Jules-Elysee, K., et al. Cytomegalovirus pneumonia after bone marrow transplantation successfully treated with the combination of ganciclovir and high-dose intravenous immune globulin. *Ann Intern Med* 109(10):777-782.

Englund, J.A., Sullivan, C.J., Jordan, M.C., et al. 1988. Respiratory syncytial virus infection in immunocompromised adults. *Ann Intern Med* 8:203-208.

Faber-Langendon, K., Caplan, A.L., McGlave, P.B. 1993. Survival of adult bone marrow transplant patients receiving mechanical ventilation: a case for restricted use. *BMT* 12:501-507.

Fay, J.W., Nash, R.A., Wingard, J.R., et al. 1995. FK506-based immunosuppression for prevention of graft versus host disease after unrelated donor marrow transplantation. *Transplant Proc* 27(1):1374.

Foot, A.B.M., Garin, Y.J.F., Ribaud, P., et al. 1994. Prophylaxis of toxoplasmosis infection with pyrimethamine/sulfadoxine (Fansidar) in bone marrow transplant recipients. *BMT* 14:241-245.

Fort, J.A., Graham-Pole, J. 1989. Pulmonary complication of bone marrow transplantation. In Johnson, F.L., Pochedlym, C. (Eds.) *Bone Marrow Transplantation in Children*, New York: Raven, 397-406.

Ginsberg, S.J., Comis, R.L. 1982. The pulmonary toxicity of antineoplaastic agents. *Semin Oncol* 9(1):34-51.

Girard, P.M., Landman, R., Gaudebout, C., et al. 1993. Dapsone-pyrimethamine compared with aerosolized pentamidine as primary prophylaxis against *Pneumocystis carinii* pneumonia and toxoplasmosis in HIV infection. *N Engl J Med* 328(21):1514-1520.

Glorieux, P., et al. 1986. Metastatic interstitial pneumonitis after autologous bone marrow transplantation: a consequence of reinjection of malignant cells. *Cancer* 58(9):2136-2139.

Goldberg, M.A., Antin, J.H., Guinan, E.C., and Rappeport, J.M. 1986. Cyclophosphamide cardiotoxicity: an analysis of dosing as a risk factor. *Blood* 68(5): 1114-1118.

Goodrich, J.M., Bowden, R.A., Fisher, L. 1993. Ganciclovir prophylaxis to prevent cytomegalovirus disease after allogeneic marrow transplant. *Ann Intern Med* 118(3): 173-178.

Granena, A., Carreras, E., Rozman, C., et al. 1993. Interstitial pneumonitis after BMT: 15 years experience at a single institution. *BMT* 13:453-458.

Gross, S.J. 1982. The pulmonary toxicity of antineoplastic agents. *Semin Oncol* 9(1):34-51.

Gross, N.J. 1977. Pulmonary effects of radiation therapy. *Ann Intern Med* 86:81-92.

Guzetta, C.E. 1984. The person with infective endocarditis. In Guzetta, C., Dorsey, B.M. (Eds.) *Cardiovascular Nursing: Body Mind Tapestry*. St. Louis: Mosby, 661-691.

Hamilton, P.J., et al. 1986. Bone marrow transplantation and the lung. *Thorax* 41(7):497-502.

Hartsell, W.F., Czyzewski, E.A., Ghalie, R., Kaizer, H. 1995. Pulmonary complication of bone marrow transplanation: a comparison of total body irradiation and cyclophosphamide to busulfan and cyclophosphamide. *Int J Radiat Oncol* 32(1):69-73.

Holland, H.K., Wingard, J.R., Beschornor, W.E., et al. 1988. Bronchiolitis obliterans in bone marrow transplantation and its relationship to chronic graft versus host disease and low serum IgG. *Blood* 72(2):621-627.

Hughes, W., Leoung, G., Kramer, F., et al. 1993. Comparison of atovaquone (566c80) with trimethoprim-sulfamethoxazole to treat *Pneumocystis carinii* pneumonia in patients with AIDS. *N Engl J Med* 328(21): 1521-1527.

Hutchison, M., King, A., 1983. A nursing perspective on bone marrow transplantation. *Nurs Clin North Am* 18 (3):511-520.

Jules-Elysee, K., Whie, D.A. 1990. Bleomycin-induced pulmonary toxicity. *Clin Chest Med* 11(1):1-20.

Kaplan, E.B., Wodell, R.A., Wilmott, R.W., et al. 1994. Late effects of bone marrow transplantation on pulmonary function in children. *BMT* 14:613-621.

Keung, Y.K., Lau, S., Elkayan, U., et al. 1994. Cardiac arrhythmia after infusion of cryopreserved stem cells. *BMT* 14:363-367.

Krowka, M.J., Rosenow, E.C., Hoagland, H.C. 1985. Pulmonary complications of bone marrow transplantation. *Chest* 87(2):237-246.

Kupari, M., Volin, L., Timonen, T., et al. 1990. Cardiac involvement on bone marrow transplantation: electrocardiographic changes, arrhythmias, heart failure, and autopsy findings. *BMT* 5:91-98.

Laszewski, M., Trigg, M., de Alarcon, P., Giller, R. 1988. Aspergillus coronary embolization causing acute myocardial infarction. *BMT* 3:229-233.

Levine, A.S. 1982. *Cancer in the Young*. New York: Masson, 735-737.

Limper, A.H., MacDonald, J.A. 1990. Delayed pulmonary fibrosis after nitrourea therapy. *N Engl J Med* 323 (6):407-409.

Link, H., et al. 1986. Lung function changes after allogeneic bone marrow transplantation. *Thorax* 41(7): 508-512.

Ljungman, P., Biron, P., Bosi, A., et al. 1994. Cytomegalovirus interstitial pneumonia in autologous bone marrow transplant recipients. *BMT* 13:209-212.

Lopez-Jimenez, J., Cervero, C., Munoz, A., et al. 1994. Cardiovascular toxicities related to the infusion of cryopreserved graft: results of a controlled study. *BMT* 13: 789-793.

Lum, L.G. 1987. The kinetics of immune reconstitution after human marrow transplantation. *Blood* 69(2):369.

Mathew, P., Bozeman, R.A., Brenner, M.K., Heslop, H.E. 1994. Bronchiolitis obliterans organizing pneumonia (BOOP) in children after allogeneic bone marrow transplantation. *BMT* 13:221-223.

Meyers, J.D., Flourney, N., Thomas, E.D. 1982. Nonbacterial pneumonia after allogeneic marrow transplantation: a review of ten years' experience. *Rev Infect Dis* 4:1119-1132.

Meyers, J.D., Flournoy, N., Wade, J.C., et al. 1983. Biology of interstitial pneumonia after marrow transplantation. In Gale, R.P. (Ed.) *Recent Advances in Bone Marrow Transplantation*. New York: A.R. Liss, 406-421.

Michel, G., Thuret, I., Chambost, H. 1994. Lung toxoplasmosis after HLA mismatched bone marrow transplantation. *BMT* 14:455-457.

Minow, R.A., Benjamin, R.S., Lee E.T., Gottlieb, J.A. 1977. Adriamycin cardiomyopathy: risk factors. *Cancer* 39:1397-1402.

Montaner, J.S.G., Lawson, L.M., Levitt, N., et al. 1990. Corticosteroids prevent early deterioration in patients with moderately severe *Pneumocystis carinii* pneumonia. *Ann Intern Med* 113:14-20.

Morrison, V.A., McGlave, P.B. 1993. Mucormycosis in the BMT population. *BMT* 11:383-388.

Ostrow, D., Buskard, N., Hill, R.S., et al. 1985. Bronchiolitis obliterans complication after bone marrow transplantation. *Chest* 87(6):828-830.

Paulin, T., et al. 1987. Variables predicting bacterial and fungal infections after allogeneic marrow engraftment. *Transplantation* 48(8):393-398.

Pecego, R., Hill, R., Appelbaum, F.R., et al. 1986. Interstitial pneumontis following autologous bone marrow transplantation. *Transplantation* 42(5):515-517.

Pihkala, U.M., Saarien, U., Lundstron, M., et al. 1994. Effects of bone marrow transplantation on myocardial function in children. *BMT* 13:149-155.

Quabeck, K. 1994. The lung as a critical organ in marrow transplantation. *BMT* 14:519-528.

Rapoport, A.P., Rowe, J.M., Packman, C.H., Ginsberg, S.J. (1991). Cardiac arrest after autologous marrow infusion. *BMT* 7:401-405.

Reusser, P. 1991. Cytomegalovirus infection and disease after bone marrow transplantation: epidemiology, prevention, and treatment. *BMT* 7(suppl 3): 52-56.

Robbins, R.A., Linaer, J., Stahl, M.G., et al. 1989. Diffuse alveolar hemorrhage in autologous bone marrow transplant recipients. *Am J Med* 87(5):511-518.

Rubin, R. 1988. Pneumonia in the immunocompromised host. In Fishman, A.P. (Ed.) *Pulmonary Diseases and Disorders*. New York: McGraw-Hill, 1745-1760.

Sale, G.E., Shulman, H.M. 1984. *The Pathology of Bone Marrow Transplantation*. Chicago: Masson, 193-194.

Saugier-Verber, P., Devergies, A., Sulahian, Al., et al. 1993. Epidemiology and diagnosis of invasive pulmonary aspergillosis in bone marrow transplant patients: results of a 5 year retrospective study. *BMT* 12:121-124.

Saunders, E.F., Olivieri, N., Freedman, N.H. 1993. Unexpected complication after bone marrow transplantation in transfusion-dependent children. *BMT* 12(suppl 1):88-90.

Schneider, M.E., Hopelman, A.I., Karel, J., et al. 1992. A controlled trial of aerosolized pentamidine or trimethoprim-sulfamethoxazole as primary prophylaxis against *Pneumocystis carinii* pneumonia in patients with human immunodeficiency virus infection. *N Engl J Med* 327:1836-1840.

Shelhamer, J.H., Toews, G.B., Masur, H., et al. 1992. Respiratory diseases in the immunosuppressed patient. *Ann Intern Med* 117(5):415-431.

Shulman, H.M., Hinterberger, W. 1992. Hepatic veno-occlusive disease: liver toxicity syndrome after bone marrow transplantation. *BMT* 10:197-214.

Spragg, R.G. 1980. Adult respiratory distress syndrome. In Bordow, R.A., Stool, E.W., Moser, K.M. (Eds.) *Manual of Clinical Problems in Pulmonary Medicine*. Boston: Little, Brown, 252-253.

Tait, R.C., Burnett, A.K., Robertson, A.G., et al. 1990. Subclinical pulmonary function defects following autologous and allogeneic bone marrow transplantation: relationship to total body irradiation and graft-versus-host disease. *Intern J Radiat Oncol* 20:1219-1227.

von Herbay, A., Dorken, B., Mall, G., Korbling, M. 1988. Cardiac damage in autologous bone marrow transplant patients: an autopsy study. *Klinische Wochenschrift* 66:1175-1181.

Weiner, R.S., Bortin, M.M., Gale, R.P., et al. 1986. Interstitial pneumonitis after bone marrow transplantation: assessment of risk factors. *Ann Intern Med 104*(2): 168-175.

Weiss, B.R., et al. 1980. Cytotoxic drug-induced pulmonary disease: update 1980. *Am J Med 68*:259-266.

Wendt, C.H., Weisdorf, D.J., Jordan, M.C., et al. 1992. Parainfluenza virus respiratory infection after bone marrow transplantation. *N Engl J Med 326*(14):921-926.

Wikle, T.J. 1991. Pulomnary and cardiac complication of bone marrow transplantation. In M. Whedon (Ed.) *Bone Marrow Transplantation: Principles, Practice, and Nursing Insights.* Boston: Jones & Bartlett, 182-205.

Wingard, J.R., Mellits, E.D., Jones, R.J., et al. 1989. Interstitial pneumonitis following autologous bone marrow transplantation. *Transplantation 46*(1):61-65.

Wingard, J.R., Melltis, E.D., Sostrin, M.B., et al. 1988. Interstitial pneumonitis after allogeneic bone marrow transplantation. *N Engl J Med 67*(3):175-186.

Wingard, J.R., Sostrin, M.B., Vriesendorp, H.M., et al. 1988. Association of hepatic veno-occlusive disease with interstitial pneumonitis in bone marrow transplant recipients. *BMT 4*:685-689.

Winston, D.J., Winston, G.H., Champlin, R.E., Gale, R.P. 1983. Treatment and prevention of interstitial pneumonia associated with bone marrow transplantation. In Gale, R.P. (Ed.) *Recent Advances in Bone Marrow Transplantation.* New York: A.R. Liss, 425-444.

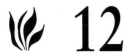

12

Renal and Hepatic Effects

Bruce Ballard, Karin Mitchell

The kidneys and liver are organs vital to the body's homeostasis. Complications of the renal and hepatic systems from high-dose radiochemotherapy and stem cell transplantation cause interrelated disruptions in this homeostasis and present unique challenges to the nurse managing a transplant patient.

RENAL FAILURE

Renal insufficiency is a significant complication of blood cell and bone marrow transplant. *Renal insufficiency* is a doubling of the baseline creatinine and occurs in approximately 40% of transplant patients early in the course of treatment (Zager, 1994). *Acute renal failure* (ARF) is a sudden onset of oliguria (<500 ml urine in 24 hours or ≤ 0.5 ml/kg per hr) (Price, 1994). ARF occurs in approximately 50% of patients with renal insufficiency primarily due to circulatory problems, drug-induced toxicities, and infection (Deeg et al., 1988; Zager, 1994). Renal insufficiency is a dynamic pathological process and exists on a continuum ranging from mild to severe. Although most cases are mild, the problem is still of consequence because it can compromise administration of optimal therapies required for the transplant patient. Even a subtle decrease in renal function can herald a more complicated clinical course

involving renal failure, fluid and electrolyte imbalance, and multiorgan failure.

Impact of Renal Insufficiency and Failure in Transplant

Renal compromise can create a great impact on the care and treatment of the transplant patient. For the patient receiving allogeneic bone marrow transplant (BMT), treatment of graft-versus-host disease (GVHD) may be impaired due to the need to decrease or withhold cyclosporin or FK506. Other drugs, such as methotrexate, antibiotics, and biological response modifiers, depend in part on adequate renal function for the best therapeutic response. Any alteration in the ability to use these agents to their full measure is challenging and could compromise the long-term health of the patient.

Renal compromise can cause or exacerbate other complications as well. Pulmonary compromise from fluid overload, cardiac compromise from excess fluid or renal hypertension, neurological symptoms from increased circulating waste products, and electrolyte imbalances, which can lead to seizures or the organ malfunction, all contribute to the morbidity and mortality of this patient population. Clinicians often wrestle with the paradox of striving to optimize their patient's renal function, while continuing therapies that impair renal function.

There is an art to this management, and astute, proactive nursing practice is a vital component of that art.

When renal failure is combined with other organ compromise, long-term survival is significantly impacted. A review of data in Seattle at the Fred Hutchinson Cancer Research Center found that when a patient had a creatinine greater than 2 and a total bilirubin greater than 4, long-term survival (defined as greater than 30 days post hospitalization) was only 2%. This sobering statistic emphasizes the need for excellent assessment and early intervention for all patients at risk for renal insufficiency and failure.

Basic renal function can be summarized as the attempt to maintain homeostasis in body water and electrolytes, and to distribute them within the body's various fluid compartments. The renal regulation of acid-base balance and hormonal functions are but some of these actions. The clearance of the metabolic waste products of cellular metabolism and the removal of therapeutic drugs are the body's attempt to maintain balance. Each of these is accomplished by altering the composition of the blood (Goodinson, 1994).

RENAL PHYSIOLOGY

Normal kidney function requires four processes to be carried on continuously by the nephrons: (1) creation of an ultrafiltrate of whole blood; (2) absorption of electrolytes, bicarbonate, glucose, and essential amino acids; (3) secretion of electrolytes, medications, and other waste products; and (4) excretion of the urine (Price, 1994) (see Figure 12.1).

The first step is filtration, which occurs at the glomerulus and Bowman's capsule of each nephron. Renal arterial blood branches down into the capillary tuft of the glomerulus. Filtering in this section occurs based on molecular size, as substances small enough move through the porous capillary walls. Blood cells, plasma proteins, and any substances bound to protein are not normally cleared by this filtration. Water, electrolytes, blood urea nitrogen (BUN), and creatinine filter easily and become part of the filtrate that moves out of the glomerulus and into the space surrounded by Bowman's capsule. The rate at which this filtrate is produced is the glomerular filtration rate (GFR), normally about 100 ml per minute in the adult. All fluid and materials not filtered at the glomerulus are passed downstream into the network of capillaries that surround the renal tubules.

From Bowman's capsule, the filtrate solution travels to the renal tubules. The purpose of the proximal and distal tubules and/or the collecting duct of the nephron is to modify the filtrate by absorption and secretion (Price, 1994). The inner lumen of each tubule is lined with epithelial cells, which perform these functions. As the filtrate passes through the renal tubules, materials and water are reabsorbed into the blood stream via the capillaries surrounding the tubules. At the same time, secretion is occurring, with the transport of the substances from the capillaries into the lumen of the tubule. Additionally, aldosterone, antidiuretic hormone, and the prostaglandins have specific functions to assist in the control of total body fluids, electrolytes, and vascular pressures (Price, 1994).

The collecting tubules continue the processes of absorption and secretion and pass the urine to the ureters, bladder, and urethra for excretion. Average urine output is 2 ml to 3 ml per minute. A decrease in urine output is one of the first signs of renal compromise. Absorption and secretion are active processes that substantially alter the character and composition of the urine. These activities provide the body with the proper balance of water, electrolytes, and acid-base balance.

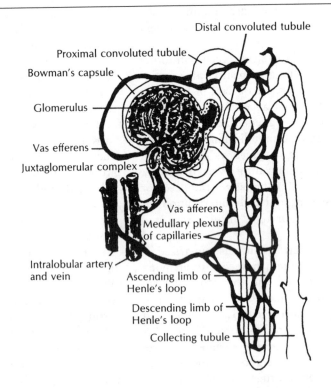

Figure 12.1
Illustration of the nephron and its associated blood supply

Sᴏᴜʀᴄᴇ: From Schottelius, B.A., Schottelius, D.D. 1973. *Textbook of Physiology, ed. 17.* St. Louis: C.V. Mosby Co. Used with permission.

Determinants of Renal Function

For the kidneys to fulfill their function, they must be able to perform each of the processes outlined above. If any determinant of renal function is impaired, renal insufficiency results (see Table 12.1). Good renal perfusion is necessary to allow enough blood to reach the glomerulus with enough force to allow filtration to occur. An adequate number of tubular epithelial cells and a tubular lumen free from obstructive debris must be present for secretion and absorption. For excretion to occur, the postrenal structures of the ureters and bladder must be patent and unobstructed.

TABLE 12.1 Determinants of renal function

Renal perfusion—filtration
  Intravascular volume
  Cardiac output
  Renal vasculature

Tubular function—secretion, absorption
  Tubular epithelial cells
  Tubular lumen

Postrenal structure—excretion
  Ureters
  Bladder
  Urethra

ACUTE RENAL FAILURE

Acute renal failure is generally classed into three types based on the etiology of the failure (Stark, 1988c). The first is termed *prerenal*. Prerenal failure has as its etiology inadequate glomerular filtration due to inadequate delivery of blood to the nephron or lack of the proper pressure differential across the capillary wall. The causes generally are not in the nephron itself but previous to it. These include clinical states common in transplantation such as hypovolemia, congestive heart failure, and septic shock.

Intrarenal failure originates at the level of the nephron. Clogged or damaged tubules or a toxic injury to the tubular epithelial cells can prevent the functions of absorption, secretion, and at times filtration. Nephrotoxicity secondary to aminoglycosides is a prime example.

Postrenal failure originates below the level of the kidney. If postrenal structures are obstructed, several processes ensue that hinder tubular filtrate processing, and renal failure is the result. Tumor masses may be a factor in this type of renal failure.

Etiology in the Transplant Patient

Renal insufficiency in the transplant patient can arise from any of the types of renal failure discussed above (see Table 12.2). Considering the clinical problems that predominate in this population, it is not surprising that the majority of renal problems have prerenal and intrarenal etiologies (Zager et al., 1989). Disruption of a normal fluid distribution in the body's compartments is a common problem, as are exaggerated sensible and insensible losses from the body. Also, nephrotoxic drugs (antibiotics and cyclosporin) are common therapy for these patients, predisposing them to acute tubular necrosis, an intrarenal class of renal failure.

Other intrarenal problems possible for this group are syndromes secondary to massive cell

TABLE 12.2 Etiology of renal failure in BMT patients

PRERENAL CONDITIONS

Hypovolemia
Dehydration
Third-spaced fluid
VOD
Hemorrhage

Impaired Circulation of Blood Volume
Septic shock
Congestive heart failure
Cardiotoxic effects

Renal Vascular Constriction
Pressor drugs

INTRARENAL CONDITIONS

Acute Tubular Necrosis
Nephrotoxic drugs
Prolonged ischemia

Tumor Lysis Syndrome
Massive tumor lysis

Postrenal Obstruction
Hemorrhagic cystitis

SOURCE: Adapted from Ford, R., Ballard, B., 1988. Used with permission.

lysis such as tumor lysis syndrome, rhabdomyolysis, and hemolysis from administration of blood components or reinfusion of autologous marrow or blood stem cells (Smith et al., 1987). Each of these problems involves the obstruction of renal tubules by the products of the cell lysis particular to them (Hou and Cohen, 1985).

PRERENAL FAILURE

The most common type of renal insufficiency seen in the patient who receives high-dose therapy is prerenal failure (Zager et al., 1989). The etiology of the prerenal state is usually multifactorial and complex to assess and diagnose. As a rule, it arises from one of the following:

hypovolemia, impaired circulation of blood volume, or vascular constriction that alters renal blood flow. It is not uncommon for several processes to coexist.

Hypovolemia

Hypovolemia results from dehydration, when body losses are greater than intake. Common etiologies of hypovolemia in this population are fever, diuresis, gastrointestinal losses from severe mucositis, diarrhea, or hemorrhage. Another cause of hypovolemia is "third spacing" of fluid. This is the shift of fluid from the vascular system to other body compartments that occurs commonly with the problems of septic shock, capillary leak syndrome, and veno-occlusive disease.

Impaired Circulation of Blood Volume

A prerenal failure can arise from impaired circulation of blood, even if an adequate volume exists. This is a common problem in septic shock resulting from profound neutropenia, where the mean arterial pressure is too low for adequate perfusion of the nephron. Congestive heart failure, which can result from myocardiotoxic drugs, is another situation in which the blood volume is more than adequate, but the ability of the heart to pump enough of it to perfuse the kidneys is impaired.

Renal Vascular Constriction

Last, during acute crises, transplant patients may be on pressor doses of drugs such as dopamine, so that the vasoconstriction of the renal arteries restricts the flow of blood to the nephron. Renal artery vasoconstriction is also seen to a lesser but significant degree with other drugs such as cyclosporin and amphotericin, both commonly administered to this group of patients. The commonality among these problems is an insufficient blood volume delivered

to the nephron or filtered at the glomerulus. Without adequate GFR, the blood-altering work of the kidney cannot be accomplished.

Determining the etiology of prerenal problems is the key to appropriate intervention. Prerenal problems are generally reversible by correcting the underlying cause of the prerenal failure. In contrast, intrarenal problems exacerbated by a profound or prolonged prerenal state result in a more severe course, both in recovery time and in the restriction of therapies necessary for these patients.

Syndrome of Inappropriate Anti-Diuretic Hormone

Although not a type of renal failure, syndrome of inappropriate anti-diuretic hormone (SIADH) is addressed here due to its common occurrence with administration of high-dose cyclophosphamide and its implications for fluid management. A transitory release of antidiuretic hormone is common during cyclophosphamide therapy. Fluid retention at this time of vigorous hydration therapy requires frequent and measured doses of furosemide or other diuretics. Careful evaluation of patients' weight gains, intake and output, and evaluation of pulmonary compromise is required. Overdiuresis is possible, giving a prerenal vascular depletion state.

ACUTE TUBULAR NECROSIS

Acute tubular necrosis (ATN) is the most common type of intrarenal failure seen in the transplant patient. ATN is caused by damage in or destruction of the renal tubules. If the insult is limited to the tubular epithelial cell layer, without damage to the underlying tissues, recovery is possible in time. Generally, the epithelial cell layer regenerates and begins functioning sufficiently in 1 to 5 weeks to carry on the demands placed on it.

Etiology of ATN in the Transplant Patient

In the transplant population, the most common cause of ATN is the use of nephrotoxic drugs. These include amphotericin B, cyclosporin, cisplatin, aminoglycosides, and acyclovir (Cooper et al., 1993; Deeg et al., 1988; Yee et al., 1985). Each of these drugs damages the tubular cells and/or tends to crystallize in a concentrated filtrate and deposit in the tissues. The tubular lumens become clogged due to the debris of tubular cell destruction and the swelling of the tubular wall caused by the insulting agent. Filtrate cannot pass through the tubule. With no movement of filtrate, GFR is reduced or stopped. Even if the debris is cleared by the healing process, it takes time for new tubular cells to become established and functional. Until this occurs, the renal functions of absorption and secretion cannot take place, necessitating therapies such as hemodialysis.

A second cause of ATN is an ischemic insult to the tubule. Since the oxygen supply to the renal tissue is the same that supplies the glomerulus, if impairment of the blood supply is profound and prolonged, renal tissues become anoxic. Severe anoxia may cause a necrosis of nephrons and their associated vasculature. The transplant patient commonly experiences fever and is often on steroidal drugs, both of which increase metabolism and, therefore, oxygen demand. Increased oxygen demand at a time of decreased supply predisposes tissue to anoxic insult. It the anoxic insult is severe, chances of recovering renal function are severely reduced.

Phases of ATN

Acute tubular necrosis has three phases: oliguric, diuretic, and recovery (Stark, 1988c).

During the oliguric phase, little if any urine is produced because the tubules are generally clogged by the edematous epithelial cell lining and debris from cell destruction. During the diuretic phase, dilute urine is increasingly produced as a result of the clearance of the tubular lumen. This clearance allows GFR to occur at a time of impaired tubular function. Concentration of the filtrate is a function of the tubules and collection ducts. Until they are functioning properly, filtration proceeds without the required reabsorption of water. This explains why the quantity of urine may seem sufficient while the quality is poor. Epithelial cells are also required for the task of secretion, which is vital for the clearance of metabolic waste products and the removal of metabolized drugs. The last phase of ATN, recovery, is characterized by the ability of the nephron to concentrate the filtrate via absorption and to clear waste products and drugs out of the blood via secretion.

Within this classification for the phases of ATN, there is variability in both timing and severity of each phase. It is not unusual for the oliguric phase to be absent. This is common for cases of ATN caused by nephrotoxic drugs. Nonoliguric ATN is often called *high output renal failure* due to the typical clinical picture of profuse urine volume at a time of poor waste product clearance (Dixon and Anderson, 1985).

RADIATION NEPHRITIS

A syndrome of late (3 to 13 months post transplant) radiation nephritis that may result from radiation damage has become evident in recent years. A clinical and pathological process affecting the kidneys has been characterized by increased serum creatinine, BUN, and GFR, along with anemia and hypertension. (Lawton et al., 1992; Lonnerholm et al., 1991; Guinan et al., 1988). The multiagent conditioning regimens combined with total body irradiation (TBI) in these patients are suspected as possible synergizers of the radiation effects to the kidneys resulting in this clinical syndrome. Lawton (1992) found that partial renal shielding reduced the incidence of late nephropathy.

ACUTE HEMOLYTIC REACTION

Rapid-onset acute renal failure has occurred following infusion of autologous marrow or peripheral blood stem cells. Investigation of this problem has centered on both the condition of the patient at the time of reinfusion and on the marrow processing and storage materials (DMSO) (Smith et al., 1987). Much is still unclear about this situation but management is similar to other forms of hemolysis. Administration of mannitol during and after the cell reinfusion, coupled with preinfusion hydration seems to prevent most of these occurrences.

The nurse should be alert for signs of hemolytic reactions by testing the urine for blood. If there is a sudden onset of hematuria and significant change in urine volume in the hours after reinfusion, prompt action must be taken. If hemolysis is determined, rapid hydration and the use of mannitol are necessary to allow the movement of hemoglobin through the renal tubules and out of the body.

In summary, the following characteristics of renal failure are common after bone marrow or blood cell transplant. Renal failure is generally acute in nature. On resolution of the problems that produced the renal insufficiency, kidney function should recover. Mild impairment is common, especially that of prerenal failure etiology. ATN is the most common type of intrarenal failure and is often of the nonoliguric type. It is most common for insufficiency to occur in the first 3 weeks after transplant, yet it can occur at any time.

NURSING ASSESSMENT OF RENAL FUNCTION

Renal insufficiency rarely exists in isolation from other clinical problems. It tends to arise at a time of multiorgan failure. If renal insufficiency is the only major clinical problem, it is generally easy to support the patient through its course. Unfortunately, this is seldom the case.

Renal insufficiency is not usually a primary toxicity to the high-dose therapy. Figure 12.2 illustrates the interrelationships of some of the toxicities and shows that the major problem in keeping the kidneys functioning properly is keeping the other organs at optimum performance. Lines from each of the toxicities may be drawn to factors that affect some element of renal function discussed here. It is the task of the nurse to understand the implications of each and to use the appropriate assessment tools to assist in the management of the patient whose renal system is impaired.

The nursing assessment (see Table 12.3) of the renal patient includes five areas:

1. blood chemistries, which help determine the fluid and electrolyte balance, the level of vital organ functions, and the acid-base balance;
2. urine assessment, which helps determine the level of renal tubular function and/or damage;
3. fluid balance assessment, which determines the compartmental distribution of fluid in the body;
4. phamacologic agents, to examine the contributors to renal dysfunction, mental status changes, and renal system demands; and
5. mental status assessment, which elucidates neurological effects of renal impairment.

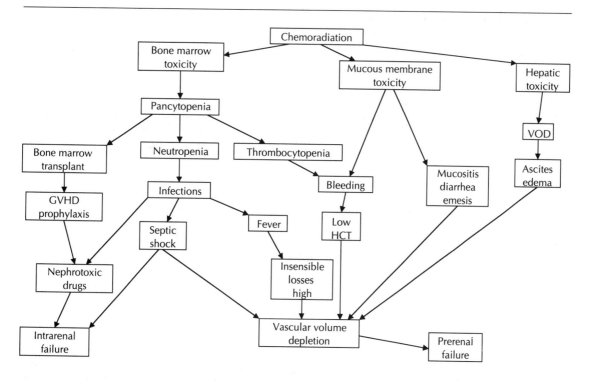

Figure 12.2 **Interrelationships of posttransplant patient problems and potential contributors to renal failure**

Blood Chemistries

Assessment of serum sodium helps calculate the patient's free water balance. Appropriate therapy of fluid quantity and quality is based on this calculation.

Assessment of serum CO_2 helps estimate the acid-base balance and determine the existence of the anion gap. If the CO_2 is low, it indicates a metabolic acidosis. If the calculated anion gap is high, it can indicate sepsis, ketoacidosis, or uremia. An acidosis without a significant anion gap is indicative of a renal tubular acidosis (RTA). This is common in patients re-

ceiving cyclosporin or amphotericin B, and is easily treatable.

Assessment of potassium is important. In renal insufficiency, hyperkalemia would be expected, but in the marrow transplant patient receiving cyclosporin or amphotericin B, potassium wasting in the urine is common. Potassium wasting results in hypokalemia, which often requires aggressive intravenous potassium replacement.

Serum blood urea nitrogen is a complex value to interpret for these patients. Because the rate of BUN production is a function of several factors, not the least of which is the

TABLE 12.3 Differential findings in acute renal failure

Test	Prerenal findings	Intrarenal findings typical to ATN
Urine		
Specific gravity	>1.015	≤ 1.010
Sodium	< 10 to 20 mEq/l	> 20 to 40 mEq/l
Sediment	MOD hyaline and finely granular casts	Dirty brown granular casts and epithelial cells
Volume output	Oliguria and anuria	Nonoliguria most common, but oliguria or anuria possible, especially if also prerenal
Blood		
BUN	Increased	Increased
Creatinine	Increased	Increased
Potassium	Increased or normal	Oliguric phase: increased
BUN/creatinine	>10/1	<10/1
Physical Exam		
Blood pressure	Low BP, often with orthostatic drop in SBP and > in HR	Varies with volume
Neck veins	Flat	Varies with volume

patient's metabolic rate, the levels may be elevated with even a slight decrease in GFR. The addition of steroids to the patient's drug profile or the presence of blood in the GI tract can significantly increase the production of BUN without any significant alteration in kidney function.

Serum creatinine is a better gauge of kidney function than is BUN. It can indicate a change in GFR, yet is not diagnostic of the etiology of the renal insufficiency.

The first important aspect of serum creatinine and BUN is the baseline measurement for that patient compared with the degree and rate of change from the baseline. A doubling of any given creatinine level means a 50% decline in renal functioning. This is an important concept. Consider the patient whose creatinine on the previous day was 1.2 mg/dl. If the morning creatinine rises to 1.5 mg/dl, the response is different than if that same patient had a creatinine the day before of 0.7 mg/dl. In the first case, we note a moderate increase in creatinine and continue to monitor the patient accordingly. In the second case, we realize that in the past 24 hours there has been a loss of more than half of the patient's renal function and a quick complete assessment and change in therapy may be needed. This follow-up should be directed at collecting information necessary to determine whether the etiology of the renal insufficiency is prerenal or intrarenal. Urine studies help in this regard.

Urine Assessment

Volume

Examination of the urine's quantity and quality indicates the adequacy of renal tubular function and the type of renal insufficiency. Assessment should include the measurement of urine volume for a single shift plus the previous 24-hour period. A decrease in this volume along with an increase in serum creatinine suggests renal insufficiency. However, other assessments are needed to determine a prerenal or intrarenal etiology of the failure.

Specific Gravity

Since the tubular functions of secretion and absorption alter the filtrate character, abnormal values can be expected for urine electrolytes and specific gravity (Stark, 1988b). Values typical of particular types of renal failure may be found. Also, urine sediment, determined by urinalysis, can be diagnostic of tubular damage.

A healthy tubule has the ability to concentrate urine if it senses inadequate intravascular volume. It does this by reabsorbing filtered water into the capillaries surrounding the tubules and creating a concentrated urine. Typically, the specific gravity is greater than 1.020. If the tubules have been sufficiently damaged, as in ATN, this ability is lost and the urine's specific gravity tends to be similar to that of the blood it filters. The specific gravity of blood is about 1.010.

As an example, consider how one might distinguish between a prerenal condition or intrarenal damage in the patient whose urine volume is decreased and the morning serum creatinine is elevated. A routine specific gravity measurement in the high range indicates that the tubules are working well and a prerenal condition would be suspected. We know this because it takes the tubular function of absorption to accomplish this state. A damaged tubule cannot concentrate urine.

Urine Sodium

In a prerenal state, the kidneys attempt to increase blood volume by resorbing sodium as well as water. This tends to deplete the tubular filtrate of sodium, yielding a low urine sodium, typically less than 20 mEq/liter. If the tubules are damaged, as in ATN, resorption of sodium is less efficient and urine sodium levels are high,

typically greater than 50 mEq/liter (Espinel and Gregory, 1980; Lam and Kaufman, 1985).

The kidneys may inaccurately sense an intravascular depletion. Sensors in the kidneys measure pressure and flow but the kidneys are unable to tell whether the low renal blood flow is a result of true volume depletion from decreased cardiac output, as in congestive heart failure, or from vasoconstrictive drugs that are restricting renal arterial blood flow. The urine sodium and specific gravity may indicate what the kidney senses is happening as well as the status of the renal tubules, but more information is necessary to complete the clinical picture. The determination of fluid distribution is helpful in this regard.

Urine Sediment

Urine casts are also diagnostic of tubular damage. If large amounts of renal tubular cell casts are passed out of the tubules, they can be seen in the urine under microscopic examination.

Fluid Balance

Fluid balance should be considered from two perspectives—the total body fluid and the distribution of that fluid in the body. Change in total body fluid is easily determined from changes in the patient's weight. For example, an overnight change in body weight is not a change in the amount of muscle or fat; it is a change in the amount of fluid in the body. Explanations for changes in weight may be found in the intake and output records and by taking into consideration insensible losses, which may be profuse in a febrile patient. Other less obvious factors causing a disturbance in fluid balance may be depletion due to the decreased intake when mucositis is present or loss due to a high volume of emesis. These are significant factors in the early posttransplant period.

Each of these assessments helps explain the amount of, or changes in, body fluid. They do not describe how that fluid is distributed in the body. From the kidneys' standpoint, it is vital to determine whether the intravascular volume is sufficient. This determination guides therapy to prevent or reverse prerenal failure and re-establish homeostasis. It may be that the replacement of an adequate blood volume is the quickest and easiest intervention for the patient. Physical assessment is key in this evaluation.

Significant depletion of the patient's intravascular volume produces significant orthostatic changes in blood pressure and heart rate. Even a patient who spends a major portion of the day in bed should be able to compensate for postural changes in vital signs within 60 to 90 seconds. Measurement of orthostatic vital signs is significant in confirming a prerenal state due to hypovolemia. A finding of significant postural changes in blood pressure and heart rate, in addition to the other findings discussed in this chapter, is generally definitive of hypovolemia, without the need for invasive monitoring.

The level of intravascular fluid can be determined by assessing the presence of distended neck veins when the patient is in Trendelenburg's position, and by a cardiac exam listening for signs of fluid overload. Pulmonary edema as a result of fluid overload may be manifested as rales in the lungs, or if severe, by frothy sputum, respiratory distress, signs of fluid on the chest X ray, or a drop in oxygen saturation. Each of these signs supports the case that fluid has left the vascular space and gone to the interstitial spaces in the lungs.

The bone marrow transplant patient, especially one who has veno-occlusive disease (discussed later), can sequester enormous amounts of fluid in the abdominal cavity, which will result in engorged organs and, at times, ascites (McDonald et al., 1986). Changes in abdominal girth and sudden weight gain indicate fluid that is not available for renal perfusion. An increase in abdominal girth without a concomitant rise in weight usually indicates a decrease in intravascular volume.

Pharmacological Considerations

Impaired renal function can be a result of drugs. In turn, the drugs we give can be affected by impaired renal function. If a change in renal function is noted, it is important to look at the patient's drug profile and make appropriate adjustments. The adjustments are aimed at preventing toxic side effects of drugs that will be poorly excreted (Bennett, 1988).

Assessment of the drug profile may also disclose a potential etiology of the renal insufficiency. If diuretics were aggressively used around the time of onset of renal insufficiency, assessment for signs of hypovolemia should occur. An elevation in BUN may reflect the increased metabolic rate seen with steroids. High-dose vasopressors such as dopamine constrict the renal arteries, causing a prerenal condition. Not all offending medications can be stopped. Some may be necessary to sustain life, but due to the presence of renal insufficiency, adjustments in drugs or doses to avoid compounding the problem may be required.

Mental Status

The patient suffering severe renal impairment often exhibits changes in mental status that must be monitored. BUN and other waste products can build up in the blood and cause uremic encephalopathy. Nonrenal etiologies for changes of mental status are common, so other causes must also be evaluated. For instance, since the kidneys metabolize many drugs, a review of the drug profile may reveal the source of mental changes. This may be true for some drugs even if the kidney is not the major site of that drug's metabolism. Many narcotics are metabolized by the liver, yet the metabolites are cleared by the kidney. It is often the case, especially if both renal and hepatic function are impaired, that the metabolites cause the changes in mental status.

MANAGEMENT OF RENAL INSUFFICIENCY

The management of renal insufficiency in the bone marrow or blood cell transplant patient requires a multidisciplinary approach that involves at least the nurse, doctor, pharmacist, and nutritionist. The goal of management is to improve or maintain renal function while allowing the other organs to function properly.

Assessment

The first step in this management is assessment. Proper diagnosis directs proper treatment. The concepts and actions discussed above give the physician the information necessary to establish the proper treatment. The nurse is often first to have the information because the nursing assessment involves the collection of weight, intake and output, abdominal girth, postural blood pressure and heart rate, lung exam, urine specific gravity, and the other indices vital to therapeutic decisions.

Correcting Vascular Volume Disequilibrium

The next management step involves the correction of any vascular volume disequilibrium. This may require diuretics or volume replacement. Whether replacement takes the form of crystalloid or colloid is determined by concurrent problems and the unique needs of the patient.

Correcting Electrolyte Imbalance

Along with this intravascular volume correction comes the correction of electrolyte imbalances.

This involves the correction of free water excess or deficit and adjustment of electrolytes in the intravenous fluids to match calculated losses and correction of any deficit of excess.

Minimizing Nephrotoxins

Adjustment or removal of nephrotoxic drugs must be attempted. This is often easier said than done in this population, given the requirements for such essential drugs as amphotericin B and cyclosporin. The decision to reduce or to maintain such therapy is based on the unique needs of the patient.

Treating Infections

To manage the renal problems that often arise in the transplant patient, infections must be adequately treated. This may seem to contradict the previous paragraph. Yet the most severely malfunctioning kidneys are those of the patient suffering septic shock and receiving pressor doses of dopamine.

HEMORRHAGIC CYSTITIS

Incidence

Hemorrhagic cystitis (HC) is reported to occur in up to 50% of BMT patients (Sencer et al., 1993; Efros et al., 1994; Miyamura et al., 1989). It is frequently a primary toxicity from the high-dose regimen due mainly to the use of cyclophosphamide. Fortunately, it is usually preventable and/or responsive to conservative treatment.

Etiology

The etiology of HC is twofold, depending on its time of occurrence. Early HC, within 48 hours of cyclophosphamide administration is felt to result from acrolein, a metabolite of cyclophosphamide that is toxic to the transitional epithelium of the bladder mucosal tissue. Small vessels in the underlying tissue hemorrhage into the bladder (Champlin and Gale, 1984; Sale and Shulman, 1984).

Later development of HC up to several months post transplant is felt to involve a super-imposed infectious agent. HC associated with papovavirus, adenovirus, cytomegalovirus, and bacteria are common in this late onset group (Miyamura et al., 1989; Sencer et al., 1993).

Presentation and Clinical Course

Hemorrhagic cystitis may present immediately with the administration of cyclophosphamide or be delayed, sometimes for months after the cyclophosphamide course. It is most commonly seen at the time of cyclophosphamide admini-stration and presents as hematuria with or without blood clots. It may also present as dy-suria or frequency. HC is generally responsive to the treatment measures instituted and re-solves within 1 or 2 days of the end of the cyclophosphamide (Champlin and Gale, 1984).

In its severe form, larger and more deeply invasive ulcerations extend into the vascular tis-sue underlying the bladder mucosa (Sale and Shulman, 1984). Bleeding may develop into a severe life-threatening problem. Also, because the blood often clots in the bladder, painful obstruction of bladder outflow may result.

Prevention

The prevention of HC involves measures to de-crease the toxicity of the metabolite. Three-way irrigation catheters are placed and 100 to 500 ml/hr of fluid continuously irrigates the bladder from the start of cyclophosphamide until at least 24 hours after the last dose or until the urine shows no evidence of blood. The goal of this intervention is to dilute and remove as fast as possible the toxic substance from contact

with the sensitive bladder tissue (Turkeri et al., 1995; Meisenberg et al., 1994).

Another preventive measure is the use of aggressive intravenous hydration with fluids at twice the usual maintenance rate (Meisenberg et al., 1994). This aggressive hydration causes a rapid and dilute filtrate to pass through the ureters, thus preventing prolonged contact of the metabolite with epithelium. Vigorous hy-dration requires monitoring of the patient's fluid. It is common for the patient to develop either an overhydrated state or, if diuretics are used to force diuresis, a prerenal state. Meas-ures discussed in the previous section of this chapter are useful in determining the appropri-ate therapies for the patient situation.

The use of drugs to prevent HC is becom-ing more common. Mesna is an example of a drug that binds acrolein to form a nontoxic compound and prevent damage (Vose et al., 1993; Shepherd et al., 1991). With the preva-lence of outpatient chemotherapy, mesna is often used as a replacement to continuous blad-der irrigation.

Treatment

Since mesna acts at the time of the cyclophos-phamide administration, there is no benefit for its use once HC has occurred. Treatment of HC involves many of the same therapies used for prevention. Continuous bladder irrigation at 500 ml to 2 liters per hour is generally sufficient to clear developing clots and prevent obstruc-tion. Infusing platelets to maintain high platelet levels is also very important. At times, cys-toscopy is required, and cautery of bleeding ulcerative areas may be attempted. Unfortu-nately this is usually not a long-term solution due to the diffuse, widespread pathology asso-ciated with the problem. The instillation of chemicals, such as mucomyst, into the bladder is also used and may benefit the patient.

VENO-OCCLUSIVE DISEASE OF THE LIVER

Veno-occlusive disease (VOD) of the liver is the most common liver problem that arises after bone marrow transplant and has serious potential effects on the patient. It is intimately involved with the disruption of normal renal function and the fluid and electrolyte balance of the patient. VOD is a distinct disease involving the blood vessels of the liver. This disease has a specific syndrome that manifests clinically with great variation in severity, affects several other organ systems, requires close attention, and alters the clinical management of the patient. In addition, it is associated with significant mortality.

Veno-occlusive disease is a complex topic and is confusing to many. Part of the reason for this is that VOD means different things to different people. To the pathologist looking at liver tissue through the microscope, VOD is distinct and specific damage to liver tissue. To the clinician, it may be the condition of a patient who is jaundiced, encephalopathic, with a distended abdomen, experiencing complex fluid and electrolyte problems. Both views are correct. Both are VOD. The pathologist looks at the cause of the clinical syndrome that nurses observe clinically.

Incidence and Risk Factors

The incidence of VOD in the BMT population is reported between 5% and 54%. This variation is due to the variability of the populations studied, the variability of diagnostic criteria, and the differing intensity of conditioning therapies (Bearman, 1995; Grandt 1989; Deeg et al., 1988; McDonald et al., 1985; Ford et al., 1983). Many incidence studies predate the current use of higher toxicity conditioning regimens. Because of this, the incidence may in-

crease as conditioning becomes more intense in attempts to prevent the recurrence of disease.

Known factors predispose a patient to VOD:

- Pretransplant liver enzyme elevation
- Fever during cytoreductive therapy
- Higher intensity cytoreductive therapy
- Mismatched or unrelated donor
- Previous radiation therapy to the abdomen

The most significant risk factor is the presence of liver abnormalities at the time of conditioning therapy. Whether the cause of abnormalities is viral hepatitis, tumor infiltrates, or infections, the finding of an elevated bilirubin and/or liver enzymes predicts an increased risk for VOD. This is such a significant finding that, if at all possible, transplant is postponed until liver function tests return to normal. Of the other risk factors for developing VOD, a higher intensity of the conditioning regimen, and the presence of infection anywhere in the body, are the most significant (McDonald et al., 1993; McDonald et al., 1984; Jones et al., 1987).

The desire to minimize risk, if possible, before proceeding with transplant results from the significant morbidity and mortality associated with the disease. About half of the patients with VOD recover. The other half with VOD die. In those who have VOD at death, VOD is the direct cause of death in the majority (McDonald et al., 1985; Jones et al., 1987).

Although the clinical symptoms of VOD arise in the time period shown in Figure 12.3, the liver insult actually occurs well before the clinical symptoms.

Etiology of VOD

The etiology of VOD is high-dose chemotherapy and radiation. Interestingly, using a single conditioning agent generally does not bring on the disease. Yet given in combination, there

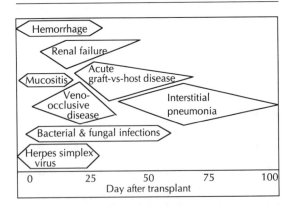

Figure 12.3 Time of occurrence of acute complications after bone marrow transplantation

SOURCE: From Ford and Ballard, 1988, with permission.

seems to be a synergistic effect producing hepatic damage well beyond that produced by any single agent (McDonald et al., 1986). Inflammatory cytokines seem to play a role in the development and severity of the disease (McDonald et al., 1993). The findings that the higher the number of febrile days during conditioning therapy results in an increased finding of severe VOD, suggests that inflammatory cytokines participate in the liver damage caused by cytoreductive therapy (Bearman, 1995).

Onset and Resolution

Veno-occlusive disease clinically appears at any time after the start of conditioning, with its peak onset in the second week after transplant. Recovery occurs about 3 weeks after the onset of jaundice (McDonald et al., 1985).

Pathophysiology

Veno-occlusive disease is a disease of the small blood vessels in the liver. It is characterized by an occlusion in the venous outflow tract of the liver, hence its name. The clinical syndrome is a logical extension of the pathophysiological changes that occur.

Normal Hepatic Physiology

Normal hepatic blood flow comes from two major courses: the majority from the portal vein, which emerges from the spleen and intestines, and most of the rest from the hepatic artery, which supplies oxygenated blood to the hepatic tissues. The blood flows down into smaller and smaller vessels and eventually into the hepatic sinuses (see Figure 12.4). The sinuses are thin-walled vessels of endothelial tissue that empty into a central collecting vein. These sinuses are lined by hepatocytes, the cells most involved in processing products in the blood as they pass through the sinuses on a path toward the venules. Blood flows out of the liver then moves from these sinusoids into central veins, which lead to larger hepatic venules and eventually into the vena cava (Kaldor, 1988).

Hepatic Venule Occlusion

The two areas of hepatic injury from VOD are the hepatic venules and the hepatocytes that line the sinusoids. As the hepatocytes metabolize and process the chemotherapeutic agents passing through the liver, the by-products, which tend to be toxic, are dumped into these small vessels. The endothelial linings of the sinuses and hepatic veins are damaged by the toxicity of these metabolites. The eventual result is impaired blood flow through the sinuses secondary to obstruction (Storek et al., 1993; McDonald et al., 1993; McDonald et al., 1986).

First, the tissue is swollen from the chemo/radiation insult. Released cytokines, like tumor necrosis factor-alpha, may result in hypercoagulabillity followed by perivascular deposition of coagulation factors with gradual

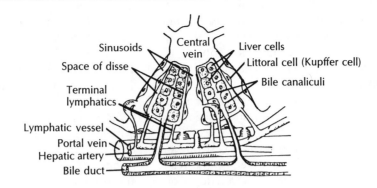

Figure 12.4
Basic structure of a liver lobule

Labels in figure: Sinusoids, Space of disse, Terminal lymphatics, Lymphatic vessel, Portal vein, Hepatic artery, Bile duct, Central vein, Liver cells, Littoral cell (Kupffer cell), Bile canaliculi

SOURCE: Reprinted from Guyton, 1986, *Textbook of Medical Physiology.* Philadelphia: W.B. Saunders, with permission.

occlusion of the vessels (Storek et al., 1993; Shulman and Hinterberger, 1992). Fibrin is deposited in the injured area in an attempt to stabilize the area. This fibrin presents an impediment to the passage of cellular debris and exfoliated hepatocytes that have died from the conditioning toxicities. The process becomes self-perpetuating as the blood flow becomes impaired and the tissue is deprived of the oxygen necessary to support the tissue. Pressure and fluid backs up into, and previous to, the sinusoids. The entire liver becomes engorged as venous outflow becomes more and more occluded. Anoxia leads to further injury and necrosis of hepatic tissue with the result that hepatic blood flow and function is even more impaired. It is from this occluded flow that all the resultant clinical problems stem (McDonald et al., 1986).

Consequences of Impaired Hepatic Blood Flow

Impaired hepatic blood flow has several consequences, summarized in Table 12.4. The liver becomes swollen. As the pressure in the hepatic vasculature exceeds its ability to keep the fluid inside the capillary bed, sodium and protein-

TABLE 12.4 Consequences of impaired hepatic blood flow and function

Pathology	Clinical symptoms/ results
Hepatic, spleenic and GI mucosal congestion	Abdominal distention, pain, respiratory comprise, third-spaced fluid
Accumulation of ascites	Abdominal distention, intravascular volume loss
Sodium/water retention by renal tubules	Total body fluid gain, edema
Serum proteins weep off liver into peritoneum	Hypoalbuminemia, edema, ascites
Ischemia, hepatocyte death, tissue necrosis	Elevated liver enzymes, impaired hepatic functions
Impaired bilirubin handling	Jaundice
Altered drug metabolism	Increased serum levels Narcotics, CSA, MTX
Impaired handling of metabolic waste production	Hepatic encephalopathy
Poor synthetic functions	Coagulopathy

rich fluid drip off the surface of the liver into the peritoneal cavity. In many patients this fluid is absorbed by the lymphatic system at the rate it is produced. If it becomes too profuse, this compensatory maneuver is inadequate, and ascitic fluid accumulates.

Restricted blood flow through the liver also causes pressure in the portal system, engorging the mucosal vessels of the small intestine. A further consequence of poor flow is strong reabsorption of sodium and water by the renal tubules (Cade et al., 1987; McDonald et al., 1985).

Each of these conditions presents its own set of problems, yet the primary effect is to shunt the vital blood away from the liver. This consequence has the most serious implications because the shunting of blood, if severe and prolonged, can prevent the delivery of oxygen to the hepatic tissue. Without oxygen and the ability to carry off the hepatically metabolized substances, liver cells start to die, tissue necroses, and this destruction adds to the problems already existent. Liver enzymes start to reflect hepatic dysfunction, and the overall metabolic capability of the liver can become severely impaired (Shulman et al., 1980).

Consequences of Impaired Hepatic Function

As hepatic function falls, the ability to remove drugs and metabolic wastes become impaired. The patient becomes jaundiced, as bilirubin is not processed out of the body. Impaired production of coagulation factors also can develop with a resultant coagulopathy.

Clinical Complications of VOD

Since VOD is set in motion at the conditioning stage of transplant treatment, the early processes occur before the clinician can see signs and symptoms. Also, VOD exists on a continuum. Some cases are very mild and some severe, depending on the degree of hepatic damage. McDonald and colleagues found 12% with mild disease, 26% with moderate disease, and 15% with severe disease (McDonald et al., 1993). These points, plus the multitude of other clinical problems potentially occurring simultaneously, makes diagnosis of VOD somewhat problematic. A definitive diagnosis is possible by tissue biopsy, but this presents risks to the thrombocytopenic patient. It is necessary and appropriate to make the diagnosis based on clinical signs and symptoms.

Clinical Diagnosis of VOD

The clinical diagnosis of VOD can be based on as few as three or four criteria. McDonald and colleagues (1984) showed that the presence of hyperbilirubinemia, hepatomegaly, or right upper quadrant pain, and significant weight gain correlated highly with the presence of VOD as confirmed by biopsy. In fact, they showed that if the patient was in the first 3 weeks after bone marrow transplant, and if these signs could not be explained by other mechanisms, the finding of any two of these three was sufficient to confirm the diagnosis 89% of the time. Conversely, McDonald and colleagues (1984) also showed that in the absence of two of the three, there was a 92% chance that VOD did not exist. Other studies have used much the same criteria and had similar results. Recent work by Shulman confirmed a correlation of the clinical and histologic findings (Shulman et al., 1994). This seems valid when one constructs a frequency chart (see Figure 12.5) of signs and symptoms in patients with VOD. The four most frequent symptoms are the ones used in the clinical diagnosis and occur in the majority of patients with the disease.

The severity of the disease may be predicted by the degree of weight gain and serum bilirubin for a given day post transplant (Bear-

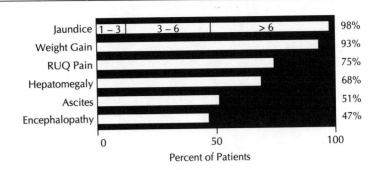

Figure 12.5
Clinical features of patients
with veno-occlusive disease
of the liver

SOURCE: From G. McDonald, et al. The clinical course of 53 patients with veno-occlusive disease of the liver. *Transplantation* 39(6):604. © Williams & Wilkins, 1985. Used with permission.

man et al., 1993). Greater weight gain and bilirubin early in the course predicted a more severe course and worse outcome.

Common Additional Clinical Findings

Multiorgan problems are more common for patients with VOD than for those without VOD. Figure 12.6 summarizes findings showing the incidence and time of onset for 190 patients who exhibited signs of VOD (McDonald et al., 1993).

Abdominal Distention

In addition to findings used in the clinical diagnosis, a vast array of other common findings are associated with VOD (see Figure 12.6). The congested GI mucosa, liver, spleen, and ascites all lead to abdominal distention. Severe enlargement of the abdomen can impair respiratory efforts such that full ventilatory movement is impaired and painful. Circulation of blood to the vital organs of the abdominal cavity can be impaired if the intraperitoneal pressure becomes too great. This is believed by some to account for at least some of the impaired renal function common in patients with VOD (McDonald et al., 1995).

Edema, Hyponatremia, Hypoalbuminemia

Water reabsorption by the renal tubules tends to produce a free water excess, which is manifest by hyponatremia. In addition, the leak of serum proteins into the peritoneal space produces hypoalbuminemia, reducing the oncotic pressure in the vascular space. This is compounded by the renal reabsorption of sodium, increasing total body sodium. The result of too much total body sodium, too much free water (which dilutes the serum sodium concentration to hyponatremic levels), and a serum oncotic pressure, invariably is the movement of water out of the capillaries into the interstitial space, or edema.

Encephalopathy

The shunting of blood away from the liver coupled with a loss of hepatic cells often causes the liver to inadequately metabolize waste products and the metabolites of drugs. These materials can build up in the blood and cause hepatic encephalopathy, which is clinically manifested as lethargy, confusion, and disorientation.

Renal Insufficiency

Several forces operate against proper renal function in the patient suffering from VOD.

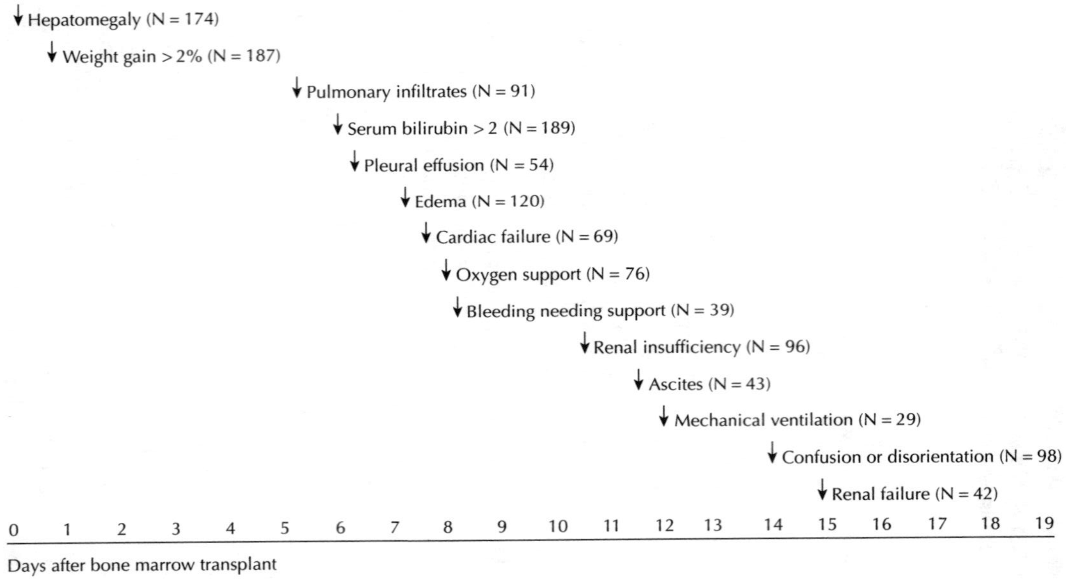

Figure 12.6 Mean day of onset of organ failure of 190 patients with liver toxicity

Source: Adapted from McDonald et al., 1993.

Although many patients with VOD never show impaired renal function, some have concomitant findings of renal insufficiency. One study of 77 bone marrow transplant patients who required hemodialysis found that all but four had a bilirubin greater than 2 mg/dl at their first dialysis. Half had a bilirubin greater than 2 mg/dl more than 10 days before first dialysis (Ballard et al., 1990).

Prerenal factors, as discussed earlier in this chapter, and the impairment of the liver's metabolism of nephrotoxic drugs seem to be the etiology of the concurrent renal failure. For instance, several prerenal factors are common to patients with VOD (see Figure 12.7). Most important is the loss of fluid from effective circulation due to an engorged liver, GI mucosa, and spleen. Ascites and edema rob the kidneys of needed intravascular volume. The use of diuretics and the restriction of IV or oral fluids, while often necessary actions, may overshoot the intended target and deplete the already tenuous intravascular status. If the intraperitoneal pressure becomes too great, venous return becomes

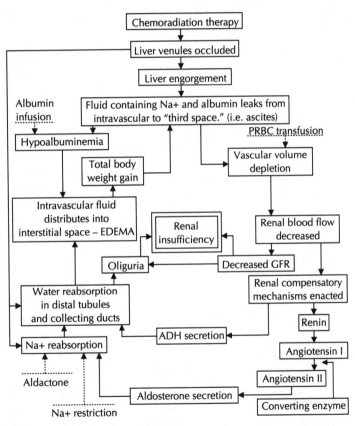

Figure 12.7
Impact of veno-occlusive disease on renal function

Dotted lines indicate the major clinical interventions used to manage this condition.

impaired and further restricts the already poor hepatic and renal blood flow.

The kidneys' response to these conditions is, in effect, to add fuel to the fire. Filtered sodium and water are reabsorbed at the renal tubules, urine output drops, clearance of metabolic waste products decreases still further, and weight gain continues.

In addition to the prerenal conditions is the potential that the kidneys may fall victim to nephrotoxic levels of hepatically metabolized drugs. Chief among these is cyclosporin, which is so commonly used in this population. (Yee et al., 1984). This close relationship between the kidneys and liver is a major concern and the focus of much of the clinical intervention directed at VOD.

Prevention of VOD

Heparin
Prophylactic medications to prevent the occurrence of VOD have been proposed and used with contradictory results. Heparin given as a continuous infusion, in low doses (100–150 U/kg per day) has been used and shown to be able to be given relatively safely. Marsa-Vila and colleagues (1991) studied 234 patients without finding a benefit to prophylactic heparin. A randomized trial by Attal and colleagues (1992) found reduced overall incidence of VOD in the group that received heparin.

Prostaglandin E₁
As a vasodilatory molecule that inhibits platelet aggregation and activates thrombolysis, prostaglandin (PGE1) may be useful to improve blood flow in hepatic venules and sinusoids. Although one study found a benefit to this therapy (Gluckman et al., 1990), severe side effects of the drug have hampered the ability to safely administer and determine the effectiveness of this drug (Bearman, 1995; Bearman et al., 1993).

Ursodeoxycholic Acid
Ursodiol, a nonhuman bile acid, protects hepatocytes from the damage caused by cholestasis by virtue of its ability to replace the more toxic bile acids (Bearman, 1995). Pilot data from Essell and colleagues (1992b) suggest that Ursodiol may decrease the incidence of VOD.

Pentoxifylline
Pentoxifylline is a drug that can inhibit TNF-alpha. Although pilot data (Bianco et al., 1991) reported positive findings, randomized trials have failed to show benefit (Clift et al., 1993; Stockschlader et al., 1993).

Treatment of Veno-Occlusive Disease

There is no definitive treatment to reverse VOD. At present, the clinical effort is generally directed toward supportive and symptomatic management of the patient until VOD has run its course and the regenerative capabilities of the liver have had a chance to repair the damage from the disease.

Recombinant tPA
Given the evidence that coagulation factors are deposited in the damaged hepatic tubules in VOD patients, thrombolytic therapy has been proposed. Recombinant tPA (r-tPA) is being used in cases of severe VOD where the benefit is worth the risk. Fatal hemorrhage is a significant potential but pilot data support that r-tPA can alter the natural course of severe VOD (Yu et al., 1994; Bearman et al., 1992).

Managing VOD Complications

The management of VOD entails preventing the extremes of the complications and maintaining of optimal vital organ function. The key is a thorough assessment that includes the knowledge of the patient's baseline information and the degree of change from this baseline.

From this knowledge base comes the plan to manage the clinical problems.

The management of VOD symptoms entails efforts to:

1. maintain fluid and electrolyte balance,
2. minimize the adverse effects of ascites,
3. adjust drugs to reflect impaired hepatic and renal function,
4. avoid compounding encephalopathy with drugs that alter mental status, and
5. attend to coagulopathy.

The overall goals of these tasks are to:

1. improve the impaired flow of blood through the liver and kidneys,
2. redistribute body fluids appropriately,
3. assist the body's compensatory efforts, and
4. counter inappropriate compensatory actions that the body institutes.

Maintaining Fluid and Electrolyte Balance

Maintenance of fluid and electrolyte balance requires a good assessment of total fluid through evaluation of weight, intake and output, and estimated insensible losses. The next task is to assess the distribution of that fluid in the body. Nursing assessment is an essential role in this task. The performance of postural blood pressure and heart rate, abdominal girth, lung exam, estimation of changes in peripheral edema, and the collection of urine for analysis are vital in determining the distribution of fluid in the body. With this information one can determine the effect of the fluid distribution on the renal, pulmonary, and cardiac status of the patient.

Optimizing Intravascular Volume

Though not a universal finding, it is common for the patient with VOD to be intravascularly depleted. Much of the crystalloid intravenous fluid given to the patient has an end point outside the vascular space. For this reason, judi-

cious use of red blood cells and/or salt-poor albumin are often recommended to maintain the volume of intravascular fluid. The infusion of these colloids is generally indicated when the patient exhibits signs of volume depletion such as orthostatic hypotension. Salt-poor albumin is used to increase the oncotic pressure in the vascular space and to replace serum proteins that are lost into the peritoneal cavity with ascites (McDonald et al., 1985).

Treating Sodium Imbalance

The treatment of elevated total body sodium levels requires a restriction of sodium intake plus the initiation of sodium diuresis. Spironolactone is effective in this regard, though it has its limitations and risks. It is only available as an oral drug, and effective sodium diuresis generally starts 36 to 72 hours after starting the drug and may persist for 24 to 36 hours after stopping doses. Spiralactone also puts the patient at risk for hyperkalemia. Care must be used if renal insufficiency develops (Conn, 1972).

Minimizing Fluids in Interstitial Compartments

The limitation of sodium intake, sodium diuresis, and colloidal support all help to minimize the movement of fluids into the interstitial spaces. This has its most important impact on the prevention or treatment of excess pulmonary fluid.

Altering Renal Hemodynamics

The use of low, renal-dose dopamine to dilate the renal arteries and improve renal efficiency has fallen out of favor at many institutions. The ability to accomplish an increase in GFR in the hepatically impaired patient has not been proved.

Minimizing Effects of Ascites

In those cases of VOD in which ascites is a significant problem, it is often the intent of clinicians to reduce ascitic fluid or to reduce the amount of fluid that has become sequestered in the abdominal organs. The removal of fluid by the aggressive use of diuretics, dialysis, or directly tapping the fluid via serial paracentesis are all effective. Yet whatever method is used, the underlying process that allowed the ascites to form in the first place persists, and the ascites inevitably reaccumulate. This reaccumulation is always at the expense of the intravascular volume and invariably leads to renal impairment (Cade et al., 1987). Whether to remove fluid, and how much fluid to remove, must be based on a careful assessment of the benefit-risk ratio for the individual situation.

Adjusting Drugs

The hepatic impairment found in VOD requires an adjustment of drugs that are hepatically metabolized. Narcotics are a common example. Changes of mental status from use of narcotics in the patient with VOD may necessitate stopping or reducing the drugs in an attempt to prevent compounding hepatic encephalopathy. Narcotics and sedatives with shorter half-lives and fewer metabolites should be considered if these drugs are needed for the patient's comfort. For example, lorazepam is preferable to valium for sedation. Also hydromorphone has a shorter half-life and requires conversion to significantly fewer metabolites than morphine.

Treating Coagulopathy

The coagulopathy associated with VOD is managed by several measures. Vitamin K replacement and regular infusions of platelets when required, are generally sufficient to prevent severe bleeding. If severe coagulopathy exists, strict attention to the prevention of bleeding is required. This includes prophylaxis against stress ulcers and avoidance of invasive procedures.

SUMMARY

The clinical issues discussed in this chapter are complex and present a challenge to the nurse caring for the bone marrow and blood cell transplant patient. Much of the required nursing assessment and action goes beyond that typical for the usual oncology patient. There is often some element of critical care nursing required for these patients, especially those who are experiencing severe renal or hepatic dysfunction. It has been the focus of this chapter to impress upon caregivers the significance of the nursing process in the overall management of these critical issues in order to improve the quality of complex care required by the transplant patient.

REFERENCES

Anscher, S., Peters, W., Reisenbichler, H., et al. 1993. Transforming growth factor B as a predictor of liver and lung fibrosis after autologous bone marrow transplantation for advanced breast cancer. N Engl J Med 328(22): 1592-1598.

Atkinson, K., Biggs, J., Golovsky, A., et al. 1991. Bladder irrigation does not prevent hemorrhagic cystitis in bone marrow transplant recipients. BMT 7:351-354.

Attal, M., Huguet, F., Herve, R., et al. 1992. Prevention of hepatic veno-occlusive disease after bone marrow transplantation by continuous infusion of low-dose heparin: a prospective, randomized trial. Blood 79(11): 2834-2840.

Azzi, A., Fanci, R., Bosi, S., et al. 1994. Monitoring of polyomavirus BK viruria in bone marrow transplantation patients by DNA hybridization assay and by polymerase chain reaction: an approach to assess the relationship between BK viruria and hemorrhagic cystitis. BMT 14:235-240.

Badr, K., Ichikawa I. 1988. Prerenal failure: a deleterious shift from renal compensation to decompensation. N Engl J Med 319(10):623-629.

Baglin, T. 1994. Veno-occlusive disease of the liver complicating bone marrow transplantation. BMT 13:1-4.

Ballard, B.D. 1989. Incidence and outcomes of renal insufficiency and renal failure after bone marrow transplant. Unpublished data.

Ballard, B.D. 1991. Renal and hepatic complications. In Whedon, M.B. (Ed.) *Bone Marrow Transplantation: Principles, Practices, and Nursing Insights.* Boston: Jones & Bartlett, 240-261.

Ballard, B.D., et al. 1990. Characteristics of bone marrow transplant patients with renal failure requiring hemodialysis. Unpublished data.

Ballardie, F., Edwards, B., Hows, J., et al. 1992. Disturbance in renal haemodynamics and physiology in bone marrow transplant recipients treated by cyclosporin A. *Nephron* 60:17-24.

Bandini, G., Belardinelli, A., Rosti, G., et al. 1994. Toxicity of high-dose busulphan and cyclophosphamide as conditioning therapy for allogeneic bone marrow transplantation in adults with haematological malignancies. *BMT* 13:577-581.

Bazarbachi, A., Scrobohaci, M., Gisselbrecht, C., et al. 1993. Changes in protein C, factor VII and endothelial markers after autologous bone marrow transplantation: possible implications in the pathogenesis of veno-occlusive disease. *Nouvelle Revue Française Hematologie* 35:135-140.

Bearman, S. 1995. The syndrome of hepatic veno-occlusive disease after marrow transplantation. *Blood* 85(11):3005-3020.

Bearman, S., Anderson, G., Mori, M., et al. 1993. Veno-occlusive disease of the liver: Development of a model for predicting fatal outcome after marrow transplantation. *J Clin Oncol* 11(9):1729-1736.

Bearman, S., Shen, D., Hinds, M., et al. 1993. A phase I/II study of prostaglandin E₁ for the prevention of hepatic veno-occlusive disease after bone marrow transplantation. *Br J Haematol* 84:724-730.

Bearman, S., Shuhart, M., Hinds, M., et al. 1992. Recombinant human tissue plasminogen activator for the treatment of established severe veno-occlusive disease of the liver after bone marrow transplantation. *Blood* 80(10):2458-2462.

Bennett, W.M. 1988. Guide to drug dosing in renal failure. *Clin Pharmacokinetics* 15:326-354.

Benya, E., Sivit, C., Quinones, R. 1993. Abdominal complications after bone marrow transplantation in children: sonographic and CT findings. *Am J Radiol* 161: 1023-1027.

Bianco, J.A., Applebaum, F., Nemunaitis, J., et al. 1991. Phase I-II trial of pentoxifylline for the prevention of transplant-related toxicities following bone marrow transplantation. *Blood* 78:1205.

Blostein, M., Paltiel, O., Thibault, A., et al. 1992. A comparison of clinical criteria for the diagnosis of veno-occlusive disease of the liver after bone marrow transplantation. *BMT* 10:439-443.

Buchsel, P. and Kelleher, J. 1989. Bone marrow transplantation. *Nurs Clin North Am* 24(4):907-937.

Cade, R., et al. 1987. Hepatorenal syndrome. *Am J Med* 82:427-438.

Carreras, E., Granena, A., Rozman, C. 1993. Hepatic veno-occlusive disease after bone marrow transplant. *Blood Rev* 7:43-51.

Carreras, E., Granena, A., Navasa, M., et al. 1993. On the reliability of clinical criteria for the diagnosis of hepatic veno-occlusive disease. *Ann Hematol* 66:77-80.

Carreras, E., Granena, A., Navasa, M., et al. 1993. Transjugular liver biopsy in BMT. *BMT* 11:21-26.

Cartoni, C., Arcese, W., Avvisati, G., et al. 1993. Role of ultrasonography in the diagnosis and follow-up of hemorrhagic cystitis after bone marrow transplantation. *BMT* 12:463-467.

Catani, L., Gugliotta, L., Mattioli Belmonte, M., et al. 1993. Hypercoagulability in patients undergoing autologuous or allogeneic BMT for hematological malignancies. *BMT* 12:253-259.

Champlin, R.E., Gale, R.P. 1984. The early complications of bone marrow transplantation. *Semin Hematol* 21(2):101-108.

Clift, R.A., Rianco, J., Applebaum, F.R., et al. 1993. A randomized controlled trial of pentoxifylline for the prevention of regimen-related toxicities in patients undergoing allogeneic marrow transplantation. *Blood* 82(7): 2025-2030.

Collins, P., Gutteridge, C., O'Driscoll, A., et al. 1992. von Willebrand factor as a marker of endothelial cell activation following BMT. *BMT* 10:499-506.

Collins, P., Roderick, A., O'Brien, D., et al. 1994. Factor VIIa and other haemostatic variables following bone marrow transplantation. *Thrombosis & Haemostasis* 72(1):28-32.

Conn, H.O. 1972. The rational management of ascites. *Progr Liver Dis* 4:269-288.

Cooper, B., Creger, R., Soegiarso, W., et al. 1993. Renal dysfunction during high-dose cisplatin therapy and autologous hematopoietic stem cell transplantation: effect of aminoglycoside therapy. *Am J Med* 94:497-504.

Deeg, H.J., et al. 1988. *A Guide to Bone Marrow Transplantation.* New York: Springer-Verlag, 123-139.

Dixon, B.S., Anderson, R.J. 1985. Nonoliguric acute renal failure. *Am J Kidney Dis* 6(2):71-80.

Efros, M., Ahmed, T., Coombe, N., et al. 1994. Urologic complications of high-dose chemotherapy and bone marrow transplantation. *Urol* 43(3):355-360.

Eltumi, M., Trivedi, P., Hobbs, J., et al. 1993. Monitoring of veno-occlusive disease after bone marrow transplantation by serum aminopropeptide of type III procollagen. *Lancet* 342:518-521.

Epstein, M. 1981. The rational approach to the management of ascites. *Drug Therapy* (Oct): 17-27.

Espinel, C.H., Gregory, A.W. 1980. Differential diagnosis of acute renal failure. *Clin Nephrol* 13(2):73-77.

Essell, J., Thompson, J., Harman, G., et al. 1992a. Marked increase in veno-occlusive disease of the liver associated by methotrexate use for graft-versus-host disease prophylaxis in patients receiving busulfan/cyclophosphamide. *Blood* 79(10):2784-2788.

Essell, J., Thompson, J., Harman, G., et al. 1992b. Pilot trial of prophylactic ursodiol to decrease the incidence of veno-occlusive disease of the liver in allogeneic bone marrow transplant patients. *BMT* 10:367-372.

Faioni, E., Krachmalnicoff, A., Bearman, S., et al. 1993. Naturally occurring anticoagulants and bone marrow transplantation: plasma protein C predicts the development of veno-occlusive disease of the liver. *Blood* 81(12): 3458-3462.

Flowers, M., Doney, K., Storb, R., et al. 1992. Marrow transplantation for Fanconi anemia with or without leukemic transformation: an update of the Seattle experience. *BMT* 9:167-173.

Ford, R., Ballard, B. 1988. Acute complications after bone marrow transplantation. *Semin Oncol Nurs* 4(1): 15-24

Ford, R., et al. 1983. Veno-occlusive disease following marrow transplantation. *Crit Care Nurs Clin North Am* 18(3):563-568.

Franco, T., Gould, D. 1994. Allogeneic bone marrow transplantation. *Semin Oncol Nurs* 10(1):3-11.

Gluckman, E., Joliveet, I., Scrobohaci, M.L., et al. 1990. Use of prostaglandin E_1 for prevention of liver veno-occlusive disease in leukaemic patients treated by allogeneic bone marrow transplantation. *Br J Haematol* 74: 277-281.

Goodinson, S.M. 1984. Renal function: an overview. *Nursing* 2(29):843-852.

Grandt, N. 1989. Hepatic veno-occlusive disease following bone marrow tranplantation. *Oncol Nurs Forum* 16(6):813-817.

Gugliotta, L., Catani, L., Vianelli, N., et al. High plasma levels of tumor necrosis factor may be predictive of veno-occlusive disease in bone marrow transplantation. *Blood* 83(8):2385-2386.

Guinan, E.C., et al. 1988. Intravascular hemolysis and renal insufficiency after bone marrow transplantation. *Blood* 72(2):451-455.

Guyton, A.C. 1986. *Textbook of Medical Physiology.* Philadelphia: Saunders, 835.

Heikinheimo, M., Halila, R., Fasth, A. 1994. Serum procollagen type III is an early and sensitive marker for veno-occlusive disease of the liver in children undergoing bone marrow transplantation. *Blood* 83(10):3036-3040.

Hommeyer, S., Teefey, S., Jacobson, A., et al. 1992. Veno-occlusive disease of the liver: prospective study of US evaluation. *Abdomin & Gastrointestin Radiol* 184:6 83-686.

Hou, S.H., Cohen, J.J. 1985. Diagnosis and management of acute renal failure. *Acute Care* 11:59-84.

Hutchinson, M.M., Itoh, K. 1983. Nursing care for the patient undergoing bone marrow transplantation for acute leukemia. *Crit Care Nurs Clin North Am* 17(4): 697-711.

Jacobson, R., Kalayoglu, M. 1992. Effective early treatment of hepatic veno-occlusive disease with a central splenorenal shunt in an infant. *J Pediatr Surg* 27(4): 531-533.

Jones, R.J., et al. 1987. Veno-occlusive disease of the liver following bone marrow transplantation. *Transplantation* 44(6):778-783.

Kaldor, P.K. 1988. Anatomy and physiology of the gastrointestinal system. In Kinney, M.R., et al. (Eds.) *AACN's Clinical Reference for Critical Care Nursing* New York: McGraw-Hill.

Kasai, M., Kiyama, Y., Watanabe, M., et al. 1992. Toxicity of high-dose busulfan and cyclophosphamide as a preparative regimen for bone marrow transplantation. *Transplant Proc* 24(4):1529-1530.

Kennedy, M.S., et al. 1983. Acute renal toxicity with combined use of amphotericin B and cyclosporin after marrow transplantation. *Transplantation* 35(3): 211-215.

Kennedy, M.S., et al. 1985. Correlation of serum cyclosporin concentration with renal dysfunction in marrow transplant recipients. *Transplantation* 40(4): 249-253.

King, C., Hoffart, N., Murray, M. 1992. Acute renal failure in bone marrow transplantation. *Oncol Nurs Forum* 19(9):1327-1335.

Kitabayashi, A., Hirokawa, M., Kuroki, J., et al. 1994. Successful vidarabine therapy for adenovirus type II-associated acute hemorrhagic cystitis after allogeneic bone marrow transplantation. *BMT* 14:853-854.

Kohno, A., Kunihiko, T., Narabayashi, M., et al. 1993. Hemorrhagic cystitis associated with allogeneic and autologous bone marrow transplantation for malignant neoplasms in adults. *Jap J Clin Oncol* 23(1):46-52.

Kone, B.C., et al. 1988. Hypertension and renal dysfunction in bone marrow transplant recipients. *Q J Med, New Series* 69(260):985-995.

Lam, M., Kaufman, C.E. 1985. Fractional excretion of sodium as a guide to volume depletion during recovery from acute renal failure. *Am J Kidney Dis* 6(1):18-21.

Lane, P., Mauer, S., Blazar, B., et al. 1994. Outcome of dialysis for acute renal failure in pediatric bone marrow transplant patients. *BMT* 13:613-617.

Lawton, C., Barbar-Derus, S., Murray, K., et al. 1992. Influence of renal shielding on the incidence of late renal dysfunction associated with T-lymphocyte–depleted bone marrow transplantation in adult patients. *Int J Radiat Oncol Biol Phys* 23:681-686.

Lawton, C., Fish, B., and Moulder, J. 1994. Effect of nephrotoxic drugs on the development of radiation nephropathy after bone marrow transplantation. *Int J Radiat Oncol Biol Phys* 28(4):883-889.

Letendre, L., Hoagland, H., Gertz, M. 1992. Hemorrhagic cystitis complicating bone marrow transplantation. *Mayo Clin Proc* 67(2):128-130.

Lin, E., Tierney, D., Stadtmauer, E. 1993. Autologous bone marrow transplantation: a review of the principles and complications. *Canc Nurs* 16(3):204-213.

Lonnerholm, G., Carlson, K., Bratteby, L., et al. 1991. Renal function after autologous bone marrow transplantation. *BMT* 8:129-137.

Mars, D.R., Treloar, D. 1984. Acute tubular necrosis—pathophysiology and treatment. *Heart & Lung* 13(2):194-201.

Marsa-Vila, L., Gorin, N., Laporte, J., et al. 1991. Prophylactic heparin does not prevent liver veno-occlusive disease following autologous bone marrow transplantation. *Eur J Haematol* 47:346-354.

McDonald, G., Hinds, M., Fisher, L., et al. 1993. Veno-occlusive disease of the liver and multiorgan failure after bone marrow transplantation: a cohort study of 355 patients. *Ann Intern Med* 118:255-267.

McDonald, G.B., et al. 1984. Veno-occlusive disease of the liver after bone marrow transplantation: diagnosis, incidence, and predisposing factors. *Hepatology* 4(1): 116-122.

McDonald, G.B., et al. 1985. The clinical course of 53 patients with veno-occlusive disease of the liver after marrow transplantation. *Transplantation* 39(6): 603-608.

McDonald, G.B., et al. 1986. Intestinal and hepatic complications of human bone marrow transplantation, part I. *Gastroenterology* 90:460-477.

Meisenberg, B., Lassiter, M., Hussein, A., et al. 1994. Prevention of hemorrhagic cystitis after high-dose alkylating agent chemotherapy and autologous bone marrow support. *BMT* 14:287-291.

Meresse, V., Hartmann, O., Vassal, G., et al. 1992. Risk factors for hepatic veno-occlusive disease after high-dose busulfan-containing regimens followed by autologous bone marrow transplantation: a study of 136 children. *BMT* 10:135-141.

Mieli-Vergani, G. 1993. Hepatic complications after bone marrow transplantation. *BMT* 12(suppl)1:96-97.

Miyamura, K., et al. 1989. Hemorrhagic cystitis associated with urinary excretion of adenovirus type II following allogeneic bone marrow transplantation. *BMT* 4: 533-535.

Moulder, J., Fish, B. 1991. Influence of nephrotoxic drugs on the late renal toxicity associated with bone marrow transplant conditioning regimens. *Int J Radiat Oncol Biol Phys* 20:333-337.

Moulder, J., Fish, B., Cohen, E. 1993. Treatment of radiation nephropathy with ace inhibitors. *Int J Radiat Oncol Biol Phys* 27:93-99.

Nattakom, T., Charlton, A., Wilmore, D. 1995. Use of vitamin E and glutamine in the successful treatment of severe veno-occlusive disease following bone marrow transplantation. *Nutr Clin Pract* 19:16-18.

Nicolau, D., Hogan, K. 1992. National survey of use of mesna for the prevention of cyclophosphamide-induced hemorrhagic cystitis in recipients of bone marrow transplants. *Mayo Clin Proc* 67:611-612.

Otheo de Tejada, E., Maldonado, M., Camarero, C., et al. 1994. Fatal hemorrhage after recombinant tissue plasminogen activator therapy for hepatic veno-occlusive disease complicating autologous BMT. *BMT* 14: 176-177.

Price, C. 1994. Acute renal failure: a sequela of sepsis. *Crit Care Nurs Clin North Am* 6(2):359-371.

Rapoport, A., Doyle, H., Starzl, T., et al. 1991. Orthotopic liver transplantation for life-threatening veno-occlusive disease of the liver after allogeneic bone marrow transplant. *BMT* 8:421-424.

Ringden, O., Ruutu, T., Remberger, M., et al. 1994. A randomized trial comparing busulfan with total body irradiation as conditioning in allogeneic marrow transplant recipients with leukemia: a report from the Nordic bone marrow transplantation group. *Blood* 83 (9):2723-2730.

Rio, B., Bauduer, F., Arrago, J., et al. 1993. N-terminal peptide of type III procollagen: a marker for the development of hepatic veno-occlusive disease after BMT and a basis for determining the timing of prophylactic heparin. *BMT* 11:471-472.

Rosenzweig, M., Schaefer, P., and Rosenfeld, C. 1994. Prevention of transplant-related hemorrhagic cystitis using bladder irrigation with sorbitol. *BMT* 14:491-492.

Russell, S., Vowels, M., Vale, T. 1994. Haemorrhagic cystitis in paediatric bone marrow transplant patients: an association with infective agents, GVHD and prior cyclophosphamide. *BMT* 13:533-539.

Sabau, D. 1992. Hematuria in bone marrow transplant patients. *J Am Soc Nephrol* 3(4):916-920.

Safwat, A., Nielsen, O., Overgaard, J. 1993. Is kidney the real dose-limiting organ after total body irradiation and bone marrow transplantation? *Eur J Canc* 29A(6): 929.

Salat, C., Holler, E., Kolb, H., et al. 1993. Monitoring of veno-occlusive disease after bone marrow transplantation by serum aminopropeptide of type III procollagen. *Lancet* 342:1062.

Salat, C., Holler, E., Reinhardt, B., et al. 1994. Parameters of the fibrinolytic system in patients undergoing BMT: elevation of PAI-1 in veno-occlusive disease. *BMT* 14:747-750.

Sale, G.E., Shulman, H.M. 1984. Pathology of other organs. In Sale, G.E., Shulman, H.M. (Eds.) *The Pathology of Bone Marrow Transplantation.* New York: Masson, 192-198.

Schottelius, B.A., Schottelius, D.D. 1973. *Textbook of Physiology,* 17 ed. St. Louis: Mosby, 604.

Schuler, U., Schroer, S., Kuhnle, A., et al. 1994. Busulfan pharmacokinetics in bone marrow transplant patients: is drug monitoring warranted? *BMT* 14:759-765.

Sencer, S., Haake, R., Weisdorf, D. 1993. Hemorrhagic cystitis after bone marrow transplantation. *Transplantation* 56:875-879.

Shaffer, S., Wilson, J. 1993. Bone marrow transplantation: critical care implications. *Coagulopath Hematol* 5 (3):531-542.

Shepherd, J., Pringle, L., Barnett, M., et al. 1991. Mesna versus hyperhydration for the prevention of cyclophosphamide-induced hemorrhagic cystitis in bone marrow transplantation. *J Clin Oncol* 9(11):2016-2020.

Shuhart, M.C., McConald, G.B. 1994. Gastrointestinal and hepatic complications. In Forman, S.J., et al. (Eds.) *Bone Marrow Transplantation.* Boston: Blackwell Scientific, 454-475.

Shulman, H., Hinterberger, W. 1992. Hepatic veno-occlusive disease—liver toxicity syndrome after bone marrow transplantation. *BMT* 10:197-214.

Shulman, H., Fisher, L., Schoch, G., et al. 1994. Veno-occlusive disease of the liver after marrow transplantation: histological correlates of clinical signs and symptoms. *Hepatology* 19(5):1171-1181.

Shulman, H.M., et al. 1980. An analysis of hepatic veno-occlusive disease and centrilobular hepatic degeneration following bone marrow transplantation. *Gastroenterology* 79:1178-1191.

Shulman, H.M., McDonald, G.B. 1984. Liver disease after marrow transplantation. In Sale, G.E., Shulman, H.M. (Eds.) *The Pathology of Bone Marrow Transplantation.* New York: Masson, 104-135.

Simpson, D., Browett, P., Doak, P., et al. 1994. Successful treatment of veno-occlusive disease with recombinant tissue plasminogen activator in a patient requiring peritoneal dialysis. *BMT* 14:635-636.

Smith, D.M., et al. 1987. Acute renal failure associated with autologous bone marrow transplantation. *BMT* 2:195-201.

Soiffer, R., Dear, K., Rabinowe, S., et al. 1991. Hepatic dysfunction following T-cell–depleted allogeneic bone marrow transplantation. *Transplantation* 52(6): 1014-1019.

Spach, D., Bauwens, J., Myerson, D., et al. 1993. Cytomegalovirus-induced hemorrhagic cystitis following bone marrow transplantation. *Clin Infect Dis* 16: 142-144.

Stark, J.L. 1988a. Renal anatomy and physiology. In Kinney, M.R., et al. (Eds.) *AACN'S Clinical Reference for Critical Care Nursing.* New York: McGraw-Hill, 843-859.

Stark, J.L. 1988b. Renal system assessment. In Kinney, M.R., et al. (Eds.) *AACN'S Clinical Reference for Critical Care Nursing.* New York: McGraw-Hill, 860-872.

Stark, J.L. 1988c. Acute renal failure. In Kinney, M.R., et al. (Eds.) *AACN'S Clinical Reference for Critical Care Nursing.* New York: McGraw-Hill, 873-885.

Stockschlader, M., Kalhs, P., Peters, S., et al. 1993. Intravenous pentoxifylline failed to prevent transplant-related toxicities in allogeneic bone marrow transplant recipients. *BMT* 12:357-362.

Storek, J., Gale, R., Goldstein, L. 1993. Analysing early liver dysfunction after bone marrow transplantation. *Transplant Immunol* 1:163-171.

Tanaka, J., Imamura, M., Kasai, M., et al. 1993. Rapid analysis of tumor necrosis factor-alpha mRNA expression during veno-occlusive disease of the liver after allogeneic bone marrow transplantation. *Transplantation* 55(2):430-431.

Turkeri, L., Lum, L., Uberti, J., et al. 1995. Prevention of hemorrhagic cystitis following allogeneic bone marrow transplant preparative regimens with cyclophosphamide and busulfan: role of continuous bladder irrigation. *J Urol* 153:637-640.

Vannucchi, A., Rafanelli, D., Longo, G., et al. 1994. Early hemostatic alterations following bone marrow transplantation: a prospective study. *Haematologica* 79:519-525.

Vose, J., Reed, E., Pippert, G., et al. 1993. Mesna compared with continuous bladder irrigation as uroprotection during high-dose chemotherapy and transplantation: A randomized trial. *J Clin Oncol* 11(7):1306-1310.

Wingard, J., Niehaus, C., Peterson, D., et al. 1991. Oral mucositis after bone marrow transplantation. *Oral Surg Oral Med Pathol* 72:419-424.

Wujcik, D., Ballard, B., Camp-Sorrell, D. 1994. Selected complications of allogeneic bone marrow transplantation. *Semin Oncol Nurs* 10(1):28-41.

Wujcik, D., Downs, S. 1992. Bone marrow transplantation. *Crit Care Nurs Clin North Am* 4(1):149-166.

Yang, C., Hurd, D., Case, L., et al. 1994. Hemorrhagic cystitis in bone marrow transplantation. *Urology* 44(3):322-328.

Yee, G.C., et al. 1984. Effect of hepatic dysfunction on oral cyclosporin pharmacokinetics in marrow transplant patients. *Blood* 64(6):1277-1279.

Yee, G.C., et al. 1985. Cyclosporin-associated renal dysfunction in marrow transplant recipients. *Transplant Proc* 17(4):196-201.

Yu, L., Malkani, I., Regueira, O., et al. 1994. Recombinant tissue plasminogen activator (r-tPA) for veno-occlusive liver disease in pediatric autologous bone marrow transplant patients. *Am J Hematol* 46:194-198.

Yuzawa, Y., Aoi, N., Fukatsu, A., et al. 1993. Acute renal failure and degenerative tubular lesions associated with in situ formation of adenovirus immune complexes in a patient with allogeneic bone marrow transplantation. *Transplantation* 55(1):67-72.

Zager, R. 1994. Acute renal failure in the setting of bone marrow transplantation. *Kidney International* 46:1443-1458.

Zager, R.A., et al. 1989. Acute renal failure following bone marrow transplantation: a retrospective study of 272 patients. *Am J Kidney Dis* 13:210-216.

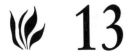

13

Neurological Effects

Deborah K. Meriney, Patricia Grimm

Neurologic and neuromuscular complications occur in 59% to 70% of patients who undergo a bone marrow transplantation (BMT) and result in a 6% fatality rate (Davis and Patchell 1988; Patchell et al., 1985a; Wiznitzer et al., 1984). The incidence of these complications in blood cell transplantation (BCT) is not yet specifically defined. However, the etiology for many neurologic complications is applicable to both BMT and BCT. In many cases, neurologic complications occur insidiously, manifesting symptoms so general that they may be easily mistaken for the sequelae of prolonged isolation, bedrest, the sedative side effects of certain medications, or as indicators of psychiatric diagnoses, particularly anxiety or depression. Many medications administered throughout the transplant process place the patient at risk for neurological side effects, particularly if concomitant changes in hepatic and/or renal function have occurred or are occurring. Delirium, the clinical picture resulting from general impairment of mental function, often occurs in hospitalized patients undergoing active treatment. This clinical state is characterized by clouded consciousness, disorientation, suspiciousness, fears, irritability, and misperception of sensory stimuli, causing delusions and visual hallucinations. While the prevalence of delirium ranges from 8% to 85%, BMT patients are at particular risk because of the frequent ad-

ministration of narcotics and steroids, and the incidence of metabolic encephalopathy (Fleishman and Lesko, 1990).

Because neurologic deficits can render individuals incapable of self-care to varying degrees, either temporarily or permanently; the impact of neurological and neuromuscular deficits on the patient, family, health team and resources, is significant. Therefore, early assessment for signs and symptoms of complications, which includes an understanding of the patient's baseline level of neurological functioning and risk factors, may help prevent or ameliorate potentially severe neurological impairment.

The neurological system is at risk for injury throughout the transplant process. Pretransplant conditioning with chemo- and radiotherapy may result in neurotoxicity. Posttransplant, neurologic, and neuromuscular effects/complications may result from infections or toxicities of antibiotics, antifungal, antiviral, and immunosuppressive agents. Therapies administered to enhance engraftment, support hematopoietic response, or control graft-versus-host disease (GVHD) may also produce neurological changes. The management of frequently experienced symptoms such as pain, nausea and vomiting, anxiety, and sleep disturbances may include pharmacologic interventions that have significant neurological side effects. Finally, system failure in other organs may lead to metabolic encephalopathy and impair neurologic function.

CHEMORADIOTHERAPY PRETRANSPLANT CONDITIONING

Neurospecific diagnostic testing prior to transplantation is limited to a lumbar puncture primarily in patients with acute lymphocytic leukemia or in those who are suspected to have central nervous system disease. Patients undergoing BMT for a malignant brain tumor may have a computerized tomography (CT) scan, but this test is not part of the routine screening for all BMT patients. Due to the lack of specific, quantitative neurological tests, it is essential that a history and physical assessment be obtained in order to establish a baseline for future comparison.

Chemotherapy used in the conditioning process places the patient at risk for neurological injury. Commonly used drugs with neurotoxic potential include etoposide (VP-16) with associated peripheral polyneuropathy in approximately 4% of cases (Imrie et al., 1994), carmustine (BCNU) with rare instances of neuroretinitis and inflammatory peripheral neuropathy (Bashir et al., 1992), and busulfan with the possible development of hallucinations, tremors, or seizures (De La Camara et al., 1991; Srivastava et al., 1993; Sureda et al., 1989), and myasthenia gravis (Arkey, 1995). Methotrexate is associated with the development of leukoencephalopathy, myelopathy and encephalopathy (Land et al., 1994; Ozon et al., 1994).

Intrathecal and standard doses of cytosine arabinoside (Ara-C) are associated with myelopathy and peripheral neuropathy (Kornblau et al., 1993; Ozon et al., 1994; Resar et al., 1993). High-dose regimens of Ara-C may cause a range of neurotoxicities, which include headache, somnolence, personality changes, memory loss, intellectual impairment, confusion, slurred speech, stupor, coma, and seizures. Other Ara-C–related neurotoxicities include cerebellar dysfunction, hearing loss, visual loss, anosmia, encephalopathy, and severe expressive aphasia (Hoffman et al., 1993; Resar et al., 1993; Vogel and Horoupian, 1993).

Antiemetic regimens containing phenothiazines, benzodiazepines, antihistamines, or cannabinoids may cause drowsiness, sedation, or other neurologic manifestations (Furlong and Gallucci, 1994). Neurologic complications of antiemetics will be discussed in further detail later in the chapter.

Total body irradiation (TBI) may cause a somnolence syndrome characterized by headache, fatigue, nausea, anorexia (Goldberg et al., 1992), weakness, and confusion, and has caused impaired cognitive function, particularly in children (Christie et al., 1994). The onset is usually 4 to 8 weeks after treatment and thought to be related to transient brain edema following irradiation (Halperin et al., 1994). Irradiation has been identified as an important contributor to the development of retinopathy (Bernauer and Gratwohl, 1992), and selective autonomic neuropathy has a suspected link to fractionated TBI (Roskrow et al., 1992). Other effects of TBI (i.e., vascular complications and leukoencephalopathy), which occur as a result of its use in combination with other treatments or as late effects are discussed subsequently in this chapter.

Total body irradiation appears to be associated with a high incidence of late onset cataracts, which are usually correctable by surgery (Fife et al., 1994; Liesner et al., 1994). It is unclear whether other factors such as the use of steroids actually cause or greatly contribute to the development of cataracts (Dunn et al., 1993; Hamon et al., 1993). Superfractionated TBI appears to be more strongly associated with cataract formation than fractionated TBI, and cataract severity appears to be decreased with fractionated rather than single-dose TBI (Locatelli et al., 1993; Tichelli et al., 1993). The risk of cataract formation appears to be increased in patients who received cranial radiotherapy prior to TBI, those receiving a higher skull dose, a TBI dose rate greater than 3.5 cGy/min, and those who receive steroids after BMT (Fife et al., 1994; Tichelli et al., 1993).

Some late onset neurological complications are thought to be due to a combination of factors, including pretransplant chemoradiotherapy, such as Lhermitte's sign (Wen et al., 1992) and high-grade pyrexia with accompanying neurological dysfunction (Murphy et al., 1994). The predisposition toward neurologic complications may also be enhanced by prior chemotherapy (for example, vincristine), which may have caused subclinical nerve damage that is magnified by the transplant and the conditioning regimen (Imrie et al., 1994).

CENTRAL NERVOUS SYSTEM INFECTIONS

Central nervous system infection is a common neurologic complication of bone marrow transplantation. Heightened susceptibility is evident during two periods of time following transplant when there is high risk of infection (Table 13.1).

The first period of risk occurs 1 month post transplant and corresponds to the period of

TABLE 13.1 Periods of risk for infection

First:	Related to granulocytopenia 0–1 month after BMT Organisms: bacteria, viruses, fungi
Second:	Related to immunosuppression 1–12 months after BMT Organisms: viruses, protozoa

granulocytopenia. During this time, bacterial, fungal, and viral infections predominate. The second period lasts from 1 month until 1 year after transplant, correlating with prolonged immunosuppression, usually the result of treatment for GVHD. Viral and protozoal infections are common (Anderlini et al., 1994; Hoyle and Goldman, 1994; Sable and Donowitz, 1994).

Bacterial Infections

The organisms responsible for infection are primarily gram-positive bacteria or *Listeria monocytogenes, Streptococcus pneumoniae, Klebsiella pneumoniae, Esterichia coli,* and alpha-streptococci (Hoyle and Goldman, 1994; Long et al., 1993; Peeters et al., 1989; Sable and Donowitz, 1994). Contiguous spread from paranasal and paratympanic areas may result in meningitis, the most common neurologic complication of bacterial infection (D'Antonio et al., 1992; Hoyle and Goldman, 1994).

Due to myelosuppression, whether from the transplant or as a result of immunosuppressive medications (Hoyle and Goldman, 1994), the body is unable to mount an inflammatory response. Therefore, meningeal inflammation is not commonly seen (Callaham, 1989). Most patients present with fever and headache, yet a substantial number may be without symptoms of CNS infection (Callaham, 1989; Francke, 1987). When present, signs of bacterial meningitis include changes in mental status, meningismus, lethargy, nuchal rigidity, increasing confusion, positive Kernig and Brudzinski signs, or seizures (D'Antonio et al., 1992; McCracken et al., 1992; Viscioli et al., 1991).

Preventive measures are those generally recommended during immunosuppression, including meticulous hand washing and a low-bacterial diet devoid of uncooked fruits or vegetables and salads (Hathorn, 1993). In addition, patients and families should be made aware that *Listeria* bacteria have been found to contaminate milk, soft cheese, paté and cook-chill prepared foods (Long et al., 1993). Antibiotic prophylaxis post transplant may prevent fatal infections (Hoyle and Goldman, 1994), but it may not be effective against encapsulated bacteria. Any upper respiratory infection in this patient population requires an early investigation for the responsible organism (D'Antonio et al., 1992).

Fungal Infections

Fungal infections account for approximately half of CNS infections in BMT recipients, and are by far most frequently caused by *Aspergillus fumigatus* (Denning et al., 1994; Milliken and Powles, 1990). The organism gains access to the CNS through hematogenous spread from the lungs, skin, or gastrointestinal tract, or by direct extension from the cranial sinuses (Denning et al., 1994). *Aspergillus* may cause brain abscesses; altered consciousness is usually the presenting sign. Focal neurologic findings like sudden hemiparesis and seizures are also associated with *Aspergillus* infection.

The *Candida* species are another common cause of fungal infection in the bone marrow transplant patient, causing meningoencephalitis, brain abscesses, and meningitis (Hiemenez and Greene, 1993; Hoyle and Goldman, 1994).

Cryptococcus, an organism ubiquitous in animals and the soil, is often acquired by patients prior to hospitalization (Deeg, 1984). Although about half of patients with cryptococcal meningitis are not immunosuppressed, infections may be opportunistic and life-threatening to neutropenic patients following BMT (Lentnek et al., 1992). The organism may become disseminated and infect the central nervous system, causing meningoencephalitis and its usual manifestations.

There are several treatments for fungal infections: oral nonabsorbable (e.g., nystatin, amphotericin B), systemic (e.g., fluconazole, amphotericin B, itraconazole, and ketoconazole), and topical (e.g., clotrimazole and amphotericin B). While each has its benefits, no agent has been proved superior to the others (Hathorn, 1993).

Viral Infections

Viral complications are most commonly due to the herpes group, notably cytomegalovirus (CMV), which occurs in about 50% of BMT patients, and the varicella-zoster virus (VZV), which occurs in 17% to 50% of BMT patients (Sable and Donowitz, 1994). Of VZV infections, 85% are due to herpes zoster and 15% are due to varicella (Sable and Donowitz, 1994). Risk factors for VZV infection include leukemias, age greater than 10 years, VZV seropositive, and pretransplant radiation (Han et al., 1994).

Herpes zoster infections are potentially severe, with great risk of dissemination, and are caused by reactivation of VZV first acquired in childhood as chicken pox. After resolution of the chicken pox, VZV may lie dormant in the posterior root ganglion of the spinal nerve or in a cranial nerve ganglion. The outbreak characteristically occurs along the dermatomes and may cause severe neuralgias.

Herpes simplex (HSV) reactivates in up to 80% of BMT recipients (Ford and Eisenberg, 1990). Fortunately, however, infection is usually localized and rarely fatal (Winston et al., 1988). Acyclovir, an antiviral agent, is often initiated prior to BMT and has been very effective against HSV (Sable and Donowitz, 1994), however, acyclovir-resistant strains of the virus are emerging (Verndonck et al., 1993).

Although acyclovir has reduced the incidence of other serious viral infections, effective prophylaxis and treatment remains elusive (Han et al., 1994; Hoyle and Goldman, 1994). Pretransplant vaccination of donor and recipient has been suggested as an efficacious means of preventing both bacterial and viral infections (Hathorn, 1993).

Viral encephalitis is associated with systemic viral dissemination. Herpes encephalitis is fatal in 70% of cases and has a morbidity rate that exceeds 90% in survivors (Whitley et al., 1992). Common clinical manifestations of encephalitis include headache, altered sensorium, behavioral disorders, seizures, and meningeal irritation (Whitley et al., 1992).

Other causative organisms of viral encephalitis include CMV and, rarely, adenovirus (Ford and Eisenberg, 1990; Whitley et al., 1992). Because these viruses may be latent in the BMT recipient prior to transplantation, encephalitis is often the result of reactivation of the virus under the conditions of immunosuppression (Meyers, 1988). Other routes of spread include the nasopharyngeal or orofecal route. Blood products have also been implicated as sources of infections of the adeno- and cytomegaloviruses (Hathorn, 1993). CMV encephalitis clinically resembles the general viral encephalitis.

Serologic screening of blood products and organ donors can reduce or eliminate transmission of CMV to those who have never been infected (Sable and Donowitz, 1994). Intravenous ganciclovir has some efficacy against CMV if administered prophylactically or before the onset of pneumonia (Winston et al., 1988).

Protozoal Infections

Once identified as a parasitic pathogen, *Toxoplasma gondii* has been reclassified as a protozoan (Sable and Donowitz, 1994). After acute infection, a competent immune system maintains the cysts of *T. gondii,* which persist in the CNS in a dormant state. Under conditions of immunosuppression resulting from BMT, the organism may be reactivated (Sande et al., 1992; Seong et al., 1993). Left untreated, the organism is fatal in virtually 100% of cases

(Sande et al., 1992). Clinically, toxoplasmosis may manifest itself as a diffuse encephalopathy or, meningoencephalitis, or as single or multiple lesions (Sable and Donowitz, 1994; Seong et al., 1994). The signs are characteristic of a progressive neurologic disorder and include bifrontal headache, nuchal rigidity, fever, disorientation, altered visual acuity, agitation, hemiparesis, and seizures (Sable and Donowitz, 1994; Sande et al., 1992; Seong et al., 1994).

Despite the fact that greater than 50% of the U.S. population may be carriers, significant infection with this organism in transplant recipients is rare (Geissmann et al., 1994; Sable and Donowitz, 1994). It is hypothesized that *Pneumocystis carinii* prophylaxis pretransplant may also protect patients from reactivation of latent toxoplasma infection. Combination therapy with pyrimethamine and sulfadiazine has been effective in treating acute toxoplasma infection (Seong et al., 1993).

Since the acquisition of toxoplasmosis is a late infection, most likely to occur long after the patient is discharged from the hospital, teaching by the inpatient nurse in anticipation of discharge, or by the clinic or the community nurse should focus on avoiding possible sources of the pathogen. Specific instructions to patients should be given. Fruits and vegetables, which may be contaminated with *Toxoplasma gondii,* should be washed carefully. Contact with cat feces or litter boxes is avoided because parasite eggs can develop in the intestines of cats.

A patient hospitalized with toxoplasmosis should be placed on seizure precautions with frequent neurologic assessments. Any changes in neurologic status should be reported to the physician. Toxoplasmosis is contagious and appropriate isolation procedures should be instituted.

A new cause of opportunistic infection in BMT patients, *Acanthamoeba,* has recently been identified. Patients develop a rapidly progressive and fatal meningoencephalitis (Anderlini et al., 1994). The organism is believed to gain access to the upper respiratory tract by inhalation or direct inoculation, and encephalitis results from hematogenous spread. Risk factors include immunosuppression, particularly in conjunction with corticosteroids, and culture-negative sinusitis (Anderlini et al., 1994). Signs of the encephalopathy include rapid mental deterioration, coma, and/or seizures. Physical examination may or may not reveal focal abnormalities (Anderlini et al., 1994). The onset may be 6 to 9 months after transplant, and infection occurs despite antibacterial and antifungal antibiotics. There is no known effective treatment for *Acanthamoeba* infections (Anderlini et al., 1994).

PROPHYLAXIS AND TREATMENT OF INFECTIONS

Many antibacterial, antifungal, and antiviral agents are neurotoxic. Aminoglycosides (amikacin, gentamicin, tobramycin) are known to adversely affect the eighth cranial nerve, which is responsible for hearing and balance. Other antibacterials, either alone or in combination with aminoglycosides, can cause neurologic deficits (Arkey, 1995). Toxicities include ototoxicity (tinnitus, hearing loss, loss of balance), acute muscular weakness, headache, dizziness, paresthesias, and fatigue (Arkey, 1995). Additional side effects may include tremors, peripheral neuropathy, mental status changes, confusion, hallucinations, twitching and, rarely, seizures. Table 13.2 lists some common antimicrobials and their neurological side effects.

Nurses who administer these therapies should be cognizant of individual and potentiated effects, appropriate neurologic assessments, and appropriate interventions to prevent or minimize toxicity. Often, the duration of treatment and dosage influence the degree and severity of the side effects. In addition, nurses should be aware of where the drug is metabolized, and concomitant conditions, such as decreased renal function, which may interfere with drug metabolism thereby exacerbating toxicity. Accordingly, serum and urine creatinine, intake and output, and daily weights need to be monitored in patients receiving antimicrobials metabolized by the kidneys. Drugs metabolized in the liver require close attention to liver function tests.

METABOLIC ENCEPHALOPATHY

Metabolic encephalopathy or coma occur in approximately 26 % to 37% of patients undergoing BMT (Davis and Patchell, 1988; Furlong and Gallucci, 1994). They are caused by multiple organ failure, and usually associated with terminal events (Davis and Patchell, 1988). Most frequently, they are caused by hypoxia or ischemia, followed by hepatic failure, electrolyte imbalance, and renal failure with associated uremia (Davis and Patchell, 1988; Snider et al., 1994).

Another encephalopathic syndrome, idiopathic hyperammonemia, is seen after high-dose chemotherapy, and its abrupt development is associated with a grave prognosis (Mitchell et al., 1988; Tse et al., 1991). Clinically, the condition is characterized by a severe, sudden alteration in mental status, lethargy, confusion, cerebellar dysfunction, seizures, and respiratory alkalosis in association with markedly elevated serum ammonia. It is usually apparent in the absence of liver dysfunction or any other identifiable cause, and progresses to coma and subsequent death in severe cases (Mitchell et al., 1988). If diagnosed early, dialysis and ammonia-trapping agents may decrease the serum ammonia and prevent irreversible brain damage (Tse et al., 1991).

In every case of encephalopathy, astute neurological assessment, monitoring of laboratory

TABLE 13.2 Neurotoxic effects of anti-infectious agents

Agents	Neurotoxic effects
ANTIBACTERIAL	
Aminoglycosides Amikacin Gentamicin Tobramycin	Ototoxicity of the eighth cranial nerve with hearing loss, loss of balance, or both; may cause acute muscular paralysis and apnea
Cephalosporins Ceftazidine Cefoperazone	Headache, dizziness, confusion, disorientation, paranoia, hallucinations; with increase in dose, twitching, seizures; paresthesias rare
Penicillins Piperacillin Penicillin G	Headache, dizziness, fatigue
Quinolones Norfloxacin	Dizziness, light-headedness, headache
Other Vancomycin	Ototoxicity with tinnitus, hearing loss, dizziness; vertigo rare
ANTIFUNGAL	
Amphotericin B	Headache, hearing loss, vertigo, peripheral neuropathy; tinnitus rare
Fluconazole	Headache
ANTIVIRAL	
Acyclovir	Nervousness, headache, clonic contractions, seizures, hallucinations, paranoia, confusion, depression; tremor rare
Ganciclovir	Headache, mental status changes, delirium

Source: Adapted from Farrington, Stoudemire, and Tierney, 1995; Ezzone and Camp-Sorrell, 1994.

values, hydration, safety precautions, dialysis, oxygen therapy, and emotional support for the patient and family are all important interventions, usually with the goal of palliation.

IMMUNOSUPPRESSIVE AGENTS

Immunosuppressive therapies are an integral part of BMT. Their role is in prevention of graft rejection and in the prophylaxis and treatment of graft-versus-host disease (Walker and Brochstein, 1988). Neurotoxic effects may be the direct effect of the immunosuppressants or the sequelae of CNS infection resulting from prolonged immunosuppression. Common agents include cyclosporin, methotrexate, the corticosteroids, antithymocyte globulin, OKT3 antibody, azathioprine, thalidomide, and tacrolimus. Table 13.3 summarizes the drugs, their actions, uses in BMT, and most common neurological complications.

TABLE 13.3 Neurologic effects of immunosuppressive therapies

Immunosuppressant	Action	Use in BMT	Neurologic Complications
Cyclosporin	Inhibits T helper cells, and T suppressor cells	Reduces the incidence and severity of GVHD	Confusion, tremors, seizures, paresthesias, muscle weakness, leucoencephalopathy, cerebellar ataxia, coma
Methotrexate	Antifolate metabolite; Immunosuppressant	GVHD prophylaxis and treatment	Aseptic meningitis, somnolence, transverse myelopathy, seizures, strokelike syndrome, confusion
Corticosteroids	Suppresses immune response at all levels	GVHD prophylaxis and treatment	Agitation, psychosis, mania, depression, delirium, cognitive deficits, tremor, sleep disturbances, seizures, euphoria, dysphoria, steroid myopathy, increased intracranial pressure
Antithymocyte globulin	Lymphocyte-specific immunosuppressant	Prevents allogeneic bone marrow graft rejection	Headache, seizures
OKT3 monoclonal antibody	Binds all immuno-components	Acute rejection treatment and GVHD prophylaxis and treatment	Headache, tremors, myalgias
Thalidomide	Mechanism of action unknown	Treatment of acute and chronic GVHD	Sedation, peripheral neuropathy, paresthesias, nocturnal muscle cramps
Azathioprine	Immunosuppressive antimetabolite	Prevents graft rejection, treatment of chronic GVHD	No direct neurotoxic effects

SOURCE: From Furlong, 1993; Vogelsang and Morris, 1993; Palmer and Toto, 1991; Walker and Brochstein, 1988; Hooks et al., 1991.

Cyclosporin

Cyclosporin (CyA) is a potent immunosuppressant, with little myelocytic toxicity, used in BMT to decrease the incidence and severity of GVHD (Furlong, 1993). CyA enhances the host tolerance of the allograft by selective inhibition of the resting T helper cells, and may secondarily also inhibit T suppressor cells (Ryffel et al., 1985; Sandoz Pharmaceuticals, 1994). Initially administered intravenously, CyA is given at doses of 2.5 mg to 5.0 mg/kg per day begin-

ning a day or two before marrow infusion. Therapy continues for several weeks until recovery from chemoradiotherapy-induced gastrointestinal toxicity (McGuire et al., 1988). At that time an oral form can be given, usually 5 mg to 10 mg/kg per day, with the dosage being tapered during the six months following transplantation (Vogelsang and Morris, 1993). The dosage of CyA may vary considerably across BMT centers.

Hepatic and renal toxicity are the most common side effects of CyA (Vogelsang and

Morris, 1993; Furlong, 1993; Palmer and Toto, 1991). Neurologic complications occur in 8 % to 29% of patients receiving this drug (Atkinson et al., 1984; Adams et al., 1987; DeGroen et al., 1987). Tremor, a reversible side effect that often appears within days of therapy initiation, occurs in 16% to 50% of patients. Seizures can occur in up to 19% of patients (Furlong, 1993); grand mal seizures have been reported in 5.5% of patients (Deierhoi et al., 1988). In addition, paresthesias have been documented in 29% of patients receiving CyA (McGuire et al., 1988), as well as quadriparesis, cerebellar ataxia, and coma (Atkinson et al., 1984; Deierhoi et al., 1988; Vogelsang and Morris, 1993). Burning dysesthesias of the palms of the hands and soles of the feet have also been documented (Berden et al., 1985). Mental status changes attributable to CyA include anxiety, confusion, amnesia, and visual hallucinations (Palmer and Toto, 1991; Katirji, 1987).

The mechanism of CyA-induced neurotoxicity is unclear (Reece et al., 1991). Factors thought to predispose to neurological symptoms, particularly seizures, include previous chemotherapy and irradiation, simultaneous administration of methylprednisolone, magnesium deficiency, concomitant hypertension, low cholesterol, and aluminum overload (Reece et al., 1991; Palmer and Toto, 1991). BMT patients receiving CyA are at risk for seizures related to previous chemotherapy and irradiation, which may lower their seizure threshold (Thomas et al., 1975; Walker and Brochstein, 1988; Ghany et al., 1991). The administration of the corticosteroid, methylprednisolone, in conjunction with CyA, in the treatment of GVHD is common practice. The neurological side effects of this drug are significant and will be discussed later.

Hypomagnesemia has been reported to be strongly associated with CyA neurotoxicity. CyA disrupts the tubular function, which re-

sults in renal magnesium wasting (June et al., 1985). The occurrence of grand mal seizures in patients on CyA is strongly associated with magnesium levels two standard deviations below normal values (Adams et al., 1987). Normalization of the magnesium levels usually results in cessation of the seizures. In addition, extremely high serum CyA levels were recorded at the onset of seizure activity (Deierhoi et al., 1988; Adams et al., 1987; Rubin and Kang, 1987).

Cyclosporin A is also documented to engender hypertension, presumably because hypomagnesemia is linked to hypertension (McGuire et al., 1988), and therefore, may result from CyA-induced hypomagnesemia (June et al., 1986). Fortunately, such hypertension may be amenable to pharmacological control. Another syndrome found in BMT patients consists of ataxia, tremor, and occasional paresis and mental status changes, in the absence of CT or EEG abnormalities (Atkinson et al., 1984). The etiology is postulated to be a reaction to CyA, either caused or enhanced by hypomagnesemia (Thompson et al., 1984).

Infrequently, a form of leukoencephalopathy (LEC) (described later) is caused by CyA. Clinical presentation shows confusion and cortical blindness, which may progress to coma (DeGroen et al., 1987). Pathologic white matter degeneration and EEG slowing are present. In summary, CyA-induced neurotoxicity remains a diagnosis of exclusion. Often multiple factors can be held responsible, as noted, as well as additional abnormal metabolic parameters and infection (Palmer and Toto, 1991).

The probability and severity of side effects are also related to CyA levels in the blood. A bolus dose of CyA, which causes a rapid increase in the serum level, will result in greater toxicity than a continuous infusion (Deierhoi et al., 1988; McGuire et al., 1988). Neurological sequelae of CyA therapy are usually not permanent. Withdrawal or reduction in dose of the drug usually results in the resolution of neurological complications, including severe encephalopathy (Walker and Brochstein, 1988). If seizure activity has been the reason for discontinuation of the drug, CyA administration can be reinstituted with careful monitoring by serial MRI examinations (Ghany et al., 1991).

Care of the patient receiving CyA includes preferably continuous administration of the drug and daily monitoring of magnesium levels, with magnesium replacement as necessary (Thompson et al., 1984). Cyclosporin levels should also be monitored at least weekly. Administration of CyA in a bolus dose, or to patients with poor renal function requires close neurological assessment, seizure precautions as necessary, and the monitoring of intake and output, weight, blood urea nitrogen, and creatinine levels.

The nurse must also be aware of drug-drug interactions, such as amphotericin B, aminoglycosides, and cisplatin, which can potentiate nephrotoxicity (Anonymous, 1988). In addition, some medications can increase (i.e., cimetidine, fluconazole, methylprednisolone, metoclopramide, verapamil) and others decrease (i.e., carbamazepine, phenobarbital, phenytoin, rifampin) serum CyA levels (Sandoz Pharmaceuticals, 1994).

Nurses are also responsible for frequent monitoring of vital signs, and administration of antihypertensive medication as needed is extremely important, because posttransplant BMT thrombocytopenia places the patient with high blood pressure at risk for intracranial bleeding. An assessment of the patient's mental state at baseline and prior to the administration of CyA is important. Continued periodic assessment of mental state, particularly if corticosteroids are also being administered, is vital to the early detection of neurologic side effects, and therefore early intervention.

Predischarge teaching should include avoiding refrigeration of oral cyclosporin, using open containers of CyA within 2 months, and preparing CyA in a glass container because the drug may stick to plastic (Arkey, 1995; Grebenau, personal communication, 1995). Additionally, eating foods high in magnesium (milk, yogurt, vegetables, nuts, and whole grains) is recommended (Ignatavicius et al., 1995). The importance of follow-up visits to monitor CyA levels, blood pressure, and renal function cannot be overemphasized.

Methotrexate

The most common agent in early clinical trials for GVHD prophylaxis, methotrexate (MTX), an antifolate metabolite, is now most often used in combination with CyA (Vogelsang and Morris, 1991). When given in combination with CyA, a short course of low-dose MTX is given which consists of 15 mg/m^2 on posttransplant day 1 and doses of 10 mg/m^2 posttransplant on days 3, 6, and 11, with CyA being continued for 6 months (Vogelsang and Morris, 1991; Ezzone and Camp-Sorrell, 1994).

Neurotoxicity is a well-documented complication, and may be acute or chronic, depending on the dose and route of administration (Balis and Poplack, 1989). Neurologic symptoms associated with intravenous high-dose methotrexate (HDMTX) include acute somnolence, fatigue, confusion, disorientation, seizures, and increased intracranial pressure during or after administration (Bleyer, 1988). Adults seem to have a higher incidence of HDMTX-induced sedation than children. Seizures have rarely been documented during infusion (Bleyer, 1977). The toxicity is thought to be mediated by lysis of tumor cells in the CNS, causing cerebral edema and is rapidly reversed by the administration of systemic corticoids (Bleyer, 1988).

High-dose MTX may also produce a strokelike syndrome in adults and children (Allen and Rosen, 1978; Bleyer, 1981; Walker et al., 1986), which typically occurs 5 to 6 days after completing a course of the drug (Walker and Brochstein, 1988). Patients present with an altered mental status, usually accompanied by hemiparesis and other focal findings, such as aphasia, dysarthria, and cranial nerve and gaze palsies (Bleyer, 1981; Walker and Brochstein, 1988). The signs may vacillate between alternate sides of the body. Without treatment, the syndrome resolves within 48 to 72 hours, and usually without residual effects or likelihood of recurrence during subsequent MTX treatments (Walker and Brochstein, 1988). The etiology and pathogenesis of this syndrome is unknown. CT scan and lumbar puncture results are normal; the only significant EEG finding is slowing (Walker and Brochstein, 1988).

Recipients of BMT for hematologic malignancy may be given a single dose of MTX intrathecally (IT-MTX) just prior to BMT (Walker and Brochstein, 1988). Acute effects of IT-MTX are manifested as aseptic meningitis, which occurs in approximately 10% of patients, and transverse myelopathy (Walker and Brochstein, 1988). Aseptic meningitis mimics bacterial meningitis but occurs soon after the injection, with symptoms of headache, photophobia, fever, meningismus, nausea and vomiting, and lethargy (Bleyer, 1977; 1981). The syndrome is self-limiting and symptoms resolve within a few days. Analgesia may be administered for headaches. Patients who develop meningitis do not necessarily experience the syndrome with subsequent injections (Walker and Brochstein, 1988). Risk factors for this syndrome have not been identified.

Transverse myelopathy occurs rarely, and is the result of multiple intrathecal injections (Bleyer, 1981; Gagliano and Costanzi, 1976). It presents within 48 hours of administration, but may be delayed for up to 2 weeks (Walker and Brochstein, 1988). CNS leukemia or prior irradiation may predispose patients to the myelopathy; other risk factors remain unclear

(Luddy and Gilman, 1973). By an unknown mechanism, the patient experiences back pain, which may or may not radiate to the legs. These symptoms are followed by a loss of sensation, bowel and bladder dysfunction, and paraplegia (Bleyer, 1981; Walker and Brochstein, 1988). Spinal cord necrosis without striking vascular or inflammatory change is seen (Skullerud and Halvorsen, 1978). While there is no treatment for this myelopathy, the symptoms are generally reversible after the drug is discontinued or the dosage reduced (Bleyer, 1988). This form of neurotoxicity appears to be related to the concentration and duration of MTX in the CNS (Pizzo et al., 1979).

Leukoencephalopathy, discussed later, is a delayed effect of MTX, and one with the most severe consequences. MTX-induced neurotoxicity seems limited to patients who undergo BMT for a hematologic malignancy who have been exposed to high CNS drug concentrations and previous irradiation (Walker and Brochstein, 1988; Balis and Poplack, 1989).

Nurses must be cognizant of the potential for neurotoxicity related to administration of MTX. Frequent neurologic assessments should be a daily part of patient care. When neurotoxicity from MTX is suspected or diagnosed, the drug should be discontinued, in favor of alternative therapies.

Corticosteroids

Glucocorticoids, including prednisone, methylprednisolone, and dexamethasone, are used to prevent and treat GVHD (Furlong, 1993). Direct adverse neurologic effects are primarily mental status changes. Indirect effects include CNS infection or superinfection and cardiovascular accidents (CVAs) related to steroid-induced hypertension (Walker and Brochstein, 1988; Furlong, 1993).

All of the drugs identified above have been implicated in causing neuropsychiatric side effects, with prednisone being most frequently implicated. The neuropsychiatric picture can range from one of mild euphoria to frank psychosis (Kershner and Wang-Cheng, 1989). The incidence of steroid-related major mental disturbances in patients without cancer ranges from 6% to 62%, with severe psychiatric reactions occurring only in about 5% of patients (Furlong, 1993). The most common clinically significant disturbances encountered are affective disorders, such as depression (40%), and mania (28%). Delirium occurs in 10% of patients with a typical picture of global cognitive impairment that may include hallucinations and delusions (Furlong, 1993). Symptoms such as anxiety, insomnia, tremor, nervousness, agitation, and euphoria/dysphoria are probably experienced by many patients and can go unnoticed by the medical and nursing team (Kershner and Wang-Cheng, 1989; Furlong, 1993).

Steroid psychosis, when present, correlates with the total dose, usually greater than 40 mg of prednisone daily (Greeves, 1984). Females are slightly more susceptible. Age, previous psychiatric illness, or previous steroid use do not suggest an increased risk for mental status changes or psychosis (Hall et al., 1979; Walker and Brochstein, 1988). These clinical manifestations can occur at any time during steroid treatment (Greeves, 1984). Withdrawal of the drug is the most effective way to treat these side effects, although the condition for which the steroids are being administered, and the necessity for a gradual tapering of the dose, might make this difficult (Walker and Brochstein, 1988). Side effects usually resolve rapidly with cessation of the steroids. If the drug must be continued, or a taper is in progress, symptoms can be treated with low-dose neuroleptics with a response usually occurring within a few days (Kershner and Wang-Cheng, 1989).

Steroid myopathy is characterized by symmetrical involvement of proximal muscles (Walker and Brochstein, 1988). Although a mild degree of weakness is seen in all patients receiving steroidal therapy for 2 to 3 weeks, prolonged administration is directly related to the severity of myopathy (Janssens and Decramer, 1989). Patients may be unable to rise from a chair, brush hair, or climb stairs, and the myopathy may progress to involve respiratory muscles (Walker and Brochstein, 1988).

Antithymocyte Globulin

Antithymocyte globulin (ATG) is a lymphocyte-selective immunosuppressant that can be used to prevent allogeneic bone marrow graft rejection (Malilay et al., 1989). ATG may also be added to the treatment regimen for GVHD when initial treatment with CyA and/or corticosteroids is unsuccessful (Vogelsang and Morris, 1991). Specific neurologic complications of ATG have not been documented. Headaches and seizures, as side effects, occur less than 5% of the time (Walker and Brochstein, 1988).

Monoclonal Antibody OKT3

Muromonab CD-3 (OKT3) is a monoclonal antibody that binds to post-thymic T lymphocytes, removing them from circulation. It is efficacious in both the prophylaxis and treatment of GVHD, as well as in the treatment of acute rejection after allogeneic BMT (Filipovich et al., 1987; Hooks et al., 1991). A complex of side effects usually occurs after the first and second injections, but subsides with subsequent doses. General neurologic side effects include headache, tremors, and myalgia. The incidence of headache and myalgia after the first exposure to OKT3 is 35% to 50% and 12% to 20%, respectively. After several exposures these incidences are 50% and 18%, respectively (Hooks et al., 1991). Tremors occur in 10% of recipients (Thistlethwaite et al., 1987; Walker and Brochstein, 1988). Premedication with methylprednisolone, acetaminophen, and an antihistamine has been administered in an attempt to avoid these early adverse effects and reactions by blocking the mediators that are released from T-lymphocyte lysis. Some patients have benefitted from this procedure (Hooks et al., 1991). The literature suggests that the doses of other immunosuppressive agents should be decreased during therapy with OKT3 (Hooks et al., 1991).

A CNS syndrome specifically associated with OKT3 has been identified (Walker and Brochstein, 1988; Hooks et al., 1991). A form of aseptic meningitis may occur 2 to 7 days after initiation of therapy (Roden et al., 1987; Thistlethwaite et al., 1987). Symptoms include fever, headache, photophobia, and meningismus. Generalized seizures have been reported (Thistlethwaite et al., 1987). This clinical syndrome resolves without residual effects or treatment in 2 to 3 days, and does not require the cessation of OKT3 therapy. The pathogenesis of the meningitis after the administration of OKT3 is uncertain (Hooks et al., 1991), and it is extremely important that it be distinguished from any serious CNS infection.

Azathioprine

Another drug used to prevent graft rejection and treat chronic GVHD is azathioprine, an immunosuppressive antimetabolite that is metabolized to mercaptopurine (Walker and Brochstein, 1988). Azathioprine suppresses cell-mediated hypersensitivities and alters antibody production as well as T-cell effects (Ezzone and Camp-Sorrell, 1994). Direct neurotoxic effects have not been seen with this drug.

Thalidomide

A new approach to the treatment of acute and chronic GVHD has been the use of thalidomide, which has an unknown mechanism of action. Patients with high-risk chronic GVHD and a projected actuarial life expectancy of

20% had an actuarial survival of 48% when treated with this drug (Vogelsang and Morris, 1991). Sedation is a common side effect of thalidomide. However, patients report adjusting to their sedation, with only a small number requiring dosage adjustment or withdrawal of the drug (Altimonte, 1993). Other neurotoxic side effects reported include peripheral neuropathy, paresthesias, and nocturnal muscle cramps (Vogelsang et al., 1992; Lopez et al., 1993).

Summary

It is evident from this discussion that transplant patients are at substantial risk for the development of neurotoxic side effects from immunosuppressive agents. These effects are magnified when the patient is receiving two or more of these therapies simultaneously. Fortunately, the majority of these complications are reversible and respond to drug withdrawal or dosage modification. Early recognition of these neurologic toxicities is paramount if unneeded physical and emotional discomfort for the patient is to be prevented or ameliorated.

NEUROLOGICAL EFFECTS OF OTHER MEDICATIONS

A variety of other medications are frequently administered to BMT patients for the purposes of symptom management and patient comfort. These include antiemetic, analgesic, anxiolytic, antidepressant, and antipsychotic (neuroleptic) agents as well as biological response modifiers (BRM). All of these classes of drugs hold potential for neurological side effects and more adverse neurotoxic reactions (*The Medical Letter*, 1993).

Antiemetic Agents

The pharmacological management of treatment-induced nausea and vomiting employs a variety of antiemetic agents. Use of these agents is not without neurotoxic effects. Prochlorperazine is a phenothiazine that blocks the chemoreceptor trigger zone, which in turn acts upon the vomiting center. Neurological side effects include sedation, fatigue, akathesia, tremors, and extrapyramidal reactions that can result in the appearance of sleeplessness and agitation (Cleri, 1995). Metoclopramide increases peristalsis without stimulating secretions. This drug has a pattern of neurotoxic side effects similar to prochlorperazine. In rare instances it can cause depression. Metoclopramide is contraindicated if the patient has a history of seizure disorder (Cleri, 1995).

The most recent development in antiemetic therapy has been the use of the serotonin antagonists ondansetron and granisetron. These drugs block the serotonin receptors in both the brain and the GI tract. They differ in their chemical structures, pharmacokinetics, and effective doses and potencies (Cleri, 1995). Headache is a side effect common to both drugs. In addition, patients who take granisetron may experience asthenia and somnolence (Cleri, 1995).

The benzodiazepine lorazepam has long been valued for its antiemetic properties. Neurologic side effects include sedation, anterograde amnesia, feelings of detachment, confusion, dizziness, weakness, unsteadiness, and disorientation. Rebound insomnia or anxiety can also occur. Headache, confusion, depression, or paradoxical rage reactions are rare occurrences (Malseed and Harrigan, 1989; Cleri, 1995; Ezzone and Camp-Sorrell, 1994). Cautious use of benzodiazepines is advised because of their addictive properties.

Analgesic Agents

Numerous analgesic agents are used in the management of pain experienced by BMT patients. Often these agents are also used as pre-

medication to manage the side effects of therapies such as amphotericin or biological response modifiers. The neurologic side effects of analgesics are well known, but worth a brief review.

The frequently used opioids (i.e., morphine sulfate, meperidine hydrochloride, and hydromorphone hydrochloride) depress the pain impulse or increase the pain threshold (hydromorphone); all act as CNS depressants (Ezzone and Camp-Sorrell, 1994). Sedation is the most common effect, although it is less profound with hydromorphone. Mental clouding, dizziness, euphoria, and changes in mood may also occur. In addition, administration of meperidine may result in anxiety, tremors, and myoclonis (Malseed and Harrigan, 1989). Many of these side effects can be dose related. An effective plan of pain management may eliminate the need for the high doses or polypharmacy that can result in the more serious neurotoxic reactions.

Anxiolytic Agents

The benzodiazepines are thought to exert their effects through potentiation of the inhibitory neurotransmitter gamma-aminobutyric acid. They reduce anxiety with less drowsiness than the barbiturates or other sedative-hypnotics. Examples include lorazepam, alprazolam, diazepam, and chlordiazepoxide. Other drugs of this class, for example triazolam and flurazepam, are frequently used for sedation at bedtime.

The most common neurologic side effects are sedation, somnolence, confusion, and motor incoordination. These are dose-dependent effects which disappear with the modification of dosage. The sedative affects can be additive when used with other CNS depressants (Massie and Lesko, 1990). Excessive doses can result in stupor, coma, and death. With long-term use, withdrawal symptoms occur if the drug is suddenly discontinued. Therefore, a tapered discontinuation of the benzodiazepines is recommended.

Antidepressant Agents

Antidepressant agents are often used for BMT patients to treat either a reactive depression (in response to the stress of the diagnosis of cancer and its treatment) or a preexisting depression. The most frequent antidepressant agents given to cancer patients are the tricyclic and second-generation antidepressants.

The tricyclics inhibit the reuptake of the neurotransmitter norepinephrine and include amitriptyline, imipramine, and nortriptyline. The common neurologic side effects of the tricyclics are drowsiness, sedation, and orthostatic hypotension. In addition, the anticholinergic effects of these drugs can worsen such conditions as stomatitis and GVHD. The possibility of lowering the seizure threshold also exists with the administration of the tricyclic antidepressants, although desipramine and doxepin are less likely to have this effect (Massie and Lesko, 1990). The neurologic side effects of these drugs are evident as soon as therapy begins, whereas the therapeutic effects do not become apparent until 2 to 3 weeks after initiation of treatment.

The second-generation antidepressants have many of the same neurologic side effects as the tricyclics. They include drowsiness, dizziness, fatigue, and orthostatic hypotension. In addition, fluoxetine, a selective serotonin reuptake inhibitor, may produce neurologic side effects of insomnia, anxiety, mania, and depersonalization (*The Medical Letter*, 1993). Trazodone and fluoxetine are second generation antidepressants.

Sympathomimetic stimulants, such as dextroamphetamine, have also been used for the treatment of depression and opioid-induced sedation in cancer patients, particularly those who are terminally ill. These drugs can provide safe, rapid relief from depressive symptoms in patients for whom tricyclic antidepressants are contraindicated (Massey and Lesko, 1990). Neurotoxic effects include anxiety, manic symptoms, agitation, paranoia, hallucinations, and bizarre behavior. These effects are dose related. Depression can occur with withdrawal of these drugs (*The Medical Letter*, 1993).

Antipsychotic Agents

The antipsychotic agents most commonly prescribed in the cancer setting are the butyrophenones (haloperidol) and phenothiazines (chlorpromazine, mesoridazine, thioridazine, perphenazine, and trifluoperazine). Primarily used to treat psychotic disorders, their use with cancer patients experiencing acute psychosis or psychoticlike symptoms with delirium has been found to be efficacious. The common neurologic side effects of these drugs include acute dystonia, akathesia, and a parkinsonian syndrome consisting of tremor and rigidity. These extrapyramidal effects rarely require discontinuation of the drug; they can be managed with the administration of diphenhydramine or benztropine (Massey and Lesko, 1990).

Biological Response Modifiers

The neurotoxic effects of biological response modifiers (BRM) have drawn increasing attention as the use of these agents in cancer treatment has continued to increase. The classification *biological response modifier* includes the interferons (alpha, beta, and gamma), erythropoietin (Epo), granulocyte-macrophage colony-stimulating factor (GM-CSF), granulocyte colony-stimulating factor (G-CSF), monoclonal antibodies, and interleukin-2. These agents, particularly the interferons and interleukin-2, have many constitutional side effects, including both acute and chronic neurotoxicities (Rumsey and Rieger, 1992). These effects may begin subtly, are cumulative and dose related (Meyers et al., 1991; Shelton and Sargent, 1990), and vary in their intensity and impairment of functioning. Minor effects include slowed thinking, decreased concentration, and memory loss; major effects include somnolence, disorientation, and confusion (Rumsey and Rieger, 1992).

One review of clinical studies of the interferons and interleukin-2 describes the cognitive dysfunction associated with these therapies (Bender, 1994). Symptoms of memory loss, disorientation, attentional and concentrational deficits, and difficulties with abstract thinking and decision making were reported. These symptoms have obvious implications for the patient's ability to participate in self-care and in treatment decision making.

Additional neurologic effects of alpha interferon and interleukin-2 have been identified. Patients receiving alpha interferon have reported loss of initiative and diminished motivation, in addition to vague feelings of anxiety and a sense of depression (Forman, 1994). The neuropsychiatric effects of interleukin-2 include severe behavioral changes that might necessitate neuroleptic treatment and physical restraints. Early indications of neurotoxicity include lethargy, memory disturbance, and irritability with variable disorientation (Forman, 1994). Seizures are a rare, though reported, occurrence. Although these symptoms usually respond to the withdrawal of the agent or dosage adjustment, neurotoxicities may persist for months after treatment is discontinued (Meyers et al., 1991). Table 13.4 identifies the common biological response modifying agents, their actions and uses, and their neurologic side effects.

Early identification and management of BRM neurotoxicities have implications for the continuation of what may be an important

TABLE 13.4 Neurological effects of biological response modifiers

Agent	Action and use	Neurologic complications
Interferon alpha beta	Biologic properties not entirely understood; have antiviral, antiproliferative and immunomodulatory effects. Alpha derived from lymphocytes; beta derived from fibroblasts.	Headache, lethargy, cognitive changes, myalgias, confusion, impaired memory, anxiety, sense depression, sleep disturbances, decreased concentration
gamma	Derived from T lymphocytes Same effects as alpha and beta	Headache, myalgias
Erythropoietin	Stimulates the mitotic activity of erythroid progenitor cells and early precursor cells in the bone marrow, increasing red blood cell production	Hypertension, seizures
Granulocyte colony-stimulating factor	Stimulates the growth of neutrophil colonies and affects mature neutrophil functions Clinical trials to study the enhancement of repopulation of bone marrow	Rare neurological side effects
Granulocyte-macrophage colony-stimulating factor	Stimulates the production of neutrophil and monocyte colonies; treatment of neutropenia	Occasional alterations of mental status, headaches, myalgias
Interleukin-2	Activates multiple classes of cytolytic leukocytes	Mental status changes, headaches, lethargy, irritability, myalgias, personality and behavior changes

SOURCE: From Weiss, 1993; Rumsey and Rieger, 1992; Forman, 1994; Bender, 1994; Meyers et al., 1991.

component of the treatment regimen. The subtle development of these effects requires close observation of patients receiving these agents, beginning with baseline and ongoing assessment of their neurological functioning. The baseline assessment should include attention to personality and coping style, substance use, sleep patterns, mental status, and headache history Ongoing assessment of mental status and sleep cycle should be conducted (Shelton and Sargent, 1990).

LEUKOENCEPHALOPATHY

Leukoencephalopathy (LEC) is a degenerative lesion occurring in the white matter of the CNS in up to 17% of patients who receive cranial irradiation and intrathecal chemotherapy (Winick et al., 1993). The onset may be within days or months of BMT. A JC polyomavirus is the suspected cause of the demyelination in immunosuppressed patients (Boerman et al., 1993; Kitamura et al., 1994).

Leukoencephalopathy is characterized by severe neurologic degeneration resulting in permanent neurologic disability or death (Sakami et al., 1993). Clinically, LEC presents as lethargy, slurred speech, ataxia, seizures, confusion, dysphagia, akinetic mutism, spasticity, aphasia, decerebrate posturing, and coma. A concomitant parkinsonian syndrome has also been described (Halperin et al., 1994; Lockman et al., 1991; Miyatake et al., 1992).

The development of LEC is most closely associated with prophylactic and/or therapeutic CNS treatment both before and after transplant. The treatment usually involves cranial irradiation in combination with intrathecal methotrexate (IT-MTX) and/or high-dose intravenous methotrexate (HDMTX) pretransplant, and usually IT-MTX post transplant (Halperin et al., 1994; Mohrmann et al., 1990; Thompson et al., 1986). Combination of these

treatments increases the risk (Halperin et al., 1994). Administration of MTX after total body irradiation contributes directly to the development of LEC (Johnson et al., 1987). In addition, cerebrospinal clearance of MTX may be altered in patients with ALL who have CNS involvement, thus increasing the risk of injury (Halperin et al., 1994).

The development of LEC is also related to the following: BMT patients who have acute lymphoblastic leukemia as the underlying disease and an age under 15 years, presumably due to brain immaturity at the time of radiation treatment (Fernandez-Bouzas et al., 1992). LEC in the patient with acute nonlymphocytic leukemia is rare (Davis and Patchell, 1988). An association with disseminated varicella-zoster infection prior to the development of progressive multifocal LEC has been reported (Hooper et al., 1982).

Benzyl alcohol was found not to be a causative factor in the development of LEC (Price and Jamieson, 1975). However, because benzyl alcohol has documented neurotoxic effects (Conrad, 1986; Norrell et al., 1974), its use in reconstituting MTX should be avoided. Alternatively, Elliott's B solution may be used (Humphrey et al., 1979). Combining MTX with hydrocortisone (Humphrey et al., 1979) and using a standard dose of MTX in patients 3 years and older may help decrease the neurotoxicity (Bleyer, 1977). A MTX dose based on body surface area is discouraged in persons older than 3 years because cerebrospinal fluid volume is constant after that age. Additionally, judicious use of radiation therapy is essential to prevent relapse and minimize the potential for development of devastating LEC (Thompson et al., 1986).

VASCULAR COMPLICATIONS

Mineralizing microangiopathy causes dystrophic calcification of CNS grey matter (Davis et al., 1986). This degeneration is usually apparent approximately 10 months after radiation and chemotherapy, and occurs much more frequently than LEC. Identified risk factors for the development of this dystrophy include a young age (less than 10 years at the time of radiation), duration of survival after chemo- and radiotherapy, and the number of CNS leukemic relapses after radiation therapy (Price, 1979). The clinical manifestations are less evident than those of LEC, and include focal seizures, poor muscle coordination, perceptual motor disability, and behavioral disorders (Packer et al., 1987).

Mineralizing microangiopathy causes permanent destructive changes in the brain, apparently affecting neuropsychological functioning. Use of IT-MTX, IV-MTX, and cranial irradiation in various combinations seem to impair short-term memory, the speed of mental processing, and the acquisition of new knowledge. IQ scores tend to be below the mean (Mulhern et al., 1992) and as the posttreatment time interval increases, drops in IQ scores may become more severe, particularly in very young children (Halperin et al., 1994).

Risk for neuropsychological impairment is increased for the youngest children treated for ALL and if whole brain irradiation is employed (Halperin et al., 1994). Because mineralizing microangiopathy is not easily controlled, neurologic examinations are important for all patients who receive radiation therapy and chemotherapy, especially those at high risk.

Cerebrovascular complications, the third most common neurologic complication, have been found in 6% to 28% of patients undergoing BMT (Mohrmann et al., 1990, 1987; Patchell et al., 1985a; Wiznitzer et al., 1984). Subarachnoid hemorrhages and infarcts occur with equal frequency. Interestingly, parenchymal hemorrhages are rare, despite extremely low platelet counts in all transplant patients (Davis and Patchell, 1988). Subdural hematomas have a relatively benign clinical outcome, in contrast to intracerebral hematomas, which tend to be lethal (Pomeranz et al., 1994).

Cerebral infarcts are most commonly associated with endocarditis (Patchell, 1985). BMT recipients have a higher incidence of developing endocarditis than those with similar diseases who do not undergo BMT, most likely resulting from the additive effects of prior chemotherapy and radiotherapy (Wiznitzer et al., 1984).

Cerebrovascular accidents due to non-bacterial thrombotic endocarditis (NBTE) are an important cause of morbidity in BMT recipients. Emboli to the CNS and heart may also manifest as seizures and focal neurologic or myocardial dysfunction (Fayemi, 1976; Kookier et al., 1976). Monitoring of the DIC screen, especially fibrinogen and fibrin degradation product, may aid in the diagnosis, and treatment with anticoagulation may prevent the associated morbidity (Jerman and Fick, 1986).

NEUROLOGIC COMPLICATIONS OF GRAFT-VERSUS-HOST DISEASE

Involvement of the CNS in GVHD has been suggested by microscopic changes in the brain and neurologic symptomatology coinciding with the development of systemic chronic GVHD (Iwasaki et al., 1993; Kajiwara et al., 1991). Acute GVHD is not associated with neurologic dysfunction, therefore, this section will be devoted to the neurologic manifestations of chronic GVHD.

Chronic GVHD is the result of a cell-mediated response of donor lymphocytes against host antigens (Iwasaka et al., 1993; Nelson and McQuillen, 1988). The cell-mediated and humoral limbs of the immune system are both impaired, and may give rise to myositis, myasthenia gravis, and Guillain-Barré syndrome.

Myositis

Myositis, like chronic GVHD, is more common in older patients (Miller, 1994; Slatkin et al., 1987). It has not been seen in autologous or syngeneic BMT recipients (Nelson and Mc-Quillen, 1988); neither are these populations at risk for developing GVHD. Those at greatest risk have undergone BMT for aplastic anemia (Slatkin et al., 1987).

The muscle is a target organ in GVHD. Autoantibodies to tRNA-associated proteins are believed to be the cause of myositis (Gelpi et al., 1994). Often symmetrical and proximal moderate to severe muscle weakness of trunk, neck, and extremities is the remarkable clinical presentation, which is indistinguishable from idiopathic polymyositis in symptomatology, pathology, and serology (Nelson and McQuillen, 1988; Plotz et al., 1995; Urbano-Marquez et al., 1986). In most cases, administration of steroids may improve strength. Azathioprine and MTX have also been used with some efficacy (Mastaglia et al., 1993).

The progression or resolution of chronic GVHD is the most important factor in determining the severity of the myositis (Nelson and McQuillen, 1988). If the chronic GVHD improves, the muscle weakness resolves proportionately; and the converse is true.

Care of the patient with myositis focuses on safety. Teaching patients and family the etiology of the weakness and ensuring that the patient ambulates or gets out of bed only with assistance is very important. Encouraging range-of-motion exercises and fostering as much independence in self-care as possible are essential for physical and psychological coping.

Myasthenia Gravis

A rare complication of chronic GVHD, myasthenia gravis is the result of an antibody-mediated response specifically against the ace-tylcholine receptor (Grau et al., 1990). The presentation is very similar to the autoimmune variety of myasthenia gravis. Symptoms include dysarthria, ptosis, diplopia, dysphagia, dysarthria, fatigue, and weakness of facial and limb muscles (Bolger et al., 1986; Hopkins, 1994; Shimoda et al., 1994). It may progress to involve the muscles of respiration, causing dyspnea and ultimately leading to failure.

Treatment with corticosteroids, immunosuppressants, and acetylcholine esterase inhibitors is appropriate (Melms et al., 1994; Shimoda et al., 1994). Respiratory failure may necessitate intubation. Plasmapheresis and continued drug therapy have been successful in reversing the condition, allowing extubation (Hopkins, 1994). The cessation of immunosuppressive therapy may precipitate a return of myasthenic symptoms (Shimoda et al., 1994). In some cases, patients can be maintained on low doses of immunosuppressive therapy.

Several risk factors for the development of myasthenia gravis in patients with chronic GVHD have been identified. These include having aplastic anemia as the underlying disease, BMT donors of the opposite sex, and the abrupt cessation of immunosuppressive therapy (Melms et al., 1994; Shimoda et al., 1994).

Nursing care for patients with myasthenia gravis includes teaching the importance of compliance with medication regimes, and encouragement to seek immediate medical attention in the event of any abnormal neurological symptoms. Safety precautions and frequent neurologic examinations are important. Psychological support for the patient and family may facilitate coping with this setback. Creative methods of communication with the intubated patient are also a necessity.

Guillain-Barré Syndrome

Guillain-Barré syndrome has been observed following both autologous and allogeneic BMT, and appears to be associated with a precipitating viral or bacterial infection and/or altered immune function (Hagensee et al., 1994; Myers and Williams, 1994; Perry et al., 1994). It is believed that Guillain-Barré syndrome, an autoimmune disorder, is initiated when EBV- or CMV-infected B cells proliferate under conditions of depressed T cell function (Myers and Williams, 1994).

The symptoms include progressive motor dysfunction in the proximal and distal lower extremities, which may result in inability to ambulate, urinary incontinence, ataxia, and stocking and glove sensory deficit (Hagensee et al., 1994; Myers and Williams, 1994; Perry et al., 1994). Immunoglobulin administration and plasma exchange are the treatments of choice, as well as ventilatory support when necessary (Hagensee et al., 1994; Myers and Williams, 1994; Perry et al., 1994).

Peripheral Nerve Complications

Peripheral nerve infections with herpes zoster have been reported (Graze and Gale, 1979; Wiznitzer et al., 1984). However, inflammatory disease of peripheral nerves is a rare, if ever, clinically recognized complication of GVHD (Nelson and McQuillen, 1988).

Reflex sympathetic dystrophy (RSD) is another infrequent neurovascular disorder that affects the joints and adjacent skin. It is believed that sympathetic nervous system irritation, together with immobilization and inadequate venous and lymphatic drainage, cause a local sympathetic axon reflex, giving rise to the syndrome. Manifestations include burning pain and swelling in the feet and ankles with dyshidrosis and an inability to walk. Treatment with pamidronate or calcitonin, osteoclast inhibitors seems to alleviate the symptoms. There is no established way to prevent RSD. In light of this, it is essential to prevent immobility in BMT patients, whether by getting out of bed, using an exercise bike, or regular physical therapy (Stamatoullas et al., 1993).

NEOPLASTIC RECURRENCE AND SECONDARY MALIGNANCY

One of the major causes of treatment failure in allogeneic BMT for acute leukemia is a recurrence of the leukemia, which occurs in 5% to 75% of patients, depending on their relative risk for relapse (Kantarjian, 1994: Kelch et al., 1990; Mohrmann et al., 1990). Generally, the risk of relapse is greatest in patients with advanced disease who undergo transplantation.

Acute lymphoblastic leukemia is associated with a higher rate of CNS relapse (approximately 13%) than acute nonlymphoblastic leukemia (approximately 2%) (Thompson et al., 1986). Relapse of leukemia after BMT generally represents a failure of the preparative chemotherapy or TBI to eradicate the patient's leukemic clone, or may be a continued leukemogenic stimuli of the patient's cells on donor cells (Ganem et al., 1989; Kelch et al., 1990). The CNS may be the site of relapse, regardless of whether the patient had previous CNS involvement. CNS leukemia may also cause systemic relapse (Bleyer, 1989; Creutzig et al., 1993).

While chemotherapy and radiotherapy are important in bone marrow ablation prior to transplantation, they impose a risk that patients will develop a secondary malignancy (Sullivan et al., 1992). The etiology seems to be multifactorial and includes the preparative chemoradiotherapy, immunosuppression, Epstein-Barr virus (EBV) infection and GVHD (Lishner et al., 1990; Lowsky et al., 1994; Ochs, 1989; Sullivan et al., 1994). The latency period of these secondary malignancies is variable, with development a short time after BMT for leukemias and lymphomas, to years for the development of solid tumors. The age-adjusted risk is nearly seven times as great as that for the general population (Milliken and Powles, 1995).

The incidence of secondary malignancy following BMT is approximately 12% (Lowsky et al., 1994) and the consequences are grave. The mortality rate exceeds 90% in patients who develop non-Hodgkin's lymphoma associated with EBV infection and 75% in those with solid tumors, despite treatment (Witherspoon et al., 1994). Following BMT for the treatment of a hematologic malignancy, patients have developed leukemia of donor cell origin, lymphoproliferative disorders including Hodgkin's disease, and solid tumors such as glioblastoma multiforme, adenocarcinoma, melanoma, and squamous cell carcinoma (Deeg et al., 1984; Lishner et al., 1990; Ochs, 1989; Sullivan et al., 1992).

Total body irradiation may play a role in the development of solid tumors following BMT (Ochs, 1989; Sullivan et al., 1992). Gliomas are the most common form of secondary malignancy following radiation therapy in children; meningiomas are the most common in adults (Ochs, 1989). Secondary gliomas are multifocal in origin and their abrupt clinical manifestation is characterized by seizures, increased intracranial pressure, or significant motor disability (Ochs, 1989). Carcinomas may develop in radiation ports (such as the thyroid, basal cell, and parotid gland) of children who have undergone previous radiation therapy (Ochs, 1989).

The development of GVHD may be both protective and a risk factor for developing a secondary malignancy. GVHD is well recognized as having a graft-versus-leukemia effect through adoptive cellular immunity and thus is responsible for preventing relapse (Horowitz et al., 1990; Sullivan et al., 1989). However, when GVHD is treated with ATG or a CD3 monoclonal antibody, the risk of a secondary malignancy is increased (Sullivan et al., 1992).

Patients and families must be made aware of the potential for secondary malignancy or relapse following transplantation, and the importance of frequent medical checkups. Emotional support must be offered to the patient and family if relapse or secondary malignancy occur. If the prognosis is poor, hospice care may be appropriate.

NURSING CARE

The nursing care of the BMT or BCT patient requires a knowledge of the actual and potential etiologies of transplant-related neurological complications. Considerations basic to the provision of nursing care are listed in Table 13.5. The patient is at risk for such complications across the trajectory of the transplant experience. By the nature of this intensive treatment approach, all aspects of the treatment itself, as well as the management of symptomatic responses to and complications of the BMT process hold neurotoxic risk. In addition, certain preexisting characteristics of the patient and cancer treatment received prior to transplant may increase that individual's risk for neurologic difficulties during the transplant process. Neuropsychologic impairment is present in a significant minority of adult BMT candidates, and the risk of further impairment increases with the number of risk factors present (Andrykowski et al., 1992). Table 13.6 identifies factors that place the patient at risk for neurologic complications.

In view of the vulnerability of BMT patients to neurologic difficulties, it is imperative that the primary focus of care be early detection of neurologic dysfunction. Early intervention with respect to those effects which are treatable is the most efficacious management of neurologic complications.

Assessment

The assessment of risk factors and neurocognitive functioning should begin at the time of admission for transplant, and continue, at regu-

TABLE 13.5 Nursing care of the BMT patient with neurologic complications

1. Knowledge of the potential etiologies of neurotoxicity, as the basis for ongoing patient assessment and evaluation, can prevent or lessen the impact of neurotoxicities.
2. Baseline neurological and mental status assessments are important aspects of the patient's admission process.
3. Continued awareness of neurotoxicities, the cumulative effects of the BMT therapy, and regimens of symptom management are imperative.
4. Ongoing assessments of neurological and mental status and behavioral change are required across the BMT trajectory.
5. Provisions must be made for the comfort and safety of patients experiencing these toxicities.
6. If toxicities are severe, exploration of modifications of therapy is needed, such as withdrawal of drugs or dosage modification.

TABLE 13.6 Risk factors for neurologic complications

Preexisting Factors
Prior central nervous system disease/events
Pretransplant therapies—cranial radiation, intrathecal chemotherapy
History of drug dependence
Older age

Pretransplant Conditioning
Total body irradiation
Chemotherapy regimen

Transplant Trajectory
Use of immunosuppressive agents
Long-term immunosuppression
Prophylactic antimicrobial therapy

Complications and/or Symptom Management
Mucositis—opioid management of pain
Nausea and vomiting—metabolic changes, antiemetics
Fluid and electrolyte imbalances
Infection
Additional antimicrobial therapy for infection
Acute renal failure—encephalopathy
Veno-occlusive disease—encephalopathy
Acute graft-vs-host disease—immunosuppressant agents, corticosteroids, possible hepatic failure, possible fluid and electrolyte imbalances
Interstitial pneumonia—hypoxia
Anxiety, depression—anxiolytics, antidepressants
Sleep deprivation—sedatives
Multisystem organ failure

SOURCE: Adapted from Ezzone and Camp-Sorrell, 1994; Freedman et al., 1990; Ford and Eisenberg, 1990.

lar intervals, throughout the transplant process. A comprehensive assessment includes review of neurologic risk factors, a comprehensive neurological examination, and a mental status examination that includes general appearance, speech, affect and mood, thought processes and content, perceptions, abstract thinking, judgment, insight, and cognitive function.

Aspects of cognitive function to be assessed include orientation, registration, attention span, short-term and long-term memory, problem-solving ability, and use of language (Wise and Rundell, 1994; Fincannon, 1995). Many screening tests exist for the evaluation of cognitive function (Baker, 1989; Hilton 1991). The Mini-Mental State Examination is widely used for baseline assessment and initial cognitive screening (Folstein et al., 1975). It is also important to interview, at the time of admission and throughout the process, the patient's family and significant others regarding their percep-

tions of this individual's behavior and any changes that occur. Family members are often the first to observe the more subtle symptoms of neurologic complications and their observations can play a vital role in the early recognition of such difficulties. A comprehensive standard of practice for the assessment of the patient with cognitive impairment has been developed (Zimberg and Berenson, 1990).

Intervention

A nursing care plan that addresses actual or potential sequelae of BMT-related neurologic complications may include potential for injury, altered thought processes, impaired communication, sensory-perceptual alterations, pain, fatigue, anxiety, impaired physical mobility, self-care deficits, low self-esteem, social isolation, and ineffective individual coping (Furlong, 1993; Rumsey and Rieger, 1992; Zimberg and Berenson, 1990; Fincannon, 1995). In addition, the family may also experience coping difficulties, and both family and patient may experience a knowledge deficit regarding the neurologic toxicities experienced (Zimberg and Berenson, 1990).

Plan of Care

If neurologic complications occur, nursing efforts must be directed at safety and teaching patients and families measures to preserve and support independence in self care. An interdisciplinary approach that involves physical and occupational therapy may be necessary to optimize the patient's functioning. Long-term follow-up consisting of ongoing intervention and emotional support is important if the patient and family are to achieve an optimal level of function and healthy adaptation to any ongoing neurocognitive limitations. It is important to develop a plan of care that represents an individualized approach to the patient with actual or potential neurologic disturbances.

SUMMARY

The process of BMT and BCT holds much neurotoxic risk for patients. Infection, vascular complications, metabolic imbalances, GVHD, CNS relapse, and secondary CNS malignancy represent potential complications or sequelae with profound neurologic implications. In addition, the therapies initiated to prevent or combat these complications and their symptoms, antimicrobial therapy, immunosuppressive agents, antiemetic, analgesic, anxiolytic, antidepressant, and antipsychotic agents and biological response modifiers, also have a high potential for neurotoxicity.

As the number of transplant recipients increases, the likelihood of neurologic complications increases. A review of the literature reveals an increase in medical and nursing research related to the biopsychosocial sequelae of transplant, some of which is focused on the neurologic sequelae (Whedon and Ferrell, 1994). Neurotoxicity can have a significant impact on an individual's ability to engage in self-care (Cammermeyer, 1983), and thus threaten that individual's independent functioning and subsequent quality of life. Nurses must be alert to these potential complications, and through assessment and nursing interventions, including patient and family teaching, prevent or diminish their effects.

REFERENCES

Adams, D.H., Ponsford, S., Gunson, B., et al. 1987. Neurological complications following liver transplantation. *Lancet* 1:949-951.

Allen, J.C., Rosen, G. 1978. Transient cerebral dysfunction following chemotherapy for osteogenic sarcoma. *Ann Neurol* 3:441-444.

Altimonte, V. 1993. Use of thalidomide for CGVHD defended. *Oncol Nurs Forum* 20(3):428.

Anderlini, P., Przepiorka, D., Luna, M., et al. 1994. *Acanthamoeba* meningoencephalitis after bone marrow transplantation. *BMT* 14:459-461.

Andrykowski, M., Schmitt, F.A., Gregg, M.E., et al. 1992. Neuropsychologic impairment in adult bone marrow transplant candidates. *Cancer* 70(9):2288-2297.

Anonymous. 1988. Cyclosporin. *Austral Nurs J* 18(1): 29-30.

Arkey, R. 1995. *Physician's Desk Reference*. Montvale, NJ: Medical Economics Co., 973.

Atkinson, K, Biggs, J, Darveniza, P., et al. 1984. Cyclosporin-associated central nervous system toxicity after allogeneic bone marrow transplantation. *Transplantation* 38:34-37.

Baker, F.M. 1989. Screening tests for cognitive impairment. *Hosp & Commun Psychiatr* 40(4):339-340.

Balis, F.M., Poplack, D.G. 1989. Central nervous system pharmacology of antileukemic drugs. *Am J Pediatr Hematol Oncol* 11(1):74-86.

Bashir, R.M., Bierman, P., McComb, R. 1992. Inflammatory peripheral neuropathy following high dose chemotherapy and autologous bone marrow transplantation. *BMT* 10:305-306.

Bender, C. 1994. Cognitive dysfunction associated with biological response modifier therapy. *Oncol Nurs Forum* 21(3):515-523.

Berden, J.H.M., Hoitsma, A.J., Merx, J.L., et al. 1985. Severe central nervous system toxicity associated with cyclosporin. (letter). *Lancet* 1:219-220.

Bernauer, W., and Gratwohl, A. 1992. Bone marrow retinitis. (letter). *Am J Ophthalmol* 113(5):604.

Bleyer, W.A. 1977. Clinical pharmacology of intrathecal methotrexate, II: an improved dosage regimen derived from age-related pharmacokinetics. *Cancer Treat Rep* 61:1419-1425.

Bleyer, W.A. 1981. Neurologic sequelae of methotrexate and ionizing radiation: a new classification. *Cancer Treat Rep* 65(suppl 1):89-98.

Bleyer, W.A. 1988. Central nervous system leukemia. *Pediatr Clin North Am* 35:789-814.

Bleyer, W.A. 1989. Biology and pathogenesis of CNS leukemia. *Am J Pediatr Hematol Oncol* 11(1):57-63.

Boerman, R.H., Bax, J.J., Beekhuis-Brussee, J.A. 1993. JC virus and multiple sclerosis: a refutation? *Acta Neurolog Scandinav* 87(5):353-355.

Bolger, B.J., Sullivan, K.M., Spence, A.M., et al. 1986. Myasthenia gravis after allogeneic bone marrow transplantation: relationship to chronic graft vs. host disease. *Neurology* 36(8):1087-1091.

Callaham, M. 1989. Fulminant bacterial meningitis without meningeal sign. *Ann Emerg Med* 8(1):90-93.

Cammermeyer, M. 1983. A growth model of self care for neurologically impaired people. *J Neurosurg Nurs* 15:299-305.

Christie, D., Battin, M., Leiper, A.D., et al. 1994. Neuropsychological and neurologic outcome after relapse of lymphoblastic leukaemia. *Arch Dis Childhood* 70(4):275-280.

Cleri, L. 1995. Serotonin antagonists: state of the art management of chemotherapy-induced emesis. *Oncol Nurs: Patient Treat & Supp* 2(1):1-19.

Conrad, K.J. 1986. Cerebellar toxicities associated with cytosine arabinoside: a nursing perspective. *Oncol Nurs Forum* 13:57-59.

Creutzig, U., Ritter, J., Zimmermann, M., et al. 1993. Does cranial irradiation reduce the risk for bone marrow relapse in acute myelogenous leukemia? Unexpected results of the childhood acute myelogenous study BFM-87. *J Clin Oncol* 11(2):279-286.

D'Antonio, D., Di Bartolomeo, P., Iacone, A., et al. 1992. Meningitis due to penicillin-resistant *Streptococcus pneumoniae* in patients with chronic graft-versus-host disease. *BMT* 9:299-300.

Davis, D., Henslee, P.J., Markesbery, W.R. 1988. Fatal adenovirus meningoencephalitis in a bone marrow transplant patient. *Ann Neurol* 23:385-389.

Davis, D., Patchell, R.A. 1988. Neurologic complications of bone marrow transplantation. *Neurol Clin* 6:377-387.

Davis, P.C., Hoffman, J.C. Jr., Pearl, G.S., et al. 1986. CT evaluation of effects of cranial radiation therapy in children. *Am J Reontgenol* 147(3):587-592.

Deeg, H.J. 1984. Bone marrow transplantation: a review of delayed complications. *Br J Haematol* 57:185-208.

Deeg, H.J., Flournoy, N., Sullivan, K.M., et al. 1984. Cataracts after total body irradiation and marrow transplantation: a sparing effect of dose fractionation. *Int J Radiat Oncol Biol Phys* 10:957-964.

DeGroen, P.C., Akasamit, A.J., Rakela, J., et al. 1987. Central nervous system toxicity after liver transplantation. *N Engl J Med* 317:861-866.

Deierhoi, M.H., Kalayoglu, M., Sollinger, H.W., et al. 1988. Cyclosporin neurotoxicity in liver transplant recipients: report of three cases. *Transplant Proc* 20:116-118.

De La Camara, R., Tomas, J.F., Daly, M.B., et al. 1991. High dose busulfan and seizures. *BMT* 7:363-364.

Denning, D.W., Lee, J.Y., Hostetler, J.S., et al., 1994. NIAID Mycoses Study Group Multicenter Trial of oral itraconazole therapy for invasive aspergillosis. *Am J Med* 97(2):135-144.

Dunn, J.P., Jabs, D.A., Wingard, J., et al. 1993. Bone marrow transplantation and cataract development. *Arch Ophthalmol* 111:1367-1373.

Ezzone, S., Camp-Sorrell, D. (Eds.) 1994. *Manual for Bone Marrow Transplant Nursing: Recommendations for Practice and Education.* Pittsburgh: Oncology Nursing Press.

Farrington, J., Stoudemire, A., Tierney, J. 1995. The role of ciprofloxacin in a patient with delirium due to multiple etiologies. *Gen Hosp Psychiatr* 17:47-53.

Fayemi, O.A. 1976. Nonbacterial thrombotic endocarditis and myocardial infarction. *Am Heart J* 97: 405-406.

Fernandez-Bouzas, A., Ramirez Jimenez, A., Vazquez Zamudio, J., et al. 1992. Brain calcifications and dementia in children treated with radiotherapy and intrathecal methotrexate. *J Neurosurg Sci* 36(4):211-214.

Fife, K., Milan, S., Westbrook, K., et al. 1994. Risk factors for requiring cataract surgery following total body irradiation. *Radiother & Oncol* 33(2):93-98.

Filipovich, A.H., Vallera, D.A., Youle, R.J., et al. 1987. Graft-versus-host disease prevention in allogeneic bone marrow transplantation from histocompatible siblings: a pilot study using immunotoxins for T cell depletion of donor bone marrrow. *Transplantation* 44(1):62-69.

Fincannon, J. 1995. Analysis of psychiatric referrals and interventions in an oncology population. *Oncol Nurs Forum* 22(1):87-92.

Fleishman, S., Lesko, L. 1990. Delirium and dementia. In Holland J., Rowland J. (Eds.) *Handbook of Psychooncology*. New York: Oxford University Press, 342-355.

Folstein, M., Folstein, E., McHugh, P. 1975. "Minimental state": a practical method for grading the cognitive state of patients for the clinician. *J Psychiatr Res* 12:189-198.

Ford, R., Eisenberg, S. 1990. Bone marrow transplant: recent advances and nursing implications. *Nurs Clin North Am* 25(2):405-422.

Forman, A. 1994. Neurologic complications of cytokine therapy. *Oncol* 8(4):105-110.

Francke, E. 1987. The many causes of meningitis. *Postgrad Med* 82(2):175-178, 181-183, 187-188.

Freedman, S., Shivnan, J., Tillis, J., et al. 1990. Bone marrow transplantation: overview and nursing implications. *Crit Care Nurs Q* 12(2):51-62.

Furlong, T. 1993. Neurologic complications of immunosuppressive cancer therapy. *Oncol Nurs Forum* 20(9): 1337-1354.

Furlong, T.G., Gallucci, B.B. 1994. Pattern of occurrence and clinical presentation of neurological complications in bone marrow transplant patients. *Canc Nurs* 17(1): 27-36.

Gagliano, R.G., Costanzi, J.J. 1976. Paraplegia following intrathecal methotrexate. *Canc* 37:1663-1668.

Ganem, G., Kuentz, M., Bernaudin, F., et al. 1989. Central nervous system relapses after bone marrow transplantation for acute lymphoblastic leukemia in remission. *Cancer* 64(9):1796-1804.

Geissmann, F., Derouin, F., Marolleau, J.P., et al. 1994. Disseminated toxoplasmosis following autologous bone marrow transplantation. *Clin Infect Dis* 19:800-801.

Gelpi, C., Martinez, M.A., Vidal, S. 1994. Autoantibodies to a transfer RNA-associated protein in a murine model of chronic graft-versus-host disease. *J Immunol* 152(4):1989-1999.

Ghany, A., Tutschka, P., McGhee, R., et al. 1991. Cyclosporin-associated seizures in bone marrow transplant recipients given busulfan and cyclophosphamide preparative therapy. *Transplantation* 52(2):310-315.

Goldberg, S.L., Tefferi, A., Rummans, T.A., et al. 1992. Post-irradiation somnolence syndrome in an adult patient following allogeneic bone marrow transplantation. *BMT* 9:499-501.

Grau, J.M., Casademont, J., Monforte, R., et al. 1990. Myasthenia gravis after allogeneic bone marrow transplantation: report of a new case and pathogenic considerations. *BMT* 5(6):435-437.

Graze, P.R., Gale, R.P. 1979. Chronic graft versus host disease: a syndrome of disordered immunity. *Am J Med* 66(4):611-620.

Greeves, J.A. 1984. Rapid-onset steroid psychosis with very low dosage of prednisolone. (letter). *Lancet* 1: 1119-1120.

Hagensee, M.E., Benyunes, M., Miller, J.A., et al. 1994. *Campylobacter jejuni* bacteremia and Guillain-Barré syndrome in a patient with GVHD after allogeneic BMT. *BMT* 13:349-351.

Hall, R.C., Popkin, M.K., Stickney, S.K., et al. 1979. Presentation of the steroid psychoses. *J Nerv Ment Dis* 167:229-236.

Halperin, E.C., Constine, L.S., Tarbell, N.J., et al. 1994. Late effects of cancer treatment. In Halperin, E.C., Constine, L.S., Tarbell, N.J., Kun, L.E. (Eds.) *Pediatric Radiation Oncology*, 2d ed. New York: Raven Press, 515-520.

Hamon M.D., Gale, R.F., MacDonald, I.D., et al. 1993. Incidence of cataracts after single fraction total body irradiation: the role of steroids and graft versus host disease. *BMT* 12:233-236.

Han, C.S., Miller, W., Haake, R., et al. 1994. Varicella zoster infections after bone marrow transplantation: incidence, risk factors and complications. *BMT* 13: 277-283.

Hathorn, J.W. 1993. Critical appraisal of antimicrobials for prevention of infections in immunocompromised hosts. *Hematol Oncol Clin North Am* 7(5):1051-1099.

Hiemenez, J.W., Greene, J.N. 1993. Special considerations for the patient undergoing allogeneic or autologous bone marrow transplantation. *Hematol Oncol Clin North Am* 7(5):961-1002.

Hilton, G. 1991. Review of neurobehavioral assessment tools. *Heart & Lung* 20(5):436-432.

Hoffman, D.L., Howard, J.R. Jr., Sarma, R., et al. 1993. Encephalopathy, myelopathy, optic neuropathy and anosmia associated with intravenous cytosine arabinoside. *Clin Neuropharm* 16(3):258-262.

Holland, G.N. 1989. Ocular toxoplasmosis in the immunocompromised host. *International Opth* 13(6): 399-402.

Hooks, M., Wade, C., Millikan, W. 1991. Muromonab CD-3: a review of its pharmacology, pharmacokinetics, and clinical use in transplantation. *Pharmacotherapy* 11(1):26-37.

Hooper, D.C., Pruitt, A.A., Rubin, R.H. 1982. Central nervous system infection in the chronically immunosuppressed. *Med* 61(3):166-188.

Hopkins, L.C. 1994. Clinical features of myasthenia gravis. *Neurol Clin North Am* 12(2):243-261.

Horowitz, M.M., Gale, R.P., Sondel, P.M., et al. 1990. Graft-versus-leukemia reactions after bone marrow transplantation. *Blood* 75:555-562.

Hoyle, C., Goldman, J.M. 1994. Life-threatening infections occurring more than 3 months after BMT. *BMT* 14:247-252.

Humphrey, G.B., Maxwell, J.D., Krous, H.F., et al. 1979. Treatment of overt CNS leukemia. *Am J Pediatr Hematol Oncol* 1:37-47.

Ignatavicius, D., Workman, M., Mishler, M. 1995. *Medical-Surgical Nursing: A Nursing Process Approach*, 2d ed. Philadelphia: Saunders, 258.

Imrie, K.R., Couture, F., Turner, C.C., et al. 1994. Peripheral neuropathy following high-dose etoposide and autologous bone marrow transplantation. *BMT* 13: 77-79.

Iwasaki, Y., Sako, K., Ohara, Y., et al. 1993. Subacute panencephalitis associated with chronic graft-versus-host-disease. *Acta Neuropathologica* 85(5):566-572.

Janssens, S., Decramer, M. 1989. Corticosteroid-induced myopathy and the respiratory muscles: report of two cases. *Chest* 95(5):1160-1162.

Jerman, M.R., Fick, R.B. 1986. Nonbacterial thrombotic endocarditis associated with bone marrow transplantation. *Chest* 90(6):919-922.

Johnson, N.T., Crawford, S.W., Sargur, M. 1987. Acute acquired demyelinating polyneuropathy with respiratory failure following high-dose systemic cytosine arabinoside and marrow transplantation. *BMT* 2:203-207.

Johnson, R.T. 1994. The virology of demyelinating diseases. *Ann Neurol* 36(suppl):S54-S60.

Kajiwara, K., Hirozane, A., Fukomoto, T., et al. 1991. Major histocompatibility complex expression in brain of rats with graft-versus-host-disease. *J Neuroimmunol* 32(3):191-198.

Kantarjian, H.M. 1994. Adult acute lymphocytic leukemia: critical review of current knowledge. *Am J Med* 97(2):176-184.

Katirji, M.B. 1987. Visual hallucinations and cyclosporin. *Transplantation* 43(5):768-769.

Kelch, B.P., Bulova, S.I., Crilley, P., et al. 1990. An unusual extramedullary relapse of acute nonlymphocytic leukemia after allogeneic bone marrow transplantation. *Am J Clin Oncol* 13(3):238-243.

Kershner, P., Wang-Cheng, R. 1989. Psychiatric side-effects of steroid therapy. *Psychosomatics* 30(2):135-139.

Kitamura, T., Satoh, K., Tominaga, T., et al. 1994. Alteration in the JC polyomavirus genome is enhanced in immunosuppressed renal transplant patients. *Virology* 198(1):341-345.

Kooiker, J.C., Maclean, J.M., Sumi, S.M. 1976. Cerebral embolism, marantic endocarditis, and cancer. *Arch Neurol* 33:260-264.

Kornblau, S.M., Cortes-Franco, J., Estey, E. 1993. Neurotoxicity associated with fludarabine and cytosine arabinoside chemotherapy for acute leukemia and myelodysplasia. *Leukemia* 7(3):378-383.

June, C.H., Thompson, C.B., Kennedy, M.S., et al. 1986. Correlation of hypomagnesemia with the onset of cyclosporin-associated hypertension in marrow transplant patients. *Transplantation* 41:47-51.

June, C.H., Thompson, C.B., Kennedy, M.S., et al. 1985. Profound hypomagnesemia and renal magnesium wasting associated with the use of cyclosporin for marrow transplantation. *Transplantation* 39:620-4.

Land, V.J., Shuster, J.J., Crist, W.M., et al. 1994. Comparison of two schedules of intermediate-dose methotrexate and cytarabine consolidation therapy for childhood B-precursor cell acute lymphoblastic leukemia. *J Clin Oncol* 12(9):1939-1945.

Lentnek, A., Sande, M.A., Whitley, R.J., et al. 1992. Evaluation of new anti-infective drugs for the treatment of cryptococcal meningitis. Infectious Diseases Society of America and the Food and Drug Administration. *Clin Infect Dis* 15(suppl 1):S189-S194.

Liesner, R.J., Leiper, A.D., Hann, I.M., et al. 1994. Late effects of intensive treatment for acute myeloid leukemia and myelodysplasia in children. *J Clin Oncol* 12(5):916-924.

Lishner, M., et al. 1990. Cutaneous and mucosal neoplasms in bone marrow transplantation. *J Infect Dis* 152:473-476.

Locatelli, F., Giorgiani, G., Pession, A., et al. 1993. Late effects in children after bone marrow transplantation: a review. *Haematologica* 78(5):319-328.

Lockman, L.A., Sung, J.H., Krivit, W. 1991. Acute parkinsonian syndrome with demyelinating leukoencephalopathy in bone marrow transplant recipients. *Pediatr Neurol* 7(6):457-463.

Long, S.G., Leyland, M.J., Milligan, D.W. 1993. *Listeria* meningitis after bone marrow transplantation. *BMT* 12(5):537-539.

Lopez, J., Ulibarrena, C., Garcia-Larna, J., et al. 1993. Thalidomide as therapy for intestinal chronic GVHD. *BMT* 11:251-252.

Lowsky, R., Lipton, J., Fyles, G., et al. 1994. Secondary malignancies after bone marrow transplantation in adults. *J Clin Oncol* 12(10):2187-2192.

Luddy, R.E., Gilman, P.A. 1973. Paraplegia following intrathecal methotrexate. *J Pediatr* 83:988-992.

Malilay, G.P., Sevenich, E.A., Condie, R.M., et al. 1989. Prevention of graft rejection in allogeneic bone marrow transplantation: I. Preclinical studies with antithymocyte globulins. *BMT* 4(1):107-112.

Malseed, R., Harrigan, G. 1989. *Textbook of Pharmacology and Nursing Care*. Philadelphia: Lippincott.

Massie, M.J., Lesko, L. 1990. Psychopharmacological management. In Holland, J., Rowland (Eds.) *Handbook of Psycho-oncology*. New York: Oxford University Press, 470-491.

Mastaglia, F.L., Laing, B.A., Zilko, P. 1993. Treatment of inflammatory myopathies. *Baillieres Clin Neurol* 2(3): 717-740.

McCracken, G.H., Sande, M.A., Lentnek, A., et al. 1992. Evaluation of new anti-infective drugs for the treatment of acute bacterial meningitis. *Clin Infect Dis* 15(suppl 1):S182-S188.

McGuire, T.R., Tallman, M.S., Yee, G.C., et al. 1988. Influence of infusion duration on the efficacy and toxicity of intravenous cyclosporin in bone marrow transplant patients. *Transplant Proc* 3(suppl 3):501-504.

1993. *The Medical Letter: On Drugs and Therapeutics*. Drugs that cause psychiatric symptoms 35(901):65-70.

Melms, A., Faul, C, Sommer, N., et al. 1992. Myasthenia gravis after BMT: identification of patients at risk. (letter). *BMT* 9(1):78-79.

Meyers, C., Scheibel, R., Forman, A. 1991. Persistent neurotoxicity of systemically administered interferon-alpha. *Neurology* 41:672-676.

Meyers, J.D. 1988. Management of cytomegalovirus infection. *Am J Med* 85(suppl 2A):102-106.

Miller, F.W. 1994. Classification and prognosis of inflammatory muscle disease. *Rheum Dis Clin North Am* 20(4):811-826.

Milliken, S., Powles, R. 1995. Bone-marrow transplantation for leukemia. In Peckham, M., Pinedo, H.M., Veronesi, U. (Eds.) *Oxford Textbook of Oncology*. Oxford: Oxford University Press, 1682-1695.

Mitchell, R.B., Wagner, J.E., Karp, J.E., et al. 1988. Syndrome of idiopathic hyperammonemia after high-dose chemotherapy: review of nine cases. *Am J Med* 85:662-667.

Miyatake, S., Kikuchi, H., Oda, Y., et al. 1992. A case of treatment-related leukoencephalopathy: sequential MRI, CT and PET findings. *J Neuro Oncol* 14(2): 143-149.

Mohrmann, R., Mah, V., Vinters, H.V. 1987. Neuropathologic findings after bone marrow transplantation: an autopsy study. *J Neuropathol Exp Neurol* 46:369 (abstr 113).

Mohrmann, R., Mah, V., Vinters, H.V. 1990. Neuropathologic findings after bone marrow transplantation: an autopsy study. *Human Pathol* 21(6):630-639.

Mulhern, R., Hancock, J., Fairclough, D. 1992. Neuropsychological status of children treated with brain tumors: a critical review and integrated analysis. *Med Pediatr Oncol* 20:181-191.

Murphy P., Parker, A., Hutchinson, R.M. 1994. High grade pyrexia following bone marrow transplantation: a neurotoxic complication of high-dose chemotherapy and radiotherapy in the UKALL XII Trial. *BMT* 13:229-31.

Myers, S.E., Williams, S.F. 1994. Guillain-Barré syndrome after autologous bone marrow transplantation for breast cancer: report of two cases. *BMT* 13:341-344.

Nelson, K.R., McQuillen, M.P. 1988. Neurologic complications of graft-versus-host disease. *Neurologic Clin* 6(2):389-403.

Norrell, H., Wilson, C.B., Slagel, D.E. 1974. Leukoencephalopathy following the administration of methotrexate into the cerebrospinal fluid in the treatment of primary brain tumors. *Cancer* 33(4):923-932.

Ochs, J.J. 1989. Neurotoxicity due to central nervous system therapy for childhood leukemia. *Am J Pediatric Hematol Oncol* 11:93-105.

Ozon, A., Topaloglu, H., Cila, A., et al. 1994. Acute ascending myelitis and encephalopathy after intrathecal methotrexate in an adolescent boy with acute lymphoblastic leukemia. *Brain and Dev* 16(3):246-248.

Packer, R.J., Meadows, A.T., Roarke, L.B., et al. 1987. Long-term sequelae of cancer treatment on the central nervous system in childhood. *Med Pediatr Oncol* 15(5):241-253.

Palmer, B., Toto, R. 1991. Severe neurologic toxicity induced by cyclosporin A in three renal transplant patients. *Am J Kid Dis* 18(1):116-121.

Patchell, R.A., White, C.L., CLark, A.W., et al. 1985a. Neurologic complications of bone marrow transplantation. *Neurology* 35:300-306.

Patchell, R.A., White, C.L., CLark, A.W., et al. 1985b. Nonbacterial thrombotic endocarditis in bone marrow transplant patients. *Cancer* 55:631-635.

Peeters, A., Waer, M., Michielsen, P., et al. 1989. Listeria monocytogenes meningitis. *Clin Neurol Neurosurg* 91(1):29-36.

Perry, A., Mehta, J., Iveson, T., et al. 1994. Guillain-Barré syndrome after bone marrow transplantation. *BMT* 14:165-167.

Pizzo, P.A., Poplack, D.G., Bleyer, W.A. 1979. Neurotoxicities of current leukemia therapy. *Am J Pediatr Hematol Oncol* 1:127-139.

Plotz, P.H., Rider, L.G., Targoff, I.N., et al. 1995. NIH Conference. Myositis: immunologic contributions to understanding cause, pathogenesis, and therapy. *Ann Intern Med* 122(9):715-724.

Pomeranz, S., Naparstek, E., Ashkenazi, E., et al. 1994. Intracranial haematomas following bone marrow transplantation. *J Neurol* 241(4):252-256.

Price, R.A. 1979. Histopathology of CNS leukemia and complications of therapy. *Am J Pediatr Hematol Oncol* 1:21-30.

Price, R.A., Jamieson, P.A. 1975. The central nervous system in childhood leukemia, II: subacute leukoencephalopathy. *Cancer* 35:306-318.

Reece, D.E., Frei-Lahr, J.D., Shepherd, J.D., et al. 1991. Neurologic complications in allogeneic transplant patients receiving cyclosporin. *BMT* 8:393-401.

Resar, L.M., Phillips, P.C., Kastan, M.B., et al. 1993. Acute neurotoxicity after intrathecal cytosine arabinoside in two adolescents with acute lymphoblastic leukemia of B-cell type. *Cancer* 71(1):117-123.

Roden, J., Klintmalm, G.B.G., Husberg, B.S. 1987. Cerebrospinal fluid inflammation during OKT3 therapy. (letter). *Lancet* 2:272.

Roskrow, M.A., Kelsey, S.M., McCarthy, M., et al. 1992. Selective autonomic neuropathy as a novel complication of BMT. *BMT* 10:469-70.

Rubin, A.M., Kang, H. 1987. Cerebral blindness and encephalopathy with cyclosporin A toxicity. *Neurology* 37:1072-1076.

Rumsey, K., Rieger, P. 1992. *Biological Response Modifiers: A Self-Instruction Manual for Health Professionals.* Chicago: Precept Press.

Ryffel, B., Tammi, K., Greider, A., et al. 1985. Effects of cyclosporin on human T cell activation. *Transplant Proc* 17(1):1268-1270.

Sable, C.A., Donowitz, G.R. 1994. Infections in bone marrow transplant recipients. *Clin Infect Dis* 18: 273-284.

Sakami, H., Onozawa, Y., Yano, Y., et al. 1993. Disseminated necrotizing leukoencephalopathy following irradiation and MTX therapy for central nervous system infiltration of leukemia and lymphoma. *Radiat Med* 11(4):146-153.

Sande, M.A., Whitley, R.J., McCracken, G.H. 1992. Evaluation of new anti-infective drugs for the treatment of toxoplasma encephalitis. *Clin Infect Dis* 15(suppl 1):S200-S205.

Sandoz Pharmaceuticals. 1994. Sandimmune® (cyclosporin) Drug Interactions. East Hanover, NJ.

Sandoz Pharmaceuticals. 1994. Sandimmune® package insert. East Hanover, NJ.

Seong, D.C., Przepiorka, D., Bruner, J.M., et al. 1993. Leptomeningeal toxoplasmosis after allogeneic marrow transplantation. *Am J Clin Oncol (CCT)* 16(2):105-108.

Shelton, B., Sargent, C. 1990. Neurologic toxicity management with BMRs. *Oncol Nurs Forum* 17(6):964-965.

Skullerud, K., Halvorsen, K. 1978. Encephalomyelopathy following intrathecal methotrexate treatment in a child with acute leukemia. *Cancer* 42(3):1211-1215.

Shimoda, K., Gondo, H., Harada, M., et al. 1994. Myasthenia gravis after allogeneic bone marrow transplantation. *BMT* 14:155-156.

Slatkin, N.F., et al. 1987. Myositis as the major manifestation of chronic graft versus host disease (GVHD). *Neurology* 37(suppl 1):205-211.

Snider, S., Bashir, R., Bierman, P. 1994. Neurologic complications after high-dose chemotherapy and autologous bone marrow transplantation for Hodgkin's disease. *Neurology* 44(4):681-684.

Srivastava, A., Bradstock, K.F., Szer, J., et al. 1993. Busulfan and melphalan prior to autologous bone marrow transplantation. *BMT* 12:323-329.

Stamatoullas, A., Ferrant, A., Manicourt, D. 1993. Reflex sympathetic dystrophy after bone marrow transplantation. *Ann Hematol* 67:245-247.

Sureda, A., Perez de Oteyza, J., Garcia Larana, J., et al. 1989. High-dose busulfan and seizures. *Ann Intern Med* 11:543-544.

Sullivan, K.M., Mori, M., Sanders, J., et al. 1992. Late complications of allogeneic and autologous marrow transplantation. *BMT 10*(suppl 1):127-134.

Sullivan, K.M., Parkman, R. 1983. The pathophysiology and treatment of graft-versus-host disease. *Clin Haematol 12*:775-789.

Sullivan, K.M., Weiden, P.L., Storb, R., et al. 1989. Influence of acute and chronic graft-versus-host disease on relapse and survival after bone marrow transplantation from HLA-identical siblings as treatment of acute and chronic leukemia. *Blood 73*:1720-1728.

Thistlethwaite, J.R., Gaber, A.O., Haag, B.W., et al. 1987. OKT3 treatment of steroid-resistant renal allograft rejection. *Transplantation 43*:176-184.

Thomas, E.D., Storb, R., Clift, R.A., et al. 1975. Bone-marrow transplantation. *N Engl J Med 292*:895-902.

Thompson, C.B., Sanders, J.E., Flournoy, N., et al. 1986. The risks of central nervous system relapse after bone marrow transplantation for acute myeloid leukemia. *Blood 67*:195-199.

Thompson, C.B., Sullivan, K.M., June, C.H., et al. 1984. Association between cyclosporin neurotoxicity and hypomagnesemia. *Lancet 2*:1116-1120.

Tichelli, A., Gratwohl, A., Egger, T., et al. 1993. Cataract formation after bone marrow transplantation. *Ann Intern Med 119*(12):1175-1180.

Tse, N., Cederbaum, S., Glaspy, J.A. 1991. Hyperammonemia following allogeneic bone marrow transplantation. *Am J Hematol 38*(2):140-141.

Urbano-Marquez, A., Estruch, R., Grau, J.M., et al. 1986. Inflammatory myopathy associated with chronic graft-versus-host disease. *Neurology 36*(8):1091-1093.

van den Broek, P.J. 1988. Infection during neutropenia. *J Hosp Infect 11*(suppl A):7-14.

Verndonck, L.F., Cornelisseu, J.J., Smit, J., et al. 1993. Successful foscarnet therapy for acyclovir-resistant mucocutaneous infection with herpes simplex virus in a recipient of allogeneic BMT. *BMT 11*(2):177-179.

Viscioli, C., Garaventa, A., Ferrea, G., et al. 1991. Listeria monocytogenes brain abscesses in a girl with acute lymphoblastic leukemia after late central nervous system relapse. *Eur J Canc 27*(4):435-437.

Vogel, H., Horoupian, D.S. 1993. Filamentous degeneration of neurons: a possible feature of cytosine arabinoside neurotoxicity. *Cancer 71*(4):1303-1308.

Vogelsang, G., Farmer, E., Hess, A., et al. 1992. Thalidomide for the treatment of chronic graft-vs-host disease. *N Engl J Med 326*(16):1055-1058.

Vogelsang, G., Morris, L. 1993. Prevention and management of graft-vs-host disease: practical recommendations. *Drugs 45*(5):668-676.

Walker, R.W., Allen, J.C., Rosen, G., et al. 1986. Transient cerebral dysfunction secondary to high-dose methotrexate. *J Clin Oncol 4*:1845-1850.

Walker, R.W., Brochstein, J.A. 1988. Neurologic complications of immunosuppressive agents. *Neurol Clin 6*(2):261-278.

Weiss, G. (Ed.) 1993. *Clinical Oncology.* Norwalk, CT: Appleton & Lange.

Wen, P.Y., Blanchard, K.L., Block, C.C., et al. 1992. Development of Lhermitte's sign after bone marrow transplantation. *Cancer 69*:2262-2266.

Whedon, M., Ferrell, B. 1994. Quality of life in adult bone marrow transplant patients: beyond the first year. *Semin Oncol Nurs 10*(1):42-57.

Whitley, R.J., Lentnek, A., McCracken, G.H., 1992. Evaluation of new anti-infective drugs for the treatment of viral encephalitis. *Clin Infect Dis 15*(suppl 1): S195-S199.

Wingard, J.R., Beals, S.U., Santos, G.W., et al. 1987. Aspergillus infections in bone marrow transplant recipients. *BMT 2*:175-181.

Winick, N.J., Smith, S.D., Shuster, J., et al. 1993. Treatment of CNS relapse in children with acute lymphoblastic leukemia: a Pediatric Oncology Group study. *J Clin Oncol 11*(2):271-278.

Winston, D.J., Ho, W.G., Gale, R.P., et al. 1988. Prophylaxis of infection in bone marrow transplants. *Eur J Cancer & Clin Oncol 24*(suppl 1):S15-23.

Wise, M., Rundell, J. 1994. *Concise Guide to Consultation Psychiatry,* 2d ed. Washington, DC: American Psychiatric Press, 31-53.

Witherspoon, R.P., Deeg, H.J., Storb, R. 1994. Secondary malignancies after marrow transplantation for leukemia or aplastic anemia. *Transplant Sci 4*(1):33-41.

Wiznitzer, M., Packer, R.J., August, C.S., et al. 1984. Neurologic complications of bone marrow transplantation in childhood. *Ann Neurol 16*:569-76.

Zimberg, M., Berenson, S. 1990. Delirium in patients with cancer: Nursing assessment and intervention. *Oncol Nurs Forum 17*(4):529-538.

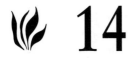

14

Psychosocial Effects
Pretransplant and Acute Treatment Phase

Susan Walch, Tim A. Ahles

The bone marrow transplantation (BMT) procedure occurs within the context of a chronic, life-threatening medical condition (most often some form of hematological or other malignancy) which carries with it many psychosocial stressors. The procedure itself is associated with additional stressors including several weeks of intensive treatment and isolation, frequent medical procedures, fluctuating medical status, treatment-related side effects, substantial financial costs, extended recuperation time, and many risks including death. While these stressors are not unique to BMT, they may be amplified as a result of the intensity of the procedure. Weighed against the many costs and risks is the potential for cure. With recent advancements in BMT technologies, potential recipients vary widely with regard to age, disease type and stage, duration of illness, and treatment history. Recent psychosocial research has indicated that several of these disease and treatment variables may result in different quality-of-life outcomes. Additionally, empirical research over recent years has resulted in expanded knowledge regarding the acute and long-term psychosocial consequences of BMT.

PSYCHOSOCIAL CONCERNS DURING THE PRETREATMENT PHASE

Several psychosocial issues arise in the pretreatment phase of BMT. They include informed decision making about the procedure and typical or common psychological responses in anticipation of the procedure once the decision to undergo transplant has been made. In addition to these common issues, some BMT candidates have special concerns resulting from the procedure. In particular, the neuropsychological effects of previous treatment and preexisting psychiatric conditions have received some attention in the psychosocial literature. Informed decision making, pretransplant psychological status, neuropsychological effects of previous treatment, and preexisting psychiatric conditions may influence the course and outcome of the transplant.

Informed Decision Making about BMT

The first biopsychosocial concern for the potential BMT recipient is the process of deciding whether to undergo BMT. Requisites for informed consent include presentation of treatment that is voluntary, comprehension of the risks, benefits, side effects, and alternative treatments, and a competent decision maker.

Although BMT is a voluntary procedure, some patients feel there are no viable alternatives and are pleased to have one more option. Others weigh the pros and cons of conventional treatments and BMT, a complex process due to the lack of clear information regarding the relative efficacy of the treatment strategies. The decision to undergo conventional treatment, if not successful, may decrease one's chances for successful BMT in the future, further complicating the decision. In addition, many patients are in remission or feeling relatively healthy and optimistic at the time BMT is considered. During a period of remission, it may be very difficult for patients to consider the risks of such a drastic treatment. Still other patients grasp at the chance for cure offered by BMT and fail to fully consider the risks.

Ideally, potential BMT recipients are considering both the risks and the benefits of the procedure and making their decisions without undue pressure. Lesko (1993) reported patients' (and parents' of pediatric patients) and physicians' perceptions of the barriers to informed consent. Patient-reported obstacles to informed consent were a perceived focus on positive aspects of the treatment, withholding questions, and the feeling that their physicians did not want them to make their own decisions. The physicians viewed the patients and parents as relatively passive, dependent, acquiescent, and preferring to defer to the physicians' recommendation. Dermatis and Lesko (1991) retrospectively assessed 39 adult BMT candidates' perceptions of the informed consent process within 48 hours of hospital admission. On average, patients could recall 41% of the risks/side effects listed on the consent form. Fifty-four percent of the sample felt that they had been sufficiently autonomous in the decision-making process; the remainder did not feel that they had made the decision autonomously. Not surprisingly, this perceived autonomy was positively associated with the perceived level of communication with the physician. Lesko (1993) noted that potential BMT candidates seek information from a wide variety of health-care sources in addition to the primary care physician, and recommended that this include a meeting with a BMT recipient and his or her family to discuss the experience.

Three small-scale studies of BMT survivors retrospectively assessed recipients' satisfaction with the information provided prior to transplant and/or their decisions to undergo BMT. Hengeveld, Houtman, and Zwaan (1988) reported that, overall, BMT survivors positively judged the preadmission information they received. However, 17 survivors interviewed reported that they did not receive adequate information regarding the psychological and sexual sequelae of BMT. Thirty-five percent of 23 survivors assessed by Andrykowski, Henslee, and Farrall (1989) at an average of 26 months after transplant reported that the treatment was "worse than expected." However, only one patient reported that he would not make the same choice (to undergo BMT) in retrospect. Belec's (1992) study of 24 BMT survivors found only one patient who would not make the same decision in retrospect. Although these patients' reports are retrospective, they indicate that patients may not be fully informed of potential negative outcomes. While most of the participants of the studies reported that they would (retrospectively) make the same decision to undergo BMT, these studies are biased in favor of BMT recipients with favorable survival outcomes; persons who had not survived until the time of the study were not available.

An additional, noteworthy issue of informed consent involves the high rates of participation in research projects by BMT recipients. Studies cited throughout this chapter had unusually high rates of agreement to participate in comparison to psychosocial investigations with other populations. Whedon and Ferrell (1994) note that this observed willingness to participate in research may actually represent a profound sense of gratitude and indebtedness that may compromise the studies of informed consent of some BMT patients.

Common Psychosocial Issues during the Pretreatment Phase

Clinical accounts and other nonempirical writings have described many of the stressors and common stress-induced responses of patients preparing for BMT. Depression and anxiety are the most commonly noted psychosocial sequelae of BMT at all phases of the process (Lesko, 1989). Several specific issues contribute to these pretreatment reactions. Patients who have to wait to find a suitable donor when timing is critical for optimal results may find the pretreatment phase precarious and uncontrollable. For all patients, many medical procedures are performed, such as tissue typing or cytapheresis. Lesko (1989) identified assessment, tissue typing, relocation, familial role shifts, vocational changes, and fending off relapse while waiting for treatment as potential stressors during the pretreatment phase of BMT. Andrykowski (1994a) noted that the period between making the decision to undergo BMT and admission to the transplant unit can be distressing, particularly when delayed. Because timing is often critical, waiting and delays can be difficult for candidates. The search for an appropriate donor can cause delays, as can other medical, financial, and logistical issues.

Two recent, investigations have examined the psychosocial status of BMT recipients prior to the initiation of the transplant procedure (Rodrigue et al., 1993; Meyers et al., 1994). Rodrigue and colleagues assessed 51 BMT re-cipients on several psychosocial dimensions including mood, coping, and personality. While significant mood disturbance was not the rule, 20% of the sample scored in the moderate to severe range on the Beck Depression Inventory and one third of the sample had elevated scores (greater than one standard deviation above the mean) on the Spielberger State-Trait Anxiety Inventory, indicating significant anxiety. Almost one quarter of recipients scored greater than 1 standard deviation above the mean on the Spielberger State-Trait Anger Expression Inventory, suggesting elevated levels of anger in a subset of patients. Coping styles were similar to those of other medical populations, with the exception of a somewhat higher tendency to use "confrontational" coping strategies. Personality assessment, as measured by the Minnesota Multiphasic Personality Inventory (MMPI), revealed an overall absence of significant psychopathology. This study was cross-sectional and did not reassess the BMT recipients throughout the hospital stay/treatment or recovery phases.

Meyers and colleagues (1994) had findings very similar to those of Rodrigue and colleagues (1993). In a sample of 21 BMT recipients (both allogeneic and autologous), scores representing significant depression were found in 22% of the sample at the prehospitalization assessment phase. Thirty-eight percent of the sample scored greater than 1 standard deviation above the mean on the State-Trait Anxiety Inventory at prehospitalization assessment. Autologous BMT recipients were significantly older, more depressed, and more anxious than allogeneic BMT recipients, a finding that is likely to reflect the type of disease for which the patients are treated. Most of the autologous BMT recipients had lymphoma and most of the allogeneic BMT recipients had CML.

Preliminary data from an investigation with a large sample of BMT recipients tends to support the findings of these smaller studies. As part of a larger investigation, Syrjala and colleagues (1995) assessed 392 adult BMT candidates for depression prior to hospital admission. The distribution of depression scores suggested that the majority of BMT candidates (67%) were not depressed just prior to hospital admission. However, scores consistent with mild levels of depression were found for 22% of the patients assessed. Eleven percent of patients had scores consistent with the presence of moderate to severe depression. Overall, the incidence of depressive symptomatology in BMT candidates does not differ substantially from that of other medically ill populations, which ranges from 12% to 36% depending on the criteria (Rodin and Voshart, 1986). However, a subset of patients does experience mood disturbance of sufficient severity to warrant careful consideration and intervention.

Preexisting Psychiatric Conditions

While psychological screening for selection of candidates for solid organ transplant is frequent due to the limited availability and high cost of donor organs, it is less common for recipients of BMT (Andrykowski, 1994b). However, given the stringent requirements for compliance, concern clearly arises in potential BMT cases with substantial psychiatric risk. The patient's ability to comply with the requirements of the procedure (e.g., exercise, mouth care, etc.) and *not* behave in ways that might be detrimental (e.g., pullout IVs or catheters, sign out AMA, etc.) are pivotal issues.

Although there has been no systematic study of the impact of premorbid psychiatric history on adjustment and adaptation to BMT procedures, Lesko (1989a, b, 1993) discusses the management of the psychiatric patient during BMT. Psychiatric consultation *prior to admission* is indicated in the presence or history of a major psychiatric disorder. Although extensive psychiatric input may be required for adequate management of patients with severe

psychopathology, even highly disturbed patients have successfully completed the BMT procedure and complied with its requirements. Denial of transplantation on the basis of psychiatric disturbance has not been reported. The use of psychopharmacological agents may be crucial to effective management of the BMT patient (Lesko, 1989a), however, some antidepressants and other psychotropic medications may increase bone marrow suppression, therefore requiring careful evaluation and monitoring with their use (Lesko, 1993).

Two published case reports have described the successful treatment of BMT patients with significant psychiatric risk factors. One report (Kaehler et al., 1989) described a woman with chronic myelogenous leukemia who required an abortion prior to BMT and had a significant family psychiatric history; her mother had bipolar affective disorder and her sister had schizophrenia. Despite the emotional trauma of the abortion and the high genetic tendency for psychiatric problems, the patient coped well medically and psychologically with BMT. In the other case (Rappaport, 1988), a 32-year-old man with chronic granulocytic leukemia underwent BMT. His psychiatric history was significant in that he was thought to have schizoid personality disorder. Despite a brief psychotic episode during BMT, the patient did very well medically and his psychotic symptoms resolved after discharge.

The basic problem with this area of study is that health-care providers must make predictions about the patients' behavior based on current functioning and/or responses to psychosocial measures. The history of research in mental health is replete with attempts to predict behavior. The consensus is that the ability to predict behavior based on psychosocial factors is very poor. Anecdotally, transplant centers have reported situations in which patients seemed psychologically healthy pretransplant yet had major compliance problems, as well as patients with poor premorbid psychosocial histories who coped well with BMT.

Neuropsychological Effects of Previous Treatment

Relatively little systematic work has been done to examine the neuropsychological effects of cancer treatments in adults. However, potential cognitive impairment due to chemotherapy, the cancer itself, and concurrently administered medications has been recognized (Silberfarb, 1983). Several related issues arise with respect to the neuropsychological effects of previous treatment and BMT. First is the impairment in cognition that may result from the neurotoxic effects of previous cytotoxic regimens, which could impair the process of informed consent and decision-making ability. Second, the presence of neuropsychological impairment from previous treatment may hinder an individual's ability to comply with the stringent self-care regimens associated with BMT. In addition, BMT may have neurotoxic effects of its own that might further debilitate cognitive abilities and could influence recipients' self-care abilities and quality of life. Because of the intensive nature of BMT, it is logical to hypothesize that if neuropsychological deficits occur during other treatments for adults with cancer, these deficits might also be seen with BMT treatments. Although the impact of neuropsychological impairment on informed consent, compliance, and quality of life of BMT recipients has not been extensively studied, several recent efforts have been aimed at describing the extent and nature of neuropsychological impairment in previously treated adults with cancer, BMT candidates, and BMT recipients.

The frequency of organic mental disorders in the general cancer population is estimated to be one quarter to one third (Meyers and Abbruzzese, 1992). However, most neuropsychological examinations are conducted on pa-

tients referred for evaluation or patients receiving CNS treatments. These two sampling methods do not necessarily represent the incidence of cognitive impairment in the general cancer population. Further, the variability of diseases and treatments within the general cancer population can limit the generalization of findings among studies. For example, while Meyers and colleagues (1991) indicated that review of the literature on prospective studies of the neuropsychological effects of systemically administered interferon-alpha generally indicates that there are virtually no persistent neurotoxic effects of this treatment, their retrospective study of 14 patients referred for neurotoxicity associated with interferon-alpha suggested that the treatment may be associated with frontal-subcortical dysfunction that may persist. The sampling method and retrospective nature of the study limit these findings but do suggest that a minority of patients may experience significant cognitive disruption from this treatment. The neuropsychological impact of interferon-alpha remains unclear, as does the neuropsychological impact of many other cancer treatments.

Some types of treatments, as well as a history of multiple treatments, appear to be associated with greater risk for neuropsychological impairment. For example, Meyers and Abbruzzese (1992) found that 32 percent of patients (N = 47) who were newly enrolled in a phase I investigational study of difluorodeoxycytidinde (dFdC) exhibited deficits in one or more of the following areas of functioning, prior to the administration of the investigational agent: memory, executive functioning, visuomotor skills, and attention. The incidence of deficits varied as a function of treatment history; patients with a history of treatment via biologic response modifiers had a 53% incidence of deficits compared to an 18% incidence of deficits in patients without such treatment history.

Similarly, Andrykowski and colleagues (1992) found that some degree of neuropsychological impairment was fairly common among BMT candidates assessed prior to initiation of BMT conditioning regimens. Some degree of memory deficit was found in approximately one third of the sample. Similar rates of impairment were detected on a task of complex attention/motor skills (Trails B). Attentional processes appeared to be relatively spared, with only 6% of the sample displaying significantly impaired scores in this area, suggesting that the other deficits are not simply a reflection of attention-impairing medication or mood states. Most interesting, this study found that the risk for neuropsychological impairment increased with the number of risk factors for disease and treatment assessed in the study, including CNS disease involvement, intrathecal chemotherapy with or without cranial irradiation, and high-dose intravenous cytosine arabinoside.

A prospective investigation evaluated 21 autologous and allogeneic BMT recipients with the administration of a neuropsychological screening tool (Dementia Rating Scale) throughout treatment and at follow-up (Meyers et al., 1994). Twenty percent of the sample demonstrated some cognitive impairment, including memory and conceptualization deficits, prior to the initiation of conditioning regimens. However, attention was virtually unimpaired. Through the BMT procedure, short-term memory problems increased during the course of hospitalization but were not significantly different from baseline measurement at follow-up after 8 months. History of treatment with interferon-alpha was unrelated to scores on the screening measure, as were type of BMT and age of recipient. A study (Ahles et al., 1996) also found that neuropsychological measures assessing higher-order cognitive functioning generally worsened over the course of hospitalization for autologous bone marrow transplant in a sample of 54 patients with hematological disorders or breast cancer. However, this investigation did not find greater impairment in patients

with a history of intrathecal therapy or cranial irradiation.

Similarly, Parth and colleagues (1989) reported on the preadmission and time-of-discharge scores of 20 BMT recipients and 9 control participants on a computerized battery of cognitive and sensory tests. They found several significant pretransplant differences between patients and controls. In addition, control participants demonstrated improvement with repeated administration whereas BMT recipients did not. The source of pretransplant differences was not discussed by the authors, however, and may represent many variables including previous treatment, disease, medication, chance, or a function of an unmatched control group. In summary, cognitive deficits may exist before BMT in some patients (although the source of these deficits is still unclear) and these may worsen over the course of hospitalization for BMT. Further, one study suggests that neurotoxic effects of BMT may arise as late effects of the procedure and not appear until months after discharge. Stemmer and colleagues (1994) noted cerebral white matter changes on MRI in 9 of 13 bone marrow transplant recipients, typically not detected until 5 or more months after transplant. The true incidence of such changes is unknown, as are the clinical ramifications.

Clinically, patients report difficulty with concentration and memory and providers observe cases of delirium. Fortunately, these major symptoms usually resolve by the time the patient is ready for discharge. It is unclear whether these problems are true cognitive deficits or are related to psychological issues such as depression, anxiety, or reintegration into a normal lifestyle. The previously discussed studies suggest that neuropsychological difficulties do, in fact, occur as a result of some treatments for cancer. They also suggest that BMT recipients may have a fair amount of risk for deficits existing pretransplant and that BMT may cause further impairment. Clearly, more investigation is needed to examine the neuropsychological effects of different neoplastic diseases and their various treatments because neuropsychological impairments may have an adverse impact on BMT recipients' capacity for informed consent, ability to comply with treatment, and long-term quality of life.

PSYCHOSOCIAL CONCERNS DURING ACUTE TREATMENT

Research examining the psychosocial consequences throughout the course of the acute treatment or inpatient hospitalization phase of BMT has begun to emerge. The need for prospective study of BMT patients has been recognized and several investigations have assessed BMT patients over the course of treatment. Such research has addressed three lines of inquiry:

1. description of the physical and psychological effects of treatment,
2. examination of the relationships between psychological factors and physical symptoms, and
3. preliminary examination of the relationships between psychological factors and survival.

In short, BMT has been associated with several adverse physical and psychological side effects, and there appear to be relationships among these psychological and somatic variables. Some preliminary evidence suggests that psychosocial factors may be related even to survival outcomes.

Psychological Factors and the Occurrence of Physical Symptoms

The prevalence and course of several somatic and psychological effects of BMT have recently been described in the literature. Pain, nausea, and emesis are the most frequently studied somatic effects of BMT, and anxiety and depression comprise the most commonly described psychological effects. Several studies suggest that there is a fairly predictable course and high incidence for each of these effects. In addition, psychological distress and physical symptoms have been correlated.

Several authors have described pain effects during BMT (Gaston-Johansson et al., 1992; Syrjala et al., 1992; Chapko et al., 1989; McGuire et al., 1993) and overall there has been remarkable consistency across investigations. Pain most frequently occurs in the oral cavity as a result of oral mucositis. McGuire and colleagues (1993) reported an 89% incidence of mucositis in a sample of 47 patients receiving either autologous or allogeneic BMT. On average, mucositis pain begins just prior to transplant, peaks during the second week after transplant, and gradually resolves, usually by day +20. Pain ratings by patients are mild overall and moderate at peak times (McGuire et al., 1993). Age and transplant type appear to be unrelated to pain (McGuire et al., 1993). However, pain is greater for patients with hematological malignancies than for those with aplastic anemia (Syrjala et al., 1992). Patients treated with total body irradiation (i.e., patients with hematological malignancies) experienced greater pain than those treated without TBI. Further, higher doses of TBI are related to higher levels of pain (Syrjala et al., 1992).

Unfortunately, pain is not fully eliminated by medication; Gaston-Johansson and colleagues (1992) reported that pain was unresolved with medication in 35% of patients. In part, this may reflect a trade-off by patients using opioids such as morphine, which may reduce pain but increase nausea. One strategy to address this problem involves the use of patient-controlled analgesia. A study comparing patient-controlled analgesia (PCA) to continuous infusion (CI) of morphine in patients undergoing BMT found that PCA resulted in one half the rate of drug use for equivalent relief, without increased side effects, tolerance, or withdrawal (Hill et al., 1990). It should be noted, however, that pain relief was incomplete with both PCA and CI morphine administration.

In addition to pain, patients undergoing BMT very often experience nausea and emesis. Although these symptoms have received less attention than pain, some descriptive information is available. Nausea and emesis follow a different time line than that of pain. These symptoms tend to begin and peak prior to transplant and then gradually subside (Syrjala et al., 1992; Chapko et al., 1989). Nausea and emesis fluctuate from day to day (Syrjala et al., 1992) and there is considerable variability among patients, which is likely to be a function of pretransplant chemotherapy regimens (Chapko et al., 1989). Again, nausea and emesis have not been completely managed with antiemetic medications (Chapko et al., 1989).

One published study has examined the incidence and course of psychological symptoms of depression and anxiety throughout the BMT procedure. Meyers and colleagues (1994) followed a sample of 21 allogeneic and autologous BMT recipients from preadmission through 8 months after discharge. At the preadmission assessment, 22% of the sample reported significant levels of depressive symptomatology. Approximately midway through the hospitalization, the percentage reporting significant levels of depressive symptoms rose to 37. By discharge, 43% of the sample reported significant levels of depressive symptomatology. Eight months after discharge, however, this figure dropped to 10%. Overall, depression increased from preadmission to discharge (highest incidence) but then returned to baseline by 8 months after discharge. Anxiety followed a different pattern. At preadmission, 38% of the sample had elevated anxiety scores. Midhospi-

talization levels of anxiety remained at 33% of the sample, but by discharge this figure dropped to 20%. By the 8-month follow-up assessment, only 10% of the sample had elevated anxiety scores. Overall, anxiety decreased from preadmission (highest incidence) to discharge to follow-up. These findings suggest that some degree of mood disturbance is not uncommon during BMT and that this mood disturbance is often temporary.

A study of serial psychological assessment of 54 autologous BMT patients found that patterns of psychological distress differed between patients with hematological disorders and patients with breast cancer (Ahles et al., 1996). While patients with hematological disorders were generally more distressed than patients with breast cancer on admission for BMT, the former became less distressed over the course of the hospitalization, while the latter demonstrated a significant increase in distress at midtreatment and returned to baseline by discharge. The authors suggest that different levels of pretransplant experience with chemotherapy between these two groups may account for the differential patterns of distress; patients with breast cancer typically have had less experience coping with intensive treatment regimens than those with hematological disorders.

Another study prospectively examined the incidence of psychological morbidity in a sample of 40 patients with a wide variety of diagnoses. Patients were assessed pretransplant and at 1 month and 6 months after BMT. While limited by an incomplete data set due to attrition (of 36 patients who underwent BMT, 32 survived to 1-month follow-up and 21 survived to the 6-month follow-up; an additional 8 patients declined further evaluation), Jenkins and colleagues (1994) found an incidence of psychological distress similar to that found by Meyers and colleagues (1994). Results of pretransplant, structured clinical interviews of 31 patients indicated that 10 patients qualified for a diagnosis of Generalized Anxiety Disorder, and 5 patients met criteria for a Major Depressive Disorder. Similarly, on a standardized pencil-and-paper measure of anxiety and depression, 30% of the 30 patients who completed the measure scored above the cutoff level at the pretransplant assessment. By 1 month after transplant, this proportion dropped to 14.5%. However, it should be noted that only 13 patients completed the measure 1 month after transplant.

Another line of inquiry that has received some attention in the study of BMT is the relationship between psychological factors and physical symptoms. Research in other areas has repeatedly demonstrated associations between pain and depression, as well as between anxiety and nausea. Pain and nausea may be influential in mood and conversely, mood may be a factor in somatic complaints. It should not be surprising, therefore, when mood and symptom reports vary. BMT is clearly associated with pain, nausea, anxiety, and depression, and some interrelationships among these variables have been found. The study by Gaston-Johansson and colleagues (1992) of pain during BMT also examined anxiety and depression. Both anxiety and depression were significantly positively associated with concurrent pain ratings. Syrjala and colleagues (1992) found that global distress scores from a psychiatric symptomatology scale predicted nausea. While suggestive, this evidence is minimal due to the small number of studies reporting such types of analyses.

Relationships among Psychosocial Factors and Survival Outcomes

As in the wider psycho-oncology literature, another area of inquiry receiving increasing attention in the BMT literature addresses the relationships among psychosocial variables and survival outcomes of BMT recipients. To date, these studies must be considered preliminary

because they have been limited in number and had small samples of patients. The findings are intriguing but must be interpreted with caution as a function of methodological limitations, inconsistency of findings across studies, and the absence of replication studies.

The earliest published report examining such relationships found a significant difference in length of survival as a function of patients' scores on the "strive for recognition and help" dimension of a personality questionnaire administered to 35 patients (mostly with diagnoses of leukemia) within 2 days of admission for BMT (Neuser, 1988). Persons who scored high on this dimension, indicating greater striving for help and recognition, survived significantly longer than those with low scores. This relationship was found after controlling statistically for age, disease, and type of transplant. The author postulated that the relationship may be mediated by behavioral factors, suggesting that patients with high scores on this dimension may have elicited help from others, possibly improving the quality of the rigorous self-care necessitated by BMT. Other dimensions of the measure, including "discipline/ impulsivity," "ascendance," and "succorance/ nurturance" did not predict survival.

Another study addressing the relationships among psychosocial factors and survival after allogeneic BMT found that depressed mood was related to decreased survival, while high family support was related to improved survival, as was first remission status/early stage of disease at time of BMT (Colon et al., 1991). While the sample was relatively large and homogeneous, including 100 adults with acute leukemia, the method employed involved retrospective review of psychiatric interviews. These clinically oriented interviews were reviewed and coded on several dimensions by the researchers, without any report of inter-rater reliabilities. Because the interviews did not appear to have been designed as part of a research project, variables were coded on preexisting data. For example, depressed mood was coded for the presence or absence of depressed mood, without quantification of the severity or duration, and family support was coded on the basis of patients' self-reported perceptions of family support. Once again, while these findings are interesting and suggestive, methodological factors limit the ability to draw conclusions with confidence.

One recent study in this area made an effort to address some of the methodological weaknesses of the former studies. Andrykowski, Brady, and Henslee-Downey (1994) prospectively assessed a homogeneous sample of 42 BMT recipients (all adult patients with acute leukemia receiving allogeneic BMT) with well-standardized measures of quality of life, adjustment to cancer, and mood. In addition, the authors included concurrent consideration of a variety of demographic, disease, and treatment-related variables that may significantly influence survival outcomes including age at BMT, marital status, gender, time lag between diagnosis and BMT, education level, extent of marrow graft match, diagnosis type, and disease state at time of BMT. Of these variables, the latter four were, in fact, related to survival outcome. Three significant predictors of survival were found: quality of marrow graft match, level of "anxious preoccupation," and quality of life. Since level of anxious preoccupation and quality of life were not significantly correlated with disease and treatment variables, they cannot be viewed as mere reflections of disease status. In contrast to findings by Colon and colleagues (1991), depressed mood was found to be unrelated to survival.

Given the growing numbers of studies examining the relationships among psychosocial factors and survival outcomes in the general cancer literature, it is likely that this trend of research will continue within BMT settings as well. Well-designed, larger scale, future studies will likely shed much more light on the nature and underlying mechanism of these relationships.

PSYCHOLOGICAL INTERVENTIONS

Neuser and colleagues (1990), Patenaude and Rappeport (1984), and Rappaport (1988) have advocated collaboration between medical practitioners and mental health professionals in caring for BMT patients. Four major areas of psychosocial intervention are (1) psychological support, (2) specific behavioral interventions, (3) support groups, and (4) psychopharmacological support.

Psychological Support

At many centers, BMT patients are evaluated and followed, as necessary, by a variety of mental health specialists such as psychiatrists, psychologists, and/or psychiatric clinical nurse specialists. The initial evaluation, ideally occurring prehospitalization, serves to identify preexisting problems (e.g., psychiatric history) that may have an impact on the patients' treatment course and nursing interventions. More commonly, however, the mental health professionals are available to provide psychological support to the patient and family as the need arises during hospitalization. Patients and family members often report feeling uncomfortable using the time with physicians and nurses to discuss psychosocial issues since they have so many medical questions. Therefore, they appreciate the opportunity to have time available exclusively for the discussion of feelings and emotions.

The staff of mental health professionals involved in BMT programs varies considerably, but ideally includes psychologists, psychiatrists, social workers, psychiatric nurses, and consult-liaison services in various combinations to provide support for patients. These resources, however, need to be integrated with the daily support and encouragement offered by the nurses and other members of the BMT team. A team approach in which there is active communication among all professionals caring for the patient is ideal.

Behavioral Interventions

Behavioral techniques are being used increasingly in the management of symptoms associated with cancer and cancer treatments, particularly pain (Ahles, 1985, 1987) and nausea and vomiting (Burish and Carey, 1986). Three specific interventions may have relevance for managing mucositis pain and nausea and vomiting: (1) hypnosis, (2) relaxation, and (3) biofeedback.

Hypnosis

Hypnosis has a long history of use as a pain control technique. Several hypnotic strategies for pain reduction have been described (Barber and Gitelson, 1980):

- direct blocking of pain from awareness through the suggestion of anesthesia or analgesia,
- substitution of another sensation (e.g., pressure) for pain,
- moving the pain to a smaller or less important part of the body,
- changing the meaning of the pain so that it becomes less threatening, thereby increasing tolerance of pain, and
- dissociating part of the body from the patients' awareness.

Spiegel (1985) described three basic principles for teaching any hypnotic technique:

1. *Filter the hurt out of the pain.* Patients are taught that there is not a one-to-one correlation between the amount of physical damage and the perceived intensity of the

pain. By separating the affective component (which amplifies the pain) from the somatic component of the pain, the suffering can be reduced.
2. *Do not fight the pain.* Patients are taught that struggling with the pain can cause an exacerbation of it either through increasing reactive muscle tension or the affective component of the pain.
3. *Use self-hypnosis.* The patients are taught self-hypnosis so that they can use the techniques apart from the therapist.

Research has supported the efficacy of hypnosis in reducing nausea and vomiting associated with traditional chemotherapeutic approaches (Redd et al., 1982). With specific regard to BMT, there has been only one randomized, controlled, treatment-outcome study of psychosocial interventions: Syrjala and colleagues (1992) demonstrated that hypnosis was effective in reducing pain, but not nausea and emesis in patients undergoing BMT. Patients receiving cognitive-behavioral intervention, an attention control group, and a standard treatment control group showed no improvement on the outcome variables measured (pain, nausea, emesis, opioid use).

Relaxation Training

Relaxation training consists of a set of techniques designed to produce physiological and mental relaxation (Taylor, 1978). Two commonly used relaxation procedures are progressive muscle and autogenic relaxation. Progressive muscle relaxation (Bernstein and Borkovec, 1973) consists of systematically tensing and relaxing various muscle groups. Additionally, patients are instructed in diaphragmatic breathing exercises and taught to associate expiration with calming words such as *relax*. Autogenic relaxation (Schultz and Luthe, 1959), on the other hand, is a relatively passive technique. Patients adopt a quiet attitude and repeat autogenic phrases, such as "my arms are warm and heavy" and "my legs feel heavy and relaxed."

Relaxation techniques have been used successfully to control chemotherapy-related nausea and vomiting (Burish and Lyles, 1981; Lyles et al., 1982; Redd and Andrykowski, 1982) and have been suggested but less well studied for the control of cancer pain (Copley and Cobb, 1984; Fleming, 1985; Noyes, 1981; Payne and Foley, 1984). However, Syrjala and colleagues' (1992) treatment-outcome study of psychosocial interventions for BMT recipients did not find support for the efficacy of a cognitive-behavioral intervention that included a strong relaxation training component. However, the authors also reported that the intervention had many components for patients to learn over a short span of time. In addition, the study design included four groups and consisted of only 45 patients. Some of these methodological difficulties may partly explain this inconsistent, negative finding.

Biofeedback

Biofeedback has been defined as "a process in which a person learns to reliably influence physiological responses of two kinds: either responses that are not ordinarily under voluntary control or responses that ordinarily are easy to regulate but regulation has broken down because of trauma or disease" (Blanchard and Epstein, 1978). Biofeedback training entails the use of special electronic devices that detect and amplify biological responses and convert these amplified responses to signals that are easily understood by the patient. For example, a common signal is a tone whose pitch varies proportionately with the level of the biological response.

One of the most common types of biofeedback is electromyographic (EMG) biofeedback. EMG electrodes are attached to major muscles such as frontalis or trapezius muscles. Patients are taught to reduce EMG activity, which is indicated by a reduction in the biofeedback sig-

nal (e.g., the pitch of the tone). Other types of biofeedback include (1) temperature biofeedback (teaching patients to raise hand temperature); (2) skin conductance level (SCL) biofeedback (teaching patients to reduce SCL); and (3) electroencephalographic (EEG) biofeedback (theta, teaching a person to produce 4 Hz to 8 Hz activity, and alpha, teaching the person to produce 9 Hz to 13 Hz activity).

Biofeedback has been used to control nausea and vomiting (Burish et al., 1981) and pain (Fotopoulos et al., 1979; Fotopoulos et al., 1983) in cancer patients. Direct application of biofeedback for somatic symptoms in BMT patients has not yet been reported. However, portable EMG and SCL units have been used with hospitalized BMT patients to enhance relaxation.

Support Groups

Patenaude and colleagues (1986) described a support group for parents and spouses of BMT patients. The issues discussed include:

- introduction to the BMT unit,
- helplessness,
- empathy versus discipline,
- family relations,
- religion and money,
- relation to the medical team, and
- preparation for discharge.

Because of the isolation requirements at certain institutions, a support group for patients is not possible during their hospital stay. However, in institutions conducting primarily autologous BMT, a patient support group may be considered.

Psychopharmacological Support

There are some situations and some patients for whom pharmacologic treatment of their psychological distress is necessary. The two most common situations are those of extreme anxiety and moderate to severe delirium; depression is occasionally treated.

Pharmacologic treatment of anxiety for BMT patients is a cost/benefit question. The distress that the anxiety causes must be weighed against the CNS depressant effects of anxiolytics. BMT patients are often sedated from antiemetics, narcotics, and hypnotics, as well as fatigued from fevers, fluid and electrolyte disturbances, hematologic derangements, and respiratory problems. Caregivers must carefully weigh the addition of any sedating medication to such a clinical picture. An added consideration is that BMT patients are long-term patients; their long-term use of benzodiazepine anxiolytics should be carefully monitored to minimize physical or psychological dependence.

In spite of these obvious concerns, however, there are times when benzodiazepines are indicated for the treatment of anxiety. Most clinicians advocate the shorter acting benzodiazepines to minimize the buildup of sedation that can occur with longer acting agents. Accompanying this regimen with behavioral techniques to assist the patient in coping with the understandable anxiety can help to decrease the use of medications as well as assist the patient to regain a sense of control and accomplishment. It is best to start this teaching well before the patient is too sick or sedated to participate. Reevaluating the use of and necessity for anxiolytics periodically throughout the hospitalization can also help to keep their use at an acceptable minimum.

Delirium poses an obvious risk to this medically ill, frail population. If delirium is kept to a minimum, basic reorientation methods as well as repetition of information and directions can often suffice to manage the patient. However, if the cause is not determined and treated, a mild delirium can progress to a more severe problem. An agitated patient can inadvertently cause a tragedy by struggling with a caregiver who is attempting to keep him or her in bed or away from whatever tubing he or she is attempting to pull out. The physical damage that such action can cause a BMT patient with thrombocytopenia is of concern. In these situations, it may be necessary to sedate and treat the patient with one of the neuroleptic medications.

The choice of neuroleptics is usually determined by evaluating the potential side effects of the specific agent. However, patients already using a neuroleptic successfully as part of their antiemetic regimen can often tolerate an increase in dose. In such cases, the increase is preferable to complicating the picture with a different neuroleptic. The extrapyramidal system (EPS) side effects associated with the neuroleptics must be monitored carefully to minimize their distressing occurrence. Sometimes switching to a different neuroleptic is possible, but some unfortunate patients react to all of the neuroleptics. In this case, clinicians must weigh the use of additional medications to treat these side effects against the necessity of using the neuroleptic. Also, the relatively rare but very serious potential of neuroleptic malignant syndrome (NMS) must be remembered, and patients' symptoms carefully monitored whenever neuroleptics (even antiemetics) are used.

In rare instances, a BMT patient's discouragement and demoralization progresses to an actual psychiatric major depression, for which antidepressant medications may be indicated. The use of tricyclic antidepressants must be weighed against their potential side effects: orthostatic hypotension, anticholinergic effects such as dry mouth, constipation, urinary retention, and delirium, and cardiac conduction effects (prolonged ventricular polarization). Agranulocytosis is rare but must be considered in these patients with prolonged periods of neutropenia. In this medically ill population, the choice of antidepressant should be heavily determined by the specific medication's side effects. Overdose of these medications can be fatal, so careful assessment of suicidality must be done before and during their use. Another major problem of the tricyclic antidepressants is the period of time that most BMT patients are NPO due to oral infections. Parenteral use of these medications is not common so clinicians should use them cautiously. Intramuscular dosing, the most common parenteral route of administration, is contraindicated in this thrombocytopenic population. This leaves only intravenous administration, which has been done only rarely.

Monoamine oxidase inhibitors (MAOIs) may help in patients who have not responded to other antidepressant medications. Their advantage over tricyclic medications is the lack of anticholinergic side effects and decreased likelihood of provoking cardiac arrhythmias. However, they can cause postural hypotension as well as hypertensive reactions associated with interactions with foods that contain tyramine and sympathomimetic drugs. Also, interactions with meperidine are exceedingly dangerous and can be fatal. Surgery on patients who are taking MAOIs must be undertaken only with great care because the chance of interaction with these medications is greatest at this time. MAOIs are not available parenterally and are therefore not appropriate for patients with significant episodes of being NPO.

Selective serotonin reuptake inhibitors (SSRIs) such as fluoxetine, sertraline, and paroxetine as a class of antidepressants have much fewer side effects and are therefore better tolerated and generally safer for the medically ill. However, these medications can interfere with the metabolism of some other medications, increasing their blood levels. Of the three, sertraline is least apt to cause these problems. SSRIs are not available parenterally, and so should not be started on patients who will soon be NPO.

All antidepressant medications require a fairly long (1 to 2 weeks) initial timeframe to see a response. The risks of side effects must be carefully weighed against the risks of untreated depression. However, pharmacological treatment of depression, even in the seriously, acutely medically ill such as bone marrow and stem cell transplant patients, can be safely achieved and contribute greatly to the patients' capability to perform essential self-care activities.

These major drawbacks to antidepressant medications, added to the necessity of starting the patient on a low dose and building up slowly in order to minimize side effects, reinforces the position that antidepressant medications are not a rapid solution to the depressed patient's problem. They are clearly not appropriate for the temporarily discouraged patient who will feel better in the near future when his or her counts come up and physical status improves. These medications should be reserved for the severely depressed patient who has consistently shown significant depressive symptoms for several weeks and/or has a significant history of major affective disorder.

Dependence and Addiction

The use of potentially addictive medications, particularly the benzodiazepines to control anxiety and nausea and use of narcotics to control pain and rigors, typically raises concerns regarding the potential for dependency and addiction. This issue has not been systematically studied in BMT patients. However, data from other medical populations suggest that the risk of developing problems of dependency or addiction is quite low when these medications are used in a medically appropriate manner to treat relatively acute problems (Porter and Jick, 1980; Angell, 1982).

MEASUREMENT OF PSYCHOSOCIAL STATUS

Standardized assessment improves comparisons across research studies and increases confidence in the reliability and validity of conclusions. For clinical purposes, standardized assessment tools allow comparison of individuals to group norms, which aids in the interpretation of an individual score. Table 14.1 provides a list of standardized psychosocial measurement tools, grouped by content area, many of which have been used in the research reviewed. Many of these tools are widely used in both research and clinical applications in BMT settings and beyond.

In addition to standardized questionnaires, investigators and clinicians have used visual analogue scales (VAS) of depression, anxiety, and distress (Ahles et al., 1984; Aitken, 1974). These scales typically take the form of 10 cm lines, anchored at the left end with "no distress" (anxiety, depression) and on the right with "extreme distress" (anxiety, depression). The patient simply places a slash along the line indicating the level of distress. The major advantage of a VAS is its simplicity and consequently, the possibility of asking patients to complete these on a daily basis. Similarly, pain can be assessed via VAS scales, as can nausea. Numerical rating scales (0–10 or 0–100) are also often used as indices of pain and nausea.

TABLE 14.1 Standardized psychosocial assessment tools for research and clinical applications in BMT settings

Content area	Name of measure	Primary reference
Psychological symptoms/mood	Profile of Mood States	McNair et al., 1971
	Brief Profile of Mood States	Schacham, 1983
	Symptom Checklist—90	Derogatis, 1977
	Brief Symptom Inventory	Derogatis & Melisaratos, 1983
	Beck Depression Inventory	Beck et al., 1961
	Zung Depression Scale	Zung, 1965
	Hospital Anxiety and Depression Scale	Zigmond & Snaith, 1983
	State-Trait Anxiety Inventory	Spielberger et al., 1970
	State-Trait Anger Expression Inventory	Speilberger, 1988
Personality	Minnesota Multiphasic Personality Inventory	Hathaway & McKinley, 1967
	Eysenck Personality Questionnaire	Eysenck & Eysenck, 1964
Coping	Ways of Coping	Folkman & Lazarus, 1987
Impact of illness	Sickness Impact Profile	Gilson et al., 1975
	Psychosocial Adjustment to Illness Scale	Derogatis & Lopez, 1983
	Mental Adjustment to Cancer Scale	Watson et al., 1988
	Manitoba Functional Living Index—Cancer	Schipper et al., 1984
Pain, nausea, and emesis	McGill Pain Questionnaire	Melzack, 1975
	Dartmouth McGill Pain Questionnaire	Corson and Schneider, 1984
	Memorial Pain Card	Fishman et al., 1987
	Morrow Assessment of Nausea and Emesis	Morrow, 1984
Other	Multidimensional Health Locus of Control	Wallston et al., 1978
	Social Adjustment Scale	Weissman & Bothwell, 1976
	Norbeck Social Support Questionnaire	Norbeck et al., 1981

SUMMARY

Although the body of empirical literature on BMT and its psychosocial effects is still relatively sparse and limited, several overall conclusions can be drawn. The decision to undergo BMT is particularly difficult because there are many unanswered questions about the procedure and outcomes. Serious psychiatric disorder and severe mood disturbance are not common responses to the pretreatment and acute treatment phases of BMT, however, a substantial proportion of patients experience some level of anxiety and/or depression during the course of the procedure. Temporary, and possibly permanent, neuropsychological impairment may occur in a proportion of BMT cases. Neuropsychological impairment can also exist as a function of pretransplant treatment. Finally, psychosocial interventions that have been useful for cancer patients undergoing other forms of active treatment may be applicable to BMT, although they may require modifications to better fit the special demands of the procedure. This type of information begins to provide valuable guidance for efforts at improving the quality of life of patients considering and receiving bone marrow transplants.

While the data reviewed here have begun to elucidate some of the psychosocial aspects of bone marrow transplant, many methodological limitations have limited the confidence with which one can apply these findings. Factors such as small sample sizes, cross-sectional and retrospective designs, absence of adequate control groups, and the use of unstandardized measures are a few examples. In such a hard-to-reach clinical population, large-scale, prospective, longitudinal, controlled designs are very difficult to implement for practical purposes. However, as the number of transplants performed increases year after year, these types of investigations may be easier to implement.

In loving memory of Jeff Necowitz

REFERENCES

Ahles, T. 1985. Psychological approaches to the treatment of cancer-related pain. *Semin Oncol Nurs 1*: 141-146.

Ahles, T. 1987. Psychological techniques for the management of cancer pain. In McGuire, D., Yarbro, C. (Eds.) *Cancer Pain Management*. Orlando: Grune & Stratton, 245-258.

Ahles, T., Ruckdeschel, J., Blanchard, G. 1984. Cancer-related pain; II: assessment with visual analogue scales. *J Psychosomat Res 28*:121-124.

Ahles, T., Tope, D., Furstenberg, C., et al. 1996. Psychologic and neuropsychologic impact of autologous bone marrow transplantation. *J Clin Oncol 14*(5): 1457-1467.

Aitken, R. 1974. Assessment of mood by analogue. In Beck, A., Resnick, H., Lettier, D. (Eds.) *The Prediction of Suicide*. Bowie, MD: Charles Press.

Andrykowski, M. 1994a. Psychosocial factors in bone marrow transplantation: a review and recommendations for research. *BMT 13*:357-375.

Andrykowski, M. 1994b. Psychiatric and psychosocial aspects of bone marrow transplantation. *Psychosomatics 35*(1):13-24.

Andrykowski, M., Brady, M., Henslee-Downey, P. 1994. Psychosocial factors predictive of survival after allogeneic bone marrow transplantation for leukemia. *Psychosomat Med 56*:432-439.

Andrykowski, M., Henslee, P., Farrall, M. 1989. Physical and psychosocial functioning of adult survivors of allogeneic bone marrow transplantation. *BMT 4*:75-81.

Andrykowski, M., Schmitt, F., Gregg, M., et al. 1992. Neuropsychologic impairment in adult bone marrow transplant candidates. *Cancer 70*(9):2288-2297.

Angell, M. 1982. The quality of mercy. *N Engl J Med 306*:98-99.

Barber, J., Gitelson, J. 1980. Cancer pain: psychological management using hypnosis. *Cancer 30*:130-136.

Beck, A., Ward, C., Mendelson, M., et al. 1961. An inventory for measuring depression. *Arch Gen Psychiatr 4*:561-571.

Belec, R. 1992. Quality of life: perceptions of long-term survivors of bone marrow transplantation. *Oncol Nurs Forum 19*(1):31-37.

Bernstein, D., Borkovec, T. 1973. *Progressive Relaxation Training*. Champaign, IL: Research Press.

Blanchard, E., Epstein, L. 1978. *A Biofeedback Primer*. Reading, MA: Addison-Wesley.

Burish, T., Carey, M. 1986. Conditioned aversive responses in cancer chemotherapy patients: theoretical and developmental aspects. *J Consult Clin Psych 54*: 593-600.

Burish, T., Lyles, J. 1981. Effectiveness of relaxation training in reducing adverse reactions to cancer chemotherapy. *J Behav Med 4*:65-78.

Chapko, M., Syrjala, K., Schilter, L., et al. 1989. Chemoradiotherapy toxicity during bone marrow transplantation: time course and variation in pain and nausea. *BMT 4*:181-186.

Cobb, S.C. 1984. Teaching relaxation techniques to cancer patients. *Canc Nurs 7*:157-164.

Colon, E., Callies, A., Popkin, M., et al. 1991. Depressed mood and other variables related to bone marrow transplantation survival in acute leukemia. *Psychosomatics 32*(4):420-425.

Corson, J., Schneider, M. 1984. The Dartmouth pain questionnaire: an adjunct to the McGill pain questionnaire. *Pain 19*:59-69.

Dermatis, H., Lesko, L. 1991. Psychosocial correlates of physician-patient communication at time of informed consent for bone marrow transplantation. *Canc Invest 9*(6):621-628.

Derogatis, L. 1977. *Administration, Scoring and Procedures Manual for the SCL-90-R*. Baltimore: Clinical Psychometrics Research.

Derogatis, L., Lopez, M. 1983. *PAIS and PAIS-SR: Administration, Scoring and Procedures Manual*. Baltimore: Clinical Psychometrics Research.

Derogatis, L., Melisaratos, N. 1983. The brief symptom inventory: an introductory report. *Psychol Med 13*: 595-605.

Eysenck, H., Eysenck, S. 1964. *Eysenck Personality Inventory*. London: University Press.

Feifel, H., Strack, S., Nagy, V. 1987. Coping strategies and associated features of medically ill patients. *Psychosomat Med 49*:616-625.

Fishman, B., Pasternak, S., Wallenstein, S. 1987. The Memorial Pain Assessment Card: a valid instrument for the evaluation of cancer pain. *Cancer 60*:1151-1158.

Fleming, U. 1985. Relaxation training for far advanced cancer. *The Practitioner 229*:471-475.

Folkman, S., Lazarus, R. 1987. *Manual for the Ways of Coping Questionnaire*. Palo Alto, CA: Consulting Psychologists Press.

Fotopoulos, S., Cook, M., Graham, C., et al. 1983. Cancer pain: evaluation of electromyographic and electrodermal feedback. *Prog Clin Biol Res 132*:33-53.

Fotopoulos, S., Graham, C., Cook, M. 1979. Psychophysiologic control of cancer pain. In Bonica, J., Ventafridda, V. (Eds.) *Advances in Pain Research and Therapy*, vol. 2. New York: Raven.

Gaston-Johansson, F., Franco, T., Zimmerman, L. 1992. Pain and psychological distress in patients undergoing autologous bone marrow transplantation. *Oncol Nurs Forum 19*(1):41-48.

Gilson, B., Gilson, J., Bergner, M., et al. 1975. The Sickness Impact Profile: development of an outcome measure of health care. *Am J Public Health 65*: 1304-1310.

Hathaway S., McKinley, J. 1967. *The Minnesota Multiphasic Personality Inventory Manual*. New York: Psychological Corp.

Hengeveld, M., Houtman, R., Zwaan, F. 1988. Psychological aspects of bone marrow transplantation: a retrospective study of 17 long-term survivors. *BMT 3*:69-75.

Hill, H., Chapman, C., Kornell, J., et al. 1990. Self-administration of morphine in bone marrow transplant patients reduces drug requirement. *Pain 40*:121-129.

Jenkins, P., Lester, H., Alexander, J. 1994. A prospective study of psychosocial morbidity in adult bone marrow transplant recipients. *Psychosomatics 35*(4):361-367.

Kaehler, S., Goodwin, J., Young, L. 1989. Bone marrow transplantation: mastering the experience despite psychological risk factors. *Psychosomatics 30*(3):337-341.

Lesko, L. 1989a. Bone marrow transplantation. In Holland, J., Rowland, J. (Eds.) *Handbook of Psychooncology: Psychological Care of the Patient with Cancer*. New York: Oxford University Press, 163-173.

Lesko, L. 1989b. Protected environments. In Holland, J., Rowland, J. (Eds.) *Handbook of Psychooncology: Psychological Care of the Patient with Cancer*. New York: Oxford University Press, 174-179.

Lesko, L. 1993. Psychiatric aspects of bone marrow transplantation, part 1: special issues during pre-transplant assessment and hospitalization. *Psycho-oncology 2*:161-183.

Lyles, J., Burish, T., Krozely, M., et al. 1982. Efficacy of relaxation training and guided imagery in reducing the aversiveness of cancer chemotherapy. *J Consult Clin Psychol 50*:509-524.

McGuire, D., Altomonte, V., Peterson, D., et al. 1993. Patterns of mucositis and pain in patients receiving preparative chemotherapy and bone marrow transplantation. *Oncol Nurs Forum* 20(10):1493-1502.

McNair, D., Lorr, M., Droppleman, L. 1971. *Profile of Mood States*. San Diego: Educational and Industrial Testing Service.

Melzack, R. 1975. The McGill Pain Questionnaire: major properties and scoring methods. *Pain* 1:277-299.

Meyers, C., Abbruzzese, J. 1992. Cognitive functioning in cancer patients: effect of previous treatment. *Neurology* 42:434-436.

Meyers, C., Scheibel, R., Forman, A. 1991. Persistent neurotoxicity of systemically administered interferon-alpha. *Neurology* 41:672-676.

Meyers, C., Weitzner, M., Byrne, K., et al. 1994. Evaluation of the neurobehavioral functioning of patients before, during, and after bone marrow transplantation. *J Clin Oncol* 12(4):820-826.

Morrow, G. 1984. Clinical characteristics associated with the development of anticipatory nausea and vomiting in cancer patients undergoing chemotherapy treatment. *J Clin Oncol* 2:1170-1176.

Neuser, J. 1988. Personality and survival time after bone marrow transplantation. *J Psychosomat Res* 32(4/5):451-455.

Neuser, J., Grigelat, G., Quabeck, K., et al. 1990. Principles of supportive psychological care for patients undergoing bone marrow transplantation. *Haematol Blood Transfusion* 33:583-586.

Norbeck, J., Lindsey, A., Carrieri, V. 1981. The development of an instrument to measure social support. *Nurs Res* 30:264-269.

Noyes, R. 1981. Treatment of cancer pain. *Psychosomat Med* 43:57-70.

Parth, P., Dunlap, W., Kennedy, R., et al. 1989. Motor and cognitive testing of bone marrow transplant patients after chemoradiotherapy. *Perceptual and Motor Skills* 68:1227-1241.

Patenaude, A., Levinger, L., Baker, K. 1986. Group meetings for parents and spouses of bone marrow transplant patients. *Soc Work Health Care* 12(1):51-65.

Patenaude, A., Rappeport, J. 1984. Collaboration between hematologists and mental health professionals on a bone marrow transplant team. *J Psychosoc Oncol* 2(3/4):81-92.

Payne, R., Foley, K. 1984. Advances in the management of cancer pain. *Canc Treat Rep* 68:173-183.

Porter, J., Jick, H. 1980. Addiction rare in patients treated with narcotics. *N Engl J Med* 302:123.

Rappaport, B. 1988. Evolution of consultation-liaison services in bone marrow transplantation. *Gener Hosp Psychiatr* 10:346-351.

Redd, W., Andresen, G., Minagawa, R. 1982. Hypnotic control of anticipatory emesis in patients receiving cancer chemotherapy. *J Consult Clin Psychol* 50:14-19.

Redd, W., Andrykowski, M. 1982. Behavioral intervention in cancer treatment: controlling aversion reactions to chemotherapy. *J Consult Clin Psychol* 50:1018-1029.

Rodin, G., Voshart, K. 1986. Depression in the medically ill: an overview. *Am J Psychiatr* 143:696-705.

Rodrigue, J., Boggs, S., Weiner, R., et al. 1993. Mood, coping style, and personality functioning among adult bone marrow transplant candidates. *Psychosomatics* 34(2):159-165.

Schacham, S. 1983. A shortened version of the Profile of Mood States. *J Personal Assess* 47:305-306.

Schipper, H., Clinch, J., McMurray, A., et al. 1984. Measuring the quality of life of cancer patients: The Functional Living Index—Cancer: development and validation. *J Clin Oncol* 2:472-483.

Schultz, J., Luthe, W. 1959. *Autogenic Training*. New York: Grune & Stratton.

Silberfarb, P. 1983. Chemotherapy and cognitive deficits in cancer patients. *Ann Rev Med* 34:35-46.

Spiegel, D. 1985. The use of hypnosis in controlling cancer pain. *Cancer* 35:221-231.

Spielberger, C. 1988. *State-Trait Anger Expression Inventory: Research Edition*. Odessa, FL: Psychological Assessment Resources.

Spielberger, C., Gorsuch, R., Lushene, R. 1970. *Manual for the State-Trait Anxiety Inventory*. Palo Alto: Consulting Psychologist Press.

Stemmer, S., Stears, J., Burton, B., et al. 1994. White matter changes in patients with breast cancer treated with high dose chemotherapy and autologous bone marrow support. *Am J Neuroradiol* 15:1267-1273.

Syrjala, K., Cummings, C., Donaldson, G. 1992. Hypnosis or cognitive behavioral training for the reduction of pain and nausea during cancer treatment: a controlled clinical trial. *Pain* 48:137-146.

Syrjala, K., Roth, S., Abrams, J. 1995. Major depression predicts survival during life threatening medical treatment. Poster presented at Society of Behavioral Medicine Annual Meeting, San Diego, March.

Taylor, B. 1978. Relaxation training and related techniques. In Agras, S. (Ed.) *Behavior Modification: Principles and Clinical Applications*. Boston: Little, Brown.

Wallston, K., Wallston, B., DeVellis, R. 1978. Development of the multidimensional health locus of control scales. *Health Ed Monogr* 6:160-170.

Watson, M., Greer, S., Young, J., et al. 1988. Development of a questionnaire measure of adjustment to cancer: the MAC scale. *Psychol Med* 18:203-209.

Weissman, M., Bothwell, S. 1976. Assessment of social adjustment by patient self-report. *Arch Gen Psychiatr* 33:1111-1115.

Whedon, M., Ferrell, B. 1994. Quality of life in adult bone marrow transplant patients: beyond the first year. *Semin Oncol Nurs* 10(1):42-57.

Zigmond, A., Snaith, R. 1983. Hospital Anxiety and Depression Scale. *Acta Psychiatr Scandinav* 67:361-370.

Zung, W. 1965. A self-rating depression scale. *Arch Gen Psychiatr* 12:63-70.

PART III
Issues of Recovery

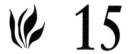

15

Fertility and Sexuality

Alyson B. Moadel, Jamie S. Ostroff, Lynna M. Lesko

One of the goals of comprehensive care is providing blood cell and marrow transplant (BCT/BMT) patients with appropriate education and rehabilitation to enable them to adjust to posttreatment changes in their function and roles. Given the high physical toxicity and psychological demands of the BCT/BMT regimen, long-term sequelae can adversely affect reproductive and sexual functioning, areas that can be particularly challenging during this adjustment process. Gonadal dysfunction and sexual impairment are commonly noted late effects of BCT and BMT (Kolb et al., 1989; Vose et al., 1992). As research and clinical study of the posttreatment adjustment of transplant survivors accumulates, it is becoming clear that these psychosexual issues are major concerns for survivors and their partners.

CANCER TREATMENT AND GONADAL FUNCTION

Patients receiving BMT or BCT are often given preparatory treatment consisting of chemotherapy and radiotherapy. Some patients also have surgery (i.e., retroperitoneal lymph node dissection for testicular cancer) prior to transplant. These three treatment modalities can all affect gonadal and sexual functioning. To quote Sherins (1993, p. 2395), "neoplastic disease and its treatment can potentially interfere with any of the cellular, anatomic, physiologic, behavioral, or social processes that contribute to normal sexual and reproductive function." The reader is referred to this excellent comprehensive review as background to material presented here. For clarity, the gonadal effects of each treatment modality will be briefly described.

Several chemotherapeutic agents profoundly influence male and female gonadal function; such chemotherapeutic agents and their toxicity are listed in Table 15.1. Similarly, gonadal dysfunction and infertility can occur in both men and women following radiation that includes the pelvic area. Further, secondary ovarian failure will likely occur from incidental hypothalamic-pituitary irradiation in women receiving radiotherapy to the brain (Bajorunas, 1980). The cumulative doses of the chemotherapeutic agent and radiation treatment, and for women, the age of the patient, are influential in the probability and severity of gonadal impairment. It appears that men and older women are less able to tolerate larger cumulative drug and radiotherapy doses before gonadal dysfunction develops and have a greater likelihood of permanent dysfunction when treatment is stopped (Sherins, 1993). For the male transplant recipient with a history of testicular cancer, the risk for gonadal impairment

TABLE 15-1 Chemotherapeutic agents associated with infertility

Risk of infertility	Drug	
	Male	*Female*
High-Definite	Chlorambucil	Cyclophosphamide
	Cyclophosphamide	Nitrogen mustard
	Nitrogen mustard	Busulfan
	Busulfan	L-Phenylalanine
	Procarbazine	
	Nitrosoureas	
Probable	Doxorubicin	
	Vinblastine	
	Cytosine arabinoside	
	Cisplatin	
Unlikely	Methotrexate	Methotrexate
	5-Fluorouracil	5-Fluorouracil
	6-Mercaptopurine	6-Mercaptopurine
	Vincristine	
Unknown	Bleomycin	Doxorubicin
		Bleomycin
		Vinca alkaloids
		Cisplatin
		Nitrosoureas
		Cytosine arabinoside

SOURCE: Adapted from Sherins, R.J. 1993. Gonadal dysfunction. In DeVita, V.T., Hellman, S., Rosenberg, S.A. (Eds.) *Cancer: Principles and Practice of Oncology,* 4th ed., vol. 2. Philadelphia: Lippincott, 2397-2398. With permission.

related to these treatments may be compounded by pretransplant surgical intervention. Retroperitoneal lymph node dissection for testicular cancer staging may injure sympathetic innervation of the pelvic viscera and result in retrograde ejaculation and inadequate emission of sperm (Sherins, 1993).

In men, gonadotoxic treatments produce a dose-related depletion of the germinal epithelium lining, which results in decreased testicular volume, oligospermia, azoospermia, and possible infertility. Low sperm count and elevated follicle-stimulating hormone (FSH) levels are physiological indicators of such germinal aplasia. (Spaulding and Spaulding, 1985, review

normal testicular development and physiology.) In women, treatment-induced ovarian failure is evident by dysfunction of ova and follicles, ovarian fibrosis, low estradiol levels, and elevated serum FSH and luteinizing hormone (LH), which results in amenorrhea and menopausal symptoms of estrogen deficiency (e.g., hot flashes, sweats, vaginal dryness). (Normal oogenesis and ovarian physiology is reviewed by Gradishar and Schilsky, 1989.)

Blood Cell and Marrow Transplantation

For the purpose of addressing sexuality/fertility issues, blood cell and marrow transplantation patients can be considered in two groups. The first group consists of individuals with hematologic malignancies, many of whom will have been previously treated with multimodal treatment (chemotherapy, radiotherapy, and/or surgery). Hence, many of these patients experience compromised gonadal function prior to even undergoing transplant. Additional high-dose chemotherapy and radiotherapy given with transplant severely complicate gonadal function and recovery. The second group consists of patients with aplastic anemia, with no previous cytoreductive treatment. For this group, the preparatory regimen for transplant usually consists of high-dose chemotherapy alone.

Men

When transplant includes total body irradiation (TBI), most men experience gonadal failure, and few experience recovery of function (Benker et al., 1989; Chatterjee et al., 1994; Heimpel et al., 1991; Keilholz et al., 1989; Sanders, 1987; Sanders et al., 1983). Further, pretransplant gonadal impairment is often exacerbated in many men following transplant (Chatterjee et al., 1994). Among prepubertal and pubertal boys transplanted after preparation with cyclophosphamide (Cy) and TBI, delayed puberty and/or abnormal gonadotropin levels have been found (Liesner et al., 1994; Sanders, 1987; Sklar et al., 1984). On the other hand, normal testicular function often follows transplant prepared with Cy and no irradiation. Such men have been found to have normal testosterone levels after transplant with most regaining normal gonadotropin levels (Sanders et al., 1983). Although limited data was available on semen analysis, 67% of patients appeared to have detectable sperm counts.

Women

Alkylating agents combined with abdominal radiation have been implicated in causing the greatest damage to the ovary (Schubert et al., 1990). Accordingly, TBI and high-dose chemotherapy given in preparation for bone marrow transplantations lead to primary ovarian failure in nearly every patient (Benker et al., 1989; Heimpel et al., 1991; Keilholz et al., 1989; Sanders et al., 1988; Schubert et al., 1990; Sklar et al., 1983). This pattern is similar among prepubertal girls who are likely to experience delayed development with absence of menarche following transplant prepared with Cy and TBI, but not with Cy alone (Liesner et al., 1994; Sanders, 1987). Transplant conditioning regimens consisting of alkylating agents (e.g., Cy) and busulfan (Bu) are equally toxic to the ovaries (Crilley et al., 1992; Vergauwen et al., 1994). On the other hand, the majority of patients who receive a regimen of Cy alone regain normal gonadal function although recovery may be transient (2 to 6 years) (Sanders et al., 1983, 1988; Sanders, 1987). Recovery of ovarian function occurred in less than 10% of women between 3 and 7 years after transplantation, all of whom were 26 years and younger at transplant. Older patient age and TBI appear to be significantly correlated with a greater probability of ovarian failure.

Blood Cell and Marrow Transplantation and Pregnancy

The outcomes of pregnancies and deliveries of normal children among transplant survivors have been described in several studies (Atkinson et al., 1994; Buskard et al., 1989; Card et al., 1980; Deeg et al., 1983; Heimpel et al., 1991; Hinterberger-Fischer et al., 1991; Jacobs and Dubovsky, 1981; Milliken et al., 1990; Russell and Hanley, 1989; Sanders, 1987; Sanders et al., 1988; Sanders et al., 1983; Wingard et al., 1992). These results are shown in Table 15.2. Transplant survivors most likely to conceive offspring are those who (1) had no previous induction or conditioning chemotherapy regi-

TABLE 15.2 Pregnancy and bone marrow transplantation

Study	Sex/Disease/Treatment	Results
Card et al., 1980	Female/aplastic anemia 29 years old at BMT Chemotherapy	Delivered normal infant 24 months post BMT
Jacobs & Dubovsky, 1981	Female/aplastic anemia 36 years old at BMT Chemotherapy	Delivered normal infant 21 months post BMT
Deeg et al., 1983	Female/aplastic anemia 25 years old at BMT Chemotherapy	Delivered normal infant 23 months post BMT
Sanders et al., 1983	31 males/aplastic anemia Chemotherapy	3 pts fathered 4 children
	41 males/leukemia Chemotherapy and TBI	1 pt fathered 2 children

Sanders et al., 1988	43 females/aplastic anemia
	Chemotherapy
	(N=27): age <26 yrs at BMT
	(N=16): age >26 yrs at BMT
		6 pts/8 pregnancies
		  5 pts delivered 7 normal infants
		  1 pt had elective abortion
		3 pts/4 pregnancies
		  1 normal delivery

	144 females/leukemia
	Chemotherapy and TBI
		9/144 ovarian recovery
		  all 13–25 yrs old at BMT
		  3 pregnancies in 2 pts at 3, 5, 6 yrs post BMT
		  no live births

Russell & Hanley, 1989	Female/leukemia 21 years old at BMT Chemotherapy and TBI	Delivered normal infant 3.5 years post BMT
Milliken et al., 1990	2 females/leukemia 16 years old at BMT Chemotherapy and Bu	Delivered 2 normal infants 4 and 5 years post BMT
	25 years old at BMT Chemotherapy and Bu	Delivered 1 normal infant 6 years post BMT
Heimpel et al., 1991	32 males/aplastic anemia or leukemia Chemotherapy and TBI/TNI	0 fathered children post BMT
	39 females/aplastic anemia, leukemia, other (N=35): chemotherapy and TBI/TNI (N=4): chemotherapy	0 pregnancies post BMT 1 pt/2 pregnancies/1 normal delivery
Hinterberger-Fischer et al., 1991	9 males/aplastic anemia, hematologic malignancy (N=7): chemotherapy and TBI/abdominal radiation (N=2): chemotherapy	0 fathered children post BMT 1 pt fathered 2 children 1 with postnatal complications

Continued

TABLE 15.2 *Continued*

Study	Sex/Disease/Treatment	Results
Hinterberger-Fischer et al., 1991 (*continued*)	14 females/aplastic anemia, hematologic malignancy (N=9): chemotherapy and TBI/abdom radiation (N=5): chemotherapy	0 pregnancies post BMT 3 pts/3 pregnancies 2 normal deliveries with postnatal complications evident
Wingard et al., 1992	82 males/53 females aplastic anemia, malignancy (N=16): chemotherapy (N=66): chemotherapy +Bu/TBI	2 males fathered infants 0 pregnancies post BMT
Atkinson et al., 1994	Female/leukemia pretransplant oocyte collection, IVF and cryopreservation 24 years old at BMT Chemotherapy and TBI	ovarian failure evident 1 of 3 transferred embryos developed normally in utero Delivered normal infant 3.5 years post BMT

KEY: pt = patient, TBI = total body irradiation, TNI = total nodal irradiation, Bu = Busulfan, IVF = in vitro fertilization

mens; (2) received only high-dose cyclophosphamide as a preparatory regimen for their transplant (i.e., no radiation); and (3) were relatively young (<26 years of age) at time of transplant. These conditions are most indicative of less gonadal damage. Consistent with this profile, many more patients treated for aplastic anemia than hematologic malignancies successfully conceive and bring to term a normal infant. However, a high incidence of pre-, peri-, and post-partum complications (e.g., newborn jaundice, persistence of fetal circulation syndrome) in the offspring has been noted (Hinterberger-Fischer et al., 1991).

SPECIFIC SEXUAL DISORDERS ASSOCIATED WITH BMT/BCT

Human sexuality is usually categorized by sex therapists and researchers according to a multiphasic sexual response cycle divided into the phases of desire, arousal, orgasm, and resolution (Kaplan, 1974, 1983). According to this model of normal human sexual response, the *desire phase* is characterized by sexual thoughts and fantasies as well as interest in having sexual activity. The *arousal phase* consists of a subjective sense of sexual pleasure and accompanying physiologic changes. For men, penile tumescence leading to erection and the appearance of glandular secretions characterize the arousal phase. For women, pelvic vasocongestion, vaginal lubrication, and swelling of the external genitalia are signs of female arousal. *Orgasm* is a period of peak sexual pleasure, with release of sexual tension and rhythmic muscular contractions. In the male, there is the sensation of ejaculatory inevitability which is followed by emission of semen. Finally, during the *resolution phase* there is a sense of relaxation. Sexual disorders can occur at one or more phases of the sexual response cycle and are categorized by the *Diagnostic and Statistical*

Manual of Mental Disorders, Fourth Edition (DSM-IV; American Psychiatric Association (1994) into sexual desire disorders, sexual arousal disorders, orgasm disorders, and sexual pain disorders.

In the following section, we will describe the impact of transplant on the sexual response cycle according to the diagnostic categories in DSM-IV, summarized in Table 15.3. Attention will also be given to plausible physical and psychological mechanisms for understanding sexual difficulties in this special population. Given the paucity of controlled research on the sexual adjustment of transplant patients, much of the material presented is based on the authors' clinical experience as Psychiatry Service consultants to the Allogeneic and Autologous Transplant Services at Memorial Sloan-Kettering Cancer Center (MSKCC) and their research examining the psychosexual adjustment of cancer survivors treated with either transplant or conventional chemotherapy.

Generally speaking, patients rarely express sexual concerns prior to or during the acute hospitalization for their transplant. This is not surprising since patients are quite debilitated by the preparatory conditioning regimen and almost uniformly preoccupied with "life and death" issues such as separation from family, "surviving the transplant," marrow engraftment and "their counts." While sexual functioning is not a primary concern for hospitalized transplant patients, standard requirements for a sterile, germ-free environment during periods of bone marrow suppression and the lengthy isolation considerations, approximately 1 to 2 months, associated with the transplant impose severe restrictions on couples' interaction, and hence, intimacy and sexuality. In addition, acute and chronic GVHD and scars from venous access catheters may increase concerns about body image, which may subsequently impair sexuality. For most patients and their partners, the transplant and im-

mediate posthospitalization convalescence represent periods of sexual abstinence due to fatigue, pain, skin rashes, and other complications secondary to the transplant as well as the acute stress of the transplant on patients and their partners.

Posttransplant convalescence is quite lengthy; physical and psychological rehabilitation may last for 6 to 12 months. Until this point, patients often complain of persistent fatigue, anxiety about infections, depression, and difficulty reentering their normal home and work activities (Lesko, 1989). Generally, transplant patients become more concerned about their sexual health as their physical health improves. Usually it is not until, at least, 6 months after transplant that sexual interest and activity are resumed. Thus, sexual concerns and disorders are usually presented to the transplant team relatively late in the transplant rehabilitation period. Preliminary reports of decreased sexual satisfaction or activity following transplant range from 16% to 86% of transplant survivors (Altmaier et al., 1991; Baruch et al., 1991; Chao et al., 1992; Vose et al., 1992; Winer et al., 1992; Wingard et al., 1992). Even 10 years or more following transplant, decreased satisfaction with sex and intimacy have been reported by up to one third of transplant survivors (N = 125) (Bush et al., 1995).

The most common sexual disorder presented by male and female transplant patients is *hypoactive sexual desire disorder*. Low sexual desire consists of persistently deficient or absent sexual thoughts, fantasies, or desire for sexual activity. This diagnosis should always be made in the context of the patient's precancer sexual desire, age, sex, and physical health status. When compared to healthy nonpatients, female patients with acute leukemia who were treated with transplants reported significantly lower sexual drive (Mumma et al., 1989). Similarly, reports of low sexual desire increased from 0% to 15% following transplant in one group of 51

TABLE 15.3 Sexual disorders with blood cell and marrow transplantation

Phase	Sexual dysfunction	Relevance to BMT/BCT patients and survivors
DESIRE Sexual thoughts, day-dreaming fantasies; finding potential partner attractive	**SEXUAL DESIRE DISORDERS** **Hypoactive sexual desire disorder** Loss of interest in sex Few or no thoughts about sex Negative ("antisexual") attitudes about sex Anxious, panicky feeling about sex Avoidance of sexual situations	Not unusual when patient is in active treatment. Prolonged separation due to lengthy hospitalization, reverse isolation. After treatment, loss of desire may be related to treatment side effects, psychological factors (depression, anxiety) and partner issues, fear of infections, body image concerns, pain, GVHD, fatigue. Often requires longer treatment of couple by sex therapist because of prominent psychological component.
AROUSAL Subjective sense of excitement and pleasure; penile erection	**SEXUAL AROUSAL DISORDERS** **Male erectile disorder** Difficulty attaining or maintaining an erection	No direct physiological link between transplant and erectile function. Treatment depends on cause. Counseling to decrease anxiety and decrease focus on performance. Rare complaint in transplant patients, unless preexisting.
Vaginal lubrication and engorement in women	**Female sexual arousal disorder** Impaired vaginal lubrication and engorement in women	Common after pelvic irradiation, or any treatment that causes women ovarian loss or failure. Patient may complain of dry, sore vagina or painful intercourse. Treatment: estrogens (local/systemic), lubricant, taking more time for foreplay, communication issues.
ORGASM Reflex muscle contractions, associated with pleasure, ejaculation and emission in men, pleasurable sensation in women	**ORGASMIC DISORDERS** **Female orgasmic disorder** Delay or absence of orgasm following normal sexual excitement phase	May be related to fatigue, depression, stress, medication, anxiety, inadequate arousal phase. Need longer or more direct stimulation of clitoris. Address need for time and relaxation, communication issues with partner.

Continued

TABLE 15.3 *Continued*

Phase	Sexual dysfunction	Relevance to BMT/BCT patients and survivors
	Male orgasmic disorder Delay or absence of orgasm following normal sexual excitement phase	May be related to fatigue, depression, stress, medication, anxiety.
	Premature ejaculation Inability to control timing of orgasm	Rare complaint in transplant patients, unless preexisting. More common in young transplant patients and after prolonged period of abstinence.
	Retrograde ejaculation Ejaculate empties into bladder resulting in "dry ejaculation"	May occur after pretransplant surgical staging of testicular cancer patients.
OTHER	**SEXUAL PAIN DISORDERS**	
	Dyspareunia: Genital pain with intercourse	Often leads to sexual avoidance unless treated promptly. Requires thorough gynecological evaluation and treatment of cause (irradiation changes, estrogen deficiency). Practice "no painful sex" rule (i.e., no intercourse unless medical cause is adequately treated).
	Vaginismus Vaginal muscle spasm, penetration painful or impossible	Response to pain or fear of pain with penetration. Good prognosis with combined relaxation and sequenced penetration treatment, done by patient herself, then with partner.

SOURCE: Adapted from Auchincloss, S.S. 1989.

men treated for hematologic malignancies (Baruch et al., 1991).

The sexual desire of transplant patients may be diminished for several direct reasons such as persistent fatigue, diminished body image (e.g. skin lesions caused by GVHD, catheter insertion), depression, and reluctance to resume sexual activity due to fear of infection with intercourse. Another factor thay may inhibit return of sexual desire is that transplant survivors may be preoccupied with more major life concerns such as reestablishing job and family roles. In addition, among female transplant patients, low estrogen levels secondary to cancer treatment also contribute to decreased sexual desire. Other indirect reasons for decreased sexual desire include patients' avoidance of sexual activity secondary to painful intercourse or decreased sexual satisfaction. Partners may inadvertently contribute to patients' low sexual desire by being reluctant to initiate sex until reassured by the medical staff that sexual activity will not interfere with rehabilitation or endanger the convalescence of the patient. In addition, low sexual desire is positively correlated with shorter time since diagnosis, more psychological distress, more illness-related problems, and poorer body image and sexual satisfaction (Mumma et al., 1992).

Male and female *sexual arousal disorder* consists of a persistent or recurrent lack of a subjective sense of sexual excitement and pleasure during sexual activity. For men, male erectile disorders are characterized by persistent or recurrent partial failure to attain or maintain erection during sexual activity. Following transplant, approximately one fourth of men report erectile difficulties (Baruch et al., 1991; Wingard et al., 1992). Although there is a lack of studies examining adverse effects of chemotherapy alone on male sexual function, radiotherapy has been shown to cause erectile difficulties (Schover et al., 1993). Although men may experience retrograde ejaculation and inadequate emission of sperm following retroperitoneal lymph node dissection, their capacity for libido, erection, and sensation of orgasm are usually not impaired. (Loescher et al., 1989; Schover and Jensen, 1988; Sherins, 1993). Therefore, most cases of male arousal disorder have a psychogenic etiology. For instance, high levels of anxiety may interfere with sexual arousal and erectile functioning. In contrast, female transplant patients are likely to experience several physiological changes that may impair female arousal. As stated earlier, ovarian failure and concomitant low estradiol levels secondary to chemotherapy and radiation are associated

with decreased vaginal blood flow and secretions, which directly affect female arousal. In addition, without these physical signs of sexual excitement, many women may not experience sexual pleasure.

Male and female *orgasmic disorder* is characterized by a persistent or recurrent delay in, or absence of orgasm following a normal sexual excitement phase that, as judged by the clinician, is adequate in focus, intensity, and duration. While clinical experience shows that male transplant patients are not likely to complain of orgasm problems, research findings indicate that ejaculatory problems (9%–13%) are experienced at a greater frequency following transplant (Baruch et al., 1991; Wingard et al., 1992). Testicular cancer patients who have undergone retroperitoneal node dissection in addition to transplant are particularly prone to orgasmic dysfunction (Schover et al., 1993). After a prolonged period of abstinence or in cases of heightened anxiety, male transplant patients may ejaculate prematurely; however, this problem is usually short-lived with reassurance and resumption of sexual activity. Women may complain of anorgasmia secondary to diminished sexual arousal. It should be evident that impairment in one sexual response phase may adversely affect another aspect of sexuality such that a more complex sexual problem develops.

Finally, sexual pain disorders are relatively common among female transplant patients. Insufficient lubrication and vaginal atrophy related to ovarian failure, radiation-induced fibrosis, or GVHD (Chiodi et al., 1991; Corson et al., 1982; Nims, 1986) often results in dyspareunia, which consists of recurrent or consistent genital pain before, during, or after sexual intercourse. Vaginismus, which is characterized by involuntary spasm of the musculature of the outer third of the vagina, can also occur. In addition, heightened anxiety, "spectatoring," or being preoccupied with extraneous thoughts during sex also reduces arousal, which in turn may lead to painful intercourse. In our clinical experience, sexual pain disorders are rare among male transplant patients.

Premature Menopause and Sexual Function

Unlike gonadal dysfunction in men, ovarian failure and subsequent premature menopause can directly and indirectly affect the sexual response cycle in woman. Low estrogen levels can result in decreased libido, vaginal atrophy, decreased vaginal secretions, and dyspareunia; all of which can have deleterious effects on desire, arousal, and orgasm. Based on clinical and research findings, prematurely menopausal women appear to be at particular risk for persistent sexual disruption (Chapman et al., 1979; Chiodi et al., 1991; Cust et al., 1989; Heimpel et al., 1991; Keilholz et al., 1989; Moadel et al., 1995; Schubert et al., 1990). In our study of 34 prematurely menopausal cancer survivors receiving hormone replacement therapy, 38% met criteria for a DSM-IV sexual dysfunction (Moadel et al., 1995). Eleven of the 13 women with a clinical sexual dysfunction suffered from hypoactive sexual desire disorder. Women with a high level of menopausal symptomatology including breast tenderness, headaches, and vaginal dryness, and general psychological distress are most at risk for sexual dysfunction.

ASSESSMENT OF SEXUAL FUNCTIONING

A comprehensive sexual history is the cornerstone of a thorough evaluation of sexual functioning. Sexual problems among cancer survivors are usually the result of both (1) the emotional and psychological distress evoked by the illness and its treatment and (2) the physiologic consequences of the type of cancer and treatments (Von Eschenbach and Schover, 1984). Certainly, this multidimensional etiology is true for transplant patients for whom sexual difficulties are often the blending of physical and psychological factors. Given that sexual difficulties are usually due to a number of psychogenic and organic insults to one's sexual health, it is imperative to place assessment of sexual functioning in the broader context of transplant patients' past and current physical, psychological, and interpersonal domains. Therefore, assessment must include the physical, emotional, and relational aspects of sexuality.

Many staff consider dealing with the sexuality of their patients to be quite challenging and they often perceive many barriers for addressing sexual issues. The initial challenge in conducting an assessment of sexual functioning is one of "communication comfort." Transplant patients rarely ask for help with a sexual problem (Schubert et al., 1990) even though research conducted with anonymous cancer patients suggests that up to 90% experience sexual concerns and difficulties (Andersen, 1985). This paradox points to the need for primary care clinicians to encourage patients to ask questions and voice concerns about their sexuality. However, few oncologists and oncology nurse clinicians have been trained to assess and treat sexual disorders secondary to cancer or its treatment. Given that transplant patients may be at particular risk for sexual dysfunction and, like most cancer patients, they may be reluctant to initiate discussions about sexual concerns, it is crucial that clinicians on the transplant team develop skill and competence in assessing the nature of patients' sexuality and making appropriate interventions or referrals, when warranted.

An important preliminary issue is when should the topic of sexuality be raised. Some patients may ask questions or raise sexual concerns during the pretransplant period. These patients are clearly indicating their interest in understanding how the transplant will affect their sexuality and want to know how they can prepare to preserve their sexual intimacy. However, it should not be assumed that patients who do not directly ask about sexual issues are not interested in the effects of transplant on sexual functioning. Health professionals who address sexual issues early in the transplant process convey a willingness to discuss these topics, provide a legitimacy to sexual health as an important aspect to quality of life, and promote sexual health as a realistic expectation for transplant survivors. Patients who are encouraged to discuss sexual concerns during the pretransplant interview will most likely feel more comfortable raising concerns during the post-transplant rehabilitation period. Therefore, we recommend asking general questions about sexuality as a routine part of the pretransplant psychosocial assessment. Open-ended questions such as "How has your sexuality been affected by your illness and its treatment?" and "What concerns do you have about the effects of the transplant procedure on your sexual or reproductive functioning?" provide an invaluable baseline to compare to posttreatment sexual functioning. Questions about sexual functioning should also be included as a routine part of follow-up care since patients often resume interest in sexual activity approximately 3 to 6 months after transplant.

When a particular sexual problem is noted, a more extensive assessment is needed. This evaluation can be done by a trained member of the transplant team or referred to a mental health professional who specializes in evaluating sexual functioning of medically ill patients. The following description of the areas of importance to be covered in a sexual history is based on clinical work conducted by Auchincloss (1989) and Schover and Jensen (1988) in adapting the evaluation model, originally proposed by Kaplan (1983), for cancer patients.

It is important to assess each phase of the sexual response cycle (desire, arousal, orgasm) so as to identify the globality of the problem. As stated earlier, loss of desire is a common complaint among male and female transplant patients. It is important to ask patients the following questions:

- How often do you have sexual intercourse?
- How often do you have sexual thoughts or fantasies?
- Have there been any changes in your sexual desire?
- What factors contribute to your loss of sexual interest?

In terms of arousal disorders (e.g., difficulty attaining or maintaining an erection, lack of vaginal lubrication and swelling), it is important to ask patients whether they feel excited and aroused during sex. Male transplant patients should be asked, "Given adequate stimulation, do you develop and maintain an erection during sex?" Females should be asked, "Do you notice signs of arousal such as vaginal swelling and wetness?" Impairments in female sexual arousal often lead to painful intercourse and subsequent avoidance of sex. Painful intercourse should be thoroughly assessed. Finally, an inability to have an orgasm or changes in orgasm can result from the psychological or physical effects of cancer treatment. Patients need to be asked whether they experience orgasms during sex.

In addition to identifying the nature of the sexual problem, it is critical to get a detailed description of the onset, severity, and frequency of sexual complaints. A careful history which highlights

- When the problem began
- How often it is a problem

- How much it interferes with either your or your partner's sexual enjoyment
- What you and your partner do when this problem arises

It is important to explore nonsexual aspects of the patient's intimate relationship and whether he or she has experienced sexual problems before.

Although many professionals and patients are unaccustomed to the private nature and explicitness of the sexual history, several techniques can facilitate the clinician's and the patients' comfort in discussing sexual issues. Conducting a sexual history in a private, professional setting after explaining the rationale of the sexual evaluation and assuring patient confidentiality are instrumental in establishing rapport and decreasing anxiety. Similarly, starting with less sensitive material and then moving to more sensitive areas is a good way to gradually increase the nurse's and the patient's comfort. In addition, "normalizing" sexual questions by prefacing them with explanations of wide variation in normal sexual practices and how common these concerns are among transplant patients will help patients feel less threatened by their fears of being perceived as aberrant. For example, it may be helpful to preface a question about frequency of sexual intercourse by stating that there is obviously no right or wrong answer and that most couples find that sexual activity depends on many factors such as energy level and the availability of a private place. As with other counseling situations, a nonjudgemental stance and a tolerance for the wide variation in expression of normal sexual functioning are critical in eliciting an honest account of sexual practices as well as in establishing a solid foundation for a therapeutic relationship. Likewise, empathy and sensitivity provide a supportive context for the exploration of sexual issues. With practice, most nurse clinicians find that they can conduct

an initial sexual functioning evaluation with comfort and confidence.

In addition to the sexual history, a complete assessment of a sexual complaint should include a medical and psychiatric evaluation. Because it is certainly plausible that transplant patients could experience sexual difficulties that are not secondary to their transplantation, the medical evaluation should be broad and targeted to the full array of organic factors associated with sexual dysfunction. Medical assessment should include a history of general health, cancer disease and treatment, and current medications. A physical examination is particularly helpful for working up dyspareunia in that a pelvic examination provides information about the extent of vaginal atrophy, stenosis, and fibrosis, which are relatively common late effects of treatment-induced menopause. Finally, in addition to serum blood levels of hormones, several laboratory procedures have been developed for the specific evaluation of male and female sexual disorders. In similar fashion to the medical evaluation, attention should be given to psychological factors (e.g., depression) that often underlie sexual symptomatology. Psychiatric evaluation should include an assessment of premorbid personality, psychiatric history (e.g., depression, phobias), and current psychosocial adjustment to illness, treatment, and other life stressors.

In summary, the goal of the sexual assessment is to gather information that enables the clinician (1) to determine the extent to which the patient's sexual functioning has been preserved, (2) to identify potential sexual problems that the patient and his or her partner are experiencing, (3) to understand the factors related to the onset and maintenance of the sexual problem, and (4) to develop an appropriate treatment plan that addresses the patient's particular needs. Most important, early identification of sexual concerns and difficulties is crucial to the prevention of sexual dysfunction secondary to bone marrow transplantation. By identifying potential problems early in the transplant, it is more likely that sexual health will be preserved following the transplant. Conducting a sexual assessment implicitly conveys a sense of importance to the goal of preserving the sexual health of transplant patients. This goal is in accordance with the more global effort to improve the quality of life for all cancer patients.

INTERVENTIONS TO IMPROVE SEXUAL FUNCTIONING

The PLISSIT Model

Once the assessment has been completed and a particular sexual problem has been identified, the nurse clinician's next step is to formulate a treatment plan that addresses the patient's specific needs. According to Annon's (1974) classic PLISSIT model of progressive intervention, depending on the severity of the problem, clinical interventions should proceed in a sequential manner beginning with permission (P), then limited information (LI) and on to to specific suggestions (SS) and intensive therapy (IT), if warranted. Each level requires a greater degree of therapeutic skill and competence. The necessary level of treatment should be determined during the sexual assessment. The PLISSIT model has been useful in oncology nursing (Cooley et al., 1986), as summarized in Table 15.4.

Permission

Permission encourages a patient to discuss a sexual concern. Giving permission to discuss sexuality often reassures patients of the normalcy of their concerns and of the appropriateness of monitoring sexual health as an important part of comprehensive cancer rehabilitation. In and of itself, permission to discuss sexual concerns with members of the transplant team often reduces fear and anxiety about sex-

ual impairment. By initiating discussions about sexual functioning, clinicians encourage transplant patients and their partners to further discuss sexual concerns with each other as well. When sexual issues are raised during an evaluation, nurses provide a useful first-step clinical intervention in preserving the sexual health of their transplant patients. When viewed in this manner, permission is seen as primary prevention of sexual disorders secondary to transplant. Giving permission to discuss sexuality sets the stage for the next level of clinical intervention.

Limited Information

Limited information includes the full range of patient education. Several informative pamphlets on male and female sexuality are available from the American Cancer Society and many transplant services have materials developed for their own patients. These guidebooks include diagrams of male and female genitalia and reproductive organs, explanations of the sexual side effects of cancer treatment, and basic advice on sexual rehabilitation. Obviously, information about the possible sexual and reproductive sequelae of transplant should be a standard part of the informed consent procedure. Accurate information about sexuality enhances patients' ability to make sound decisions about preserving sexual health. In addition, education helps to dispel misconceptions regarding sexual activity. Patients are often reluctant to engage in sexual activity after a period of abstinence due to medical treatment. Reassurances about the safety of resuming sexual functioning are often helpful to patients and their partners.

Specific Suggestions

The next level of intervention involves making specific suggestions about sexuality. At this stage, a specific sexual concern or disorder has been identified. These specific suggestions may

TABLE 15.4 Treatment strategies for sexual disorders: the PLISSIT model

		Sexual disorder
P	Assess and encourage discussion about treatment with staff and partner	Desire, arousal, orgasm, pain
LI	Patient and partner education about common causes of low desire; explain reproductive sexual side effects of transplant; reassure patients and partners of safety of post-transplant sex	Desire
	Patient education about impact of radiation and chemotherapy on sexual arousal	Arousal
	Patient/partner education	Pain/orgasm
SS	Plan "romantic" evening with partner; plan sexual activity when rested and relaxed; make time for sexual activity	Desire
	Water-based genital lubricant; increase time and intensity of clitoral vaginal stimulation	Female arousal
	Encourage prolonged nondemand penile stimulation; discourage performance anxiety	Male arousal
	Alter position during sexual intercourse; water-based lubricant; encourage adequate arousal prior to penile penetration; discourage sexual intercourse until cause of painful intercourse has been treated	Pain
	Recommend longer or more direct clitoral stimulation; encourage communication with partner; plan sex when rested and relaxed	Female orgasm
	Encourage adequate penile stimulation; plan sexual activity accordingly during time of maximum relaxation and energy	Male orgasm
IT	Refer to sex therapist	Desire[a]
	Relaxation techniques; refer for hormone replacement therapy	Female arousal
	Refer to sex therapist and urologist for thorough work-up of possible organic causes	Male arousal
	Refer to sex therapist and gynecologist; hormone replacement therapy	Dyspareunia[b]
	Relaxation techniques combined with vaginal dilation exercises	Vaginismus
	Refer to sex therapist or gynecologist	Female orgasm
	Refer to sex therapist or urologist	Male orgasm

[a]May require more intensive treatment by sex therapist due to prominence of illness-related and global psychological factors

[b]Needs to be treated promptly in order to prevent impairment in all sexual phases

involve a combination of medical and psychosexual recommendations.

For instance, as stated earlier, radiation-induced vaginal changes (e.g., stenosis, fibrosis, and decreased lubrication) can diminish arousal and excitement, thereby increasing the likelihood of dyspareunia and decreased orgasmic response. Hormonal imbalance can further reduce vaginal secretions and lead to painful intercourse. These impairments, in turn, may lead to a pernicious cycle of avoidance by the patient and/or partner of sexual activity and lowered desire. Treatment for radiation-induced vaginal changes should include support and education. Specific suggestions such as trying different positions for sexual intercourse and using an external, water-based lubricant along with finger dilation of the vagina during foreplay can ease entry of the penis. Many women find that the female superior position offers greater control over the rate of thrusting and the depth of penetration and therefore they feel less anxious about pain and respond more easily during intercourse. Given that radiation-induced vaginal changes often slow a female's excitement response, couples should be encouraged to engage in adequate foreplay to intercourse so as to enable the female transplant patient to be fully aroused.

For most transplant patients, separations due to prolonged hospitalization, preoccupation with medical decisions, and fatigue often diminish sexual desire. Some patients reporting diminished sexual desire respond to specific suggestions to plan a "date" with their partner, which often promotes sexual intimacy.

Intensive Treatment

It is important to remember that the etiology of sexual disturbances is often quite complex and that more intensive psychological and/or medical treatment may be necessary for some patients. Intensive therapy requires a highly trained and competent professional who specializes in treating sexual disorders among medically ill patients. There is a growing cadre of mental health professionals with advanced training in sexual and marital therapy. While many transplant centers have identified appropriate referrals in their area, an additional source for identifying a competent sex therapist is the American Association of Sex Educators, Counselors and Teachers (AASECT, Washington, D.C.).

In recent years, the subspecialty of sex therapy has established itself as a well-researched and highly effective treatment for many sexual disorders. Detailed information about the principles and practices of sex therapy is available in recent books by Kaplan (1974, 1979, 1983), Leiblum and Pervin (1989), LoPiccolo and LoPiccolo (1978), and Schnarch (1991).

The following three clinical vignettes illustrate many of the psychosexual issues expressed by patients undergoing transplant. Two cases are women, who more often than their male counterparts express such issues, but who may actually exhibit more problems by our clinical and research experiences. The one male case illustrates the issues around couples-based erectile dysfunction. These cases reveal that patients never exhibit just one complaint nor are as "clear cut" as DSM-IV; many issues multiply and compound sexual and psychosocial functioning.

Case Vignette I

A 37-year-old married woman who was status posttransplant for 9 months and in remission from Hodgkin's disease was referred to the sex counseling clinic for treatment of low sexual desire. She complained of being too tired for sex and not experiencing sexual pleasure with her husband during sexual intercourse. She wondered whether she was normal and worried that her husband was angry, sexually frustrated and found her less attractive.

She also stated that she often experienced pain during sexual intercourse and added that it was worse during prolonged and deep penile penetration.

When interviewed, her husband stated that he was not comfortable with sexual activity due to his concerns about hurting his wife, not wanting to tire her, and feeling that sex was less of a priority following her cancer treatment. He stated that he initiated sex much less than he used to and that when he did he tried to get it over with as soon as possible. Neither of them had discussed current preferences for sexual activity with each other.

The first step in the treatment plan involved providing information about the causes of their multiphase sexual difficulties. This patient was referred for a thorough endocrine work-up, which revealed ovarian failure secondary to chemotherapy and radiation treatment. She was started on estrogen replacement therapy and encouraged to use a water-based vaginal lubricant prior to sexual intercourse and experiment with various positions that would reduce discomfort during intercourse. She found that the female superior position afforded her maximum comfort and control over the rate and depth of penile penetration. She and her husband were encouraged to plan at least one evening per week when they did something enjoyable together. This particular suggestion was initially quite difficult for them and it became apparent that they were quite out of practice discussing and doing non–cancer-related activities. At 1-year follow-up, this patient and her partner reported improved sexual relations.

Case Vignette II

A 22-year-old single woman was referred to the psychiatric service during her autologous bone marrow transplant for lymphoma. A psychiatric consultation at that time was requested to rule out depression during her convalescence in the hospital. She was followed weekly as an outpatient for the first 6 months after discharge. During this time, she was living by herself and complained of extreme fatigue, malaise, and difficulty adjusting to being outside of the hospital because of these physical problems. After 6 months she obtained her first job as an architect in a small firm. Since she had gone to school previous to her cancer diagnosis, this was her first "real" job after graduating with her degree. During this time she continued in psychotherapy and related many adjustment problems concerning "who she should tell at work about her illness," "what would happen if she became ill again," "how much time would she have to take off," "how she would manage her numerous outpatient visits," and "would her supervisor at work allow her such time."

During subsequent psychotherapy sessions she revealed that she felt quite uncomfortable about her body. She had many visible minor scars from venous catheters and an episode of herpes zoster and also had lost a considerable amount of weight. She felt extremely uncomfortable about her body and felt that it was damaged in some way by her illness and her transplant. Many of her sessions revolved around how she could ever meet any young men her own age and if she did, how would she tell them about her illness; let alone her issues of infertility. Prior to the patient's illness in college she had been engaged to a fellow student and they were living together and she was sexually active.

Over the several months she subsequently was very successful at work, began to go on several blind dates and dated several young men. One man she became particularly interested in was approximately 3 years younger than herself and very sexually naive. Upon meeting this new gentleman, she had many worries telling him about her cancer diagnosis, the transplant itself, the physical sequelae that she experienced, and her inability to have children. "Who would have someone like me who is half a woman?" It became quite evident the patient was extremely anxious about initiating any long-term relationship, let alone engaging in a physical relationship. She finally became comfortable with this boyfriend only after he told her that both his parents have had episodes of cancer and they were doing quite well. With that she felt more comfortable in revealing much of her history. Slowly, as she became psychologically more comfortable in this relationship, she began to develop a physical relationship with him. He was extremely naive and due to both of their anxieties, his because of the newness of initiating intercourse and hers because of feeling uncomfortable about her body and not having engaged in any sexual activity in approximately 4 years, their whole physical relationship was shrouded and surrounded in much psychological turmoil and anxiety. It also became quite evident that the anxiety was contributing to a problem with sexual desire and also arousal. However, it became much more apparent that arousal and actual orgasm was inhibited due to decreased vaginal secretions and most likely low estrogen levels secondary to the radiation and chemotherapy both from her original Hodgkin's treatment and the bone marrow transplant procedure.

She was referred for a thorough endocrine work-up, which revealed ovarian failure secondary to radiation treatment. She was started on estrogen replacement therapy and encouraged to use water-based vaginal lubricants prior to sexual intercourse and also experiment with various positions that would reduce discomfort during intercourse. She subsequently discontinued her endocrine replacement because of weight gain and headaches. She continued a physical relationship with this young man and because the relationship deepened, he became more experienced and her anxiety decreased because she felt comfortable with him. Issues of lack of sexual desire and arousal disappeared over the next couple of months.

She subsequently broke up with this young man 6 months into the relationship but has continued to meet other men through work associates and has felt extremely comfortable engaging with them in various relationships. She has continued to be quite successful at work and is in the process of changing jobs so that she will have better health benefits and vacation leave. She is considering adopting a child as a single parent.

Case Vignette III

A 34-year-old married man who underwent bone marrow transplant complained of difficulty maintaining an erection. Prior to his transplant, he had banked sperm for cryopreservation. At the time of the consultation, 1 year following transplant, he described often feeling anxious about disappointing his wife. He reported frequent thoughts about being "less attractive and masculine" and noted that he had diminished strength and had not regained his pretransplant weight. Initial attempts to resume sexual activities had not gone exceptionally well and he was embarrassed by the unpredictability of his erections. These early posttransplant sexual encounters were frustrating to him and he approached physical contact with his wife with much hesitation and dread.

Though outwardly supportive, his wife was at a loss for how to help. She neither wanted to pressure him nor become "sexually retired." She was worried about his health and the small scars at the previous catheter sites reminded her of her husband's vulnerability. During the assessment, he reported that he was able to maintain an erection during masturbation. The situational specificity of his erectile difficulties along with the information that all laboratory hormonal tests were within normal limits indicated that his sexual dysfunction most likely was psychogenic. The primary treatment goal of their brief, conjoint sexual counseling was to shift the emphasis of intimate contact from performance to pleasure. Initially, he and his wife were encouraged to make time for touching and to focus on enjoying physical intimacy without the added pressure of intercourse. Sensate focus and massage were helpful for this couple. In addition, greater communication about persistent illness-related concerns and sexual issues enhanced their feelings of closeness.

Combining Sexual Counseling and Medical Treatments

Given the complex etiology and manifestation of sexual and reproductive problems, a multidisciplinary approach is often necessary to evaluate treatments such as hormone replacement therapy, pharmacotherapy for sexual disorders, sperm banking, and pharmacologic and surgical means of protecting fertility.

Hormonal Replacement Therapy

Hormone replacement may be effective in several situations with patients undergoing transplant. Some adolescent or prepubertal boys receiving radiation may need testosterone replacement in order to promote the development of secondary sexual characteristics. Second, all women who have undergone premature menopause after treatment for transplant need hormonal replacement. Although combinations of low-dose estrogen and progesterone and topical estrogen ameliorate many menopausal symptoms including hot flashes, sweats, and vaginal dryness (Chiodi et al., 1991; Heimpel et al., 1991; Moadel et al., 1995), sexual desire appears less responsive to exogenous estrogen (Bancroft, 1984; Segraves, 1988). Recent investigations indicate that androgens (i.e., testosterone) more than estrogen alone, can increase desire in surgically menopausal women without a history of cancer (Ganger and Key, 1993; Greenblatt, 1987; Sherwin and Gelfand, 1987; Sherwin et al., 1985) and should be examined as a potential treatment in prematurely menopausal cancer survivors.

It has been suggested that hormonal replacement during chemotherapy may suppress germ cell proliferation, thereby preventing antineoplastic therapy associated gonadal toxicity (Chapman and Sutcliffe, 1981; Redman and Bajorunas, 1987; Redman et al., 1986). Gonadal protection during chemotherapy has included administering testosterone to men, oral contraceptives to women, and gonadotropin releasing hormone analogues to both sexes. Despite encouraging preliminary results, none of these approaches has proved efficacious (Sherins, 1993). One possible explanation is the lack of adequate time to suppress germ cell proliferation prior to initiation of cancer therapy.

Pharmacotherapy

A number of nonhormonal drug therapies have been used to improve sexual response in men (Riley and Riley, 1993). Intracorporeal injection of vasoactive drugs (e.g., papaverine, PGE_1) has shown success in inducing erection in many men. Yohimbine, an indole alkaloid derived from the yohimbine tree, is effective in restoring erectile function in some men. Other treatments under investigation for the management of erectile difficulties include opioid antagonists, nitrites and nitrates, and pentoxifylline. There are fewer known nonhormonal drug treatments of sexual dysfunction in women. Antidepressants and anxiolytics may offer secondary benefits in sexual function disrupted by psychological factors including depression and anxiety (Auchincloss, 1994). In addition, for women who decline estrogen replacement, clonidine may help relieve severe menopausal symptoms (i.e., hot flashes with resultant insomnia) that may interfere with sexual response.

Sperm Banking

An appropriate and relatively effective method of protecting fertility in men undergoing transplant is sperm banking. Unfortunately, semen from pretreated cancer patients and treated patients about to undergo transplant may reveal low sperm count and poor or inadequate sperm mobility (Redman et al., 1987). Approximately half of the men with testicular cancer or lymphoma have abnormal sperm specimens, which prevents sperm banking prior to any cancer treatment. However, cryobanking should be encouraged for all male patients, even if sperm counts are low. Multiple ejaculates can increase the number of viable sperm for storage. This procedure involves sensitive encouragement by transplant staff for patients to bank sperm, a receptive patient who has undergone little or relatively nontoxic cancer treatment, a local sperm bank, and enough time and financial resources for travel and banking. These last factors are critical and often unavailable. Many insurance companies do not currently reimburse the costs associated with this procedure and financial constraints may present a barrier for some men who wish to take advantage of this technique.

Other Fertility Options

Techniques that have been used to protect fertility during gonadotoxic treatment include oophoropexy in women and testicular shielding in men. In oophoropexy, the ovary is shielded from radiation by surgically placing the ovaries midline behind the uterus. This procedure appears to lower the risk of ovarian failure from a range of 70% to 100% to 50% of women (Sherins, 1993). The testicular shield has been shown to reduce radiation exposure in men to less than 10% of the patient's prescribed dose (Sherins, 1993).

An experimental fertility option available to women prior to bone marrow transplantation is in vitro fertilization (IVF). Several fertility centers have developed highly innovative programs in which women ending chemotherapy for their cancers are stimulated with hormonal therapy in order to collect ova for fertilization and then storage. Possible use of these fertilized ova after transplantation is a new and highly ethically and emotionally charged area of patient concern, particularly for the potential father of a woman who has unsuccessfully proceeded through the transplant procedure. To date, there is one known report of a successful pregnancy with an embryo that had been cryopreserved prior to transplant (Atkinson et al., 1994).

Alternatively, female transplant survivors may carry a child conceived by a donor oocyte with the husband's sperm (Hubner and Glazer, 1993). Although its costliness, limited success

rate, and risk to egg donors are important considerations, ovum donation can potentially offer women the experience of pregnancy, labor, and delivery.

RECOMMENDATIONS FOR FUTURE RESEARCH

A thorough review of the literature reveals a paucity of empirical studies examining the impact of bone marrow transplantation on sexual functioning. Clinical experience and research findings borrowed from the general literature of cancer survivors serves as a foundation for current clinical practice. However, further clarification of the incidence, nature, and risk factors associated with sexual dysfunction among transplant patients is needed in order to develop and refine prevention and rehabilitation efforts geared towards maintenance of sexual health among cancer survivors treated with transplant. This call for further specificity in our research efforts is reflected in Andersen's (1985) overall recommendation that we need to answer the question "What disease/treatment contexts produce what kind of sexual difficulties for which subgroups of cancer patients over what time course, and what are the etiologic components?"

Considering the growing use of BMT and BCT as curative treatment for many neoplastic disorders, it is important to consider whether the addition of transplant to the treatment protocol for a specific disease produces effects different from those found in patients who had been treated with conventional treatment only. For instance, Mumma and his colleagues (1992) compared the sexual functioning of acute leukemia survivors treated with either conventional chemotherapy alone or conventional chemotherapy followed by allogeneic bone marrow transplantation. They found no significant differences in sexual desire, satisfaction, and body image between these two subgroups of long-term leukemia survivors. They concluded that leukemia survivors treated with BMT experienced no greater psychosexual sequelae than those who received conventional treatment, who noted significant decline in sexual satisfaction. This research protocol was also conducted with chronic leukemia patients treated with either conventional chemotherapy alone or followed by allogeneic BMT; and the results were similar in that BMT patients fared no worse in terms of their sexual health.

The age at which a patient undergoes transplant is another important factor to be examined in relation to psychosexual adjustment. More and more, BCT and BMT are used to treat various childhood and adolescent cancers (e.g., leukemia, lymphoma, neuroblastoma) (Abramovitz and Senner, 1995). Extended separation from school and one's peer group during treatment for pediatric cancer may result in alterations in sexual self-image (Smith, 1992). The specific impact of transplant on the psychosexual development of childhood and adolescent cancer patients is being examined in ongoing research at the Memorial Sloan-Kettering Cancer Center.

There are several methodological suggestions that would help researchers in the field to develop a data base for expanding our knowledge of the sexual functioning of transplant patients. Prospective studies of patients with the various diagnoses (e.g., acute leukemia, Hodgkin's disease, testicular and breast cancer) currently treated with BMT/BCT must be conducted. Careful attention needs to be paid to subject selection so as to ensure comparability of treatment groups. Given the multiplicity of disease and treatment-related factors related to sexual functioning, it is important for investigators to gather patients that are homogeneous with regard to disease site, treatment regimen, phase of treatment (e.g., active treatment, post-treatment), age at treatment, and prognosis. The issue of differences in sexual morbidity among male and female transplant patients must also be addressed, in light of the differential effects of transplant on gonadal function.

In addition, research findings based on psychometrically robust questionnaires developed to study sexual functioning and physiological indices of sexual response (e.g., estrogen and gonadotropin levels) will advance our knowledge in this area. For instance, Derogatis's Sexual Functioning Inventory (Derogatis, 1975) measures three dimensions of sexual functioning: degree of sexual interest, sexual satisfaction, and body image. Several semistructured interviews have been developed to assess sexual functioning (Schover and Jensen, 1988). It is quite helpful to include both self-report questionnaires and clinical interviews in an assessment battery to account for patients' preferences in disclosing sensitive information. Including patients' spouses in data collection will enable a more dyadic perspective of how couples maintain sexual and global satisfaction in relationships. Longitudinal studies will allow researchers to observe when, during the course of treatment, patients experience sexual dysfunction as well as the process of posttransplant sexual readjustment. Finally, research that assesses multidimensional indices of quality of life, including sexual functioning, will help professionals understand factors necessary for optimal adjustment among posttransplant cancer survivors and will facilitate appropriate clinical intervention.

REFERENCES

Abramovitz, L.Z., Senner, A.M. 1995. Pediatric bone marrow transplantation update. *Oncol Nurs Forum* 22 (1):107-115.

Altmaier, E.M., Gingrich, R.D., Fyfe, M.A. 1991. Two-year adjustment of bone marrow transplant survivors. *BMT* 7:311-316.

American Psychiatric Association. 1994. *Diagnostic and Statistical Manual of Mental Disorders,* 4th ed. Washington, DC: American Psychiatric Association.

Andersen, B. 1985. Sexual functioning morbidity among cancer survivors: current status and future directions. *Cancer* 55:1835-1842.

Annon, J. 1974. *Behavioral Treatment of Sexual Problems, vol. 1, Brief Therapy.* Honolulu: Enabling Systems.

Atkinson, H.G., Apperley, J.F., Dawson, K., et al. 1994. Successful pregnancy after allogeneic bone marrow transplantation for chronic myeloid leukaemia. *Lancet* 344:199.

Auchincloss, S. 1994. Sexual dysfunction after cancer treatment: an overview. *Nederlands Tijdschrift Voor Obstetrie & Gynaecologie* 107:76-79.

Auchincloss, S. 1989. Sexual dysfunction in cancer patients: issues in evaluation and treatment. In J. Holland, J. Rowland (Eds.) *Handbook of Psychooncology: Psychological Care of the Patient with Cancer.* New York: Oxford University Press.

Bajorunas, D.R. 1980. Disorders of endocrine function following cancer therapies. *Clin Endocrinol & Metabol* 9(2):405-412.

Bancroft, J. 1984. Hormones and human sexual behavior. *J Sex & Marital Ther* 10:3-27.

Baruch, J., Benjamin, S., Treleaven, J., et al. 1991. Male sexual function following bone marrow transplantation. *BMT* 7(suppl 2):52.

Benker, G., et al. 1989. Allogeneic bone marrow transplantation in adults: endocrine sequelae after 1–6 years. *Acta Endocrinol* (Copenh) 120:37-42.

Bush, N.E., Haberman, M., Donaldson, G., et al. 1995. Quality of life of 125 adults surviving 6–18 years after bone marrow transplantation. *Soc Sci Med* 40(4):479-490.

Buskard, N., Ballem, P., Hill. R., et al. 1989. Normal fertility after total body irradiation and chemotherapy in conjunction with a bone marrow transplantation for acute leukemia. *Conference Proceedings of the 15th Annual Meeting of the EBMT,* Badgastein, Austria (abstr 76).

Card, R.T., et al. 1980. Successful pregnancy after high dose chemotherapy and marrow transplantation for treatment of aplastic anemia. *Exper Hematol* 8(l):57-60.

Chapman, R., Sutcliffe, S. 1981. Prediction of ovarian function by oral contraception in women receiving chemotherapy for Hodgkin's disease. *Blood* 58:849-851.

Chapman, R.M., Sutcliffe, S.B., and Malpas, J.S. 1979. Cytotoxic-induced ovarian failure in Hodgkin's disease II: effects on sexual function. *JAMA* 242: 1882-1884.

Chatterjee, R., Mills, W., Katz, M., et al. 1994. Germ cell failure and leydig cell insufficiency in post-pubertal males after autologous bone marrow transplantation with BEAM for lymphoma. *BMT* 13:519-522.

Chao, N.J., Tierney, K., Bloom J.R., et al. 1992. Dynamic assessment of quality of life after autologous bone marrow transplantation. *Blood* 80:825-830.

Chiodi, S., Spinelli, S., Cohen, A., et al. 1991. Cyclic sex hormone replacement therapy in women undergoing allogeneic bone marrow transplantation: aims and results. *BMT* 8(suppl 1):47-49.

Cooley, M., Yeomans, A., Cobb, S. 1986. Sexual and reproductive issues for women with Hodgkin's disease: application of PLISSIT model. *Canc Nurs* 9:248-255.

Corson, S.L., Sullivan, K.M., Batzer, F., et al. 1982. Gynecologic manifestations of chronic graft-versus-host disease. *Obstet Gynecol* 60:488-492.

Crilley, P., Styler, M., Topolsky, D., et al. 1992. Late complications of allogeneic bone marrow transplant for leukemia following busulfan (Bu) and two days of cyclophosphamide (Cy2). *Exper Hematol* 20(6):713 (meeting abstract).

Cust, M.P., Whitehead, M.I., Powles, R., et al. 1989. Consequences and treatment of ovarian failure after total body irradiation for leukaemia. *Br Med J* 299: 1494-1497.

Deeg, H.J., Kennedy, M.S., Sanders, J.E., et al. 1983. Successful pregnancy after marrow transplantation for severe aplastic anemia and immunosuppression with cyclosporin. *JAMA* 250(5):6471.

Derogatis, L. 1975. *Derogatis Sexual Functioning Inventory.* Baltimore, MD: Clinical Psychometrics Research.

Ganger, K., Key, E. 1993. Individualising HRT. *Practitioner* 237:38-360.

Gradishar, W.J., Schilsky, R.L. 1989. Ovarian function following radiation and chemotherapy for cancer. *Semin Oncol* 16(5):425-436.

Greenblatt, R.B. 1987. The use of androgens in the menopause and other gynecic disorders. *Obstet Gynecol Clin North Am* 14:251-268.

Heimpel, H., Arnold, R., Hetzel, W.D., et al. 1991. Gonadal function after bone marrow transplantation in adult male and female patients. *BMT* 8(suppl 1):21-24.

Hinterberger-Fischer, M., Kier, P., Kalhs, P., et al. 1991. Fertility, pregnancies and offspring complications after bone marrow transplantation. *BMT* 7:5-9.

Hubner, M.K., Glazer, E.S. 1993. Now on common ground: cancer and infertility in the 1990s. *Infertil & Reproduct Med Clin North Am* 4(3):581-596.

Jacobs, P, Dubovsky D.W. 1981. Bone marrow transplantation followed by normal pregnancy. *Am J Hematol* 11:209-212.

Kaplan, H. 1974. *The New Sex Therapy: Active Treatment of Sexual Dysfunctions.* New York: Brunner/Mazel.

Kaplan, H. 1979. *Problems of Sexual Desire.* New York: Brunner/Mazel.

Kaplan. H. 1983. *The Evaluation of Sexual Disorders.* New York: Brunner/Mazel.

Keilholz, U., Korbling, M., Fehrentz, D., et al. 1989. Long-term endocrine toxicity of myeloablative treatment followed by autologous bone marrow/blood derived stem cell transplantation in patients with malignant lymphohematopoietic disorders. *Cancer* 64:641-645.

Kolb, H.J., Bender-Gotze, C., Haas, R.J., et al. 1989. Late effects in marrow transplanted patients—results of the AG-KMT Munich. *BMT* 4(suppl 3):31.

Leiblum, S., Pervin, L. 1989. *Principles and Practice of Sex Therapy.* New York: Guilford Press.

Lesko, L. 1989. Bone marrow transplantation. In Holland, J., Rowland, J. (Eds.) *Handbook of Psychooncology: Psychological Care of the Patient with Cancer.* New York: Oxford University Press, 163-173.

Li, F. 1977. Follow-up of childhood cancer survivors. *Cancer* 84:1776-1778.

Liesner, R.J., Leiper, A.D., Hann, I.M., et al. 1994. Late effects of intensive treatment for acute myeloid leukemia and myelodysplasia in childhood. *J Clin Oncol* 12:916-924.

Loescher, L., Welch-McCaffrey, D., Leigh, S., et al. 1989. Surviving adult cancers; part 1: physiological effects. *Ann Intern Med* 111:411-432.

LoPiccolo, J., LoPiccolo, L. 1978. *Handbook of Sex Therapy.* New York: Plenum.

Milliken, S., Powles, R., Parikh, P., et al. 1990. Successful pregnancy following bone marrow transplantation for leukaemia. *BMT* 5:135-137.

Moadel, A.B., Ostroff, J.S., Lesko, L.M., et al. 1995. Psychosexual adjustment among women receiving hormone replacement therapy for premature menopause following cancer treatment. *Psycho-Oncology* 4:273-282.

Mumma, G., Mashberg, D., Lesko, L. 1992. Long-term psychosexual adjustment of acute leukemia survivors: impact of bone marrow transplantation vs. conventional chemotherapy. *Gen Hosp Psychiatr* 14:43-55.

Nims, J. 1986. Late effects of cyclophosphamide, total body irradiation (TBI) and marrow transplantation on human sexuality. *Oncol Nurs Forum* 13:121.

Redman, J.R., Bajorunas, D.R. 1987. Suppression of germ cell proliferation to prevent gonadal toxicity associated with cancer treatment. *Proceedings of the Workshop on Psychosexual and Reproductive Issues affecting Patients with Cancer.* American-Cancer Society Pub. 87-5M-4515, pp. 90-94.

Redman, J.R., Bajorunas, D.R., Goldstein, M.C., et al., 1987. Semen cryopreservation and artificial insemination for Hodgkin's disease. *J Clin Oncol* 5:233-238.

Redman, J., Davis, R., Evenson, D., et al., 1986. Prospective, randomized trial of testosterone cypionate to prevent sterility in men treated with chemotherapy for Hodgkin's disease: preliminary results. *Proceedings of the 14th International Cancer Congress,* Budapest, Basel: S. Kargen, p. 440.

Rieker, P., Edbril, S., Garnick, M. 1985. Curative testis cancer therapy: psychosocial sequelae. *J Clin Oncol* 3:1117-1126.

Riley, A.J., Riley, E.J. 1993. Pharmacotherapy for sexual dysfunction: current status. In Riley, A.J., Peet, M., Wilson, C. (Eds.) *Sexual Pharmacology.* New York: Oxford University Press, 211-226.

Russell, J.A., Hanley, D.A. 1989. Full-term pregnancy after allogeneic transplantation for leukemia in a patient with oligomenorrhea. *BMT* 4:579-580.

Sanders, J.E. 1987. Ovarian and testicular function following marrow transplantation. *International Conference on Reproduction and Human Cancer.* Bethesda, MD: National Cancer Institute.

Sanders, J.E., Buckner, C.D., Amos, D., et al., 1988. Ovarian function following marrow transplantation for aplastic anemia or leukemia. *J Clin Oncol* 6:813-818.

Sanders, J.E., Buckner, C.D., Leonard, J.M., et al. 1983. Late effects of gonadal function of cyclophosphamide, total body radiation and marrow transplantation. *Transplantation* 36(3):252-255.

Schnarch, D.M. 1991. *Constructing the Sexual Crucible: An Integration of Sexual and Marital Therapy.* New York: Norton.

Schover L., Jensen, S. 1988. *Sexuality and Chronic Illness: A Comprehensive Approach.* New York: Guilford Press.

Schover, L.R., Montague, D.K., Schain, W.S. 1993. Sexual problems. In DeVita, V.T., Hellman, S., Rosenberg, S.A. (Eds.) *Cancer: Principles and Practice of Oncology,* 4th ed., vol. 2. Philadelphia: Lippincott, 2464-2480.

Schubert, M.A., Sullivan, K.M., Schubert, M.M., et al. 1990. Gynecological abnormalities following allogeneic bone marrow transplantation. *BMT* 5:425-430.

Segraves, R.T. 1988. Hormones and libido. In Lieblum, S.R., Rosen, R.C. (Eds.) *Sexual Desire Disorders.* New York: Guilford Press, 271-312.

Sherins, R.J. 1993. Gonadal dysfunction. In DeVita, V.T., Hellman, S., Rosenberg, S.A. (Eds.) *Cancer: Principles and Practice of Oncology,* 4th ed., vol. 2. Philadelphia: Lippincott, 2395-2406.

Sherwin, B.B., Gelfand, M.M. 1987. The role of androgen in the maintenance of sexual functioning in oophorectomized women. *Psychosomat Med 49:*397-409.

Sherwin, B.B., Gelfand, M.M., Brender, W. 1985. Androgen enhances sexual motivation in females: a prospective, crossover study of sex steroid administration in the surgical menopause. *Psychosomat Med 47:*339-351.

Sklar, C.A., Kim, T.H., Ramsay, N.K.C. 1984. Testicular function following bone marrow transplantation performed during or after puberty. *Cancer 53:*1498-1501.

Sklar, C.A., Kim, T.H., Williamson, J.F., et al. 1983. Ovarian function after successful bone marrow transplantation in postmenarcheal females. *Med Pediatr Oncol 11:*361-364.

Smith, K.C. 1992. Measurement of self-concept in adolescent cancer survivors (Doctoral dissertation, University of Texas Southwestern Medical Center at Dallas, 1992). *Dissertation Abstracts International 53*(6B): 3168.

Spaulding, M.B., Spaulding, S.W. 1985. Chemotherapy and gonadal function. In Higby, D.J. (Ed.) *The Cancer Patient and Supportive Care.* Boston: Martinus Nijhoff, 31-55.

Vergauwen, P., Ferster, A., Valsamis, J., et al. 1994. Primary ovarian failure after prepubertal marrow transplant in a girl. *Lancet 343:*125-126.

Von Eshenbach, A., Schover, L. 1984. The role of sexual rehabilitation in the treatment of patients with cancer. *Cancer 54:*2662-2667.

Von Eschenbach, A.C., Schover, L.R. 1984. Sexual rehabilitation of cancer patients. In Gunn, A.E. (Ed.) *Cancer Rehabilitation.* New York: Raven, 155-173.

Vose, J.M., Kennedy, B.C., Bierman, P.J., et al. 1992. Long-term sequelae of autologous bone marrow or peripheral stem cell transplantation for lymphoid malignancies. *Cancer 69:*784-789.

Winer, E., Lindley, C., Hardee, M., et al. 1992. Quality of life assessment in patients with breast cancer surviving twelve months or more following high dose chemotherapy with autologous bone marrow transplant. *Proc Am Soc Clin Oncol 11:*1328.

Wingard, J., Curbow, B., Baker, F., et al. 1992. Sexual satisfaction in survivors of bone marrow transplant. *BMT 9:*185-190.

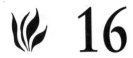

16

Quality of Life after Transplantation

Elaine DeMeyer, Marie Whedon, Betty Ferrell

Advances in transplantation such as blood stem cell transplants, marrow purging, hematopoietic growth factors, graft-versus-host disease (GVHD) prevention, and gene therapy have improved survival rates and expanded the indications for this treatment. The evolution of transplantation from an experimental treatment to a conventional treatment modality has been accompanied by an evolution of outcomes research. The majority of research regarding clinical outcomes of transplantation has focused on morbidity and mortality, reported in terms of "disease-free survival," "tumor response," or "toxicity." In the 1970s, research studies began to include quality-of-life (QOL) measures of clinical outcome. Long-term complications such as chronic graft-versus-host disease, pulmonary complications, cataracts, and secondary malignancies have been well described. Recently, research data has documented the complex, long-term, psychosocial impact of transplantation on patients' lives. The majority of available information focuses on the quality of life of patients receiving allogeneic transplants. Little information is available about the influence of autologous or blood cell transplant on patients' perceived quality of life.

One of the greatest challenges transplant teams are encountering today is economics or cost of transplantation. The transplant procedure is intense, high-tech, and high cost. Payers are establishing their own guidelines to determine indications for treatments and criteria for exclusion. Outcomes-oriented research such as quality-of-life research is increasingly used to develop such guidelines. Lacking acceptable quality-of-life outcomes, provider-institutions or third-party payers might choose to eliminate transplants as covered treatments on the basis that "there is no evidence BMT is of any great benefit" (Morreim, 1992). Increasing our knowledge about the quality of life of transplant survivors is critical to support the usefulness of transplant as a treatment modality and to ensure that it remains a treatment option for patients.

WHY QUALITY-OF-LIFE RESEARCH IS IMPORTANT

Several reasons support the premise that QOL information about bone marrow transplant survivors is critical. First, improving QOL has always been a central goal of health care.

When only morbidity and mortality outcomes are described, health-care providers are overlooking one of their most important clinical goals—to make life better, not merely longer (Morreim, 1992). With more information about QOL outcomes, patients can be better informed prior to consent for transplant. Knowing the effect of transplant on patients' QOL can help patients and practitioners to decide if alternative treatment options would be more satisfactory for the patient (Schmidt et al., 1993; Andrykowski et al., 1990; Whedon and Ferrell, 1994).

Assessment of long-term complications and QOL helps identify which problems might be transient, related to the original disease, or a result of the conditioning regimen and transplant. Identification of long-term physical and psychological complications experienced by survivors might also suggest areas for improvement in the transplant procedure or for additional patient and family education (e.g., sexuality and fertility problems) (Andrykowski et al., 1990). Many transplant programs' continuous quality improvement (CQI) efforts originated from information gained from transplant survivors and their families.

Research on QOL can help evaluate differences in patients' perceived outcome related to treatment, and how these differences are influenced by socioeconomic, educational, and ethnic or cultural factors. QOL measurement can help to identify which patients would benefit from early rehabilitation or counseling interventions. QOL information can also be used to develop needs-based programs to assist future BMT patients and their families (Schmidt, 1994; Whedon and Ferrell, 1994).

Quality-of-life end points are being used to compare treatments with similar disease outcomes. QOL outcomes are especially important in phase III clinical trials that compare the efficacy of a new therapy against the current standard of care. For example, QOL information is crucial when comparing marrow or blood cell transplant for breast cancer to conventional chemotherapy, assuming the disease outcome is equivalent. When comparing treatment options, a QOL framework also allows a more thorough analysis of the treatment costs and benefits. QOL information is used to determine "cost per additional year of life" or quality-adjusted life years (QALYs) to compare treatment options (Moinpour et al., 1995).

Finally, QOL findings can help patients formulate realistic expectations of life after transplant. Health-care professionals can develop resourses to match survivors' quality-of-life needs. Undoubtedly employers and third-party payers will also be interested in this aspect of recovery. In summary, QOL research in BMT is important because "the ultimate success of cancer treatment is not only the absence of disease, but is also the patient's perceived quality of life" (Whedon and Ferrell, 1994).

DEFINING QUALITY OF LIFE

Quality of life must be clearly defined to be clinically useful. How to define health-related QOL and whether to use an all-encompassing or population-specific definition remains a topic of debate. QOL is a complex, multidimensional concept. Many terms such as *quality of life, health status, well-being, meaning of life, value of life,* and *functional status* are used synonymously (Stewart, 1992). Health status and functional status often focus on disease progression and physical functioning. Quality of life is a broader concept that encompasses an individual's ability to function and derive satisfaction from doing so (Grant et al., 1990). Quality of life encompasses multiple dimensions of well-being—physical, psychological, social and interpersonal, financial, and spiritual.

Quality of life has been defined in both subjective and objective terms. As Frank-Stromborg (1988) suggests:

> The major challenge to the use of the term quality of life . . . is that the term is too broad and inclusive to be meaningful. Central to this position was the definitional problem, that is, the term is operationally defined in very different ways by different investigators. Thus, the failure to achieve a shared definition results in the use of measures that are assessing different things. (p. 80)

Although there is no "gold standard" definition of QOL, there is strong agreement that QOL is a subjective phenomenon and should be based on patients' self-reports. Therefore, perhaps QOL can best be defined as "the degree of satisfaction with present life circumstances as perceived by the individual" (Belec, 1992).

TOOLS TO MEASURE QUALITY OF LIFE

A variety of instruments have been used to measure QOL of transplant recipients. There is no single ideal QOL tool. Haberman (1994) summarized issues to consider when measuring quality of life, including:

- incorporating data triangulation, combining qualitative and quantitative methods;
- selecting instruments specific to the population;
- separating instruments to measure each QOL dimension or using a multidimensional tool; and
- choosing instruments with established reliability and validity.

Forman (1994) suggests that in grouping tools or designing a new QOL tool the following factors should be considered.

- The tool should be in the patient's language.
- The tool should be varied enough to obtain information on all facets of QOL.
- The tool should be scientifically reliable and easy to administer.

Both Haberman (1994) and Schmidt (1994) concur that QOL research should not cause a burden to subjects, emotionally or financially.

Traditionally, QOL measurement has been unidimensional. Information about treatment toxicities and improvement in disease-related symptoms was usually from the perspective of the physician. For example, physicians frequently use the Karnofsky Status, developed in 1948, to evaluate the functional aspect of quality of life. However, measures of physical function alone do not define the patient's physical and psychological well-being. Unidimensional measurements include single items to assess particular areas of QOL. Unidimensional measures are easy to develop and use, yet they provide limited information about the multiple domains of quality of life.

Researchers have used several approaches to a comprehensive assessment of QOL of transplant survivors. A combination of standardized questionnaires, each measuring one aspect of QOL (e.g., symptom distress) can be used in an attempt to capture all aspects of QOL. Another approach is to use a single instrument designed to measure a range of QOL dimensions. Yet another approach is to use multidimensional QOL models that can be adapted to the specific population under study (Grant, 1992).

There is a lack of agreement about how and when to measure QOL in conjunction with other evaluations of treatment (Gill and Feinstein, 1994). However, there seems to be general agreement in two important areas: (1) the patient's report of quality of life is the *most* valid measure of quality of life and (2) quality of life is a *dynamic, multidimensional* construct that includes more than just physical functioning. It is important that the QOL instrument selected reflects the definition of QOL, evaluates the perception of the individual whose quality of life is being assessed, captures the broad concept of quality of life, and addresses individual differences (Mast, 1995). Table 16.1 lists tools frequently used to measure aspects of quality of life for BMT patients.

QUALITY-OF-LIFE RESEARCH

An evolving body of studies have begun to describe QOL following transplantation. Methods and results of investigations to date are summarized in Table 16.2 and briefly discussed below.

Wolcott and colleagues (1986) were some of the first researchers to study health status and psychosocial functioning as perceived by

TABLE 16.1   Tools to measure aspects of QOL of BMT survivors

Instrument	Description
Beck Depression Inventory (BDI)	21-item measure comprises severity ratings for 13 cognitive-affective and 8 somatic symptoms of depression
Functional Living Index—Cancer (FLIC)	22-item questionnaire answerable in Likert format with a 1 to 7 range. The FLIC has five factors: physical well-being, psychologic state, family situational interaction, social ability, and somatic sensation.
City of Hope Quality of Life—BMT Instrument	Specific to BMT (e.g., GVHD, cataracts); assesses four domains of QOL: physical, psychological, social, and spiritual well-being; uses demographic data questions and 63 Likert scales.
Karnofsky Performance Status	Objective scale rates physical activity from 1% to 100% in increments of 10
Medical Outcomes Study	36-item short form assesses physical, role, social, and emotional functioning
Profile of Moods Status (POMS)	65-question self-report checklist of adjectives with six subscales including tension/anxiety, depression, anger, fatigue, vigor, and confusion/bewilderment
Sickness Impact Profile (SIP)	136 items in 12 categories of life activities including physical dimension, psychosocial dimension, sleep and rest, taking nutrition, usual daily work, household management, leisure, and recreation
Simmons Scale	9-item self report of self-esteem adapted from the Rosenberg Self-Esteem Scale
Sleep, Energy, and Appetite Scale (SEAS)	9-point Likert scales rate level of energy, quality of sleep, and appetite
Symptoms Experience Report (SER)	Assesses the presence of 20 symptoms during the past week; if present, respondents rate the severity of symptoms using a 7-point Likert scale
Weissman Social Adjustment Scale—Self-Report	54-item questionnaire with seven role function subscales: work, social/leisure, marital, parental, economic, family, and extended family

TABLE 16.2 Quality-of-life studies in BMT

Investigators/ subjects	Study goals	Measures	Results
Wolcott et al. (1986)/ allogeneic patients and their donors (N = 26)	Describe adaptation post BMT for both recipients and donors	Investigator-developed survey, profile of moods status, Simmons Scale, social adjustment scale, self-report	75% were doing well; 15-25% reported significant emotional distress
Hengeveld et al. (1988)/allogeneic patients (N = 17)	Study psychosocial aspects of BMT	Investigator-developed survey, Symptom Checklist-90, Beck depression inventory, Karnofsky performance status	Close link between physical condition and psychological state; 50-100% reported fertility and sexual problems
Andrykowski et al. (1989a)/allogeneic patients (N = 23)	Document function and psychosocial aspects	Functional living index, profile of moods status	Younger age (<30 yrs) was only variable associated with better physical outcome and better psychological function
Andrykowski et al. (1989b)/allogeneic patients (N = 16)	Explore function and psychosocial aspects over time	Functional living index, profile of moods status, sickness impact profile	Little change in psychosocial functioning over time
Andrykowski et al. (1990)/allogeneic patients (N = 29)	Compare BMT with renal transplant patients	Functional living index, profile of mood status, sickness impact profile, sleep, energy, and appetite scale, psychological adjustment to illness scale, symptoms experience report, perceived health questionnaire	QOL about the same; both groups perceived their health as poorer than others their age; higher education associated with less dysfunction and higher QOL
Syrjala et al. (1990)/allogeneic patients (N = 100)	Assess function and psychosocial aspects prior to BMT and 1 year later	Sickness impact profile, Beck depression inventory, BMT events scale	Functioning returned to normal at 1 year except for areas of work, recreation, and pastimes; 22% reported mild to severe depression at 1 year
Baker et al. (1991)/ allogeneic, autologous and syngeneic patients (N = 135)	Study role retention and quality of life of BMT survivors	Role checklist, satisfaction with life domains scale, Cantril self-anchoring ladders, profile of mood states, positive and negative affect scales	Roles of worker, home maintainer, friend, and family member were most important
Wingard et al. (1991)/allogeneic autologous and syngeneic patients (N = 135)	Determine the health, functional ability, and employment status of adults who survive BMT	Medical outcomes study (short form), Karnofsky performance status	93% reported they could do normal activities; 23% reported job discrimination; 39% had problems obtaining insurance
Altmaier et al. (1991)/allogeneic patients (N = 23)	Compare BMT survivors to patients undergoing maintenance chemotherapy	Investigator-developed survey	Objectively, QOL in BMT patients was lower; but subjectively BMT survivors do not view their situation as any different from that of chemotherapy patients

TABLE 16.2 *Continued*

Investigators/ subjects	Study goals	Measures	Results
Belec (1992)/allogeneic and autologous patients (N = 24)	Describe the QOL of BMT survivors	Quality of Life Index—Cancer	92% acceptable QOL; QOL was influenced by number of physical problems and family functioning
Chao et al. (1992)/ autologous patients (N = 58)	Study QOL in autologous BMT survivors	Investigator-developed survey	88% reported above-average to excellent QOL at 1 year; 36% dissatisfied with sexual function
Ferrell et al. (1992)/ allogeneic patients (N = 119)	Define QOL by BMT survivors; develop BMT-specific QOL tool	Qualitative BMT instrument	QOL defined by allogeneic BMT survivors; BMT-specific QOL tool proposed
Grant et al. (1992)/ allogeneic patients (N = 179)	Assess reliability and validity of QOL-BMT instrument	City of Hope QOL-BMT instrument	BMT-QOL tool measuring physical, psychological social, and spiritual well-being
Haberman et al. (1993)/allogeneic, autologous and syngeneic patients (N = 125)	Document systematically how BMT survivors perceive their QOL	Investigator developed survey	Long-term survivors perceive themselves as leading meaningful lives; 5% reported poor physical and mental health
Syrjala et al. (1993)/ allogeneic patients (N = 100)	Prospectively study physical and psychological functioning after marrow transplantation	Sickness impact profile, Beck depression inventory, BMT events scale	At 1 year physical and psychological functioning returned to normal except in areas of work, recreation, and stamina
Schmidt et al (1993)/ allogeneic patients (N = 162)	Study long-term survivors' issues of QOL	City of Hope/Stanford long-term BMT survivor index, Karnofsky performance status	Reported QOL at 8 on scale of 1 to 10; younger patients had fewer physical complications
Whedon et al. (1994)/autologous patients (N = 37)	Extend knowledge of post-BMT QOL from survivors of allogeneic BMT to survivors of autologous BMT	City of Hope QOL-BMT tool	Few physiologic disruptions and above-average QOL reported
Andrykowski, et al. (1995b)/allogeneic, autologous and syngeneic patients (N = 28)	Assess the impact of BMT on long-term physical and psychosocial functioning	Profile of mood states, functional living index, subscales of the psychological adjustment to illness scale, and sickness impact profile, symptom experience report, sleep energy, and appetite scale	Males and older age at BMT reported largest decline in physical and psychosocial health

Continued

TABLE 16.2 Quality-of-life studies in BMT *Continued*

Investigators/ subjects	*Study goals*	*Measures*	*Results*
Andrykowski et al. (1995b)/allogeneic and autologous patients (N = 200)	Further explore QOL following BMT	Profile of mood states, subscales of the psychological adjustment to illness scale, and sickness impact profile, recovery of function scale, perceived health questionnaire, symptoms experience report	Allogeneic recipients reported poorer QOL than autologous recipients. Greater age, lower level of education, and more advanced disease at BMT were risk factors for poorer QOL
Haberman et al. (1995)/allogeneic autologous, and syngeneic patients (N = 125)	Assess QOL of long-term survivors of BMT	Descriptive study of QOL, late medical complications, psychological distress, demands of long-term recovery, and health perceptions	74% of long-term BMT survivors reported their QOL as the same or better than before transplantation
Kanabar et al. (1995)/children receiving autologous BMT rescue (N = 28)	Assess QOL in survivors of childhood cancer who received megatherapy followed by autologous BMT	Investigator-developed survey	96% respondents judged their QOL to be good; pain and depression remained ongoing problems for approximately 30% of respondents
King et al. (1995)/ BMT nurses (N = 150)	Capture BMT nurses' perceptions of patients' QOL and compare their perceptions to survivors' perceptions	City of Hope BMT-QOL tool—Nurses' version	BMT nurses perceived patients as having poorer QOL than patients reported

long-term adult BMT survivors. At approximately 3½ years after BMT, 25% of the survivors reported chronic physical symptoms, high rates of infections, and high use of medical care. The majority of BMT survivors (75%) were doing well psychosocially, while 15% to 20% experienced increased emotional stress, low self-esteem, and suboptimal life satisfaction. A parallel study was performed simultaneously with these patients' marrow donors. Twenty-six (72%) patients and 18 (50%) of the donors completed the study. Four of 18 (22%) of the donors reported having physical problems they attributed to donating marrow. The relationship between recipient and donor was highly related to the recipient's health status. This study recommended that both recipients

and donors might benefit from psychosocial support, particularly for the 10% to 20% who experience chronic physical illness.

A retrospective study was conducted by Hengeveld (1988) to examine the psychological adaptation of 17 adult survivors 1 to 5 years after allogeneic BMT. Forty to fifty percent of them reported sexual or fertility problems, occupational disability, and/or daily life hindered by physical complications. Researchers concluded that patients need more preparation for the emotional and sexual problems of survivorship.

Andrykowski has contributed to QOL research after BMT in five studies. In 1989, Andrykowski and colleagues studied the physical and psychosocial functioning of 23 adult survivors of allogeneic BMT between 3 and 52 months after BMT. Compared to other cancer survivors, BMT survivors reported greater physical problems but similar overall functioning. Better physical and psychological functioning was reported by patients who received transplants before age 30. Survivors were also asked whether they would still decide to have a transplant, and whether their course of transplantation corresponded to their expectations. Only one patient indicated that he would not make the same choice again. However, one third perceived their course of transplantation and its side effects as *worse* than expected. The authors concluded that information about the long-term functioning of BMT survivors is critical for the process of informed consent. Additionally, once health-care providers develop a better understanding of why patients differ in post-BMT functional status, they can better assist patients to resume normal, productive lives.

In a follow-up study, Andrykowski and colleagues (1989) reassessed survivors on two separate occasions, at post-BMT intervals of 1 year, to determine if perceptions of physical and psychosocial functioning changed with time. Of the 23 patients in the original study, 16 participated in all three assessments. BMT survivors experienced long-term difficulties in physical, occupational, emotional, and cognitive functioning. Little change in psychosocial functioning occurred over time. This study suggests that some survivors might benefit from post-BMT rehabilitation programs that include physical, psychological, sexual, occupational, and marital counseling.

In a third study, Andrykowski and co-workers (1990) compared QOL of BMT recipients with QOL of renal transplant recipients. Twenty-nine recipients in each group completed the study. Results indicated few differences between the two groups. As with previous findings, an older age at BMT was associated

with poorer post-BMT QOL. Increased doses of total body irradiation and less education were associated with poorer status and poorer QOL. The authors concluded that the similarity of BMT and renal transplant recipients' post-transplant QOL can help justify reimbursement of BMT procedures.

One-hundred adult BMT survivors were assessed pretransplant and 1 year after transplant for physical and psychological functioning by Syrjala and colleagues (1990). At 1 year only 3 out of 12 areas of functioning were impaired for more that 25% of the population. Impairments included work (41%), recreation and pastimes (37%), and ambulation (26%). Physical impairment at 1 year was not predicted by pretransplant diagnosis, type of BMT, conditioning regimen, or age. Twenty-two percent of survivors reported mild to severe depression at 1 year. The most common concerns of survivors included uncertainly about the future (86%), worry about relapse (83%), feeling tired or worn out (81%), having to slow the pace of life (79%), thoughts about dying (78%), thoughts about things that could go wrong (77%), and worry about their families (76%). More than 33% indicated these concerns caused them moderate to severe distress. The authors concluded that although most survivors return to normal functioning at 1 year after BMT, distress related to consequences of the disease and transplant persisted for a small subgroup.

In a study by Wingard and colleagues (1991), 135 adult BMT survivors 6 to 149 months after BMT were asked to complete a survey to determine their health, functional ability, and employment status. Most survivors (93%) reported they could do normal activities with minor or no physical problems. Global health was described as good to excellent by 67% of recipients. Three fourths were employed or enrolled in school. Job discrimination

(23%) and problems obtaining insurance (39%) were reported. Loss of employment was associated with lower social functioning, chronic graft-versus-host disease, greater job discrimination, and female gender. These investigators concluded that despite the intensity of BMT, eventually high rates of recovery were achieved. These outcomes are comparable to outcomes in survivors of cancer who receive less intensive therapy.

Altmaier and colleagues (1991) compared 12 BMT survivors transplanted for leukemia at least 2 years after BMT with 10 leukemia patients undergoing maintenance chemotherapy. BMT survivors reported more symptoms and side effects, and poorer marital/intimate relationships and sexual functioning. Half of the BMT survivors experienced job discrimination compared to only 20% of patients receiving maintenance chemotherapy. Although BMT survivors experienced greater difficulties in several areas, BMT survivors did not view their QOL differently than did the patients on maintenance chemotherapy.

Belec (1992) studied 24 adults who were 1 to 3 years after BMT regarding their perceptions of their QOL. Approximately 92% of the scores were in the upper half of the possible range of scores, suggesting that the majority of BMT recipients perceived their QOL to be acceptable. More than 61% stated that their families provided them the greatest life satisfaction. For approximately 75%, health continued to be a major source of concern. Belec noted that recipients underwent a period of adjustment and adaptation that was influenced by the BMT experience. During this period, a reappraisal or reassessment of life values occurred that positively affected their overall QOL.

Although many studies have been conducted on the QOL of recipients of allogeneic transplants, Chao and colleagues (1992) conducted one of the first studies on QOL of adult survivors of autologous BMT. Survivors were assessed at 90 days and again at 1 year after BMT. The mean QOL at 90 days was 7.8 on a scale of 1 to 10, with 10 being the best. At 1 year, the mean QOL had increased to 8.9. Seventy-eight percent were employed. Fourteen percent reported difficulties with sexual activity. These results suggest that by 1 year, QOL returns to a reasonable and acceptable degree in the majority (88%) of BMT survivors.

Haberman and colleagues (1993 and 1995) surveyed 125 adult survivors who had survived 6 to 18.5 years after transplant. Seventy-four percent reported their quality of life was the same or better than it had been before BMT. Eighty-eight percent said the benefits of BMT far outweighed the treatment side effects. Overall, 77% of the long-term survivors surveyed ranked their current health as good to excellent. Although survivors identified a variety of physical and psychological problems, most described them as only mild or moderate. The problems cited most frequently were emotional distress, followed by fatigue, eye problems, sleep disturbances, pain, and cognitive deficits such as memory lapses and difficulty concentrating. The study findings suggest that nursing interventions focus on providing accurate and timely information about the known long-term complications of BMT.

Syrjala and colleagues (1993) conducted the first prospective study documenting the physical and psychosocial functioning of patients before and after BMT. In this study, 67 allogeneic transplant patients were assessed before transplant, 90 days and 1 year after transplant. Physical function returned to pretransplant levels by 1 year in most cases. Psychosocial functioning remained stable at the three points measured. Investigators found that a measure of family conflict obtained prior to BMT was a significant predictor of physical functioning 1 year following BMT. This study concluded that family relationships were important determinants of physical and emotional recovery.

Brief, simple interviews were conducted by Schmidt and colleagues (1993) to obtain QOL information in 212 allogeneic BMT survivors. The investigator-designed survey included three domains of QOL: productive activity and functioning, health status and treatment-related physical symptoms, and qualitative aspects of daily life. Survivors rated their overall quality of life on a scale of 1 to 10, with 1 representing the worst and 10 representing the best. The median score was 9, with 21% reporting a score of 8 and 57% reporting a QOL score of 9 or 10. In addition, 74% of survivors who were employed at time of diagnosis returned to work and 95% of survivors in the pediatric group were attending school. Older patients had a higher incidence of physical symptoms and a lower Karnofsky status. Researchers concluded that the majority of adult and pediatric survivors, who had survived 3 years or longer after BMT, appeared to be doing well in the domains evaluated.

More recently, Andrykowski and colleagues (1995a) compared physical and psychosocial status of 28 adults 1 year after BMT to their physical and psychosocial status before BMT. Two questions were investigated: (1) what is the impact of BMT on physical and psychosocial functioning? (2) what demographic, disease-, and treatment-related factors predict change in physical and psychosocial status following BMT? Analysis of group means suggested little difference between pre- and posttransplant assessments. However, when individual scores were examined, many patients showed substantial improvements or declines in physical or psychosocial status following BMT. Males and older patients reported the largest decline in physical and psychosocial functioning. The investigators concluded that since BMT may have long-term effects on physical and psychosocial functioning, patients need to

be aware that these effects may exceed pretransplant complications.

In 1995, Andrykowski and colleagues also conducted a multisite (N = 5 centers) study. Two hundred survivors, 46% of allogeneic BMT and 54% of autologous BMT, completed the study. Allogeneic recipients reported poorer QOL than autologous recipients. Greater age at BMT, lower level of education, and more advanced disease at BMT were consistent risk factors for poorer QOL. Significant differences were found in recovery of function between autologous and allogeneic recipients regarding "working outside the home" and "personal appearance." More autologous recipients returned to work and reported a better personal appearance than allogeneic recipients. The researchers concluded that more in-depth studies of sexual functioning, employment, fatigue, and sleep disturbance would be useful.

Little research data is available about the QOL of children who have survived BMT. Kanabar and colleagues (1995) studied QOL in childhood survivors of autologous BMT. Ninety-six percent of the respondents judged their QOL to be good. No disability was noted in 40%; an additional 33% reported minimal disability. Approximately 30% of patients had moderate to severe disabilities, with pain and depression as ongoing problems. Some adolescents felt unable to cope with everyday life or with interactions their peers.

Only one study has examined BMT nurses' perception of the meaning of QOL for BMT survivors. King and colleagues (1995) explored the nurses' perceptions of the impact of QOL of survivors and compared them to patients' responses on the same item. Six hundred fifty (650) questionnaires were mailed to BMT nurses in the United States and Canada; 150 responded (23%). Findings reflect that transplant nurses generally perceive patients as having a poorer QOL than the patients actually report. Nurses' perceptions of QOL concerns were compared to those of survivors identified by Ferrell and colleagues (1992). Nurses' perceptions were consistent with those of BMT survivors, yet nurse respondents described several additional factors they perceived as affecting QOL. King and colleagues concluded that QOL should be a component of professional BMT education, and that survivors need greater access to psychosocial and spiritual support services.

CITY OF HOPE QUALITY-OF-LIFE CONCEPTUAL MODEL

Based on the responses of BMT survivors to six open-ended questions, researchers at the City of Hope National Medical Center in Duarte, California, adapted a model of quality of life for the bone marrow transplant patient. The interview questions were:

1. What does the term *QOL* mean to you?
2. How do you think that BMT has affected your QOL?
3. What makes your QOL better?
4. What makes your QOL worse?
5. What do you think that the physicians and nurses could do to improve your QOL?
6. Are there other thoughts you would like to share about your experiences as a BMT patient or about QOL?

Nine themes were identified from the responses to "What does QOL mean to you?"

1. having family and relationships
2. being independent
3. being healthy
4. being able to work, having financial success
5. having a heightened appreciation for life
6. being alive
7. being satisfied

8. feeling fulfilled with life
9. being normal

Nine themes were also identified from responses to "How do you think BMT has affected your QOL?"

1. numerous side effects
2. infertility
3. fear of relapse
4. strength and stamina decreased
5. work and activities are limited
6. a second chance was given
7. an opportunity to improve my QOL was given
8. spirituality increased
9. increased appreciation of life

In order to assess reliability and validity of the City of Hope QOL-BMT instrument, Grant and colleagues (1992) surveyed 179 allogeneic BMT recipients. Psychometric analysis indicates that the instrument has beginning reliability and validity and can be useful in the evaluation of BMT survivors. The study findings demonstrated the unique aspects of QOL in BMT survivors and the value of QOL assessment in clinical practice and research. This model was based on the investigators' previous research on quality of life of patients with cancer. The City of Hope model has been refined and specifically adapted to the population of BMT survivors (see Figure 16.1). The model identifies the four domains of quality of life: physical, psychological, social, and spiritual well being. BMT is thought to affect all four domains, presenting unique challenges (e.g., GVHD) as well as challenges similar to those of other illnesses.

Physical Well-Being

Physical well-being is the most extensively documented domain of survivorship. After high doses of chemotherapy and/or total body irra-

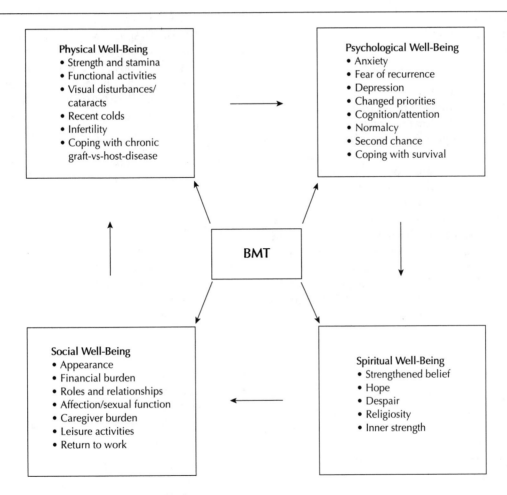

Physical Well-Being
- Strength and stamina
- Functional activities
- Visual disturbances/ cataracts
- Recent colds
- Infertility
- Coping with chronic graft-vs-host-disease

Psychological Well-Being
- Anxiety
- Fear of recurrence
- Depression
- Changed priorities
- Cognition/attention
- Normalcy
- Second chance
- Coping with survival

BMT

Social Well-Being
- Appearance
- Financial burden
- Roles and relationships
- Affection/sexual function
- Caregiver burden
- Leisure activities
- Return to work

Spiritual Well-Being
- Strengthened belief
- Hope
- Despair
- Religiosity
- Inner strength

Figure 16.1 BMT impacts the dimensions of quality of life.

SOURCE: From B. Ferrell et al. 1992a. The meaning of quality of life for bone marrow transplant survivors. Part 1. The impact of bone marrow transplant on quality of life. *Cancer Nursing* 15:159. Copyright © 1992 by Raven Press. Reprinted with permission of Lippincott-Raven Publishers..

diation, the immune system can take up to a year after transplant to recover and in some cases may never regains full functioning. Physiological effects can be attributed to the transplant, the chemotherapy, radiation therapy, or immunosuppressive agents, or a relapse of the original disease. Ferrell and colleagues (1992) listed seven factors that may influence physical well-being:

- strength and stamina
- functional activities
- visual disturbances/cataracts
- recurrent colds

- infertility
- chronic GVHD
- nutrition

Of these, only cataracts and GVHD are unique to the BMT survivor.

The physiologic effects of chronic GVHD may occur in all major organ systems. Other long-term complications not related to GVHD effects include sterility, bladder shrinkage, cataracts, memory, attention, and concentration difficulties, hypothyroidism, and aseptic necrosis of the bone. In many survivors, the physical effects of treatment resolve over time, and the majority of debilitating symptoms subside within the first year. However, some survivors continue to experience life-long physical disabilities that may interfere with normal activities of daily living (Webster, 1995) Additional long-term complications may be identified as BMT survival rates increase.

Psychological Well-Being

Psychological well-being after BMT is influenced by the fear of recurrent disease, the desire for normalcy, and coping with survival (Copeland, 1996). Ferrell and colleagues (1992a, b) list eight factors that may affect psychological well-being:

- anxiety
- fear of recurrence
- depression
- changed priorities
- cognition/attention
- normalcy
- second chance
- coping with survival

Some early studies of psychological well-being of BMT survivors reported significant emotional distress, low self-esteem, and less than optimal life satisfaction (Wolcott et al., 1986; Altmaier et al., 1991). Later studies have shown only mild to moderate psychological distress in

BMT survivors (Haberman et al., 1993; Syrjala et al., 1993). Despite the complications of BMT, some survivors report an unexpectedly high quality of life, possibly due to being "glad to be alive" or to having a "second chance" (Whedon and Ferrell, 1994). Despite the long-term complications, very few survivors later regretted their decision to have a BMT and would change their decision (i.e., not consent to have a BMT) (Andrykowski et al., 1989; Belec, 1992; Haberman, 1993).

Social Well-Being

Social well-being encompasses issues of intimacy, relationships, family, employment, and social reintegration. Ferrell and colleagues (1992) described seven factors that influence social well-being:

- appearance
- financial burden
- roles and relationships
- affection/sexual function
- caregiver burden
- leisure activities
- return to work

BMT poses a potential for significant loss in one's ability to retain important roles and relationships. Baker and colleagues (1991) found that after BMT employment, home responsibilities, and relationships with friends and family members became more important to BMT survivors. Other studies have focused on whether the survivor returns to work or school. Relationships and intimacy are often in terms of sexuality. More in-depth research is needed to define how alterations in body image, fatigue, and medications contribute to loss of libido, physical changes such as vaginal dryness, and partners' anxiety (Andrykowski et al., 1995a).

Family relationships may strengthen as a result of BMT or relationships may grow apart.

Close relationships and support of family correlates with patients' perceived QOL. Syrjala and colleagues (1993) found that a measure of family conflict obtained prior to BMT was a significant predictor of physical functioning 1 year after BMT. Many people who have not been through the BMT experience find it difficult to discuss with survivors. Survivors often seek new relationships with other individuals who have experienced BMT. Support groups or one-on-one counseling may help BMT survivors and their families and friends.

In allogeneic transplants, the long-term psychological effects of the donor-recipient relationship are of interest, including the long-term impact of the transplant experience on the relationship and how this relationship changes depending on the patient's physical well-being. Only one published study has examined the psychological adjustment of adult BMT donors in which the recipient survived (Wolcott et al., 1989). Overall, donors reported little change in their relationship with their recipients after BMT. For most donors, the opportunity to give a person a second chance at life is very rewarding. Either the recipient or donor may feel obligated to maintain a relationship when there may not have been a relationship prior to BMT. One who had received a matched unrelated BMT shared his disappointment after 1 year when he stated, "I don't understand why my donor didn't want to meet me." The donor can feel guiltly or responsible if the transplant fails. If the recipient deteriorates or dies, the donor may feel a sense of failure. Health-care professionals should assess not only the psychological needs of the patient and family, but also the needs of the donor.

Spiritual Well-Being

Spiritual well-being is the least defined and least studied area of the BMT survivor. Spiritual well-being is influenced by altered beliefs, hope, despair, and religiosity (Copeland, 1995).

Themes often incorporated into the overall theme of spiritual well-being by BMT survivors include global spirituality (inner strength, conviction, and life goals); religiosity (faith in God, trust, indebtedness to God); and life appreciation (overall priorities, valued relationships) (Ferrell et al., 1992a). Ferrell and colleagues (1992) described five factors that influence spiritual well-being:

- strengthened belief
- hope
- despair
- religiosity
- inner strength

Organized religion may play a role in a person's spiritual well-being. Survivors frequently describe changes in priorities and values and a search for the meaning of life. Ten of twelve survivors interviewed for the *BMT Newsletter* (Stewart, 1993) stated that religion played a major role in their recovery. The effect of spiritual well-being on overall survivorship and QOL is a fertile ground for more research, especially since many survivors identify spirituality as an important coping mechanism.

Survivors sometimes describe feelings of guilt about having lived when others did not. Instead of asking "Why me?" some survivors ask "Why not me?" The term *survivorship guilt* has been coined to describe these feelings. Survivorship guilt was first reported in 1942 in a study of individuals who escaped a Boston fire. Survivorship guilt is so widely accepted as a symptom of posttraumatic stress disorder that it is included in the *Diagnostic and Statistical Manual of Mental Disorders* (DSM-IV) category. Maxwell and Aldredge-Clanton (1994) identify characteristics of survivorship guilt at the deepest level of spiritual concerns. Survivorship guilt raises issues related to search for meaning, feelings of responsibility, and need for restitution. Support groups can help BMT survivors understand and accept survivorship guilt. Chaplains are key in guiding the survivor who struggles for meaning of or feelings of responsibility for someone's death. Once survivorship guilt is recognized, health-care professionals can help survivors work through their grief. Survivorship guilt is often a neglected concern of BMT survivors and deserves the attention of health-care professionals.

The City of Hope-BMT QOL model addresses the interrelationships of the four domains of well-being: physical, psychological, social, and spiritual. A disruption in one domain affects one or multiple domains and quality of life in general. Understanding these relationships enables the health-care professional to assess the impact of BMT on the QOL of the patient and family in order to meet his or her needs in a comprehensive manner. This model allows for assessment of QOL throughout the BMT continuum from pretransplant to recovery. One patient's comments on QOL summarizes the interrelationships of the four domains of this model: "I feel tired often, but I get stronger each day. I felt like I had a second chance in life. I am closer to my family and to prayer. I learned that life is precious and how blessed I was to get to enjoy life with my grandchildren and family."

SPECIAL CONSIDERATIONS

Cultural Considerations

Although the U.S. population is a multitude of racial and ethnic groups, BMT quality-of-life research has focused on the majority of survivors, who are Caucasian Americans (Stewart, 1992). Cultural and ethnic background influence every aspect of quality of life: physical, psychological, social, and spiritual well-being. Assessment of quality of life must be understood within the survivor's cultural boundaries. Members of minority groups often have a lower socioeconomic status and less education,

which is consistent with reports of poorer QOL (Andrykowski et al., 1989; 1995b). Perhaps a higher level of education is associated with better pre-BMT physical status, better access to health care, and a wider variety of coping or rehabilitative resources. More educated individuals may even have a more realistic expectation of the outcome of BMT. Additional information is needed about the impact of cultural beliefs on patient's perceived QOL.

Quality of Life as an Outcome Measure

Findings from outcome-oriented research is increasingly used to develop guidelines for allocating funds for BMT or donor charges. Conflicts occur regarding BMT because the benefit and cost-effectiveness have not been proved. Will quality of life be used as a means to justify treatment options such as BMT? Using quality of life as justification for allocating resources raises many ethical questions. Ethical questions evolve from issues of sanctity of life vis-à-vis quality of life, conflict between individual good and good of others, and autonomy versus beneficence. For example, "Should BMT be denied so that more babies can be immunized?" With a lack of agreement on QOL definition and measurement, QOL cannot be a valid criterion for decision making regarding health-care policy. As QOL becomes more defined and assessed with more valid and reliable measures, it may be used in guiding health-care decision making.

The majority of clinical trials have focused on the cancer response "benefit" of BMT rather than the QOL "benefit" of BMT. The FDA now suggests that QOL be assessed in clinical trials related to new drugs. How QOL is defined or measured is not clearly stated in the FDA guidelines. Quality-of-life researchers can help determine how the concept will be defined and measured so that treatment end points can be compared in clinical trials.

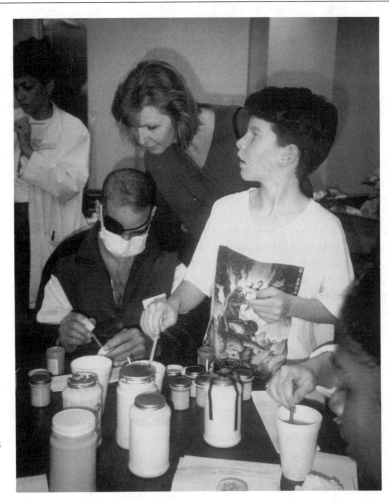

Figure 16.2
Activities such as ceramics
encourage interaction
among BMT patients and
their families.

SOURCE: Courtesy of the Physical Medicine and Rehabilitation Department of Baylor Rehabilitation Services at Baylor
University Medical Center, Dallas, Texas.

Quality of life can also be an outcome measure for examining related variables, for example, in pain research (Ferrell, 1989). Like pain, QOL is an individual experience that can best be evaluated by the person experiencing it. A QOL tool enables health-care professionals to evaluate not only a given treatment such as the effect of an analgesic on pain, but also the effect of the treatment on overall QOL.

Caregiver Burden and Quality of Life

Transplant recipients may feel guilty because they perceive that they are an emotional or financial burden on their families. How do families feel? The caregiver (parent, spouse, or significant other) is usually very involved in the patient's care throughout the course of BMT. Reducing the period of neutropenia results in earlier discharge of BMT patients. With the shift from inpatient to outpatient treatment, the burden of care is shifting from the health-care professional to the lay caregiver. Health-care providers rely heavily on caregivers to assist in the management of patients who are at risk for physical and psychological complications. In these situations, caregivers are challenged to learn new skills, new roles, self-care management, and ways to relate and communicate. Like QOL, caregiver burden is difficult to define. What may be a burden for one caregiver may not be a burden for another. Little research is available on the caregiver's response to BMT or the impact of BMT on the caregiver's QOL. More information is needed to determine how caregivers define the survivor's QOL and how that compares to the survivor's perception of QOL. The issues of caregiver burden and QOL span the continuum of BMT (before BMT, BMT, after BMT, and long-term recovery). How these demands change with time and the demands of long-term recovery are unknown. Knowledge is needed of what variables influence the family's psychosocial functioning and strategies families use to achieve optimal QOL across the BMT continuum. With more information about demands on caregivers and the relationship between a caregiver's burden and the patient's QOL, nurses can better address the needs of caregivers.

Finances and Quality of Life

One of the long-term stressors associated with BMT is the financial burden. Some BMT patients have sold their homes and used all their savings to pay for the transplant. One of the themes identified by survivors when asked "What makes QOL better?" was having a job, money, or finances (Ferrell et al., 1992). Financial issues were one of the three concerns survivors listed as difficult to deal with upon returning home (Haberman et al., 1993). Survivors

also identified dealing with medical/life insurance companies as a concern. This problem is best described by Stewart (1992): "There's a tug of war going on between some insurance companies and hospitals with BMT patients caught in the middle. Insurance companies are fighting to contain escalating health care costs. The patients are simply fighting to stay alive." Survivors report irritation associated with finding a new insurance carrier, maintaining existing insurance policies, or paying barely affordable premiums. More information is needed about the financial burden of BMT, including out-of-pocket costs, and how this affects the patients' and families' perceived QOL.

Fatigue and Quality of Life

Several studies have indicated that fatigue is identified by survivors as a common problem that impacts quality of life. (Whedon et al., 1995; Haberman et al., 1993; Andrykowski et al., 1990). Feeling tired was the most frequent and severe symptom experienced by BMT survivors before BMT (76%) and at 1 year after transplant (89%) (Andrykowski et al., 1990; Andrykowski et al., 1995). Two of the most common concerns of survivors were feeling tired or worn out (81%) and having to slow the pace of life (79%) (Syrjala et al., 1990). When Haberman and colleagues (1993) asked survivors "What things are you currently unable to do as a result of transplant?" the response was that activities were limited by "less energy/stamina."

Altmaier and colleagues (1991) found that BMT survivors at 2 years after BMT reported more fatigue (33%) than patients receiving maintenance chemotherapy (20%). Fatigue is associated with age at time of transplant, suggesting that younger patients experience less fatigue and function better overall (Andrykowski et al., 1988). With the increasing age of eligibility for most BMT protocols, fatigue could become more prevalent than previously reported. Belec (1992) reported that 50% of survivors mentioned a lack of energy and increased fatigue since transplant. This concerned survivors because it limited their ability to perform their jobs, exercise, and participate in sports. Even routine everyday activities caused them to tire easily.

Fatigue becomes a significant problem when it begins to affect the person's well-being, daily activities, lifestyle, social and work-related activities, familial and sexual relations, and compliance with therapy. Having the energy to carry out these activities of daily living is crucial to participating in life (Willingham et al., 1994). For many individuals, the limitations imposed by fatigue are unacceptable. The side effects of fatigue are multiple and have a direct impact on quality of life. The goal of nursing care for the survivor who is experiencing fatigue is to facilitate adaptation, thereby minimizing it and maintaining or enhancing QOL. Willingham (1994) has identified four strategies to help manage fatigue:

1. *Balance activity and rest.* Schedule both activity and rest periods, and adhere to the schedule. On stressful days, plan for more rest the day before and the day after.
2. *Plan ahead.* Anticipating events and planning ahead can help an individual adapt to increased energy demands. Not all events can be anticipated, but some stressful events are predictable such as physician visits and holidays.
3. *Just say no!* Realizing limitations and permitting the use of the word *no* can help conserve energy for more important activities. However, some individuals are not good at saying no; so practice is necessary.
4. *Keep active.* Too much rest can have a detrimental effect on energy production and may actually increase fatigue. Even

short periods of activity are essential for management of fatigue.

INTERVENTIONS TO IMPROVE QUALITY OF LIFE

In the QOL survey developed by Ferrell and colleagues (1992), BMT survivors were asked, "What makes your QOL better?" "What makes your QOL worse?" and "What do you think that physicians or nurses could do to improve your QOL?" Table 16.3 compares the themes identified for making QOL better or worse.

When BMT survivors were asked what physicians or nurses could do to improve their QOL, "being accessible" was the most common response. Survivors also said that discov-

TABLE 16.3 Themes identified by survivors for making QOL better or worse and frequency of responses

What makes QOL better?	What makes QOL worse?
Having good health (N = 81)	Physical losses (N = 92)
Having family and friends (N = 77)	Losing relationships (N = 10)
Having a job/money/ finances (N = 15)	Being financially distressed (N = 6)
Having a positive attitude and peace of mind (N = 30)	Losing spiritual strength and hope (N = 5)
Being able to enjoy life (N = 25)	Being psychologically distressed (N = 31)
Having goals/being productive (N = 8)	Having unfulfilled goals (N = 8)
Being alive/having appreciation for life (N = 38)	

SOURCE: Data from Ferrell et al., 1992b.

ering a cure, providing support groups, reinforcing current education, increasing patients' participation in decision making, and providing patients information about additional coping strategies would be helpful. The survivors' comments carry implications for nurses:

Be Accessible. Although BMT is a "high-tech" field, it needs to also be a high-touch field. Touching is important to help patients overcome the feeling of isolation often associated with BMT. Foot and back massages can be incorporated into the treatment plan because they are often comforting and relaxing for patients. Nurses must remember that this treatment is completely new for nearly all patients. Caring requires much patience and proactive sharing of information to minimize fears or concerns (Decker, 1995). Patients need to be able to express their concerns in an open, nonthreatening setting. A nonjudgmental attitude is especially important when patients are expressing concerns about sexuality. Often, the best thing that nurses can do for patients is to "just be there."

Reinforce Current Education. Transplant technology changes daily. It is important for nurses to keep current about BMT to provide accurate and timely information by drawing on the latest research that describes the long-range medical and psychosocial complications (Haberman et al., 1993). Educating patients can increase their adherence to the plan of care, satisfaction, ability to manage symptoms, and sense of control (Jassak and Porter, 1995). Even BMT survivors who live 6 to 18.4 years after transplantation continue to need answers to questions regarding sterility, prognosis of health in later years, long-term effects of total body irradiation, and future impact on family or society (Haberman et al., 1993).

Provide Support Groups. According to survivors, support groups provide vital information

that helps them cope with their disease, face the challenges of their treatment, and improve their quality of life (Stewart, 1993). The need for support groups is evident through all phases of BMT: pretransplant through long-term rehabilitation and adjustment to life as a BMT survivor (Ferrell et al., 1992). Nurses can assist with arranging former patients to talk with current ones, facilitating inpatient support groups or post-BMT support groups. If support groups are facilitated by a social worker or chaplain, nurses can be invited guests to provide information on topics of concern to the group.

Increase Patients' Participation in Decision Making. Allowing patients as much autonomy as possible in decision making gives them a sense of control over their well-being (Webster, 1994). Enhancing the perceived self-control of the patient is a key component in the patient's psychological well-being (Syrjala, 1995). As personal control over health increases, so does the sense of purpose or meaningfulness. Reinforcement of control over life can positively affect the patient's self-esteem and help decrease anxiety (Lewis, 1982). Some strategies to increase patients' participation in decision making include:

Providing Information The more information patients receive, the more involved they can be in making informed decisions. Information should be proactive, advising survivors of possible consequences of disease and treatment and providing strategies to address these consequences (Webster, 1994). Decision making is linked to maintaining control in a perceived "out of control" situation (Ferrell et al., 1992). Nurses can give accurate and complete information to help minimize BMT patients' feelings of "loss of control."

Empowering Patients An example of a tool to empower patients is the "Caring for Yourself" video used at Baylor University Medical Center. This 25-minute video is viewed by BMT patients and families within 24 hours of hospital admission to empower them to be involved in their own care. Carepaths™, or Caremaps™, another intervention that can empower patients, guide the clinician in the steps that provide the best care for patients. Carepaths are usually designed in a grid fashion with outlines of interventions and outcomes by all disciplines against a timeline (see Figure 16.3). In order to include the patient as part of the team, professional caregiver carepaths can be translated to "patient carepaths," simplified versions of the professional carepaths. The patient's version uses lay terms and personalization with the word *I*. Patients can post their carepaths in their rooms or keep them as a diary. Spaces can be incorporated for information such as laboratory values and daily weights, and for activities such as physical therapy or oral care. Patients and families can actually chart their progress. As patients become active participants in their care, they can visualize the results that the team is working toward for their benefit and understand that they are an important member of the team.

Giving Choices When patients are hospitalized, many things, including choices, are taken away from them. Even small choices (e.g., when to take a shower, arranging bedside table) can help patients feel in control. Once discharged, patients can make choices regarding the day and appointment time of visits to the clinic.

Encouraging Exercise A comprehensive exercise program promotes a sense of normality and gives the patient a feeling of control. Patients often react with anger to the loss of control. Exercise can help diffuse patients' anger and frustration. Group exercise can help BMT patients overcome feelings of isolation and withdrawal (James, 1987).

Provide Additional Coping Strategies. Patients had suggestions for both patients and family members about helpful "coping strategies."

Stewart (1992) summarized tips for BMT patients and tips for support persons caring for them based on interviews with patients. Nursing interventions related to these tips include encouraging patients and families to ask questions and to discuss their concerns with their healthcare team. Nurses have the opportunity to explore previous coping strategies with patients and families. For patients and families who desire new strategies, the nurse can offer information through formal and informal educational programs; assistance in problem solving through counseling; role modeling techniques such as deep breathing and music therapy; and referral to support systems (Clark, 1992).

Nurses are in a position to coordinate multiple resources to improve QOL for patients and families. Through education, the nurse can influence the survivor's perception of QOL (King et al., 1995). Future research is needed to determine if coping skills and self-care strategies taught by nurses during the early phases of BMT therapy actually span the continuum of care to long-term survival. Further research will also help identify specific nursing interventions that enhance long-range QOL (Haberman et al., 1993).

REHABILITATION AND QUALITY OF LIFE

It is important to assess the quality of life of an individual patient so that directions for rehabilitation become clear. Padilla and colleagues (1992) state that one of the reasons nurses should pursue quality-of-life research is to demonstrate the effect of specific rehabilitative approaches. The increasing number of BMT survivors necessitates increased attention to their rehabilitation. Andrykowski and colleagues (1989) state:

> It is imperative that rehabilitation be recognized as a significant long-term concern fol-

	Day 1 −6 BMT	Day 2 −5 BMT	Day 3 −4 BMT	Day 4 −3 BMT
Assessment	My weight is _____ kg	My weight is _____ kg	My weight is _____ kg	My weight is _____ kg
Tests Procedures	Catheter Placement _____	WBC _____ HCT _____ PLT _____ T POLY _____ ANC _____	WBC _____ HCT _____ PLT _____ T POLY _____ ANC _____	WBC _____ HCT _____ PLT _____ T POLY _____ ANC _____
Medications IVs	IV fluids start at 10 PM	Blood products	Blood products	Blood products
Hygiene	Oral care every 2 hours: 1___ 2___ 3___ 4___ 5___ 6___ 7___ 8___ 9___ 10___ 11___ 12___ Catheter care ___ Skin care products: Eucerin lotion ___ Lever 2000 ___ Natural Tears ___ Nasal spray ___	Oral care every 2 hours: 1___ 2___ 3___ 4___ 5___ 6___ 7___ 8___ 9___ 10___ 11___ 12___ Catheter care ___ Shower _____ Wash #1 _____ Wash #2 _____	Oral care every 2 hours: 1___ 2___ 3___ 4___ 5___ 6___ 7___ 8___ 9___ 10___ 11___ 12___ Catheter care ___ Shower _____ Wash #1 _____ Wash #2 _____	Oral care every 2 hours: 1___ 2___ 3___ 4___ 5___ 6___ 7___ 8___ 9___ 10___ 11___ 12___ Catheter care ___ Shower _____ Wash #1 _____ Wash #2 _____ Diarrhea protocol

Education	Admission orientation:
	• Blood counts
	• Refrigerator policy
	• Neutropenic precautions
	• Thrombocytopenic precautions
	• Oral care
	• Skin care protocol
	• Preparative regimen schedule
	• Pain scale
	• Daily routine
	Support group information
	Catheter care book ___
		"Caring for Yourself" video ___
		Watched:
		  catheter dressing change ___
		  ports flushed ___
		Demonstrated:
		  oral care ___
		  skin care ___
		  hygiene ___
		Read the catheter care book ___
		I understand my chemotherapy and its side effects ___
			Watched:
			  catheter dressing change ___
			  ports flushed ___
			I know:
			  bleeding precautions ___
			  lab values ___
			Met the rehab therapists ___
			Written information on exercise and activities ___
				Demonstrated catheter dressing change ___ and flushing ports ___ on the mannequin
				I know the function of WBCs, platelets, and red blood cells ___

	Day 1 −6 BMT	Day 2 −5 BMT	Day 3 −4 BMT	Day 4 −3 BMT
Psychological Social Emotional Spiritual	Chaplain visit ＿＿ Social worker visit ＿＿ "Looking Forward" group on Tuesday ＿＿	Set schedule ＿＿ Set goals ＿＿ Chaplain visit ＿＿ Social worker visit ＿＿	Chaplain visit ＿＿ Social worker visit ＿＿	Chaplain visit ＿＿ Social worker visit ＿＿
Activity	Activities: Rehab group every Wednesday and Thursday	Activities:	Activities:	Activities:
Nutrition	Dietitian visit Foods not allowed on my diet	Dietitian visit ＿＿ General diet with neutropenic precautions	Dietitian visit ＿＿ General diet with neutropenic precautions	Dietitian visit ＿＿ General diet with neutropenic precautions
Discharge Planning		After discharge I plan to stay at ＿＿＿＿＿＿＿ ＿＿＿＿＿＿＿ ＿＿＿＿＿＿＿ My caregiver will be ＿＿＿＿＿＿＿		

Figure 16.3 A two-page excerpt from a patient carepath. Courtesy of Baylor Institute of Transplantation Sciences at Baylor University Medical Center, Dallas, Texas.

lowing BMT. The development of structured rehabilitation programs, similar to those commonly employed with stroke or cardiac trauma patients, needs to be seriously considered.

The goal of rehabilitation is to help BMT survivors reduce the extent to which the disability affects their ability to function in everyday life. Mayer (1975) noted that the concept of cancer rehabilitation includes the theme of quality of survival—not how long a person lives but how well he or she lives within the restrictions of the disease (Welch-McCaffrey, 1992). Patients, family members, and health-care professionals need to have realistic expectations of functional recovery following BMT, especially of allogeneic recipients. Although the majority of patients expect to return to "normal" following their transplants, a minority actually do. "Being normal" was one of the themes identified when survivors were asked, "What does QOL mean to you?" Survivors consistently referred to the lack of normalcy and the differences between themselves and those who had not undergone a BMT (Ferrell et al., 1992). Unrealistic hope of returning to "normal" can result in disappointment, disillusionment, and depression. Survivors, especially those with significant complications, often describe a "new normal" after BMT.

Similar to quality of life, several domains of rehabilitation for long-term survivorship include physical, emotional, sexual, social, vocational, and economic (Welch-McCaffrey, 1992). A comprehensive rehabilitation program for BMT survivors should include:

1. mechanism for rehabilitation to span the continuum of care,
2. budget for development of plan and for follow-up cost/benefit analysis,
3. program to monitor continuous quality improvement, and
4. documentation in order to measure progress through the rehabilitation plan.

When designing a rehabilitation program, it is important to keep in mind that individual needs vary. *Rehabilitation* means different things to different people. A rehabilitation program focusing on the physical domain may include interventions such as an exercise program or symptom management approach. Occupational therapy aimed at role adjustment and coping mechanisms focuses on the emotional and social domains. Other interventions may concentrate on the sexual, vocational, economic, or spiritual domains of rehabilitation. Roles of physical therapy, occupational therapy, and therapeutic recreation are summarized in Table 16.4.

An example of a comprehensive rehabilitation program with physical therapy, occupational therapy, and therapeutic recreation is in place at the marrow transplant program at Baylor University Medical Center in Dallas, Texas. In 1992, the FOCUS/PDSA model and process tools of a continuous quality improvement program was utilized to improve rehabilitation therapy for BMT patients. The purpose of rehabilitation therapy is to improve patients' ability to function physically, mentally, and socially. The program includes preadmission assessment of rehabilitation needs, physical precautions and treatment considerations, treatment and discharge criteria to facilitate patients' independence and cost containment, and continued outpatient BMT rehabilitation services to provide continuity of care.

Marrow transplant candidates meet with the rehabilitation team—physical therapist, occupational therapist, and recreational therapist—during their pretransplant workup. The team assesses strength, endurance, coping skills, leisure skill, support systems, and everyday functional roles. Patients are asked introspective questions such as, "How do you deal with anger?" and "How do you know when you are stressed?" All domains (physical, psychological, social, and spiritual) are assessed by questions such as, "What things do you enjoy?" and

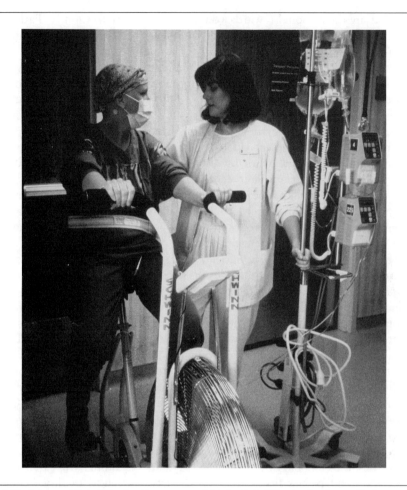

Figure 16.4
A physical therapist
supervises a patient exer-
cising on a stationary bike,
which helps build patient's
endurance.

SOURCE: Courtesy of the Physical Medicine and Rehabilitation Department of Baylor Rehabilitation Services at Baylor
University Medical Center, Dallas, Texas.

TABLE 16.4 Physical medicine and roles of rehabilitation therapy

Physical therapy (PT)	Occupational therapy (OT)	Therapeutic recreation (TR)
Assists patients with strength, mobility, balance, coordination, endurance, posture, safety, gait, stairs	Focuses on patient's ability to perform tasks related to activities of daily living, life roles, socialization, and leisure activities	Addresses patient's community resources, support sources, self-concept, self-awareness, leisure skills and interests, social-interpersonal skills, stress management, emotional and physical outlets, and clarification of values

"What are the personal rewards you get?" The therapists inquire about the patients' treatment goals or goals for rehabilitation. Information gained during the pretransplant rehabilitation evaluation is used to help keep patients motivated during their BMT experience.

Once admitted to the hospital, patients are given a packet of information regarding stress management, entertainment videos, and energy conservation. Patients who live more than 60 miles from the transplant center are also given a resource guide to local activities, restaurants, and services. An exercise routine, usually containing Theraband exercises, is developed for the patient based on interests and needs that were identified pretransplant. Patients are given a calendar of activities that includes the weekly inpatient support group facilitated by the chaplain and social worker and the rehabilitation groups offered two afternoons per week. The most popular rehabilitation groups are the adaptive sports activities such as "bowling for platelets" (bowling) and "serving up stem cells" (volleyball). Other rehabilitation groups include self-help activities such as scarf creations, stress management, and time management. Massage therapy and music therapy are offered once a month. Group activities consist of games like Pictionary or Bingo. Holiday parties and event parties (e.g., Super Bowl party) also provide opportunities for social interaction among patients and families as well as entertainment.

Rehabilitation therapy after hospital discharge is tailored to individual patient needs. Patients are encouraged to continue their inpatient exercise routines, particularly the strength and endurance exercises. Individual counseling, outpatient physical and occupational therapy, and a monthly post-BMT support group are some options for patients and families. Members of the rehabilitation team are often invited to the post-BMT support group to discuss stress management, body-image changes, and "nor-malization." Patients dealing with chronic GVHD often require more rehabilitative interventions to help manage contractures, role changes, and body-image changes. Outlets for anger often need to be explored by the rehabilitation team for patients dealing with a lengthy illness such as chronic GVHD.

FUTURE RESEARCH

The Oncology Nursing Society ranks quality of life and closely related areas of symptoms management among their highest research priorities (Stetz et al., 1995). Only two prospective studies to date have assessed the impact of BMT on physical and psychosocial well-being (Syrjala et al., 1993; Andrykowski et al., 1995). It is important to survey BMT candidates prior to BMT to obtain baseline QOL data to determine the effect of BMT on the patient's perceived quality of life. Although some studies suggest that patients report a decrease in QOL after BMT, it is difficult to assess outcomes without prior measures of QOL to assess effects of conventional cancer treatment or the disease.

With the exception of Chao and colleagues (1992), other QOL studies have not used longitudinal, repeat measures of the patient's perceived quality of life. There is some evidence that certain aspects (e.g., physical) of quality of life show an improvement with time while others (e.g., psychological and social) do not (Chao et al., 1992; Whedon and Ferrell, 1994). A longitudinal study assessing QOL before transplant and at specific time intervals after transplant could give a better perspective of the post-BMT QOL. With baseline data, prospective, longitudinal studies can more accurately describe QOL throughout the continuum of care and recovery. Longer follow-up is necessary to determine whether QOL, when compared to pretransplant QOL, improves or declines over time.

Studies are also needed of cultural influences on QOL after BMT. Some QOL tools have been translated to Spanish. The influence of culture and ethnicity on patients' perceived quality of life is unknown. Multicenter, cross-cultural investigations of quality of life are needed to provide a sufficient sample size to evaluate differences in perceived quality of life due to cultural and ethnic beliefs. Based on these differences, nursing interventions aimed at improving QOL can be selected to meet individual needs.

King and colleagues (1995) concluded that BMT nurses view QOL differently from patients, and they may focus on physical aspects more than psychological, social, and spiritual health when providing care. Further research is needed to determine which interventions nurses commonly use to enhance QOL and what is the outcome of these nursing interventions. Research is needed to evaluate interventions for unresolved psychological needs of patients who have recovered physically from transplantation. It is unclear whether nursing interventions such as self-care strategies and information about additional coping strategies taught during the early phases of BMT actually assist the long-term BMT survivor. Research about caregiver burden is definitely lacking. Research is needed regarding family and quality of life to answer some of the following questions:

- How do families define their QOL after BMT?
- How do families define the survivor's QOL and how does that compare to the survivor's perception?
- What are the family's demands across the continuum of BMT (before BMT, BMT, after BMT, and long-term recovery)?
- What are the family's demands associated with long-term recovery?
- What variables influence the family's psychosocial functioning?

- What strategies have families used to achieve optimal QOL across the BMT continuum?

Finally, further research is needed on psychological issues such as hope and depression related to QOL. Hope has been found to be a key element in coping with and adaptation to illness. Six dimensions of hope have been described: confidence in outcomes, relationships with others, possibility of a future, spiritual beliefs, active involvement, and hope from within (Clark, 1992). Many of the dimensions of hope overlap with the domains of quality of life. Hope is often correlated with a higher quality of life. Depression, on the other hand, often occurs due to a lack of hope. Both depression and hope can influence the quality of life of survivors. The spiritual domain and the role of nurses in instilling, maintaining, and restoring hope to enhance QOL and overcome depression are important areas for further investigation.

SUMMARY

Tools (e.g., Karnofsky scores) that measure a patient's functional ability fail to measure all the factors that survivors feel contribute to "quality of life." QOL information is essential when evaluating the success of BMT. QOL related to BMT is a dynamic, highly individualized process. After BMT, many survivors find new value to life. Attitudes, priorities, goals, and coping responses change. Time becomes "precious." No longer do survivors worry about the distant future, but now concentrate on living in the present (Haberman et al., 1993). One patient stated, "I no longer sweat the small stuff; I realized big problems were really little ones."

REFERENCES

Altmaier, E., Gingrich, R., Fyfe, M. 1991. Two-year adjustment of bone marrow transplant survivors. *BMT* 7:311-316.

Andrykowski, M., Altmaier, Barnett, R., et al. 1990. The quality of life in adult survivors of allogeneic bone marrow transplantation. *Transplantation 50*(3):399-406.

Andrykowski, M., Bruehl, S., Henslee-Downey, P. 1995a. Physical and psychosocial status of adults one year after bone marrow transplantation: a prospective study. *BMT 15*:837-844.

Andrykowski, M., Greiner, C., Altmaier, E., Burish, T., et al. 1995b. Quality of life following bone marrow transplantation: findings from a multicentre study. *Br J Canc 71*:1322-1329.

Andrykowski, M., Henslee, P., and Barnett, R. 1989. Longitudinal assessment of psychosocial functioning of adult survivors of allogeneic bone marrow transplantation. *BMT 4*:505-509.

Andrykowski, M., Henslee, P., Farrall, M. 1989. Physical and psychosocial functioning of adult survivors of allogeneic bone marrow transplantation. *BMT 4*:75-81.

Baker, F., Curbow, B., Wingard, J. 1991. Role retention and quality of life of bone marrow transplant survivors. *Soc Sci Med 32*:697-704.

Belec, R. 1992. Quality of life: perceptions of long-term survivors of bone marrow transplantation. *Oncol Nurs Forum 19*(1):31-37.

Bush, N., Haberman, M., Donaldson, et al. 1995. Quality of life of 25 adults surviving 6–18 years after bone marrow transplantation. *Soc Sci Med 40*(4):479-490.

Chao, N., Tierney, D., Bloom, J., et al. 1992. Dynamic assessment of quality of life after autologous bone marrow transplantation. *Blood 80*(3):825-830.

Clark, J. 1992. Psychosocial dimensions: the patient. In Groenwald, S., Frogge, M., Goodman, M, Yarbro, C. (Eds.) *Cancer Nursing: Principles and Practice.* Boston: Jones & Bartlett, 346-362.

Communicore. 1995. The issue of survival and quality of life. *Supportive Therapies for Cancer Chemotherapy Patients: The Intersection of Quality of Life and Economics.* Newport Beach, CA: Communicore, Inc., 1-16.

Copeland, D. 1996. The effect of exercise on the quality of life of the bone marrow transplant patient. Ph.D. Thesis Baylor Univ., Dallas, TX. August.

Dean, H. 1990. Political and ethical implications of using quality of life as an outcome measure. *Semin Oncol Nurs 6*(4):303-308.

Decker, W. 1995. Psychosocial considerations for bone marrow transplant recipients. *Crit Care Nurs Q 17*(4):67-73.

Dickerson, A., Oakley, F. Comparing the roles of community-living persons and patient populations. *J Occupational Therapy 49*(3):221-228.

Ferrans, C. 1990. Quality of life: conceptual issues. *Semin Oncol Nurs 6*(4):348-354.

Ferrans, C. 1994. Quality of life through the eyes of survivors of breast cancer. *Oncol Nurs Forum 21*(10):1645-1651.

Ferrans, C., Ferrell, B. 1990. Development of quality of life index for patients with cancer. *Oncol Nurs Forum 17*(3):15-21.

Ferrell, B., Dow, K., Leigh, S., et al. 1995. Quality of life in long-term cancer survivors. *Oncol Nurs Forum 22*(6):915-922.

Ferrell, B., Grant, M., Schmidt, G., et al. 1992a. The meaning of quality of life for bone marrow transplant survivors; part 1: the impact of bone marrow transplant on quality of life. *Canc Nurs 15*(3):153-160.

Ferrell, B., Grant, M., Schmidt, G., et al. 1992b. The meaning of quality of life for bone marrow transplant survivors; part 2: improving quality of life for BMT survivors. *Canc Nurs 15*(4):247-253.

Ferrell, B., Wisdom, C., Wenzl, C. 1989. Quality of life as an outcome variable in the management of cancer pain. *Cancer 63*:2321-2327.

Frank-Stromborg, M. 1988. The achievement of excellence in cancer nursing practice. *J Assoc Ped Oncol Nurs 5*:22-23.

Gill, T., Feinstein, A. (1994). A critical appraisal of the quality of quality-of-life measurements. *JAMA 272*:619-626.

Grant, M., Ferrell, B., Schmidt, G., et al. 1992. Measurement of quality of life in bone marrow transplantation survivors. *QOL Res 1*:375-384.

Grant, M., Ferrell, B., Schmidt, G., et al. 1992. Researching quality of life indicators: their impact on the daily life of bone marrow transplant patients. *Cancer Nursing: Changing Frontiers, Proceeding of the Seventh International Conference on Cancer Nursing.* Harrow, England: Scutari Projects, pp. 80-84.

Grant, M., Padilla, G. Ferrell, et al. 1990. Assessment of quality of life with a single instrument. *Semin Oncol Nurs 6*(4):260-270.

Haberman, M. 1988. Psychosocial aspects of bone marrow transplantation. *Semin Oncol Nurs 4*:55-59.

Haberman, M. 1994. Quality of life as an outcome for oncology nursing. *Fighting Fatigue: Resolving Issues for the Cancer Patient.* Beachwood, OH: ProEd Communications, 30-36.

Haberman, M., Bush, N., Young, K., et al. 1993. Quality of life of adult long-term survivors of bone marrow transplantation: a qualitative analysis of narrative data. *Oncol Nurs Forum 20*(10):1545-1553.

Haberman, M., Donaldson, G., Sullivan, K. 1995. Quality of life of 125 adults surviving 6–18 years after bone marrow transplantation. *J Soc Sci Med* 40(4):479-490.

Hengeveld, M., Houtman, R., Zwaan, F. 1988. Psychological aspects of bone marrow transplantation: a retrospective study of 17 long-term survivors. *BMT* 3:69-75.

Holtsman, L. 1989. Physical therapy intervention following bone marrow transplantation. *Clin Manage* 8(2): 6-9.

Jalowiec, A. 1990. Issues in using multiple measures of quality of life. *Semin Oncol Nurs* 6(4):271-277.

James, M. 1987. Physical therapy for patients after bone marrow transplantation. *Phys Ther* 67(6):946-952.

Jassak, P., Porter, N. 1995. Strategies for education of the BMT patient. In Buchsel, P., Whedon, M. (Eds.) *Bone Marrow Transplantation: Administrative and Clinical Strategies*. Boston: Jones & Bartlett, 353-363.

Juttner, C., Fibbe, W., Nemunaitis, J., et al. 1994. Blood cell transplantation: report from an international consensus meeting. *BMT* 14:689-693.

Kanabar, D., Attard-Montalto, S., Saha, V., Kingston, J., et al. 1995. Quality of life in survivors of childhood cancer after megatherapy with autologous bone marrow rescue. *J Pediatr Hematol Oncol* 12(1):29-36.

King, C., Ferrell, B., Grant, M., et al. 1995. Nurses' perceptions of the meaning of quality of life for bone marrow transplant survivors. *Canc Nurs* 18(2):118-129.

Lewis, F. 1982. Experienced personal control and quality of life in late-stage cancer patients. *Nurs Res* 31(2): 113-119.

Lindley, C., Hirsch, J. 1994. Oncology nurses' attitudes, perceptions, and knowledge of quality-of-life assessment in patients with cancer. *Oncol Nurs Forum* 21(1): 103-110.

Marshall, P. 1990. Cultural influences on perceived quality of life. *Semin Oncol Nurs* 6(4):278-284.

Mast, M. 1995. Definition and measurement of quality of life in oncology nursing research: review and theoretical implications. *Oncol Nurs Forum* 22(6):957-964.

Maxwell, T., Aldredge-Clanton, J. 1994. Survivor guilt in cancer patients: a pastoral perspective. *J Pastoral Care* 48(1):25-31.

Mayer, N. 1975. Concepts in cancer rehabilitation. *Semin Oncol* 2:1527-1535.

Mellette, S., Blunk, K. 1994. Cancer rehabilitation. *Semin Oncol Nurs* 21(6):779-782.

Moinpour, C. 1994. Measuring quality of life: an emerging science. *Semin Oncol Nurs* 21(5):(suppl 10):48-63.

Moinpour, C., Chapko, M., Sullivan, K., et al. 1995. Cost issues for BMT. In Buchsel, P., Whedon, M. (Eds.)

Bone Marrow Transplantation: Administrative and Clinical Strategies. Boston: Jones & Bartlett, 427-442.

Morreim, E. 1992. Medical ethics and the future of quality of life research. *Prog Cardiovasc Nurs* 7(1):12-17.

Nims, J. 1991. Survivorship and rehabilitation. In Whedon, M. (Ed.) *Bone Marrow Transplantation: Principles, Practice, and Nursing Insights*. Boston: Jones & Bartlett, 333-345.

Nims, J., Strom, S. 1988. Late complications of bone marrow transplant recipients: nursing care issues. *Semin Oncol Nurs* 4(1):47-54.

Padilla, G., Grant, M. 1985. Quality of life as a cancer nursing outcome variable. *Adv Nurs Sci* 8(1):45-60.

Padilla, G., Grant, M., Ferrell, B. 1992. Nursing research into quality of life. *QOL Res* 1:341-348.

Padilla, G., Presant, C., Grant, M., et al. 1983. Quality of life index for patients with cancer. *Res Nurs Health* 6:117-126.

Presant, C., Klahr, C., Hogan, L. 1981. Evaluating quality-of-life in oncology patients: pilot observations. *Oncol Nurs Forum* 8(3):26-30.

Schipper, H., Clinch, J., McMurray, A., et al. 1984. Measuring the quality of life of cancer patients: The Functional Living Index—Cancer: development and validation. *J Clin Oncol* 2(5):472-483.

Schmidt, G. 1994. Assessment of quality of life following bone marrow transplantation. In Forman, S., Blume, K., Thomas, E. (Eds.) *Bone Marrow Transplantation*. Boston: Blackwell, 572-580.

Schmidt, G., Niland, J., Forman, S., et al. 1993. Extended follow-up in 212 long-term allogeneic bone marrow transplant survivors: issues of quality of life. *Transplantation* 55(3):551-557.

Stetz, K., Haberman, M., Holcombe, J., et al. 1995. 1994 Oncology Nursing Society research priorities survey. *Oncol Nurs Forum* 22:785-789.

Stewart, S. 1992. *Bone Marrow Transplants: A Book of Basics for Patients*. Highland Park, IL: BMT Newsletter.

Stewart, S. 1993. Long-term BMT survivors . . . *BMT Newsletter* 15.

Stewart, S. 1993. Support groups offer help, hope. *BMT Newsletter* 18.

Syrjala, K. 1995. Meeting the psychological needs of recipients and families. In Buchsel, P., Whedon, M. (Eds.) *Bone Marrow Transplantation: Administrative and Clinical Strategies*. Boston: Jones & Bartlett, 283-301.

Syrjala, K., Gerorgiadour, F. Hazelwood, L., et al. 1990. Recovery from marrow transplantation (MT): physical and psychological functioning at one year posttransplant. *Exper Hematol* 18:660 (abstr).

Syrjala, K., Chapko, M., Vitaliana, P., et al. 1993. Recovery after allogeneic marrow transplantation: prospective study of predictors of long-term physical and psychosocial functioning. *BMT* 11:319-327.

Thomas, E., Lochte, H., Lu, W., et al. 1957. Intravenous infusion of bone marrow in patients receiving radiation and chemotherapy. *N Engl J Med* 257:491.

Webster, J. 1995. Survivorship issues in post-induction therapy. In Wujcik, D. (Ed.) *Nursing Care Issues in Adult Acute Leukemia.* Huntington, NY: PRR, Inc., 28-32.

Welch-McCaffrey, D., Leigh, S., Loescher, L., et al. 1992. Psychosocial dimensions: issues in survivorship. In Groenwald, S., Frogge, M., Goodman, M., Yarbro, C. (Eds.) *Cancer Nursing: Principles and Practice.* Boston: Jones & Bartlett, 373-381.

Whedon, M., Ferrell, B. 1994. Quality of life in adult bone marrow transplant patients: beyond the first year. *Semin Oncol Nurs* 10(1):42-57.

Whedon, M., Stearns, D., Mills, L. 1995. Quality of life of long-term adult survivors of autologous bone marrow transplantation. *Oncol Nurs Forum* 22(10):1527-1535.

Wingard, J., Curbow, B., Baker, F., et al. 1991. Health functional status, and employment of adult survivors of bone marrow transplantation. *Ann Intern Med 114*: 113-117.

Winningham, M. 1994. New concepts in the nursing care of fatigue. *Fighting Fatigue: Resolving Issues for the Cancer Patient.* Beachwood, OH: ProEd Communications, 13-19.

Winningham, M., Nail, L, Barton Burke, M., et al. 1994. Fatigue and the cancer experience: the state of the knowledge. *Oncol Nurs Forum* 21:23-36.

Wolcott, D., Wellisch, D., Fawzy, F., et al. 1986. Adaptation of adult bone marrow transplant recipient long-term survivors. *Transplantation* 41(4):478-183.

Wolcott, D., Wellisch, D., Fawsy, F., et al. 1986. Psychological adjustment of adult bone marrow transplant donors whose recipient survives. *Transplantation* 41(4): 484-488.

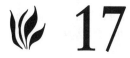

17

Patients' Perspectives

Susan Stewart

Surviving a bone marrow transplant is a challenging experience, both physically and emotionally. Patients leave the hospital physically changed, emotionally drained, and uncertain about whether they've bought a little more time or have actually been cured. Survivors ride an emotional roller coaster as days of improvement are often followed by complications that require the patient to be rehospitalized. For the first year following a BMT, survivors measure the "future" a day at a time, unable to commit with certainty to anything longer.

The following six survivors have written about various aspects of their transplants and survival experiences. They hope that these narratives will provide some insight into what it's like to undergo and survive a BMT.

Following a second relapse of acute lymphocytic leukemia in 1992, 27-year-old Lisa Powell underwent an allogeneic BMT with marrow from a matched unrelated donor. She is currently disease free.

BEATING THE ODDS

Lisa Powell

In 1977, when I was 11 years old, I was diagnosed with acute lymphocytic leukemia (ALL).

I achieved a remission and underwent 3 years of chemotherapy, looking forward to that magic 5-year mark when I would be considered cured. Four years and 9 months later I relapsed.

Fortunately, I was able to attain a good remission that lasted 9 years. During those years I attended college, earned a degree in finance and international business, married my husband Rick, and began working as a claims adjuster at an insurance company. Life was great.

In the fall of 1991 I began getting excruciating headaches. I felt listless and sick all the time. The thought never crossed my mind that the cancer had returned. I thought leukemia was a thing of the past, something I had put behind me.

When my doctor told me I had relapsed I was devastated and felt betrayed. But I told myself I had beaten leukemia twice and could do it again. At age 26, I underwent chemotherapy again and immediately went into remission. However, my doctor told me my only real chance for a cure was a bone marrow transplant.

Deciding to undergo a BMT was the hardest decision of my life. The odds of survival were not in my favor and the fact that I would be infertile, could never bear a child of my own, following the transplant tore me apart. I finally decided I had too much to live for and too much more to accomplish to give up. I agreed to undergo a BMT.

Unfortunately, no one in my family matched my marrow type and could serve as my donor. One week after contacting the National Marrow Donor Program, an unrelated donor was found. On September 3, 1992, new life was transplanted into me. On October 19, my husband's birthday, I was released from the hospital and spent 3 months recuperating in an apartment close to the hospital.

Today I am considered cured of this dreadful disease, thanks to a wonderful man in California who donated his marrow to me, the transplant team at Shands Hospital, and my oncologist who gave me the strength and encouragement to proceed. Granted, life was not rosy during my hospitalization and recuperation—I had lots of ups and downs with infections and graft-versus-host disease. I still have some weakness in my legs and knees but I hope to resolve that problem by working out every day.

I have been back to work for a year and am exuberant. My hair grew back thicker after the BMT and best of all, my new immune system is in peak condition. I hardly ever get sick. Other than minor skin rashes due to graft-versus-host disease, I feel as healthy as ever.

I believe the secret to my success was the support I received from my husband and parents—they were incredible. There wasn't a moment during the day when I was alone. They were always there to keep my spirits up.

I found it helpful to get ready emotionally for the BMT by reading books on imagery and visualization, developing a positive attitude, and praying. Each night before I retired, I would envision the radiation and chemotherapy attacking the cancer cells and then I would pray. I tried not to dwell on the negative or the possibility of not having a successful BMT. Today, I take one day at a time, live for today, and appreciate life more than ever.

Margaret Steslicki underwent an allogeneic BMT for myelodysplasia in 1990. Five years later (1996), she is disease free.

I'M BACK ON MY FEET AGAIN

Margaret Steslicki

In 1990 my world fell apart. I was diagnosed with myelodysplastic syndrome (MDS) and was told that I needed a bone marrow transplant. Even though I'm a Registered Nurse, the only experience I'd had with BMTs was through a medical resident who had worked with me on a medical-surgical unit 9 to 10 years earlier. He had had leukemia, gone through chemotherapy, and then a BMT. He had made it through the BMT but died several weeks later. At age 33, I was told I too would need a BMT if I wanted to survive long term.

It took a while for everything to sink in—facing a life-threatening blood disorder that could only be cured with a medical procedure that was also life-threatening. I prayed a lot, and with the support of my husband, family, and friends, I developed a strong will to live. A BMT was my only chance for survival. I thought "If 50 people out of 100 can survive a BMT, I can be one of those 50 people."

After researching BMT centers and their experience with MDS, I chose to have my BMT at Harper Hospital in Detroit. We were impressed with the BMT team, and being treated at Harper allowed me to remain close to my family, something I felt was very important.

The hardest part of the transplant was leaving my two small children. I remember thinking that if I died, 5-year-old David would remember me but 2-year-old Rachel would not. My children gave me the strength and willpower to fight the disease. A quotation from one of Bernie Siegel's books stuck in my mind: "He who has a *why* to live can bear almost any *how.*" I had every *why* in the world to live and I was going to do just that.

Being an avid gardener, I and my husband explained the BMT process to our children using gardening metaphors. We compared the chemotherapy to a weed killer that would destroy my bad marrow or bad seeds. We then explained that new seeds in the bone marrow that Uncle Bill would give me would produce new blood cells and make my bone marrow and blood flower once again.

Before my hospitalization, I collected several small gifts for my children including books, candy, balloons, small figurines, and toys. The gifts were not costly, just little things from the dime store. I also collected special cards and stationery. Each day in the hospital, I sent a letter or special card home to my children with a little surprise. It was a way that they could connect with me, and I with them.

On the morning of September 17, 1990, I left my in-laws' house to enter the hospital. It was one of the most difficult moments of my life. I said good-bye to my children and left the house with tears in my eyes. I had an overwhelming fear that I might never see them again.

The transplant wasn't easy. The 8 days of intensive chemotherapy were difficult for me. I was sedated most of the time and remember little except sleeping and vomiting. I remember that toward the end of my conditioning regimen I had awful feelings and hallucinations. I saw the room spinning and people melting into the floors and walls. A few days after my BMT, I figured out that the Ativan was causing these feelings, and I refused to take it, preferring to control the nausea and vomiting with ice chips and crackers.

The day of transplant was an emotional, exciting day. This would be my new birthday, a day of new life. The actual transplant was anticlimactic. I tolerated the procedure well, although the nausea and vomiting persisted and

I was started on total parenteral nutrition (TPN).

Days passed as I lay in protective isolation, listening to the hum of the large room filter. Being separated from my children was the most difficult thing at this point. My physician helped me cope with my loneliness by telling me, "These days and weeks away from your children may seem like a long time now, but it will mean a lifetime with them."

During my hospitalization I tried to phone my children daily, although sometimes I just wasn't up to it. My husband and family always made sure the children understood why I couldn't call, and gave them one of the presents I had collected for them. Sometimes my husband would bring the video camera into my hospital room so I could talk to the children and show them where I was. I'd read stories while my husband videotaped me. I was told that my daughter would carry the video around with her all day and watch it over and over. Videos of the kids were also done and brought to me in the hospital room.

On October 19, 1990, I was discharged to my in-laws' home. It was the happiest day of my life! I had survived the BMT! I knew there were potential complications and I wasn't yet free and clear, but I hoped and prayed that all would go well.

Twenty-four hours later I had a cerebral hemorrhage and ended up back in the hospital. I had been prepared for the BMT but not the stroke. I had survived one life-threatening disease and its treatment, only to face another. I had paralysis of my left arm, a left facial drop, weakness in my left leg, and difficulty with balance. "Why me?" I asked. My own little miracle was that had the hemorrhage occurred 1 week earlier I probably would have died, since my bone marrow had just started producing platelets.

As the days passed in the hospital, I saw a multitude of doctors and underwent a variety of tests. I developed symptoms of graft-versus-host disease and cytomegalovirus (CMV). After a few weeks, my abdomen was so swollen I looked like I was pregnant with twins. I developed a paralytic ileus and many high fevers. There were many days when I thought I wouldn't make it. I had hit an all-time low.

I needed to work on getting well, but didn't have much physical strength. I needed help with all my personal needs: dressing, bathing, going to the bathroom, walking, and preparing food. It was devastating and humiliating. I've always been the caregiver and very independent, and now my independence had been taken away.

With the help of physical therapy (PT) and occupational therapy (OT) I gradually learned to walk with a walker, then a four-pronged cane, and then a cane. Six weeks after entering the hospital for the stroke, I was discharged home, where I continued PT and OT for several weeks.

Post-BMT complications continued. I was admitted two more times with viral meningitis. The first time was 2 days after Christmas. After being admitted for observation, I had a grand mal seizure while undergoing a spinal tap. I had a respiratory arrest and had to be resuscitated. I vividly remember going into the seizure; it is a feeling I will never forget. I woke up on a ventilator, the spinal tap was completed, and I was rushed to the intensive care unit.

Five years later (1995) I'm doing very well and am considered cured. I still follow-up with a neurologist regularly due to the stroke, and will probably be on Dilantin for the rest of my life. My mobility is about 95% normal; I occasionally get clumsy when I'm tired, but it's a manageable problem. I'm back to nursing and raising my two children, and am working on my master's degree in health promotion and health care management.

My BMT experience has changed my life forever. I have gained wisdom I never knew possible, both as a human being and as a nurse.

I will never take life or people for granted, and I cherish my time with family and friends. I counsel patients who are about to go through a BMT to keep a positive attitude, and to be prepared for the ups and downs. With hope, they will find the end of the rainbow.

I found that emotional support, for both me and my family, was extremely important throughout my illness and treatment. While in the hospital, my mind was at ease knowing my children were well cared for, and my husband had the support of many family members and friends. Since recovering from my BMT, I have tried to support others facing a BMT or other life-threatening disease or treatment. I volunteer with groups such as the National Bone Marrow Transplant Link, the Red Cross and Saginaw Valley Blood Program, and the Central Michigan Gift of Life Bone Marrow Program. I believe that things happen for a reason. The BMT experience has helped me find one of my purposes in life.

Judith Miller at age 32 underwent an allogeneic BMT for acute myelogenous leukemia in 1993. She is currently disease free.

LIVING IN THE POST-BMT "SNAKEPIT"

Judith A. Miller

A recent BMT survivor recently asked me, "Is it normal to feel as mean as a snake after a BMT?" I could only nod my head, remembering the first few months after my allogeneic BMT for AML in January 1993. "Oh yes," I told her, "your feelings are normal. The drugs, stress, and emotional upheaval of a BMT can throw anyone into snakedom." I look back on the first few months after BMT with a mixture of wonder, sorrow, laughter, and enormous pity for anyone who had to put up with me.

My BMT at Emory University Hospital went smoothly: I was very lucky. My donor was my brother and his marrow engrafted quickly. I had some graft-versus-host disease, and an infection or two, but no real trauma. My family and friends were terrific, caring for me throughout. To my great joy, I was released on day 32. And then, to my great shock, I crashed and entered full-blown "snakehood."

Throughout the BMT I had operated on adrenaline. My experience before being diagnosed has colored my response to the disease: I had been sick for almost 2 years, but no physician had taken me seriously and so there had even been some relief when I finally found out what was wrong. I embarked on treatment in a fairly aggressive frame of mind. I was 32, very independent, career oriented (I am a professor of French history at Emory), and liked a good challenge. I had a deep, durable network of friends, and incredible physicians and nurses.

My parents canceled a cruise to care for me after I was released from the hospital, and they pulled my cluttered apartment into shape. A dear friend, Melinda, arrived from Houston the following week to stay with me, and even planned a delayed birthday party for me with 30 people. So far, so good. Then I was on my own.

The first obstacle was to learn to ask for help and to accept it. I live alone, so that meant scheduling friends to help me with housekeeping, resisting the urge to entertain when they came to help, and most vexing, anticipating what I might need days in advance. On Mondays, one friend put laundry in the washer; on Tuesdays, another friend put it into the dryer; on Wednesdays, another friend folded it. (I couldn't bear to be around anyone, or to inflict myself on them, long enough to do a load from start to finish). Often, I felt it was harder to schedule things than to do them myself. I had never realized how independent I had been used

to being, and it was excruciating to have others helping me.

For months after my BMT I was the "nausea queen." You name it, I could throw it up. My daily prayer became, "Let me make good choices." At first, that meant food, then slowly it expanded to cover the rest of my life. My selections were very odd, but finally some worked. For awhile, all I could handle was Carnation™ Instant Breakfast. Then, in the fourth and fifth months it was Capt'n Crunch™—box after box of it—then coffee and beer and finally, in the eighth month, a normal diet. I took Ativan to relieve the nausea but it didn't help too much and made me feel down. What a terrific choice: have a quieter stomach but feel blue, or keep throwing up and be slightly more cheerful. Now I can laugh about the situation, but at the time it really tested me.

I also experienced obsessive thoughts and irritability caused by the Ativan and the cyclosporin I was taking to control graft-versus-host disease, and the general emotional trauma that comes with months of illness. One day, for example, I read that car timing belts need to be replaced at 60,000 miles. I thought I had replaced my belt the year before, but couldn't bring myself to check my car diary to confirm this. So I tooled around Atlanta for almost 6 months, worrying that the belt was going to snap and strand me, and feeling that the world was far too complicated.

Another day I gazed at a construction site and realized I didn't understand what held up buildings. I became depressed every time I was in a tall building and felt it shake. I wasn't afraid it was going to collapse, but instead saw it as a further sign that the world was too complex.

After a while almost every decision I had to make seemed too complicated. Even filling the gas tank or taking the cats to the vet was overwhelming. "How would I get them in the cat carrier?" I wondered, "How could I drive them to the vet and get the carrier back out the car? What seat should I put the carrier in?" When I finally read the cyclosporin and Ativan packaging and found irritability and depression listed as side effects, I felt much better about these crazed thoughts. When the drugs tapered off, the obsessions ended as well.

A few weeks after my release from the hospital, I simply decided I was tired of being sick and was ready to get on with life. On day 53, I signed up for a two-hour tennis lesson, suited up, scarf on my very bald head, mask on, and headed to the courts. I stayed until the very end of the session on a bitterly cold March night, and trotted home, quite pleased that my backhand was still intact.

The next morning I could not move. Terrified, I called the hospital. I was sure I had relapsed. When I told them I had spent the prior night playing tennis, they read me the riot act. I was to depend more on friends, do less, and give my body a chance to recover, they said. I had no choice. My muscles were so sore I could only flop on the sofa for the next 3 weeks, playing with the TV remote control.

After the tennis debacle, depression hit hard. I hated sitting home alone, but was too cranky and tired to deal with people, even my family and dearest friends. And to make it even more frustrating, everyone was being wonderful. They were infinitely sympathetic, offering help, cassettes, videos, books, and visits, none of which I wanted in the least.

I couldn't concentrate. I couldn't read. I hated junk TV (but got hooked on Wheel of Fortune and MTV). I couldn't keep food down. I was tired of scheduling help and saying thank you. I hated being away from home, but hated being cooped up. I hated people who tried to cheer me up. I felt guilty that I wasn't radiantly happy to be in good health. "After all," everyone said, "think how terrific your blood counts look!" That argument left little leeway for

whining. The days stretched endlessly into monotonous, more-or-less silent, self-pity. I even got to the point where I thought it might be easier to relapse than put my life back together. I feared the depression would continue, yet tried to take it on faith that it would ease as I became stronger and time passed.

There is, however, a cheerful ending to this tale. At about the 100-day mark I began to improve, albeit haltingly, and by the fourth month I could feel week-by-week progress. My hair started to look like just a very bad styling choice. I kept down a bit of food and even, wonderfully, coffee, which gave me a bit more energy. Friends at the Leukemia Society support group helped me rediscover my sense of humor.

By the fifth month, I decided I was running a fun deficit and began going out a bit with friends. Slowly, reading came back, along with listening to music. I started working out, and by the seventh month was walking a brisk 3.5 miles per day, although I couldn't run until the ninth month.

I began teaching again in August. One of my happiest moments was the first day back teaching. I got to talk for 2 hours about French history—something, at last, that had nothing to do with leukemia. In the tenth month, I rushed back to France for a 2-week research trip and sat in my favorite cafe as if nothing had ever happened. On New Year's Day, 1994, I retackled my research, although concentration was very difficult. In the fourteenth month I finally recovered my craving for chips and dip, a taste I thought had disappeared entirely (a terrific side benefit of the BMT, I had hoped!). And in the eighteenth month, I began to take stock, grieve some, and put things into perspective.

Putting my life back together has been a bit-by-bit process. I hadn't realized the various components that made it up: hair, fingernails, book chapters, my morning rhythm of coffee, the *New York Times* and National Public Radio, my niece, Garth Brooks played very loudly with my car windows rolled down, conference organizing, "my" seat in the French archives, dinner parties for 30 on the spur of the moment, pulling all-nighters, and driving very fast. New pleasures: a black leather jacket (paid for with the money I didn't spend on a wig), on the first anniversary of my transplant skiing with my brother Robert (who was my donor) and his family, and my baby nephew. Of course, one has to add time for grieving about the years lost to illness, nearly overwhelming sadness for friends who didn't make it, frustration with colleagues who still can't understand what happened, and time for extra sleep, rebuilding, and letting go. I would not have guessed this would be the outcome during my "snake days."

I am thankful I survived the "snake days" and was able to return to my usual chaotic existence. And sometimes I crash, and sleep, and stare at a wall for a few hours when there is no adrenaline left, and I tire of proving I'm back.

I offer this story not to discourage anyone, but rather as a tale of what happened to one person, and as encouragement for both patients and caretakers to carry on. While the snakes are out there during the recovery period, so too are miracles, all part and parcel of returning to the life you love.

At age 39 Mike Eckhardt underwent an allogeneic BMT for chronic myelogenous leukemia in 1992. He is currently disease free.

COMING OUT OF THE FOG

Mike Eckhardt

It's been more than 2 years since my BMT for chronic myelogenous leukemia. I'm just now gaining some perspective on its repercussions on my life. I've wanted and needed to write about it for some time to sort it out. One thing's for sure—catastrophic illness is tremendously invasive and pervasive. It touches every facet of one's existence both in the short and long term. Though it may seem hard to believe, there are even some positive aspects of the experience.

I still find it almost bizarre that I would be the one to get so sick. I was very physically active. I rode my bike 2,000 miles a year, swam about 100 miles, and was active in my children's lives. Leukemia happens to people you read about in the newspaper during their appeals for donors or money for transplants. It doesn't strike enormously healthy, happy, and vital 39-year-old family men.

I had been having trouble with my hip. It was very stiff and painful and was absolute hell on my golf game. I was due for my biennial company physical and a colleague was going in for his, so I made an appointment with his doctor. I went in, the doctor walked me through the paces, and I then went on the road for a few days. When I got back, I found messages from the doctor waiting for me all over town. He told me I needed to repeat the blood test. I didn't think much of it until I saw his nurse running my blood sample over to the hospital across the street for testing. He told me that my white cell count was significantly elevated and suggested I see a hematologist.

There was never any cataclysmic moment when I discovered I had leukemia. I knew early on that leukemia was suspected. The genetic confirmation was almost an anticlimax. My wife, Karen, and I decided to be up front with our boys, so we told them that night. The fact that my 11-year-old son's appendix ruptured exactly at the moment we told them only makes the day more memorable. Gannon only paused from his pain long enough to ask me if he was going to lose his dad. I told him I didn't think so, and after he decided I was telling the truth, he went right back to clutching his stomach and groaning. At that moment, I learned something about unqualified love and acceptance. Our 14-year-old, Donovan, really didn't say much. Still waters run pretty deep with Don, and I was a little concerned about how he would deal with this.

I mentioned there are some silver linings to this particular cloud. The best for me was the response by our two boys. They dealt with the situation in their own ways and each contributed greatly to my recovery in different ways. Gannon is a real live wire. His natural enthusiasm for life energized me whenever I got to see him. Gannon's story was and is about unqualified love and support, which is exactly what a recovering cancer patient needs.

Our older son, Donovan, is a big strong kid. Now 16, at 6'4" and 210 football-playing pounds, I never felt more secure than when he had hold of me. He never hesitated to pitch in, even for an instant. He was a rock for both Karen and me. I think my illness robbed him of some of the innocence of youth, for which I am truly sorry. If I die tomorrow, I know he will grow up to be a good man because I've already seen that he is.

Karen and I have been married for 19 years. The vows read "in sickness and in health" but I'm not sure the author had this kind of sickness in mind. I have a lot of respect for Karen and her strength. Over the years I've come to expect a lot from her. And she has never let me down. Karen really, really persevered and I wouldn't have survived if it weren't for her. It never occurred to me that Karen wouldn't be there for me, which was probably unfair.

I have three bothers and two sisters. Fortunately, my younger brother, Bill was a perfect 6 out of 6 antigen match. I had the BMT in April 1992. From then until March 1993, I was in and out of the hospital on seven occasions, in-cluding the initial 5-week stay. The remaining six were due to problems related to graft-versus-host disease. At one point, I was in for about 3 months.

Although I still deal with some GVHD, my family considers my leukemia a thing of the past, which is good. I'm not quite ready to give it up until I'm sure I've wrung everything I can out of the experience. Catastrophic illness and recovery offers a unique perspective on life that is too precious to waste. It's a physical and emotional roller coaster and I want and need to understand what it's done to me and how it has changed me.

I talk to as many patients as possible because cancer is very isolating. Although each person's cancer experience is different, it's important to know that one need not go through it alone. It's a pretty exclusive fraternity, even if I don't wish membership on anyone.

Brenda Herman at age 52 underwent an autologous BMT for stage IV breast cancer in 1992. Three years later she relapsed. Her first essay was written 1 year after transplant. Her addendum was written 6 months after her relapse.

INSIDE THIS PATIENT THERE IS A PERSON

Brenda J. Herman

I love to travel. Adventure travel. Leningrad by commuter train from Helsinki. Australia, snorkeling in The Great Barrier Reef. New Zealand, flying to the peak of Mt. Cook in a three-passenger plane, landing on a glacier and stepping out into snow above my knees. Climbing inside an Egyptian pyramid. The Far East—Japan, Hong Kong, Thailand, and Singapore. Having just returned from the Galapagos Islands and the Amazon, I am in the process of planning my next trip—China. My oncologist is clutching his chest. Mea culpa.

You see, I have breast cancer. By the time I was diagnosed in 1987 my disease had advanced to stage IV. Mammograms had revealed nothing, and breast exams every 3 or 4 months by competent physicians had revealed nothing. Caution was the watchword since my mother had had breast cancer 20 years earlier. A chance encounter with a new lump prompted me to have a biopsy. The lump was benign but the surrounding tissue contained cancerous cells; there was cancer in both breasts.

There was no choice but to have a bilateral mastectomy. I agreed to it, along with immediate breast reconstruction. Twenty-five cancerous lymph nodes were removed. Breast cancer had spread to my bone marrow. The picture was bleak.

The disease took over my life. I was sick and bald from the chemotherapy for almost a year. Watching my red hair wash down the shower drain was a shock. But time and lots of TLC (tender loving care) heals. After a few years, I thought I was home free and began to relax. No such luck.

In 1991 I started having painful stomach problems. I was told I had ulcers caused by stomach cancer. Those breast cancer cells had spread once again. This was a warning. Next it could be a major organ. Drastic action was required. After much soul-searching and hand-holding, I decided on high-dose chemotherapy and an autologous bone marrow transplant.

Where to go? Rejected by several hospitals because of my advanced condition, I was finally accepted for treatment by the University Hospital in Denver, Colorado. They had a young, brilliant team of doctors and nurses, and a specially designed high-tech environment. What more could I ask for? I just wanted another chance at life, to be myself again.

I will never forget the summer of 1992. My husband and I moved to Denver—he to an apartment and I into the hospital. I spend half my time there in isolation. My oncologist had told me that this treatment would probably be the closest experience to death that I would ever encounter without dying. He was right. After leaving the hospital, there were lots of problems over the next 8 months—fevers, infections, anemia, scarred lungs, and neurological damage.

Was it worth it? I don't know yet but I am grateful that 1 year later, against my doctor's best advice, I have just returned from a great adventure—a trip celebrating the renewal of life.

Inside this patient there is a person who wants to live life to the fullest according to her own rules. None of this would have been possible without a caring support team of family, friends, and physicians. I will be forever grateful to all of them. They will always receive my postcards from distant, exotic places.

Inside This Person There Is a Patient—Addendum

It has been 3 years since I had my BMT. During this time I have tried to resume my normal lifestyle, my piano, volunteering, traveling, and so on.

Last year, 1994, I had the opportunity to travel to Moscow and China. In Moscow, I was invited to perform in the International Music Festival. My family accompanied me. It was a wonderful experience.

We lived with families in the House of Composers. We met musicians, composers, artists, singers, and actors. We shared meals, communicating in Russian and English. Our hosts provided unique activities for us including a private outdoor concert on the banks of the Moscow River. A group of folk singers performed medieval songs a cappella. We all learned about a culture different but so much like our own.

Six weeks later, my husband and I toured China for nearly a month. Another group of interesting experiences—climbing the Great Wall, the hustle-bustle of Shanghai, the small towns, cruising the rivers, the ballet, opera, observing great artisans at work, Tiananmen Square. We learned about a completely different culture.

A lot of travel for a relatively brief period so I decided to postpone any further travel for a while and enjoy my own home and beaches. A fortuitous decision. Things did not go exactly as planned.

Six months later my mother died unexpectedly. Shortly afterwards, my cancer recurred. My breast cancer had once again metastasized, but this time to my bones. My ribs, rampant with tumors, were continuously breaking. With almost every turn, pull, squeeze, and bend I could hear and feel them crack. Excruciating pain. Once again I was on chemotherapy and radiation. After about 30 radiation treatments, much of the pain was finally relieved.

How can this be happening? I have gone through so much treatment—surgery, chemotherapy, radiation, hormone drugs, and a BMT. It seems that every few years I am back to square one, back to 1987. How can I still survive mentally and physically?

What have I done wrong? Why does this keep happening? Intellectually, I know the answer. Emotionally, I do not. These experiences are not unique. Breast cancer is a chronic disease. It almost always returns.

Even though my current treatment is working, survival seems to become more and more difficult. I am trying to help myself in every way. I see a psycho-oncologist and participate in art therapy. Although I have not painted in 30 years, vivid images are exploding on my canvasses. I am engrossed in my music and learning the most difficult compositions I have ever attempted.

I don't know why all this is happening, but I feel there is a deadline. The privilege of old age has been revoked. I am a young woman in my sunset years. I have accepted that but there is much to do, much to see.

My perspective on life is clear. I am grateful to my family, friends, and doctors for their ongoing support. It is difficult for them as well. Every moment with my dear husband and daughters is precious. We will be traveling together again soon to Alaska. I will be involved in every detail, knowing it is important for me to plan for the future.

When my quality of life is no longer acceptable and no other treatment is appropriate, it will be time for me to let go. I hope I will be strong enough to realize that. I want my family and friends to remember me as the person they have grown with, not the patient they watched disintegrate. Meanwhile, I still remain optimistic and hopeful. My body will not leave here without a struggle. My soul will remain forever.

At age 33 Jim King underwent an allogeneic BMT for primary myelofibrosis in 1994. He is currently (1995) disease free.

IT'S A MARATHON, NOT A 10 K

Jim King

On March 17, 1994, I saw a physician for a simple ear infection. After noticing that my left abdomen was enlarged, he ran a few tests. Ten days later I was diagnosed with primary myelofibrosis. An oncologist told me I probably would not survive. My only hope was a bone marrow transplant, which had been successful in a few isolated cases.

I was in shock. I felt fine. I had completed the Chicago Marathon only 4 months earlier. I couldn't be that sick. The denial phase lasted only a couple of days. Then I entered a state of despair. I was angry and confused. I had a wonderful wife and three small children whom I adored. I was going to die and leave them alone. I felt like my family was being cheated. I had dreamed of seeing my sons graduate from college, but now kindergarten was a stretch.

After a week of despair I roared into action. I knew I was in for the fight of my life and I needed a plan and support team. The first thing I did was take a 2-week vacation with my family and trade in my conservative Volvo for a Miata. Now was as good a time as any to have a mid-life crisis. I read every book I could on survival and support. One of the books talked about building a support team. My wife was the coach (a Lou Holtz type). My brothers and sister were the dependable line, my old college roommates were the running backs, and a few great friends who had endured personal tragedies were the defense. As my transplant day grew closer, many other people joined the support team and were crucial to my ability to maintain a positive attitude.

I planned for the worst. I finalized a will, set up educational trusts for my children, finalized a buy/sell agreement with my business partner, and even picked out the songs and prayers for my funeral. I didn't actually expect them to be used, but wanted to get all the prudent planning out of the way so I could focus on winning. I was scared, but anxious to get on with it. My motto was "Bring it on"—false bravado, probably, but I wanted others to catch my optimism.

I was amazed at the number of people who flocked to help my family. Friends would ask what they could give me. I asked for platelets, and for them to put a collection of their favorite songs together on a cassette tape to remind me of them and keep me fired up during the transplant. I got a lot of great tapes but not a lot of platelets.

On June 28 my 8-pound spleen was removed. I recovered in a couple of weeks and felt ready for the transplant. I felt lucky—lucky to have had such a great life so far, lucky to have a wife who loved me, lucky to have my sons, and lucky to have an interesting career. I

was mentally prepared for the transplant and ready to go.

I entered the BMT unit on a sunny day in August, full of optimism. The first thing I did was shave my head. It was my way of establishing who was in charge of this contest. I wasn't going to let radiation take my hair, I took it first. I decorated my hospital room with pictures of family and friends, a stereo, CD player and VCR, a small basketball hoop, Nintendo, and some books. The books proved to be worthless because I quickly lost my ability to concentrate, but the tunes really helped. Whenever I was down or a new drug or procedure was to start, I would crank REM's song "Superman" as loud as possible. Great songs helped keep me pumped.

After I got my room set up the nurses introduced themselves. They were great. Nurses are a pretty special breed to begin with, but the BMT nurses were incredible. They bent over backwards to help me, comfort me, and educate me.

The first procedure was an intraspinal injection of methotrexate. It didn't hurt, especially when compared to a bone marrow biopsy, but I had to lie flat on my back for 6 hours. It was pretty boring so I counted all the dots on the ceiling.

The next morning the real fun began. At 7:30 A.M. I went for my first round of radiation and then had a Hickman catheter installed. I developed a love-hate relationship with my Hickman. I loved it because I was no longer stuck with needles all the time, but hated having it stick out of my body.

After 5 days of radiation therapy, I was given a chemotherapy drug called VP-16. I tolerated it well with few side effects. A week later my brother Kevin's marrow was transplanted into me. It was an emotional day, but the process itself was a yawner. It took 3 hours to infuse the new marrow and I felt great. I started to think that the stories I'd heard about how tough it is to undergo a BMT were exaggerations. I felt a little weak, but was doing fine. I went to sleep that night feeling on top of the world.

The hammer came down the next morning. It was not gradual. I woke up feeling sicker than I had ever felt in my life. My hair was all over the sheets and my own spit made me nauseous. I had a fever, diarrhea, and could barely hold my head up. The next 10 days were terrible. I had trouble eating because of the nausea and sores in my stomach and mouth. I lost 30 pounds, got several rashes and infections, and had continuous fevers. This was the crucial period. I was getting packed red cells, TPN, antibiotics, Neupogen, fluids, and steroids. At one point I counted 15 bags on my IV pole. I was also given a wonderful little button that allowed me to self-dispense morphine every 5 minutes. I pushed it a lot. I don't remember much more about that week—I've blocked it out. It's a fog and I'm glad.

I began to feel better about 10 days after the transplant and was anxious to go home. I asked the doctor what I had to do to get out of there. He said my blood counts had to improve and I had to have solid stools. I couldn't control my counts, but I could control my eating and stools. That night I ate a ham sandwich—bad choice. It hurt a lot, but I was determined to hold it down no matter what. It came up a few times but I closed my mouth and swallowed—gross, but effective. My superstar nurses gave me hot packs to put on my stomach and encouraged me to keep fighting. I did, and soon I was eating regularly. Eating wasn't pleasant, but I was doing it. Finally, a solid stool. I still can't believe how excited I got when it happened.

At last the head of the transplant team said the four words I thought I'd never hear: "You can go home." I was ecstatic. I packed up my "war room," hugged any nurse I could find, and was heeled out of the hospital. The air outside smelled wonderfully dirty and I took in all the sights. I was discharged just in time to get stuck in Chicago's rush-hour traffic and I enjoyed every minute of it.

My family had decorated our house with balloons and a big sign that said "Welcome Home Daddy." I felt like a grade-school kid whose long year had just ended and whose summer vacation was just beginning. I thought the tough part was over. Now I would rest a bit and then resume a normal life.

I had never been so wrong. The inpatient stay was the easiest part of the BMT process. I was focused and fired up for the inpatient phase of the battle. All the worldly things such as my role as a husband and father were secondary to winning my inpatient battle. Other routine things such as house payments, medical bills, career, and church weren't even on my mind. Nurses and doctors took care of me. It wasn't easy, but I felt I was making significant progress toward beating my disease.

The clarity of purpose and sense of progress was lost when I came home. Instead of feeling like a successful patient, I felt like a failed person. All those worldly things that I had ignored in the hospital, such as my role as husband and father, came roaring back. They were once again important and I felt I was woefully inadequate in those roles. We had three children, ages 4 and a set of 8-month-old twins, and I couldn't help at all with their care. I wasn't allowed to change a diaper, and didn't have the strength to carry any of my boys upstairs. All my self-esteem and self-confidence was gone. I couldn't imagine ever functioning like a normal person again.

The steroids and cyclosporin made me extremely emotional and irrational. I would cry because I had too much milk on my cereal. I couldn't sleep (steroids), couldn't shower (Hickman), couldn't read (no concentration), couldn't drink coffee in the morning (nausea), couldn't exercise (no strength), and couldn't get close to my children (might get an infection).

Even taking my medicine was confusing and overwhelming. I spent a lot of time worrying about things I couldn't control. I was convinced I was going to run out of money, lose my house, my dog, and so on. There was no measured progress anymore. I felt I was regressing.

To get out of my emotional rut, I began setting myself up for small victories, and treating myself to tastes of normal life. I would see how fast and accurately I could flush my Hickman catheter and change my dressing. If I did it in record time or could safely eliminate a step, I'd reward myself with a nap. I added an additional lap to my walk around the neighborhood every other day and felt like a winner. I'd drive my car to Burger King, get a drive-through breakfast, and cheer when I didn't throw up. Not a big achievement, but it seemed huge then. I shampooed and conditioned my bald head so that I'd feel normal. I forced myself to read a whole section of the newspaper without giving up in frustration. I even called a restaurant and had them set up a table in an empty banquet section for me and my wife. I couldn't eat much but the fact that we were going out for dinner made me feel normal again, at least for an evening.

The number of small victories increased as the doses of steroids and cyclosporin tapered off. I began to feel normal around Christmas, 120 days after transplant.

Currently, I'm 14 months post transplant. I celebrated my 1-year transplant anniversary by climbing a mountain in Colorado and getting second row, center section seats for a Jimmy Buffet concert. Lots of people celebrated with me and gave me inspirational messages, gifts, and support. My favorite gift came from Dr. Daugherty of the BMT unit—an interpretation of my latest bone marrow biopsy report. The interpretation pretty much describes my life today—normal.

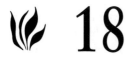

18

Family Issues and Perspectives

June G. Eilers

Over time clinicians and researchers have gained an increased understanding about the profound impact illness, disease, and treatment can have on the entire family involved with the patient. The extent of the impact varies, related partially to extrinsic factors such as the specific illness or disease and the treatment administered, and partially to intrinsic factors regarding the family itself and the individuals that make up the unit. Bone marrow transplant (BMT) is a procedure with promise for the individuals involved, because it offers hope where other treatments are less effective. But, it is not without risk. The stress of this risk is experienced not only by the patient, but is shared by family of the patient and thus, BMT has the potential to impact the family. In fact, as early as 1979, Patenaude, Szymanski, and Rappeport (1979) reported on the intensity of the potential stress for the family of individuals undergoing BMT and indicated that it can be one of the most stressful events for families to experience. More recent literature regarding psychosocial factors in BMT supports this early warning (Atkins and Patenaude, 1987; Patenaude, 1990; Andrykowski, 1994a, b).

As BMT has become a more widely accepted treatment for many types of cancer and marrow-related disorders, the numbers of

transplants have escalated rapidly. Consequently, the number of family members affected by BMT has also escalated. In order to provide optimum care to patients and their families, it is important to be aware of the potential stress associated with BMT and view this stress and the related risks from the family's perspective. Futterman, Wellisch, Bond, and Carr (1991) included family in the rating scale of emotional difficulties related to BMT. The importance of nursing attending to the family was indicated by Tomlinson, Kirschbaum, Tomczyk, and Peterson (1991): "The client is dependent on an environment organized to provide highly specific technological interventions, the acuity of illness is often of crisis proportions, and nursing care, though highly specialized, must incorporate family needs unique to this setting" (p. 246).

FAMILY FRAMEWORK

"What is family?" is a question that has been addressed over the years in the social sciences and psychology. Family can be understood as the social matrix within which we live and function. For some individuals, this family unit is very clearly delineated along traditional lines of formal marriage and offspring. In other situations, family units do not follow these legal definitions of family. The last several decades have seen multiple changes in what was formerly viewed as the "typical" family. There are increasing numbers of single-parent families, second marriages, and blended families, as well as individuals who are cohabitants, but not married. All contribute to the wide diversity of family units today. This chapter will not attempt to identify and address each of the multiple options, but will address family generically as emotionally bonded individuals committed to the well-being of the BMT patient. These individuals may or may not be related by bloodlines or law, yet they function in such a way that they consider themselves family.

In addition, it is worthwhile to note that family is one of the few social organizations in which membership is based strictly on who you are, rather than what you can do. This can provide comfort and security for individuals who do not have to work to earn membership in a family, but simply become members by birth or marriage. However, it can add stress when individuals are not performing in the expected manner, but cannot be denied membership in the family. For the most part in this chapter, family will be presented as a single entity. Specific identities and relationships such as spouse-partner and parent-child will be indicated only to enhance the content.

Sociologists and psychologists have long attempted to gain an increased understanding of the family. Although we frequently hear about the impact of changing times on the family, and questions if the family can survive, the family unit has been in existence since the beginning of recorded history and is probably the longest standing social institution. As such, the family serves critical functions for society and the individuals involved in the family unit.

Ogburn (1933) identified seven major functions of the family in our society:

1. economic
2. protective
3. recreational
4. educational
5. religious
6. status placement
7. affectional

Over time some of these functions have been shared with various institutions, and others have been essentially assumed by institutions in society. Therefore, more recently these functions have been grouped into three categories: affection, economic cooperation, and socialization of children (Bahr, 1989).

If the family is to accomplish these functions efficiently and successfully, certain roles must be fulfilled by the individuals within the family unit. Awareness of the roles of the family members in terms of essential tasks that must be completed for successful family life increases the clinician's ability to assess the impact of illness and treatment or the family. Nye (1976) identified the key roles as provider, housekeeper, child care, child socialization, recreational, kinship, sexual, and therapeutic. Families establish their own system for the roles based on the skills, talents, and abilities of the individuals. A family member may assume primary responsibility for a role, the roles may be shared by two or more individuals, or family members may share the roles with others outside the unit. Once the family has established a system for the roles, normal interactions and functions will be affected if individuals do not fulfill their respective roles (Turner, 1970). Illness and treatment can interfere with an individual's ability to perform the expected roles in the family. Adjustments must be made for the family to continue functioning in these situations. When a member of a family is ill and undergoes a life-threatening procedure such as transplant, the rippling effect can be felt throughout the family.

Family Units in Transplant

Because the age of BMT patients extends from infancy to adults older than 60 years, a wide range of family situations and relationships are represented in the transplant population. Therefore, it is difficult to describe the "typical" family in BMT. Family may be the parents of a child of any age, from infancy to adult; this adult child may be married or single, launched and independent or remaining at home. Family may be the spouse or other partnered significant other. The partner relationship with the patient may have been in existence for years or for only a relatively short period of time. Children may be the siblings of the patient or they may be children or grandchildren of the patient. They may be young and require significant direct care, nurturing, and supervision or may be older and function essentially independently.

The family units may be any of the multiple types defined by Schlesinger (1979) in Table 18.1. Two types of families should be added to Schlesinger's list: nonmarried couples with children and homosexual couples.

Transplant family units present a varied picture not only in terms of types and number of members, but also in terms of the ages of the members and duration of time as a family unit. *Family life cycle* is the term used to refer to a set of stages that a family unit typically passes through over the course of existence as a family (Glick, 1977).

The idea of a family life cycle to refer to the various stages of family development was pioneered by Duvall and Hill in 1948. The stages are similar in concept to the developmental stages of individuals as presented by Erickson (1950). The stages were further defined by Duvall (1977). Since that time, various other family theorists have commented on the specific number of stages and the importance of the different stages. As with the developmental stages for the life cycle of individuals, successful

TABLE 18.1 Family types

Nuclear family: husband, wife, and children
Childless couple: husband and wife only
One-parent families: widowed, divorced, separated, and deserted spouses and never-married mothers
Adopted families: husband, wife, and adopted child(ren)
Reconstituted families: second marriages and blended families
Communal families: group of families living together with or without children

SOURCE: Data from Schlesinger, B., 1979.

fulfillment of the tasks that commonly occur at each of the stages promotes satisfaction and facilitates the likelihood of smooth transition through the life cycle. The beginning of each stage is a time of critical transition that requires change in roles and tasks (Barnhill and Longo, 1978; Bahr, 1989). See Table 18.2 for two examples of proposed stages and the tasks at the transition points.

The inclusion of the unattached young adult who is between families in Carter and McGoldrick's (1980) model is an important component for BMT, because these individuals are frequently involved in transplant either as a patient or as an adult child of an older patient. Duvall's (1977) delineation of family with children into more components based on ages of the children allows clearer differentiation of families in these stages because of the unique needs of children in the identified age groups. Therefore, for application in transplant it may be beneficial to utilize a combination of the two models. The transitions (Barnhill and Longo, 1978) can be seen as the changes the family must accomplish for smooth progression through the stages of the life cycle.

Numerous factors including illness, treatment, death, separation, divorce, and financial disaster impact movement through the life cycle

TABLE 18.2 Stages of family life cycles and transitional tasks

Carter and McGoldrick	Duvall	Transitions
Unattached young adult between families	Not addressed	
New marriage	Married couple without children	Commitment of couple to each other
Family with young children	Childbearing family in which the oldest child is younger than 30 months of age	Developing new parental roles, as husband and wife become mother and father
	Family with preschool children, in which the oldest child is from 2 ½ to 6 years of age	Accepting the new personality as the child grows up
	Family with school children, with the oldest child between 6 and 13 years of age	Introducing the child to institutions outside the family such as school, church, scouts, guides, sports groups, and so on
Family with adolescents	Family with teenagers, with oldest child between 13 and 20	Accepting adolescence, with the changed roles associated with this and the parents' need to come to terms with the rapid social and sexual changes occurring in their son or daughter
Launching the children and moving on	Family launching young adults, starting with the first child's departure from the home and ending when the last one goes	Allowing the child to experiment with independence in late adolescence and early adulthood Preparations to launch child
	Middle-aged parents, from the "empty nest" to retirement	Come to accept their child's independent adult role, including starting his or her own family Letting go—facing each other again, husband and wife alone
Later life	Aging family members, period from retirement to death	Accepting retirement and/or old age, with the changed lifestyle involved

SOURCE: Data from Carter and McGoldrick, 1980; Duvall, 1977; Barnhill and Longo, 1978.

for families. Stress and strain from previous events in the life of the family can have a lasting effect and affect future coping ability. Thus, a family's current status may be influenced by previous events such as the initial diagnosis and treatment. Clinicians should also be aware of normative transitions that are occurring simultaneous to BMT and those that may have been affected by previous stressful events.

Since a large portion of these models is based on the presence of children in the family, they do not always provide a direct fit for childless families or families with a wide span of ages among children. In addition, diseases requiring transplant may have actually interfered with plans for marriage and/or children. Thus, individuals and couples may not be at the stage they had intended for themselves prior to the illness and treatment. Although the diversity in families today and preexisting circumstances preclude stringent application of the stages and tasks as mandatory for all families to follow, the concept of family life cycles fosters increased understanding of family stressors that may occur at a given period in time for the family unit. Awareness of the family life cycle stage and accompanying responsibilities will increase clinicians' sensitivity to additional stressors the family unit may be experiencing during transplant.

Involvement of Family in Transplant

Although family involvement is not new to transplant, the focus has changed over time as advances in BMT have allowed increased family participation and as our knowledge in the area has expanded. To date, the majority of the literature regarding BMT focuses on the patient. Articles make general references to families, but seldom address their specific needs. Research focusing on families in BMT is also limited and primarily pediatric and/or retrospective in nature (Lee et al., 1994; Nelson, 1994; Sormanti, Dungan, Rieker, 1994).

Family members have served as donors in allogeneic BMT since the time of the early transplants. After giving informed consent, these individuals were expected to be available for the transplant and to donate blood components if indicated. However, due to the isolation restrictions early in transplant history, direct family involvement with the BMT patient was very limited. Family members were physically separated from their loved one with limited, if any, direct contact or activity in the patient's room. At the same time, families were frequently disrupted for an extended period of time by the expectation that the patient, frequently a young person, remain in the transplant center city for 100 days after transplant to allow for monitoring and treating graft-

versus-host disease (GVHD). Thus, at least a portion of the family would temporarily relocate to the transplant city. Because only a limited number of centers were doing transplants, these family members frequently had to travel a great distance.

With gradual changes in transplant protocols and increased sensitivity to the potential benefit to family members and to the patient, more direct family involvement was allowed. During this time, transplant isolation procedures also became less restrictive, and BMT expanded to include autologous transplants. Autologous BMT extended the number of transplant candidates and the age range of patients. The expanded availability of pharmaceuticals for infections and the use of growth factors to decrease the length of neutropenia facilitated this increased involvement by family members. With earlier dismissal from the inpatient unit, family involvement has now become essential so that the patient has a caregiver present as recovery continues in the outpatient setting. Increasing numbers of centers are expanding into the new frontier of performing outpatient BMTs (Cavanaugh, 1994). As family involvement continues and even increases, there is a definite need for further study in this area.

Nurses are usually aware when family members are with the patient during transplant and frequently indicate their presence in documentation. However, the role the family plays in providing support and assistance to the patient, and the impact of the transplant on the family present remains unclear (Winters, 1994). Larson's (1995) interviews with patients found that they wanted their family members present to assist with nonmedical needs, assist with management of side effects, and to provide emotional support.

Clinicians have learned to value family involvement as a benefit for support and encouragement of patients. However, the ability of families to handle the situations encountered varies, as does the approach taken. At times incorporation of the family may actually increase the time required to care for the patient. Lesko (1994) describes family as second-order patients for nursing staff. BMT does not occur in isolation from the other activities and transitions of family life. Families come to transplant with various prior experience and resources. Especially in the case of long-term illness, families are seldom dealing with a single illness-induced stressor. An increased understanding of the interrelatedness of the multiple factors facilitates the clinician's ability to work effectively with the family.

Family Response to Stress

McCubbin and McCubbin (1993) use the concept of "pileup" to describe the accumulation of stressors, strains, and transitions that families bring with them into new situations. In their Resiliency Model of Family Stress, Adjustment, and Adaptation, the McCubbins have identified six broad categories of stressors and strains that influence how a family adapts to an illness-related situation:

1. the illness and related hardships over time,
2. normative transitions in the life cycle of individuals and the family unit,
3. prior family strains accumulated over time,
4. situational demands and contextual difficulties,
5. consequences of family efforts to cope, and
6. intrafamily and social ambiguity, which leaves the family and individuals with inadequate guidelines for how to act or cope with the situation.

Bone marrow transplantation is not the first major stressor for most of the families in transplant. Each has had to deal with the patient's initial diagnosis and the life-threatening aspect of that individual's condition. In addition, families frequently have encountered other

stressful situations in their lives such as natural disasters, job losses, accidents, and difficulties within the family. Sensitivity to the potential pileup of stressors and strains from any of the six categories identified is important for a more accurate picture of the family during transplantation.

According to the Resiliency Model by McCubbin and McCubbin (1993), family resources, strengths, and capabilities vary. A capability for family is the potential it has for meeting the demands of a given situation. Resources to aid in this process may be tangible or intangible, and may come from the individual family members, the family unit as a whole, or from the community. The family's resources, strengths, and capabilities moderate the impact of the crisis of BMT for the family.

Therefore, just as it is important not to view the patient and exclude family, the current episode in the family's life doesn't tell the whole story of a family. A family's experience with illness, treatment, and general life crises can have two effects. Families could have learned from experience and can use it as stepping stones for future growth as they meet the challenges of BMT, or memories of experiences could be stumbling blocks and interfere with the family's ability to cope with their current situation.

FAMILY ASSESSMENT— CLINICAL IMPLICATIONS

Direct involvement of the family in transplant can increase the support available to the patient (Larson, 1995), allow family to better understand what the BMT patient experiences, and assist the family in coping with the stressor. However, this involvement could actually increase the immediate stress experienced by the family, so it is important that clinicians also provide family-focused care.

Conducting a family assessment is a critical component of caring for families in the transplant environment. The specific form or format is not so crucial as the information obtained. This assessment may be performed by the nursing staff or may be provided by team members from other professional psychosocial support services such as psychology or social work. As an initial step, knowing the patient's type of family unit (see Table 18.1) facilitates the continued assessment and the planning of care. Families come to transplant with varied histories and abilities to cope (Wolcott and Stuber, 1992) and cannot be regarded or treated as a homogenous group.

A theoretical model such as McCubbin's Resiliency Model of Family Stress and Coping (1993) can provide a framework for assessment and then guide use of the information to plan care. The basic information to be aware of includes:

- Who is in the patient's family unit?
- What stage of the family life cycle is the family in at this time?
- What is the developmental stage of children (if any) in the family?
- Who is planning to be present during the transplant?
- What is the relationship of these individuals to the patient? Are there underlying reasons that some members of the family will not be present?
- What other critical incidents has the family experienced? When did these occur?
- How did the family cope with previous crises?
- Are there other preexisting or current stressors in the family?

It is also important to be aware of how the patient's illness has affected the family to date. Because transplant is performed at various stages of disease, depending on the specific disease, families proceed through stages of adjustment to the diagnosis. If the diagnosis is fairly new, a family may be in the state of initial shock. Another family may have thought it was free of worry of the disease because the patient had been in remission for an extended time, and now the disease has come back! Such recurrence can be extremely stressful for families who thought they had already dealt with all of the issues related to the disease. Still other families have been living with the patient's diagnosis for an extended time, with little break from the continual stress on the patient and family. Families may see themselves as having a very large support system ready to provide support or may see themselves as all alone in the process. Distance from home influences the availability and importance of some resources for the family.

Although identification of this initial family-related information does not necessarily provide a whole picture of the family, it can aid the clinician in designing a family-focused approach to care. It can also help nurses determine if more in-depth assessment is necessary and can provide the rationale for making referral(s). Although we do not have sufficient research to predict family response to transplant, by collecting the previously identified information, clinicians can begin to identify families who may be at risk for high levels of stress during transplant.

A word of caution, when multiple family members are present to support the patient during transplant, clinicians may obtain varying views of the family system from different family members. Clinicians must be careful not to get "caught up" in the family's struggles. Transplant is not a time to attempt to alter the "normal" functioning of the family system, unless their pattern of function will be detrimental to the well-being of the patient. If families require such counseling, clinicians should refer them to an appropriately qualified therapist. In most situations it is better to have the family seek such counseling after the current transplant crisis is past.

POTENTIAL STRESS OF BMT FOR FAMILY MEMBERS

Multiple BMT-related factors contribute to the stress of the patient and family. Uncertainty is emerging as a common theme in literature regarding the psychological stress associated with transplant (Atkins and Patenaude, 1987; Eilers, 1992, 1993a, 1993b; Lesko, 1994; Haberman, 1995). Mishel's (1988, 1990) work regarding uncertainty in illness provides a potential framework for increasing our understanding of this phenonemon. Another theme characteristic of BMT is the combination of the high-technology environment, the high potential for complications, and the hope for positive outcomes (McConville et al., 1990; Eilers, 1993a; Lesko, 1994).

Prior to coming to transplant, the patients have usually been informed that, based on current knowledge, the disease will likely lead to premature death unless a different, more aggressive treatment is pursued. Thus, families have been confronted with the potential death of their loved ones secondary to the disease process. BMT is offered as a treatment option, and at times, as the only hope to reverse the disease process. (Eilers, 1992, 1993a; Stensland, 1993; Haberman, 1995). However, they are soon informed that BMT is not without significant risk, and if complications arise, may result in the patient's death even sooner than would have been expected secondary to the disease. The family must deal with considering an immediately life-threatening procedure while not fully comprehending the life-threatening nature of the current condition. Parents of minor children struggle with the additional stress of having to make such life-and-death decisions for their children. Frequently patients

and families have stated that they felt as though they had no choice—if they wanted a chance for longer life, BMT was the best option. The uncertainty triggered at the time of the initial discussion about BMT continues throughout the transplant process, and can be perceived as anxiety-provoking or as presenting hope and promise for the future.

Once the family has accepted the hope for their loved one via transplant, issues of insurance coverage, financial eligibility, and acceptance to a BMT program may become stressors. Insurance coverage for transplant is not guaranteed in many policies. Families without adequate insurance coverage may shift their focus from the stress related to the risks of transplant, to a fight with the insurance company, or to a massive fund-raising campaign. Some families struggle with not knowing whether their loved one will be eligible for BMT based on disease-related factors. Families who have experienced stressors in these areas prior to transplant may come to BMT with a weariness or may have been energized by the success of overcoming barriers. The needs of the families who do not make it into transplant programs for reasons related to insurance coverage, financial eligibility, and programs' criteria for acceptance have received limited attention in the literature, and are beyond the scope of this chapter, but deserve future study.

Although at times patients and families are offered a choice of transplant programs, some patients and families may not find themselves in the anticipated location for transplant. Preferred provider contracts, program experience/specialty, and physician referral patterns influence selection of a transplant program (Patenaude, 1990; Eilers, 1993). This could mean using a transplant center other than the one closest to home and in an unfamiliar community. When offered a choice, patient and families may struggle with uncertainty regarding how to select the "right" program. Some families conduct extensive information-gathering missions; others select the program that is most convenient. If the patient develops complications, the issues of program selection may resurface.

Because the majority of transplants are performed at large cancer treatment facilities, patients and families frequently have to travel considerable distances for BMT. Thus, families find themselves far removed from usual supports, in an unfamiliar environment, encountering one of the most stressful events in their lives. This is particularly important for staff to remember when the patient becomes critically ill and the spouse or significant other is left to make major decisions without the aid or support of their loved ones. For some, this is the first time they have had to make critically important decisions alone.

The impact of the distance from home has been noted to actually have a varied effect on family members (Eilers and Stensland, 1990; Eilers, 1993). The greater distance may or may not be an additional stressor. When the transplant center is close to home, family members often try to maintain their usual schedules, plus visit and support the patient. If the center is too far away to allow frequent short trips back and forth, family members are more likely to separate from their usual daily responsibilities. These family members have to do more extensive preparation prior to leaving home and at the time of the BMT have commented that once at the transplant site they had to "let go" of those home-maintenance concerns.

The fact that other aspects of the family's life goes on while the patient is having the transplant can cause additional stress for families. The normal functional responsibilities of the family continue even if the family is separated due to the transplant. Responsibility for practical tasks such as mail, bills, lawn care, and home maintenance may need to be delegated. The ability to accomplish this depends on family and community support. The ease with which families are able to do this varies. Family members also struggle with child-care responsibilities and their inability to maintain involvement in other family activities such as children's sports, birthdays, and special events at school.

If there are dependent children in the family, decisions regarding their care must be made prior to the transplant. This must include the range of responsibilities from nurturing and affection to planning for and transporting to activities. Children left at home in the care of others may experience stress related to adjusting to the parent substitutes. In addition, they experience normal developmental struggles and may want to know when their parents are returning home. Family members have to strive to find the right balance of time at the transplant center and time at home. They often struggle with the need and desire to be in two places at once, although attempts to do so adds to the stress and may lead to exhaustion.

Although there may be adequate insurance coverage for the transplant, it usually does not include financial coverage for transportation, housing, food, and living expenses for the family member(s) spending time with the patient. Maintaining regular phone contact with family members who are not at the transplant center can add greatly to the expenses. Families' stress increases due to these additional out-of-pocket expenses that occur at a time when their income is most likely decreased.

Transplant centers usually recommend that families consider having someone accompany the patient to the transplant city and remain available to support the patient. This has become particularly true as transplant centers have moved more of their services to the outpatient setting. However the ultimate decision regarding which family members accompany the patient to the transplant facility are made by family.

As discussed previously, families in transplant cover a wide spectrum in terms of age, relationship, and stage of family life. In some instances, multiple nuclear families who make up an extended family for the patient share responsibility for being present and supporting the patient. These families may take turns being present or may alternate and attempt to "pass the baton" from one to another.

Financial demands on the family, work-related regulations, individual coping abilities, and personal commitments influence which family members are able to be at the transplant site. Because membership in families is based on who one is and not on satisfaction of relationships and role performance, clinicians should be aware that the gathered family members may not be accustomed to being together and may not always find their relationships mutually supportive. The stress of BMT can contribute strain to previously stressed relationships as well as affect supportive relationships.

Parents of adult children who have been independent face unique challenges as they accompany their children to transplant settings (Eilers and Stensland, 1989). Although the patients are adults who are able to and required to make their own informed decisions and sign consent forms, to the parents, adult patients are still their children. These parents struggle with concerns about their children's well-being. Since their children have been independent and in some instances married, the closeness of their relationships vary. In addition, parents may not have been present during the patient's pretransplant education and process of informed consent. Thus, parents may not be adequately informed regarding the indications for transplant and the potential side effects.

Preparing families for what to expect in transplant is not a straightforward process (Lesko, 1994). There are many BMT scenarios. Families must be prepared for the possible complications, yet be able to maintain a positive attitude and support the patient. A common theme from family members interviewed prior to the transplant of a loved one was identified as "preparing for the worst, and hoping for the best" (Eilers, 1993a).

Because the normal expected course for BMT varies widely, it is difficult to tell family members precisely what to expect. Among the factors that influence the course are the type of transplant, the preparatory regimen, and the overall condition of the patient prior to transplant. Some patients have relatively simple courses of short duration and return to a normal level of function fairly soon. Others experience multiple life-threatening complications and repeated setbacks, have extended stays in the hospital, and require extremely long recovery periods. Unfortunately, others do not survive the multiple life-threatening complications. Because clinicians cannot predict the precise BMT course for a given individual, family members must deal with an inherent amount of uncertainty.

Once patients have been accepted into the transplant program and start the preparatory regimen, family members' concerns focus on the preparative regimen (Eilers, 1993). Depending on the patient's diagnosis, stage of disease, and their involvement with the patient's previous treatment, family members have varying levels of knowledge regarding chemotherapy and radiation therapy. Based on pretransplant information, they often regard the current doses as "super high" and very dangerous. In fact they sometimes use the term *supralethal* to describe the chemotherapy. At times family members mention how many times higher the current dose is compared to doses for normal chemotherapy. Although appropriate use of medications can control the majority of the patient's nausea and vomiting, family members' anxiety and recall of this portion of the transplant is intense. They struggle with knowing that high doses are essential to overcome the disease, and not wanting to see their loved one suffer.

Family members' responses to transplant day also vary (Eilers, 1993). Literature has often identified the day as anticlimactic for the patient (Lesko, 1994). This same sense is seen in a portion of family members. For others, it is a highly charged, highly emotional day. Because this day signifies a new start and hope for the future, they are very concerned that everything go well. These individuals become concerned if the staff's attitude does not indicate adequate attention to detail. Some have indicated that transplant day takes on almost a religious connotation of rebirth. A portion of family members actually find it physically and emotionally difficult to be in the room during the transplant. They want to be kept informed of the progress, and then want to know as soon as it is over and that all has "gone well." Once the day of the infusion is over, family members become anxious for engraftment and recovery. The uncertainty of this time contributes to the impact of transplant on them.

The need for isolation and the risk of life-threatening infections contribute further to the stress of BMT. Families struggle with the fear of causing a serious infection and frequently assume the role of "guard" to watch others around their loved one. At the same time patients and family members alike often need closeness, touch, and affection. Thus they struggle with what is "allowed," and what is "too risky." Although technically under isolation precautions of various intensities, they often feel bombarded with excess stimuli. Transplant routines and the involvement of multiple team members limits the amount of private uninterrupted time. In addition, patients and family members often struggle with the fact that due to the necessary sharing of information among the transplant team's members, it seems that everyone knows them but they don't even know the names of many of the team's mem-

bers. This can especially be problematic in large transplant units and teaching centers.

Making plans and recommendations for visitors while the patient is at the transplant center can also be problematic. Visitors to the transplant center may be allowed as a source of support for the family member who is staying with the patient. However, family members often feel guilty that they need emotional support (Andrykowski, 1994a, b). Families may allow visitors in an attempt to provide additional support to the patient or to allow the visitor to remain connected with the patient (especially children of an adult patient). When patients suffer complications and are at risk of dying, allowing children to visit may be especially important to prepare them emotionally for the loss.

Family members staying with the patient may have mixed feelings regarding visitors (Eilers, 1993a). They need to decide if they will assume the role of entertaining the visitors or separate from that responsibility. The condition of the patient and the willingness of the family member to leave the patient influence this decision. Some family members want breaks from the facility, and others are not comfortable physically leaving.

Monitoring visitors to be certain they don't place the patient at risk for life-threatening infections places additional responsibility on the family members. Some families decide not to allow visitors in an attempt to decrease risk of exposure to infections. Allowing young children to visit, while beneficial for parents and children, stimulates concerns regarding exposure to contagions and the ability of the child to report symptoms.

When treatments that are integral to transplant cause disfigurement and pain, family members struggle emotionally and in an almost helpless state with the physical impact of the treatment on their loved ones (Eilers, 1993a; Lesko, 1994). Such changes include severe mucositis, jaundice, fluid retention, and skin alterations including rashes, blisters, and peeling. Not only do family members experience the stress related to these problems occurring in their loved one, due to the intensity of the environment and close identification with other family members, just knowing that other patients are experiencing difficulty can add to the stress (Wolcott and Stuber, 1992). Although their loved ones may have experienced side effects with previous chemotherapy treatments, the extremely high doses used in BMT heightens concern. Often these side effects alter the patient's ability to interact in a pleasant, meaningful manner. Thus, family members may feel all alone and at times rejected by their loved one. Since most family members have not experienced transplant previously, they are uncertain if the side effects they are witnessing are normal or an indication of the severe complications that can lead to death.

Decision making when the patient becomes critically ill is of particular concern for family members. For the spouse of the patient, it may be the first time in their relationship that a major decision is made without discussing the situation as a couple. When the family members responsible for making the decisions for the adult patient are his or her parents, they may feel they didn't realize just how critical the situation was for their child. If the adult patient's spouse and parents are at the transplant facility, it requires careful discussions with all family members present. Parents of young children also struggle with making decisions for their children, and may question their earlier decision for a transplant. Families with multiple adult children sharing the responsibility of being with their parent during transplant often find it difficult to keep everyone informed. Regardless of the family configuration, members struggle with not wanting to see their loved one suffer, yet not wanting to give up hope if there is a chance for recovery. The patient must make

the initial decision regarding the transplant, but if severe complications occur family members have the burden of critical decisions regarding specific aspects of life support measures. This is the first time some families have had to make such critical decisions regarding another individual's life.

Knowing that the patient's condition can change very quickly has been identified as being even worse than the roller-coaster existence discussed by families with cancer. Family members have said it is "more like a yo-yo, it can change so quickly." They never know quite what to expect from morning to afternoon and are uncertain when they leave the patient's room at night what it will be like when they return in the morning. Although family members have been informed of potential side effects and complications, it is difficult for them to ascertain if what they are seeing is "normal" for transplant. Family members usually find it easier to cope with what the patient is experiencing if the particular changes are within the "normal range." Not only are such rapid changes stressful for family members present, it makes it difficult to keep informed those who are not at the transplant center. In addition, BMT remains a poorly understood treatment process by those who have not been directly involved. Families are asked by others back home such questions as "Is the surgery is over yet?" and "Now that he has had his transplant, is he better?" Dealing with these individuals can add to family stress at a time of little reserve.

Because the length of time for engraftment varies greatly, family members again face the uncertainty of not knowing (Eilers, 1992, 1993a, b). For those who have been actively involved in coaching the patient's active participation in care to prevent complications, the inability to affect the return of white cells may be difficult. In transplant in general, growth factors have decreased the length of aplasia, however, not all cell lines respond consistently well to the growth factors currently in widespread use. The patient may experience flulike symptoms and other side effects secondary to the growth factors, thus although the growth factors are seen as potentially beneficial, once again family members struggle with knowing that the patients "have to tolerate bad to get better." In addition, not knowing how long engraftment will take makes it difficult for family members to plan their length of stay at the transplant center. This then makes it difficult for them to plan and make arrangements for their own posttransplant lives.

NEW ISSUES FOR FAMILY IN BMT

Two changes in BMT have resulted in decreased number of inpatient days for transplant—earlier dismissals and moving portions of transplant care to the outpatient setting. Whereas families used to be informed they should prepare for 6 to 8 weeks of hospitalization, stays for most BMT patients are now considerably shorter. This move toward shorter length of inpatient stay and increased outpatient care has had a mixed impact for families. Patients and families alike are frequently anxious for the patient's discharge from the hospital. This gives them the opportunity to be in a more homelike atmosphere in outpatient housing and to regain some sense of control and independence. However, it can also be frightening. In the hospital they knew highly skilled staff were always available to assist if anything should change. Confidence in the staff helped decrease concern regarding potential side effects. Family members may find themselves being prepared to administer treatments and care that were formerly provided by staff. Family caregivers are often uncertain if they will know what to do if something should change, or if they will notice important changes (Eilers,

1992, 1993a, b). Thus family members question their ability to assume the responsibility being placed on them by the transplant center. For some, the dismissal to outpatient care has been equated to "cutting the umbilical cord."

Continuing care in the outpatient setting can have a mixed effect. Patients enjoy knowing they no longer require hospitalization and like being away from the constant reminders of the transplant that are presented by the hospital room. Family members appreciate knowing that the BMT patient is well enough to leave the hospital but are often concerned about the risks that remain. They are very anxious regarding their skill as care providers and monitors of symptoms. Long hours in the outpatient treatment setting for continued care can also contribute to family stress during this phase of transplant. When immediate side effects decrease with time and engraftment continues, thus decreasing the risk of infections, family members become more at ease and anticipate a return to normal. As BMT continues to change and increasing numbers of patients have outpatient transplants (Cavanaugh, 1994), its impact on patients and families will require close monitoring.

Families of patients who develop graft-versus-host-disease experience new uncertainties. When GVHD persists, the situation encountered by the family is not unlike that reported by cardiac transplant families (Mishel, 1987). They find they may have traded one disease and its treatment for another, and thus need to "redesign their dream." Fear and uncertainty persist as they realize the GVHD may become life threatening. Family response in these situations requires further study.

As families return home after transplant and the immediate concerns of the acute-phase side effects subside, their focus changes. Questions regarding the success of the transplant and how to keep the cancer from returning surface at this time. Sormanti, Dungan, and

Rieker (1994) found that although most parents coped well after transplant, financial strains and fears of relapse remain. Families express a new appreciation for life and a realignment of priorities. Further study will be necessary to better understand the long-term impact of BMT on families.

Acknowledgment

I thank my family and all the families that have added to my life during my experience in cancer care. Family is, has been, and always will be an important component of my personal and professional life. My parents, Donald and Elise Fechtner, provided for me a sense of the importance of family and the core values that guide my life. I dedicate this chapter to them. It was as I stood by their hospital beds that I truly learned the impact that watching a loved one during health-related life-threatening situations has on family. My personal family experience will live on forever and increased my empathy for the families involved in transplant.

REFERENCES

Andrykowski, M.A. 1994a. Psychosocial factors in bone marrow transplantation: a review and recommendations for research. *BMT* 13:357-375.

Andrykowski, M.A. 1994b. Psychiatric and psychosocial aspects of bone marrow transplantation. *Psychosomatics* 35(1):13-24.

Atkins, D.M., Patenaude, A.F. 1987. Psychosocial preparation and follow-up for pediatric bone marrow transplant patients. *Am J Orthopsychiatr* 57(2):246-252.

Bahr, S.J. 1989. *Family Interaction*. New York: Macmillan.

Baker, F. 1994. Psychosocial sequelae of bone marrow transplantation. *Oncology* 8(10):87-92, 97.

Barnhill, L.H., Longo, D. 1978. Fixation and regression in the family life cycle. *Fam Proc* 17:469-478.

Carter, G.A., McGoldrick, M. 1980. *The Family Life Cycle: A Framework for Family Therapy*. New York: Gardner Press.

Cavanaugh, C.A. 1994. Outpatient autologous bone marrow transplantation: a new frontier. *Quality of Life—A Nursing Challenge* 3(2):25-29.

Duvall, E.M. 1977. *Marriage and Family Development*, 5th ed. Philadelphia: Lippincott.

Duvall, E.M., Hill, R.L. 1948. Report of the committee on the dynamics of family interaction. Washington, DC: National Conference on Family Life.

Eilers, J. 1992. Qualitative research: an approach to increase our understanding of the impact of BMT on family members. *Oncol Nurs Forum* 19(2):311.

Eilers, J. 1993a. The experience of family members of bone marrow transplant patients. Presentation at International Bone Marrow Transplant Symposium. Seattle, WA.

Eilers, J. 1993b. Measurement of uncertainty in family members of bone marrow transplant patients. *Oncol Nurs Forum* 20(2):334.

Eilers, J., Stensland, S. 1989. Parents of adults with cancer—an initial look at the experience. Unpublished paper.

Eilers, J., Stensland, S. 1990. Survey of patients' and family members' perceptions of bone marrow transplantation. *Oncol Nurs Forum* 2(suppl 17):211.

Erikson, E.H. 1950. *Childhood and Society*. New York: Norton.

Futterman, A.D., Wellisch, D.K., Bond, G., Carr, C.R. 1991. The psychosocial levels system—a new rating scale to identify and assess emotional difficulties during bone marrow transplantation. *Psychosomatics* 32(2): 177-186.

Glick, P.C. 1977. Updating the life cycle of the family. *J Marriage & Family* 39:5-13.

Haberman, M. 1995. The meaning of cancer therapy: bone marrow transplantation as an exemplar of therapy. *Semin Oncol Nurs* 11(1):23-31.

Larson, P.J. 1995. Perceptions of the needs of hospitalized patients undergoing bone marrow transplant. *Canc Prac* 3(3):173-179

Lee, M.L., Cohen, S.E., Stuber, M.L., Nader, K. 1994. Parent-child interactions with pediatric bone marrow transplant patients. *J Psychosoc Oncol* 12(4):43-60.

Lesko, L.M. 1994. Bone marrow transplantation: support of the patient and his/her family. *Support Care Cancer* 2:35-49.

McConville, B.J., Steichen-Asch, P., Harris, R., et al. 1990. Pediatric bone marrow transplants: psychological aspects. *Can J Psychiatr* 35:769-775.

McCubbin, M.A., McCubbin, H.I. 1993. Families coping with illness: the resiliency model of family stress, adjustment, and adaptation. In Danielson, C.B., Hamel-

Bissell, B., Winstead-Fry, P. (Eds.) *Families, Health, and Illness*. St. Louis: Mosby, 21-63.

McCubbin, H.I., Thompson, A.I. 1991. *Family Assessment Inventories for Research and Practice*. Madison WI: University of Wisconsin-Madison.

Mishel, M.H. 1988. Uncertainty in illness. *Image: J Nurs Sch* 20(4):225-232.

Mishel, M.H. 1990. Reconceptualization of the uncertainty in illness theory. *Image: J Nurs Sch* 22(4): 256-262.

Mishel, M.H., Murdaugh, C.L. 1987. Family adjustment to heart transplantation: redesigning the dream. *Nurs Res* 36:332-338.

Nelson, A. 1994. Parents' responses when their child has a bone marrow transplant. *Oncol Nurs Forum* 21(2): 371.

Nye, F.I. 1976. *Role Structure and Analysis of the Family*. Beverly Hills, CA: Sage.

Ogburn, W.F. 1933. The family and its functions. In *Recent Social Trends in the United States*. New York: McGraw-Hill, 661-708.

Patenaude, A.F. 1990. Psychological impact of bone marrow transplantation: current perspectives. *Yale J Bio Med* 63:515-519.

Patenaude, A.F., Levinger, L., Baker, K. 1986. Group meetings for parents and spouses of bone marrow transplant patients. *Soc Work Health Care* 12(1):51-65.

Patenaude, A.F., Szymanski, L., Rappeport, J. 1979. Psychological costs of bone marrow transplantation. *Am J Orthopsychiatr* 49(3):409-422.

Schlesinger, B. 1979. *Families: Canada*. Montreal: McGraw-Hill Ryerson, 8.

Sormanti, M., Dungan, S., Rieker, P.P. 1994. Pediatric bone marrow transplantation: psychosocial issues for parents after a child's hospitalization. *J Psychosoc Oncol* 12(4):23-42.

Stensland, S. 1993. Bone marrow transplant patient responses to admission interview questions: a descriptive study. National Association of Oncology Social Work Annual Conference, New York.

Tomlinson, P.S., Kirschbaum, M., Tomczyk, B., Peterson, J. 1993. The relationship of child acuity, maternal responses, nurse attitudes and contextual factors in the bone marrow transplant unit. *Am J Crit Care* 2(3): 246-252.

Turner, R. 1970. *Family Interaction*. New York: Wiley.

Wingard, J.R., Curbow, B., Baker, F., Piantadosi, S. 1991. Health, functional status and employment of adult survivors of bone marrow transplantation. *Ann Intern Med* 114:113-118.

Winters, G., Miller, C., Maracich, L., Compton, K., Haberman, M.R. 1994. Provisional practice: the nature of psychosocial bone marrow transplant nursing. *Oncol Nurs Forum* 21(7):1147-1154.

Wolcott, D., Stuber, M. 1992. Bone marrow transplantation. In Craven, J., Rodin, G.M. (Eds.) *Psychiatric Aspects of Organ Transplantation*. Oxford: Oxford University Press, 189-204.

PART IV
The Care Environment

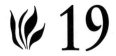

19

The Bone Marrow and Blood Stem Cell Transplant Marketplace

Marilyn K. Bedell, William T. Mroz

The boundaries between the business strategy of a health-care organization and the actual production of patient care are blurring. Cost reduction is a health-care management priority and clinicians find themselves practicing in a competitive and uncertain world.

This chapter provides an overview of the financial aspects of bone marrow transplantation (BMT) and blood cell transplantation (BCT). As the operating environment becomes more complex, a seamless integration of overall organizational strategy and transplantation-specific business strategy will be essential for success. This integration will require that clinicians have a working knowledge of the environmental factors that affect patient care. In this way, they will be able to participate in the formulation of strategy, and function to enact it. It is assumed that the era of operating programs as pure research endeavors without concern for the generation of revenue and patient volume is ending. As cost pressures force provider organizations to consider carefully the portfolio of services they provide, transplant programs will come under scrutiny as an area of potential savings. Several questions will be considered:

- How do reimbursement models affect the delivery of health care?

- What are the most important factors in the external environment that are influencing the direction of transplantation?
- What critical information should be gathered to decide whether to start a new transplant program?
- What opportunities exist for improvement of program performance?

HISTORICAL PERSPECTIVES

The 1940s to 1980s

As World War II (WWII) ended, health-care technology was developing rapidly. At the same time, many WWII veterans were reentering the workforce, and they began raising families. Memories of the Great Depression of the 1930s stimulated this generation of workers to explore ways to secure an income and their family's future. Because health care could quickly deplete savings, systems to decrease economic risk due to illness were desired. Hospitals were also interested in developing a revenue system that would ensure a steady stream of income. Hospitals began to sponsor pre-payment plans, which eventually became know as Blue Cross plans (Anderson, 1985). During the war years the government had placed a freeze on wages but at the same time passed legislation which determined that health insurance coverage was a tax-exempt business expense. Providing health insurance, as a fringe benefit, became an economically sound investment for corporate America. It wasn't long before provisions for health-care insurance were identified as a desired component of corporate benefits packages. By 1952, more than 50% of the U.S. population was covered by some form of health insurance (Anderson, 1985).

In 1965, Medicare legislation was passed, along with Medicaid funding for the poor. Americans were beginning to believe that health insurance was no longer just a benefit but a right. Insurers gave implicit support to cover all hospital and physician charges.

The National Cancer Act, signed by Richard Nixon in 1971 (Devita, 1993), provided researchers with dollars to create new, sophisticated treatments. Many that were found to be beneficial also carried high price tags. Health-care costs rose at a rate greater than the rate of inflation, which caused the public and employers to complain bitterly about premiums for health insurance. Third-party payers looked for ways to control costs. At the same time providers of cancer care were trying to demonstrate how much could be done for a person with cancer. Providers and payers were on a collision course.

The Late 1980s and 1990s

By the late 1980s, it could no longer be assumed that procedures such as transplantation would be paid for by insurers. Third-party payers adopted the position that transplantation was an experimental procedure and had not been proved effective. Critics of BMT believed that bone marrow transplantation did not represent a cost-effective use of limited health-care dollars. Providers of care argued that it gave many patients their only chance for long-term survival.

As third-party payers began to deny coverage for high-cost treatment, individual patients were able to obtain media attention and public sympathy for their situations. Lawsuits were filed by patients denied coverage because transplantation was deemed experimental (Saver, 1992). As transplantation evolved into a treatment option for women with breast cancer, women activists worked to have payment for this treatment modality legislated (Wynstra, 1994). However, approvals for transplantation coverage continued to vary widely among insurance companies. Peters and Rogers (1994) examined the consistency of predetermination decisions by insurance companies for 533 patients enrolled in grant-supported clinical trials for transplantation for breast cancer. Requests for insurance coverage for transplantation was approved in 77% of cases. Patients who had payment denied were told the therapy was deemed experimental. The frequency of approval did not appear to be influenced by the patient's pretreatment clinical characteristics. There was substantial inconsistency in frequency of approval of coverage among insurers and among decisions made by some individual insurers, even for patients within the same study protocol. This type of variation has helped patients win large settlements and public attention. A California court awarded $89 million in damages to the family of a woman who died after her health maintenance organization refused to pay for her BMT (Meyer and Muir, 1994).

Health-care reform became the centerpiece for the 1992 presidential campaign. Clinton's election set the stage to move this agenda forward. A legislative compromise was not reached at that time. But as Baird (1995) states, marketplace reform has gathered strength and influence.

REIMBURSEMENT

The blending of the business and clinical domains in health-care delivery is very evident when the progression of change in reimbursement is examined. To meet the basic organizational objective of positive financial performance, managers and clinicians are working more closely to eliminate inefficient operations and identify the most appropriate therapeutic interventions in the proper clinical setting. Reimbursement is an excellent example of how market forces are influencing dramatic changes in the delivery of clinical care. It would be a gross oversimplification to suggest that reimbursement is the only factor forcing change. Issues beyond the scope of this chapter, such as cost benefit/effectiveness analysis, quality-of-life issues, litigation by patients, analysis of clinical outcomes, and the definition of experimental treatments, are at the heart of a very difficult public policy debate. Reimbursement, however, provides an anchor for understanding a complex and volatile BMT/BCT operating environment.

Figure 19.1 demonstrates that the health-care reimbursement landscape is moving from fee for service toward capitation. These reimbursement methods will be explained later. The central concept to consider in this progression is sharing financial risk: Should the provider or the payer assume the financial risk for a high-technology, high-cost procedure? Payers are reluctant to reimburse for procedures they consider experimental because such high-cost, and potentially low-benefit, procedures deplete their financial reserves and limit their ability to meet all the needs of their members. Providers are more convinced of the benefit of transplantation, and many are of the opinion that it is both a necessary and cost-effective therapy. As this debate continues, and a point on the continuum is determined, radical changes in the delivery of care will be needed to meet reimbursement levels, and to maintain safe, effective patient care.

Fee for Service

Historically, third-party payers reimbursed hospitals retrospectively for services provided. A structure of charges was set by the hospital and often reviewed for appropriateness by a regulatory commission. No preauthorization or clearance for treatment from the payer was required prior to hospitalization. At the completion of the patient's encounter, a bill for physician and hospital services was submitted to the insurer. As long as the bill agreed with the approved charging structure, the payment was made. In this scenario, the provider organization was rewarded for long hospital stays and high use of ancillary services. The more tests ordered on a specific patient, the greater the potential revenue generated for the physician and hospital. This type of cost-plus (cost of the

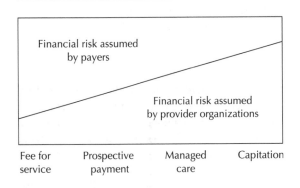

Figure 19.1 Reimbursement continuum

procedure plus some percentage for profit) has been a pivotal issue driving the restructure of health-care reimbursement. Here, all of the risk is assumed by the payer, who has minimal input into the process of care. Retrospective cost-reimbursement/fee-for-service systems still exist, but are quickly becoming extinct.

Prospective Reimbursement Systems

Many payers have developed prospective reimbursement systems. The first prospective reimbursement system was introduced by Medicare in 1983. This system was based on diagnosis related groups (DRGs) with preestablished reimbursement rates. In this scenario, payment for service is fixed and providers of care are not rewarded for high use of services or long hospitalizations. In fact, the opposite is true. The system rewards efficient processes of care with early discharge and limited clinical intervention. This is the first example of a large payer forcing providers to think about how a service is provided. Overuse of services in this patient population erodes profitability.

Payers have also forced competition among health-care providers by negotiating discounts directly with hospitals and providers. For many high-cost, high-technology treatments such as BMT/BCT and solid organ transplantation, contractual agreements are made between the hospital and the payer for provision of services (Cleverly, 1986). Health-care providers compete for these contracts and winners are selected on the basis of service value (Arford and Allred, 1995). Service value is measured by using both cost and quality of outcomes. Bids are evaluated based on technical aspects, qualification of the personnel, and cost. If technical merits and personnel are deemed equal, the low bid will likely win the contract. This payment system is used more and more by health maintenance organizations and preferred provider organizations to fund bone marrow transplantation.

Managed Care

In the managed care setting, primary care physicians (PCPs) direct how and when a population of patients will receive health-care services. Managed care organizations establish criteria to assist the PCP in the decision to use specialty and tertiary-care services. Systems such as case management are designed to monitor adherence to the criteria and limit overusage of more costly tertiary care. In this way, the risk-bearing organization (the managed care organization) can be managed.

Managed care systems have evolved as processes for managed care organizations to verify and participate in the care of their members. Again, financial risk plays an important role in a payer's desire to understand what it is purchasing because the insurer is financially responsible for all of its members' health-care needs. Therefore, it is assuming the risk for providing services to all members. If an insurer has a high proportion of older, sicker members, it is exposed to high risk for associated hospitalization and physician costs. A small health maintenance organization (HMO) with limited financial reserves might be financially devastated by several transplantation patients who have complicated hospital courses with long lengths of stay and intensive care unit admissions.

Many HMOs have developed case management systems. Case management is a systematic, planned approach to patient care that emphasizes individual care planning and resource management to produce high-quality, cost-effective outcomes within and across settings. Case management personnel literally "manage the care" of the patient in concert with the transplantation program's staff to make certain there is agreement on the appropriateness of the care prior to allowing a patient to begin transplantation, as well as over the continuum of care. This hands-on process combined with payment strategies that include discounted payments helps to ensure that some risk is shifted to the provider organization.

Capitation

Capitation refers to the per capita payment a managed care organization or provider organization receives from a payer for the provision of specified clinical services to members (Grimaldi, 1995). The capitation payment is a per member per month (PMPM) rate: the provider will receive a rate for each month that each patient is a member (Grimaldi, 1995). In simplistic terms, a hospital may negotiate with a payer to receive a payment of $50 PMPM for all of the lives that the payer covers. Assume the plan covers 95,000 lives. The hospital will receive $57,000,000 (95,000 lives × $50 × 12 months) over the course of one year for provision of all services negotiated in the contract between the organizations. The health plan, in turn, determines a premium to charge its members that covers the cost of the PMPM and the health plan's administrative costs. In general, payers prefer capitation because most of the risk is shifted to the providers of care who are then rewarded for keeping patients healthy and out of the hospital or away from costly procedures. Providers are making the transition to risk-sharing arrangements to help ensure viable referral patterns. Contracts can be quite complex and involve the use of actuarial data to determine the types of services that will likely be required by the members of the health-care plan. In many instances, reimbursement for transplantation is a separately negotiated contract based on clinical, program, and price criteria.

To protect against high financial risk, many hospitals and physician groups are joining to form health-care alliances. This allows a health-care system to manage care across the entire continuum from prevention to end-of-life care. The benefit of this type of arrangement is added control over the development of cost-effective operations and programs that limit high use of services. A large system of care is in a better competitive position than a single provider organization because of its ability to assume higher financial risk. Implicit in this type of network is the influence of a capitated reimbursement structure on the way in which transplantation is performed. Peters and colleagues (1994) described a method of performing outpatient BMT/BCT for breast cancer that has lower associated costs than traditionally performed inpatient BMT/BCT. All things being equal, in a capitated marketplace programs with outpatient transplantation capability may become more competitive and financially successful than programs capable only of inpatient transplantation because less of the PMPM will be used by the outpatient provider, which will create more positive profit margins.

At the present time, the BMT/BCT marketplace is a mixture of reimbursement methods. This presents organizations with the dilemma of how to organize clinical care to maximize reimbursement. Should the emphasis on reduced length of stay and limited use of services be implemented in the patient populations that are fee for service? Clearly, this would reduce overall financial performance of the program. Or, should the program organize its care to assume capitation? The clear market trend is toward reduced reimbursement as a result of managed care strategies and competition. Program managers need to take the long view with respect to reimbursement and program operations and assume that capitation, or something similar, will predominate the reimbursement landscape in the future.

THE CURRENT ENVIRONMENT

Figure 19.2 illustrates that all products progress through a life cycle from introduction to decline (Wasson, 1978). Cues in the marketplace sug-

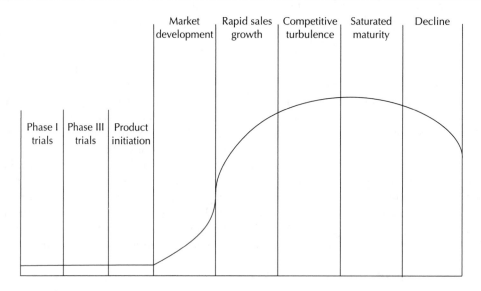

Figure 19.2 **The product life cycle**

SOURCE: Adapted with permission from Bonoma and Kosnick, 1990.

gest that BMT is headed toward maturity. For example, Bennett and colleagues (1995) have documented a reduction of procedure cost from $96,000 to $55,000 over a period of 5 years as experience has been gained treating Hodgkin's disease with transplantation. Proprietary companies are providing on-site stem cell collection and processing to organizations that do not have the capability or the capital to initiate such a service. This type of outsourcing places high-dose chemotherapy with stem cell rescue within the realm of many potential market entrants. Further, consider the work done by Duke University to move transplantation from the traditional inpatient setting to the outpatient setting (Peters et al., 1994). This type of procedural refinement could not have been considered without the experience of treating women with breast cancer in the traditional inpatient setting. Finally, new research efforts are suggesting that perhaps placental/umbilical cord blood can be used successfully in unrelated bone marrow transplantation (Beatty, 1995).

These examples are in direct contrast to the transplantation market of 10 to 15 years ago, which was characterized by long hospitalizations, resource-intense delivery of care, high cost, and relatively few centers performing the treatment. There are now more than 250 BMT sites ranging from large academic programs to mobile (traveling) units (Beatty, 1995). Simply put, the research and design necessary to provide BMT has come to the point where market entrants have the potential to copy the technology, price the product to the market, and produce a process of care that may be as effective as that of entrenched providers. This type of external threat is characteristic of a maturing marketplace. It is also safe to assume that during this period of maturation, purchasers of transplantation have become more savvy about what they are paying for, and more demanding of documented high-quality outcomes. The proliferation of transplant centers has altered market forces and raised concern within the transplant community about defining self-imposed regulations to ensure appropriate program structure and function (Beatty, 1995). Within this volatile context, organizational and program effectiveness can only occur when the internal characteristics of an organization match and support the demands of the external marketplace.

SITUATION ANALYSIS: PREPARING FOR THE FUTURE

Analyzing the External Environment

Michael E. Porter (1979) developed a model to describe how competition in an industry can shape strategy. Porter's model (Figure 19.3) provides a good framework to contemplate the forces influencing BMT. The model considers five specific factors in the marketplace:

- the bargaining power of buyers
- the threat of substitute products
- the bargaining power of suppliers
- the threat of new entrants
- rivalry among existing firms

By examining the current BMT/BCT operating environment using this framework, environmental opportunities and threats can be contemplated.

The Bargaining Power of Buyers
Third-party payers are by far the largest purchasers of BMT. They have exerted significant influence in the health-care marketplace, and

the transplantation community has not been immune. As Figure 19.1 points out, reimbursement to providers from third-party payers is progressing from fee for service toward capitation. Each step in the progression has forced the market price for transplantation downward, and created a shift of financial risk from payer to provider. Pockets of fee-for-service reimbursement remain, but they are dwindling rapidly as the concept of payer designated centers of excellence begins to dominate the transplant reimbursement landscape (Evans and Bengel, 1994).

A *center of excellence* is a transplant center that has been designated for use by a payer-based selection process. Generally, designation of centers is based on three hypotheses concerning the interrelationships among volume of cases, outcomes, and costs (Evans, 1992). Selection can also depend on other facets of program design and function such as quality improvement programs, the experience of practitioners, a demonstration of user-friendly systems for communication with the payer and referring physician, the level of organizational commitment to transplantation measured by the amount and type of support allocated to the transplant effort, and the types of services available to patients who must travel long distances to the designated center. Patient-specific services may include, for example, discounts from airlines and lodging for patients and families forced to travel.

An important aspect of the selection process, and an area in which payers exert significant influence, is negotiation of a "case rate" or "global" price. Financial risk is shifted to the provider by pricing a bundled package of the services required to provide the process of transplant care, and determining a preset length of stay (LOS) for which the price will apply. Figure 19.4 is an example of a typical contract that a health-care provider might negotiate with a health plan. Table 19.1 is an example of

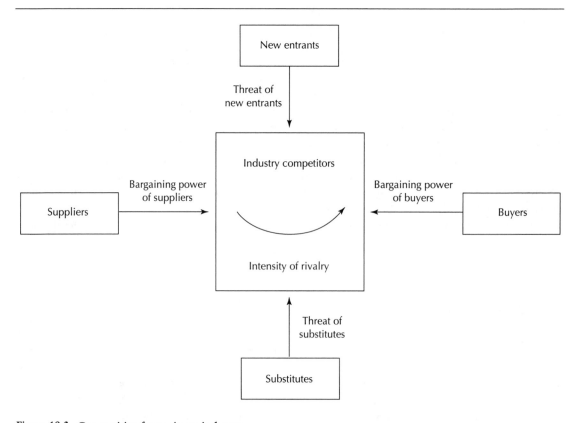

Figure 19.3 Competitive forces in an industry

SOURCE: Adapted from Mintzberg and Quinn, 1996.

how this pricing structure would impact reimbursement, and demonstrates the fact that providing efficient low-cost care is critical to success in the marketplace of managed care.

This example points to the need for appropriate patient selection, the need for a process of care that limits readmission rates, the need for an internal case management process that monitors use of services, and the benefit of such tools as critical pathways to provide consistency in practice. It also points to the benefits of creating good contracts and knowing the cost of producing the BMT process of care from referral through 100 days post-transplantation.

By forcing transplant centers to compete with each other with respect to price, program structure and function, and clinical outcomes, payers can create networks of preferred centers. Transplant centers participating in these networks are the beneficiaries of directed referrals.

Opportunity. Seeking contracts with payers can increase the number of covered lives that a given transplant program can access. By becoming part of a transplant network, a type of directed referral system is established that places the transplant program in a corps of elite

	Fixed fee (1)	LOS outlier cutoff	% Charges in outlier range (2)
AUTOLOGOUS BONE MARROW (3)			
Acute Myelogenous Leukemia (AML)	$102,300	50	80%
Breast Cancer, Hodgkin's Disease, Non-Hodgkin's Lymphoma	$92,070	38	80%
ALLOGENEIC BONE MARROW	$130,000	50	80%

1. (A) Fixed price includes pretransplant evaluation and maintenance that occurs during the transplant admission, organ acquisition (including repeat harvests, tissue typing, harvest hospitalization for live donors, marrow processing and storage, and inpatient days of convalescence associated with organ acquisition), transplant stay, and all transplant-related readmission for thirty (30) days following discharge from transplant admission.
   (B) Pretransplant outpatient evaluation and pretransplant hospitalization (excluding bone marrow harvest admission) will be paid at 80% of billed charges.
   (C) Posttransplant care provided on an outpatient basis or an inpatient basis for admissions after thirty (30) days after transplant discharge will be paid at 80% of billed charges.
   (D) Retransplants will be considered a new procedure.
2. If the cumulative inpatient stay, including inpatient days for entire transplant admission and all transplant-related readmission within 30 days of transplant discharge, are greater that the LOS cutoff, then days beyond the cutoff shall be paid at 80% of billed charges.
3. When the autologous bone marrow harvest for AML occurs during a separate hospital admission from the transplant admission, payment will be at 80% of billed charges. The subsequent transplant for the patient will be subject to a $5,000 credit off the fixed fee.
4. In the event the patient dies during the transplant admission or discharge from the transplant admission occurs prior to the LOS cutoff, payment will be the lesser of the fixed fee or 80% of billed charges.
5. Fixed fees for bone marrow transplants for diagnoses other than those listed above shall be negotiated on a case-by-case basis.

Figure 19.4 Sample center of excellence pricing contract for hospitals and physicians

centers from which health plans can choose. An opportunity exists to develop internal case management systems that work in conjunction with managed care organizations. This type of willingness to collaborate on managing the care of transplant patients recognizes the inevitable future operating environment, and can be instrumental in winning contracts with payers.

Threat. Competitors for BMT service can come from any part of the country. Payers are willing to negotiate travel as part of a package price with a provider, and offer members the opportunity to obtain therapy at a center that meets their thresholds for price and clinical outcomes. Securing local access for a program's catchment area means, in many cases, securing local payer contracts. Price negotiation can have an adverse financial impact on an organization if the cost of treatment is not known. Meeting the market price may increase program volume, but hurt the financial health of the organization when operating costs exceed revenues. The actual mix of payers that a transplant program attracts will have a profound impact on its financial performance. For example, a large pool of Medicare (prospective payment system) and uninsured patients would

TABLE 19.1 Financial impact of center of excellence pricing on provider organizations

What would be the impact of the contract in Figure 19.4 be on reimbursement for the hospitalization of two allogenic bone marrow transplants? Case 1 is an uneventful transplant discharged before the length of stay (LOS) cutoff of 50 days. Case 2 is an outlier case, complete with intensive care unit days, and unfortunately, death. In the first case the inlier clause (statement 4) applies and reimbursement is at 80% of gross charges. Statement 2, in this case, would be interpreted to mean that the patient has a balance of 22 days that could be applied toward the global rate in the first 30 days after discharge. In Case 2, the inlier clause applies again since the patient died prior to the LOS cutoff of 50 days.

	LOS	Total hospital and professional charges	Impact of 80% inlier	Total reimbursement	Discount from charges
Case 1	36 days	$155,479	−$31,149	$124,600	20%
Case 2	32 days	$224,786	−$44,957	$130,000	58%

quickly create a poor financial picture. Conversely, a mixture of fee-for-service, minimal free care, and well-conceived managed care contracts could create a more positive financial performance. Organizations able to accurately determine the cost of providing BMT/BCT will be in a better position to negotiate financially robust contracts.

Threat of Substitute Products

The transplant community and the insurance community is moving past the issue of whether transplantation has a place in the care of cancer patients (Beatty, 1995). Progression to this point has not been without intense interaction between payers and providers. In many early cases, lawsuits were filed by patients denied coverage because transplantation was deemed experimental (Saver, 1992). Peters and Rogers (1994) in their examination of the consistency of predetermination decisions by insurance companies found that only 77% of 533 patients enrolled in grant-supported clinical trials were approved for treatment. Analysis of cost-effectiveness provides systematic information about the consequences, both positive and negative, of allocating resources to perform a specific therapy (Arford and Allred, 1995). Re-

search to evaluate cost-effectiveness has been attempted in BMT (Bennett et. al., 1995; Faucher et al., 1994; Hillner, Smith, Desch, 1992; Uyl-de Groot, Richel, Rutten, 1994). These studies demonstrate that evaluating economic outcomes is becoming just as important as evaluating clinical outcomes. These studies are a beginning attempt to match outcomes to cost. The use of this analytic methodology is now helping payers and providers to consider such issues as the timing and prognostic factors that will result in the best survival for a population of patients treated with BMT, and least use of this high-cost treatment in patients who would have no benefit (Beatty, 1995). However, while these issues are being debated, some patients who are eligible for transplantation may not be referred for consideration.

Opportunity. Continuing medical education (CME) of referring providers can give providers the opportunity to make more informed referral decisions. CME has been documented as a marketing methodology that can improve referral rates (Van Harrison et al., 1990). Since many primary care providers now work in concert with managed care companies, marketing to the medical directors of health plans can augment participation in transplantation networks by highlighting the benefit of transplantation to an entire staff of primary care providers. An ongoing effort needs to be made to understand the cost-effectiveness of transplantation.

Threat. Clinical trials are under way to compare the effectiveness of standard therapy and autologous BMT or BCT for breast cancer. The findings of this research will have a profound impact on the transplantation community. This will be especially true if the costs of transplantation and standard therapy are significantly different but the outcomes are not.

As the current process of care is refined, a new process that is substantively different may evolve. This type of change in production may make current facilities obsolete. Finally, without ongoing continuing medical education of referring physicians, referrals for transplantation can be lost to standard chemotherapy.

Bargaining Power of Suppliers

The transplant program must consider the payer, referring physician, and patient as a triad in the referral decision. In most cases there is a relationship among the patient's insurance plan, the insurance company's negotiated contract with specific transplant centers, and the restrictions this negotiated contract places on the patient's physician concerning to which transplant center he or she can be referred. The structure of the transplant program must meet the needs of these stakeholders, especially in areas where competition offers an alternative choice to any member of this referral triad. As the process of care becomes more commonplace in a maturing marketplace, programs must focus on operational aspects other than direct clinical care (France and Grover, 1992). The concerns of the patient-payer-physician dynamic can exert significant influence on programmatic function by forcing competition among transplant centers. Some

examples of the bargaining power of suppliers include:

- Payers can demand that hospitals and providers produce an invoice that incorporates all appropriate terms of the contract. This may seem like a small issue, but it usually means more administrative hours to individually track and calculate the patient's bill because the contract is complex, and different from others the organization may have.
- Managed care organizations can demand prior authorization for all aspects of treatment from referral through posttransplantation, and insist on regular communication during the course of care to assess the appropriateness of care.
- Managed care organizations can assess a program's ability to measure effectiveness and document clinical outcomes through analysis of quality improvement activities.
- Referring providers can demand rapid turnaround time of written and oral follow-up communication, and base referrals on that criterion.
- Patients and referring physicians can demand rapid access to referral appointments, and convenient hours of operation especially if travel is involved.

Opportunity. Developing systems for smooth interactions with payers and referring physicians can sometimes mean the difference between seeing an increase in referrals and losing market share. As the marketplace matures, and outcomes begin to homogenize, suppliers will be drawn to transplant centers that make billing and communication easiest and most cost effective. Assessing patients' satisfaction and designing systems to meet and exceed the expectations of patients can influence the selection process of referring physicians and insurers. Anticipating payers' questions of quality and devising a well-conceived quality improvement program can demonstrate organizational commitment to transplantation. One method of achieving this type of care planning is development of practice guidelines.

Practice guidelines have been defined as systematically developed guidelines to assist practitioner and patient with decisions about appropriate health care for a specific clinical circumstance (Field and Lohr, 1990). Winn (1995) has identified three categories of practice guidelines: Path Guidelines, Boundary Guidelines, and Critical Care Pathway Guideline (Table 19.2). Guidelines can outline either what care should be delivered or how the care should be delivered. Many grassroots efforts are under way to develop guidelines and pathways for transplantation (Field and Lohr, 1990). A systematic plan to evaluate guidelines must be put into place to understand significance of variation.

Threat. Clinical outcomes will always be the primary concern of providers. However, a lack of respect for a changed operating environment that is sensitive to all aspects of transplantation can limit the growth of a transplant center. If one considers the actual procedure as the center of the transplant product, referrals will be influenced by issues that are at the margins of the production process. In short, the many customers of transplantation must be satisfied. Additionally, because payers are negotiating with the competition, they are obtaining a database of comparative information that positions them to make informed decisions about which program offers patients the most value for their insurance premium.

Threat of New Entrants

New entrants to an industry bring new capacity, the desire to gain market share, and often substantial resources (Porter, 1979). The motive of a potential entrant may be academic such as a new research initiative of an academic

TABLE 19.2 Categories of practice guidelines applicable to oncology

Category	Description
Path guideline	Step-by-step management of a particular tumor type; usually done on stage-specific basis
Boundary guideline	Evaluation of modalities and procedures so as to define range and appropriate use
Critical care pathway guideline	Delineation of how to deliver care once clinical decisions are reached; focuses on sequence and timing of intervention

SOURCE: Winn, R.J. 1995. Current status of practice guidelines in oncology. *Oncology,* 9(7): 601-610. Reprinted by permission of PRR, Inc.

cancer care effort. One cannot assume that the formidable barriers to entry such as the volume thresholds of payers or capital-intense investment in transplant-trained physicians will deter all interested parties. The potential exists, too, for oncology practices to outsource to stem cell collection agencies, and duplicate transplantation services. Constant assessment of the marketplace is required to remain certain that the a program is current in its approach to clinical practice and to its many customers.

Opportunity. Careful assessment of developments in BMT on a national and local level can ensure that a BMT program remains well positioned in the marketplace. Working to force down the cost of BMT, for example, can create an insurmountable entry barrier for a new program. Constant assessment of the needs of the payer-referring physician-patient triad will help prevent loss of market share by ensuring that a program has a product that can be differentiated from that of the competition.

Threat. As the available BMT cases are spread to more centers that do not participate in clinical trials, answers to overarching questions such as documentation of good outcomes in certain diseases and cost-effectiveness will be more difficult to research. Established programs that are not prepared for rivalry from new competition will be forced to react quickly. In most cases, the reaction will take the form of a reduction in price of service without a reduction of production cost, which may lead to poor financial performance.

Rivalry among Existing Firms

Porter (1979) suggests that rivalry among existing competitors takes the familiar form of tactics such as price competition, new product introduction, and advertising campaigns. The transplantation industry is no different. In the highly academic setting of transplantation, competition to write and manage groundbreaking clinical trials in which many centers will agree to participate is fierce. Academic medical centers and medical schools invest huge sums in research endeavors with the hope that significant grants will result. These same organizations recruit the brightest minds in transplantation to lead programs and attract research dollars and patients to their centers. Price competition comes in the form of aggressive price cutting by competitors attempting to gain market share in new areas. The transplantation consumers (patients, payers, and referring physicians) are better informed about their options and are willing to look for the best care for the most reasonable price.

Transplantation is taking place in a very volatile setting. Offering a safe, effective clinical service no longer guarantees that patients will receive care. Marketing at the margins of the production process for transplantation, offering attractive packages to payers, and constant assessment of the actions of rival transplant programs are necessary to ensure that a program remains viable. Despite this complex situation and a sense that many of these obstacles are too great to overcome, opportunities abound for existing programs to take advantage of their experience.

SUMMARY

Clinicians can no longer be concerned solely about the science and patient care aspects of transplantation. They must learn to blend these aspects of transplantation with the appropriate strategic thinking of senior leadership to develop a successful operating plan for the transplantation program. This chapter presented some of the global issues in the external marketplace that influence the direction of BMT/BCT. Certainly, many local influences exert pressure on the operations of a specific program. However, it should be stressed that the external environment was emphasized in the preceding pages. The key to success is matching or structuring the internal environment to meet the needs of stakeholders in the external environment.

An assessment of the strengths and weaknesses of the program in the context of a complex operating environment is a challenging endeavor, but critical as a foundation for change. Some questions to consider might be:

- Do the management reports generated for the transplantation program allow management to accurately position the program in the marketplace?
- Does the financial reporting include accurate cost information?
- Can the management information system help to respond rapidly to managed care contracts by providing data to understand the impact of many pricing scenarios?

- Do the administrative, physician, and nursing leaders possess the skills necessary to lead in a complex and volatile environment?
- Do the staff of the BMT unit have the skills necessary to develop internal case management or continuous quality improvement efforts to reduce operating cost?

Once an understanding of how to structure a program to compete in a given marketplace is gained, it is critical to make certain that BMT/BCT is a product that is important to senior leadership of the organization. This can be accomplished by constantly assessing the external environment, making programmatic adjustments to meet the needs of customers, and keeping senior leaders informed of developments.

REFERENCES

Anderson, O.W. 1985. *Health Services in the United States: A Growth Enterprise Since 1875.* Ann Arbor, MI: Health Administration Press.

Arford, P., and Allred, C.A. 1995. Value = quality + cost. *J Nurs Admin* 25(9):64-69.

Baird, S. 1995. The impact of changing health care delivery on oncology practice. In Hubbard, S.M., Goodman, M., Knobf, T. (Eds.) *Oncology Nursing: Patient Treatment and Support* 2(3):1-13.

Beatty, P.G. 1995. Clinical and societal issues in blood and marrow transplantation for hematological diseases. *Biology of Blood and Marrow Transplantation* 1:94-114.

Bennett, C.L., Armitage, J.L. Armitage, G.O., et al. 1995. Costs of care and outcomes for high-dose therapy and autologous transplantation for lymphoid malignancies: results from the University of Nebraska 1987 through 1991. *J Clin Oncol* 13(4):969-973.

Bonoma, T., Kosnik, T. 1990. *Marketing Management, Text and Cases.* Homewood, IL: Irwin, 311.

Cleverly, W.O. 1986. *Essential of Health Care Reform.* Rockville, MD: Aspen.

Desch, C.E., Smith, T.J. 1995. Defining treatment aims and end-points in older patients with cancer. *Drugs & Aging* 6(5):351-357.

Devita, V.T. 1993. *Cancer Principles and Practice of Oncology.* Philadelphia: Lippincott.

Evans, J., Bengel, M. 1994. National center of excellence can have an impact on reform. *Modern Health Care* 24(3):27.

Evans, R.W. 1992. Public and private insurer designation of transplant programs. *Transplantation* 53(5):1041-1046.

Faucher, C., le Corroller, A.G., Blaise, D., et al. 1994. Comparison of G-CSF-primed peripheral blood progenitor cells and bone marrow auto transplantation: clinical assessment and cost-effectiveness. *BMT* 14:895-901

Field, M., Lohr, K.N. (Eds.) 1990. *Clinical Practice Guidelines: Directions for a New Agency.* Institute of Medicine. Committee on Clinical Practice Guidelines. Washington, DC: National Academy Press.

France, K.R., Grover, R. 1992. What is health care product? *JAMA* 12(2):31-38.

Grimaldi, M. 1995. Capitation savvy a must. *Nurs Manage* 23(2):33-34.

Hillner, B.E., Smith, T.J., Desch, C.E., 1992. Efficacy and cost-effectiveness of autologous bone marrow transplantation in metastatic breast cancer. *JAMA* 267(15):2055-2061

Meyer, M., Muir, A. 1994. Not my health care: insurers beware, consumers are going to court to protect benefits. *Newsweek* January 10:36-38.

Mintzberg, H., Quinn, J. 1996. *The Strategy Process, Concepts, Contexts, Cases,* 2d ed. Englewood Cliffs, NJ: Prentice-Hall, 62.

Peters, W.P., Rogers M.C. 1994. Variation in approval by insurance companies of coverage for autologous bone marrow transplantation for breast cancer. *N Engl J Med* 330(7):473-477.

Peters, W.P., Ross, M., Verdenburgh, J.J., et al. 1994. The use of intensive clinic support to permit outpatient autologous bone marrow transplantation for breast cancer. *Semin Oncol* 21(4 suppl 7):25-31.

Porter, M.E. 1979. How competitive forces shape strategy. *Harvard Bus Rev* (Mar-Apr):137-146.

Saver, R.S. 1992. Reimbursing new technologies: why are the courts judging experimental medicine? *Stanford Law Review* 44(1051):1095-1131.

Uyl-de Groot, C.A., Richel, D.J., Rutten, F.F. 1994. Peripheral blood progenitor cell transplantation mobilized by r-metl-lug-CSF (Filgrastrim): a less costly alternative to autologous bone marrow transplantation. *Eur J Canc* 30A(11):1631-1635.

Van Harrison, R., Gallay, L, McKay, N.E., et al. 1990. The association between community physician's attendance at a medical center's CME courses and their patients referrals to the medical center. *J Contin Ed Health Prof* 10:315-320

Wasson, C.R. 1978. *Dynamic Competitive Strategy and Product Life Cycles,* 3d ed. Austin, TX: Austin Press.

Winn, R.J.. 1995. Current status of practice guidelines in oncology. *Oncology* 9(7):601-610,

Wynstra, N.A. 1994. Breast cancer: selected legal issues. *Canc Suppl* 74(1):491-511.

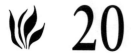 # 20

Transplant Networks and Standards of Care
International Perspectives

Susan A. Ezzone, Monica Fliedner

Over the past 30 years, bone marrow transplantation has evolved into a conventional treatment modality for a variety of malignant and nonmalignant diseases and its use continues to evolve. In the past 10 years, blood stem cell transplantation has been introduced as a treatment option for persons otherwise ineligible for marrow transplantation. The use of autologous transplantation following high-dose chemotherapy for aggressive treatment of solid tumors is a major focus in the 1990s. Rapid changes in the specialty have made it difficult for healthcare professionals to become or keep up-to-date on current practice and trends in transplantation. Published standards of care or recommendations for practice are few, but several organizations have identified the need to develop such documents. Futhermore, transplant teams have found many ways to collaborate informally. These resources and networks are described to give newer clinicians a broad picture of transplantation internationally. This chapter will review the known networks and standards of care established in marrow and/or blood stem cell transplantation at this time.

HISTORY OF TRANSPLANT NETWORKS

International Nursing Networks

For many years, nurses working in bone marrow and blood stem cell transplantation have exchanged ideas and knowledge related to the specialty through participation in conferences offered in the United States, Canada, and Europe. The following is a review of known networks, but is not an exhaustive description. Probably networks exist in transplant nursing that are undiscovered or not published.

Nursing Networks in the United States
The Oncology Nursing Society (ONS) is an internationally recognized organization of more than 25,000 members whose mission is to promote excellence in oncology nursing. In the early years of marrow transplantation, the ONS provided a forum for networking among transplant nurses through attendance at the ONS Annual Congress. Many of the initial educational offerings focusing on bone marrow

transplant nursing were provided through the ONS Annual Congress and in later years through the Fall Institute. Since ONS members' needs are very broad and reach all aspects of oncology nursing, transplant nurses searched for ways to meet their needs related to education, practice, administration, and research issues in transplantation.

In 1989, ONS approved the development of special interest groups (SIGs) to provide a forum for nurses working in oncology specialty areas to network and collaborate in education, practice, administration, and research. The Bone Marrow Transplant SIG was formed in 1989, and the first strategic plan was developed in 1992 to direct SIG activities toward accomplishing the stated mission and strategic goals (see Table 20.1). The BMT SIG, as an organization of more than 380 members within ONS, collaborates with other ONS committees or SIGs to promote to oncology nurses an expanded knowledge base regarding marrow and blood stem cell transplantation. Some of the activities of the BMT SIG include providing educational offerings at ONS Congress and Fall Institute, publishing a newsletter, disseminating new information, distributing a BMT nursing resource directory, publishing a manual of recommendations for education and practice, conducting nursing research, and offering regional workshops. The BMT SIG meets yearly at the annual ONS Congress to discuss and plan activities, and communicates throughout the year via a newsletter, mailings, and phone contact.

Other nursing networks in marrow and stem cell transplantation are in geographic locations where several transplant centers collaborate to meet the educational and networking needs of transplant nurses in the area. In 1983, the Seattle Marrow Transplant Nursing Consortium (SMTNC) was formed through collaboration of five transplant programs in the Seattle area: Department of Veteran Affairs

TABLE 20.1 BMT SIG stategic plan mission and goals

Mission Statement

BMT nursing exists to provide optimal care to persons who undergo BMT. Therefore, the mission of the BMT SIG is to promote excellence in BMT nursing by

- promoting the highest professional standards of BMT nursing
- studying, researching, and exchanging standards of BMT nursing
- encouraging nurses to specialize in the practice of BMT nursing
- fostering the professional development of BMT nurses, individually and collectively
- maintaining an organizational structure and function that is responsive to the changing needs of BMT SIG members, and populations they represent.

Strategic Goals

I. To develop products, services, opportunities, and a knowledge base that promotes excellence in BMT nursing.
   A. Develop and implement educational strategies that provide and integrate state-of-the-art knowledge and new technological trends in the care of the BMT patient.
   B. Continue to enhance the quality and versatility of the BMT newsletter.
   C. Facilitate collaboration and networking between BMT centers and/or SIGs.
II. To increase resources in order to ensure the continued growth and strength of ONS.
   A. Explore and implement strategies of recruitment and retention.

SOURCE: Data from ONS BMT SIG Strategic Plan, 1992.

Medical Center, Fred Hutchinson Cancer Research Center, Swedish Medical Center, University of Washington Medical Center, and Virginia Mason Medical Center. The founding members developed the purpose of the organization, which is to promote the highest professional standards in marrow transplant nursing through education, networking, research, and support. The SMTNC coordinates a biannual international bone marrow transplant nursing symposium, which provides educational and research presentations on advanced topics in transplantation focusing on practice, new technologic advances, administrative issues, and the changing indications and use of marrow and blood stem cell transplantation. In addition, the symposium provides an opportunity for networking among transplant nurses from a variety of practice settings and countries. Similarly, the University of Minnesota and University of Nebraska transplant programs have collaborated to offer an international bone marrow transplant nursing symposium on alternate years, which allows nurses the opportunity to attend an annual symposium. Due to the expanded use of blood stem cell transplantation, a growing number of transplant programs are emerging in the Seattle area and other areas of the country. The increased number of transplant programs presents new issues for educational and program development of the transplant nurse.

Five southwestern states—Arizona, Louisiana, New Mexico, Oklahoma, and Texas—formed the Southwest Marrow/Stem Cell Transplant Nursing Consortium in 1993 as a forum for professional nurses committed to the advancement of excellence in the rapidly evolving field of marrow and stem cell transplantation. Organizational goals include to promote networking, provide educational opportunities, encourage and support collaborative research, and provide representation from the southwest area to the National Marrow Transplant Nursing Consortium. The southwest consortium meets at least annually during a spring and/or fall meeting to conduct business as well as participate in an educational offering. Offering associate memberships for other health-care profes-

sionals is being considered. Similar regional networks or consortiums have been developed in other regions including northern California, Los Angeles, central Texas, New England, and Chicago.

Nursing Networks in Europe and Canada

The European Bone Marrow Transplant (EBMT) Nurses Group began in January 1985 with encouragement and support of physicians working in transplantation. Because most European countries have small transplant centers, the need to share information grew rapidly. The first meeting of the EBMT Nurses Group was held in Bad Hofgastein, Austria, as a 1-day conference, which later expanded to a 2-day conference. At present a 3-day nursing conference is held in conjunction with the physician conference and offers many concurrent abstract and instructional sessions. The joint conference provides a forum for nurses and physicians to network and share information about new developments in treatment modalities. The conference has been lengthened over time to allow nurses opportunities to share expertise and clinical knowledge among European countries. Over the years, learning needs of conference attendees have changed and currently reflect an increased need for sessions on pediatric nursing and care of the BCT patient.

The first speakers in 1985 were from four European countries including Great Britain (Jean Edwards, Royal Marsden, London; Linda Ward, Hammersmith Hospital, London; Carien Pot-Mees, Westminister Children's Hospital, London; Imelda Dillon, Royal Marsden, London), Austria (Monica Seltenheim, University Hospital, Vienna), The Netherlands (Graziella Lantrua, Leiden; Ineke Bartijn, Utrecht; Jenny Snoek-Liefrink, Rotterdam; Els de Boer, Leiden), and Switzerland (Annerose Herzog, Basel). Every year the board of the EBMT nurses group, which consists of the president, vice president, secretary, treasurer, and delegates from the country hosting the conference, invites keynote speakers. In the past, speakers included not only physicians who gave updates on developments in transplantation, but also nurses who have performed important work related to nursing care of the transplant patient.

Approximately 26 countries participate in the EBMT. Because they represent many languages, there are difficulties in communication. Many nurses speak only their native language and have difficulty communicating in English. Therefore, it is not always possible to translate protocols or research studies into the primary language of the country. Each country brings its culture, meaning of nursing care, status of nurses, educational preparation of nurses, and health-care systems. Especially with new treatment modalities like transplantation, it is difficult to translate and transcribe nursing care strategies to another language. With these challenges, nurses need an effective communication network to be able to exchange new ideas.

To facilitate networking in Europe, the EBMT nurses group established a group of contact persons from every country. These contact persons receive announcements for the next conference and distribute them in their countries. Also, the contact persons meet at the conference to receive an update on the work of the board and then report important information to their countries in their languages. Many transplant centers in a country can be located so far apart that nurses do not communicate regularly throughout the year. These countries organize meetings of their fellow nurses during the conference to exchange information. The EBMT Nurses Group holds a national nursing group meeting during the conference to facilitate networking. Some countries, such as France, Great Britain, and the Netherlands, are organized in national BMT/BCT working par-

ties. Many topics have been discussed during the past 12 EBMT meetings. Overviews of the oral presentations are published as abstracts in the EBMT proceedings and as complete manuscripts in an EBMT nursing monograph (see Table 20.2).

In the beginning of the EBMT nurses group, the presentations at the conferences were published in the proceedings and sent to all attendees of the conference, which allowed distribution of the information only to a limited number of nurses. Since 1992, the EBMT nurses group develops and distributes an EBMT journal in which the presentations of the conferences are published along with other important information. The journal is published twice a year and is received by all attendees of the conference and all nurses who are members of the EBMT nurses group. Publication of the journal provides the opportunity to nurses who did not attend the conference to acquire information presented. In the future, the EBMT nurses group will encourage more multicenter nursing research, which can be coordinated by an EBMT research coordinator. It will be very interesting for centers from many countries to work together on several specific topics.

In Canada, the Canadian Association of Nurses in Oncology (CANO) promotes excellence in oncology nursing practice and education. In recent years, marrow and stem cell nurses who attend the annual CANO conference meet to network and share ideas related to transplant nursing. For three consecutive years a transplant workshop was offered during the CANO conference in an effort to meet the educational needs of transplant nurses. Because transplant centers in Canada are separated by hundreds of miles, networking is difficult. The formation of special interest groups within CANO is under consideration and may provide a more effective networking opportunity among Canadian transplant nurses.

TABLE 20.2 Subjects presented at the EBMT Nurses Group meetings

Subject	Year of presentation	Author and country
Mismatch transplants and matched unrelated donor transplants	1985	J. Edwards, UK
	1989	N. Morel et al., F (poster)
	1991	C. Boyd, UK
	1992	M. Smit-Hannot, NL; N. de Heusden et al., NL
	1994	I. Hirsch et al., F
Complementary therapy	1994	S. Hallisey et al., UK; C. Simonds et al., F; M. Monteiro et al., UK
Monoclonal antibodies and growth factors	1989	C. Thain et al., UK
	1990	W. E. Fibbe, NL; C. Davis, UK
Patients' own stories	1987	N. Naylor, UK
Unit presentations	1987	H. Giger et al., CH
Ethical aspects	1988	L. Posner, Israel
	1989	M. Seltenheim, NL
	1993	S. Alvarez et al., F
	1994	M. Goldberg et al., Israel
Care for the dying	1988	E. Baier, D
	1991	R. Vecchi et al., I
Outpatient care, post-discharge, continuity of care	1988	E. Dannie, UK
	1988	J. Fryer, UK
	1989	A. Toy, UK
	1991	J. Bieleveldt et al., NL
Patient information	1989	M. Smit et al., NL; J. Larsen, DK; K. Haupt et al., CH (poster); C. Saudubray et al., F (poster)
	1991	J. Kersteman et al., NL
	1994	R. Keskimaeki, Fin
Transcultural nursing aspects	1988	F. I. Wilson, Saudi Arabia
	1990	E. de Boer, NL
Relapse after BMT/BCT	1991	M. Smit-Hannot, NL
	1994	E. Dannie, UK
Sexuality and fertility	1989	J. Pugh et al., UK (poster)
	1990	E. Goren, Israel
	1993	M. Fliedner, NL
Care for the donor	1990	E. Dannie, UK
	1993	C. Andersson et al., S
Support groups	1988	L. Ilves, Fin
	1990	L. Ilves, Fin
Conditioning regimen	1985	L. Ward, UK
	1987	C. H. Huisman, NL
	1988	H. Afroy, F
Preparation of the pediatric BMT/BCT patient	1989	J. Dennis, UK
	1991	E. Lorenz et al., D

TABLE 20.2 *Continued*

Subject	Year of presentation	Author and country
Involvement of family in care	1987	U. Nilsson, S
	1988	K. Hulme, UK
	1989	A. Casey, UK; F. Gibson, UK
	1991	C. Andersson, S
	1992	L. Goldberg et al., Israel; E. Hucklesby, UK
Pediatric diseases and BCT/ BMT procedures	1987	M. Bater, UK
	1988	E. de Boer, NL
	1989	W. Emminger, A; E. de Boer, NL; J. Omolara, UK
	1992	J. O. O. Oyesiku et al., UK; I. Hirsch, F
BMT nursing in general, nursing collaboration, and safe handling	1985	A. Herzog, CH
	1988	T. van Boxtel, NL
	1989	T. van Boxtel, NL; H. van Wezel et al., NL; C. Charley, UK
	1990	J. Kelleher, USA; A. Asunmaa, Fin; C. Mentink, NL; I. Hirsch, F; M. Evans, UK; E. Garland, UK
	1991	R. Vecchi, I; S. Thomas, UK; G. Morgan, UK; C. Charley, UK
	1992	M. Bakitas Whedon, USA; C. Coenen et al., NL
	1993	J. Claisse et al., F
	1994	M. Evans, UK; H. Porter, UK; W. Bowden et al., UK
Antiemetic	1987	C. P. Mentink et al., NL
	1989	K. Shaw, UK (poster)
	1990	M. Smit-Hannot, NL
	1992	B. Benamo et al., F; C. Maraninchi et al., F
	1993	J. Norcott et al., UK; L. Stirrup, UK
	1994	R. M. W. Anderson et al., UK; T. Morgan et al., UK
Mouth care	1990	N. Morel, F
	1991	M. Stamato, NL; M. Stotts et al., Can
	1992	C. Correia et al., Portugal
	1993	G. Bass et al., UK
	1994	R. Sandford et al., UK
Rehabilitation	1987	M. Planzer, CH
	1991	P. Harbin et al., UK
	1993	J. L. Harris et al., UK
	1994	D. A. Kretzer et al., UK
Cell separator and blood products and supportive care	1987	E. Dannie, UK; A. Wagner, A
	1988	A. Wagner, A
	1989	A. Wagner, A; P. Hoecker, A
	1991	A. Wagner, A
	1993	E. Freeman et al., UK; S. A. Jones et al., UK
	1994	C. G. Boyd, Australia

Continued

TABLE 20.2 Subjects presented at the EBMT Nurses Group meetings *Continued*

Subject	Year of presentation	Author and country
Graft-versus-host disease and medication	1985	M. Seltenheim, A; L. Ward, UK
	1989	E. Dannie, UK; M. Williams, UK
	1990	H. F. L. Guiot, NL; S. Andersson, S
	1992	A. Entonen, Fin
	1994	S. Andersson et al., S; M. Seltenheim et al., NL
Psychosocial aspects and quality of life after BMT/BCT	1985	C. Pot-Mees, NL; I. Dillon, UK
	1987	E. Baier et al., D; F. M. P. van de Loo et al., NL
	1988	M. G. C. Evans et al., UK
	1989	S. Wilke et al., D
	1990	G. Hansson, S; A. Inder, NZ; W. Yang, NL; K. Haupt et al., CH (poster)
	1991	K. Wendel et al., NL; E. Dannie, UK; N. Morel et al., F
	1992	A. Gloriod et al., F; M. Fliedner, NL; K. Haupt et al., CH
	1993	R. Wiren et al., Fin; N. Tazelaar et al., NL
	1994	A. Molassiotis et al., UK; E. Fradique et al., Portugal; C. Boyd, Australia; N. Tazelaar et al., NL; M. Jensen Hjermstad, N; A. Molassiotis et al., UK; M. Fliedner, NL
Isolation, decontamination, and infection control	1985	G. Lantrua, NL; E. de Boer, NL
	1987	M. Neyens, B; E. de Boer, NL
	1988	K. Shaw, UK; H. F. L. Guiot, NL; M. Baumgartner et al., CH
	1990	O. Lanselle, F; R. Wagner, D; M. Baumgartner, CH; E. Benitah, F; S. de Sanctis, I
	1991	S. Andersson, S; M. Jansen et al., NL; F. Weinreich et al., D; M. Stotts et al., Can; T. van Boxtel, NL; P. Cushing et al., UK; G. Kiefer et al., D; F. Amrane et al., F
	1992	T. van Boxtel, NL; E. Dannie, UK; G. van Nierop, NL
	1993	A. Dumont et al., F; J. Harrisingh et al., UK; J. Antrum, UK; J. Perrin, F
	1994	E. Jux, D; P. Vickers, UK; C. Defendini et al., F
Venous access devices and dressing management	1985	I. Bartijn, NL
	1988	S. van Workum et al., NL
	1990	T. van Boxtel, NL; C. Savini et al., F
	1991	D. Bressan et al., I; G. Horrau et al., F
	1992	L. Steegen et al., B; U. Foetsch, A
	1994	E. Fessard et al., F
Nutrition	1985	J. Snoek-Liefrink, NL
	1987	I. Schloesser, NL
	1990	J. Iestra, NL; J. Swire et al., UK; I. Schloessner et al., NL
	1991	G. Ferrarello et al., I; A. Entonen et al., Fin; L. Pozzo, I
	1994	F. Perry et al., UK
Pain control	1989	N. Bennett-Rees, UK
	1993	Y. Ben David, Israel

International Medical Networks

Medical Networks in the United States

For many years physicians in the United States and other countries have participated in specialty organizations such as the American Society of Clinical Oncology (ASCO), the American Society of Hematology (ASH), and Regional Cooperative Oncology Groups. These organizations provide physicians the opportunity to share information related to the treatment of persons with cancer and/or hematologic diseases and collaborate on developing and conducting research. Advancements in technology and knowledge as well as research findings are presented at annual conferences. In the past, ASCO's annual conference has been held immediately following the ONS annual congress, which facilitates collaboration among physicians and nurses, and offers a joint session coordinated by ASCO and ONS members. Presentations on marrow and BCT are given during the annual conferences.

The American Society for Blood and Marrow Transplantation (ASBMT) was recently formed to advance the science and practice in transplantation through promoting education, research, and medical development of transplantation. Three levels of membership are offered, which allows individuals who demonstrate expertise in transplantation as well as individuals who are completing fellowship training programs to join ASBMT. Nurses, PhDs, and other non-MD professionals are encouraged to join as affiliate members (Sullivan and Antman, 1995, communication inviting members).

Cooperative oncology groups were formed in 1955 by the National Cancer Institute (NCI) for the purpose of developing and coordinating controlled clinical trials jointly among researchers to expand the science and treatment of cancer (Cheson, 1991). As of 1991, 13 cooperative oncology groups were conducting research in many oncology centers. The clinical trials are funded by the National Cancer Institute through cooperative agreements and clinical trials are conducted at several centers in an effort to expedite patient accrual and development of new knowledge and treatments for cancer. Many cooperative groups (e.g., CALGB, ECOG) are conducting investigative studies evaluating the effectiveness of bone marrow and/or BCT for a variety of diseases.

The International Bone Marrow Transplant Registry (IBMTR) was formed in the 1970s for the purpose of collecting, organizing, and analyzing all data on allogeneic and syngeneic bone marrow transplantation. Transplant centers are encouraged to participate in the IBMTR by submitting data to the registry on every transplant performed. The international data collated through the IBMTR provides a large data base for analyzing trends or changes in practice and outcomes of transplantation. The results of the IBMTR data are published in medical journals and presented at international scientific meetings. In 1990, the Autologous Blood and Marrow Transplant Registry (ABMTR) was formed to facilitate efforts in international data collection on autologous transplant, in a way similar to the IBMTR. The first meeting of the ABMTR was held in January 1995 prior to the American Society for Blood and Marrow Transplantation conference in Keystone, Colorado. The IBMTR and ABMTR are coordinated through the Medical College of Wisconsin in Milwaukee, Wisconsin. Uniform data reporting forms are provided by the IBMTR/ABMTR to transplant centers that submit data. Data reporting forms are available in handwritten and/or computerized format. Physicians, transplant coordinators, nurses, and data managers are encouraged to attend the IBMTR/ABMTR conferences. Concurrent sessions for nurses, data managers, and coordinators are offered and provide practical information on data collection and management responsibilities. Disease-specific committee meetings are held to discuss in detail the trends, outcomes, and changes in practice of transplantation.

A unique network is the Ohio Bone Marrow Transplantation Consortium (OBMTC). This consortium was founded in 1992 to ensure excellence in patient care, enhance and support timely access by patients, promote fiscal responsibility, and develop cooperation and collaboration among transplant centers in Ohio (Ohio, 1992). The OBMTC has developed membership standards and conducts annual reviews of transplant programs, as well as maintains a statewide registry of patients to track outcomes. The consortium is available to assist third-party payers in determining selection criteria for transplantation, providing expert reviews, and developing funding strategies to provide care to the indigent. Efforts are made to avoid duplication of services and support reasonable use of health-care dollars through appropriate selection of patients. An annual scientific meeting promotes collaborative research among Ohio transplant centers.

Medical Networks in Europe and Canada

In 1975, the first working party meeting was held in St. Moritz, Switzerland, where 10 physicians from Switzerland, France, and The Netherlands met to exchange experiences and knowledge on clinical aspects of BMT. Two years later, in 1977, three other countries (United Kingdom, Germany, and Italy) joined the working party and together formed the EBMT with their first president Professor B. Speck, M.D., from Basel, Switzerland. Over the years, the physicians formed 10 working parties to address acute leukemia, chronic leukemia, lymphoma, solid tumors, aplastic anemia, immune biology, inborn errors, infectious diseases, late effects, and pediatric diseases. The EBMT working parties publish regular reports on their collaborative activities. The number of transplant centers that participate in the EBMT increases every year. In 1992, 203 centers from

26 countries submitted data on BCT (Gratwohl and Hermans, 1994).

The Canadian Bone Marrow Transplantation medical organization is comprised of physicians primarily, but allows participation by transplant coordinators and transplant laboratory personnel. Traditionally the organization's biannual conference has been targeted to physicians, transplant coordinators, and research laboratory personnel. Recently, the organization has expanded its offer of membership to nurses and a nurses' group meets during the biannual conferences.

DEVELOPMENT OF STANDARDS OF CARE

Nursing Standards in Transplantation

Bone marrow transplant nursing has been recognized as a subspecialty of oncology nursing for many years. Initially, transplant nurses derived guidelines for practice from other nursing specialty areas such as hematology, oncology, critical care, burn care, infectious disease, transfusion therapy, and ambulatory care. Although similarities in practice between transplant nursing and these specialties exist it was evident that marrow and blood stem cell transplantation was a unique practice area. Many of the initial publications on marrow transplantation originated from nurses in the Seattle area and focused on describing the process of transplantation, complications, and specific practice issues (Hutchinson and Itoh, 1982; Stream, Harrington, Clark, 1980). In 1981, de la Montaigne and colleagues at Memorial Sloan-Kettering Cancer Center published standards of care for the patient with graft-versus-host disease; they still provide the basis of nursing management for this unique complication. Over the past 10 years marrow transplant nursing practice has been integrated into oncology nursing textbooks (Davis, 1991; Wikle, 1992; Buchsel, 1993). In addition, professional journals have dedicated an issue or part of an issue on marrow transplantion (Hutchinson, 1983; Buchsel and Ford, 1988; Buchsel and Kelleher, 1989; American Association of Blood Banks, 1990; Ford and Eisenberg, 1990; Wujcik, 1994). In recent years, papers on nursing research, practice, quality of life, and patient education appear frequently in professional journals. All of these and other publications assist to define the standards of practice of marrow and blood stem cell transplantation.

In 1991, the first transplant nursing textbook was published (Whedon, 1991). This book provides an essential reference for the nurse caring for transplant recipients and donors. Basic concepts of marrow transplantation are presented including a description of the types of transplant, acute and long-term effects, psychosocial and ethical issues, and program development. The second edition (this book) has been retitled to reflect the changing field of transplantation. A second transplantation textbook (Buchsel and Whedon, 1995) provides a valuable focus on administrative and management issues of transplant programs as well as new clinical issues. An attempt is made to provide basic critical pathways for the medical care of the transplant recipient through the continuum of care. Both textbooks are used by nurses in a variety of practice settings and internationally as a guide for understanding and practicing in marrow and blood stem cell transplantation.

Publications specifically developed as standards of care for marrow and stem cell transplant nursing are few. In 1992, Eisenberg and Maracich, published a manual through the Fred Hutchinson Cancer Research Center (FHCRC). This manual, developed for use as a practice guide for nurses caring for transplant patients at FHCRC, was made available to be purchased by nurses at other transplant programs. The content of the manual is organized by

physiologic system in a nursing care plan format and identifies the problem, expected outcome, assessment criteria, interventions, and rationale. Although the information is specific to practice at the FHCRC, the manual provides basic guidelines for management of common symptoms or complications experienced by the transplant recipient.

From its beginning, the ONS BMT SIG identified a need to develop guidelines for education and practice in marrow and stem cell transplant nursing. The BMT SIG identified important issues that challenged the development of these guidelines:

- The field of transplantation was rapidly growing and changing.
- The use of blood stem cells for transplantation was emerging.
- Indications and learning needs of both the novice and expert transplant nurse needed to be addressed.
- A growing demand for skilled nurses caring for transplant nurses and recipients exists.

After more than 2 years of work, in 1994, a manual was published by the ONS (Ezzone and Camp-Sorrell, 1994). In collaboration with the ONS Clinical Practice Committee, the manual was written by 17 BMT SIG members and reviewed by many others. The purpose of the manual was to present an overview of BMT nursing practice and provide a framework for developing orientation courses or educational programs for transplant nursing. A scope of practice was written to provide a definition of the specialty of transplant nursing and a basis for the nursing practice across the continuum of care through the transplant process. Six recommendations for education and practice were written and provide guidance for developing education programs, policies, procedures, and standards of quality care (see Table 20.3). Course objectives and detailed content are provided on general principles of transplantation,

TABLE 20.3 **Recommendations for education and practice**

Recommendation I
Nursing care, services, and resources related to BMT should be available to meet the physical, psychological, social, cultural, spiritual, ethical, and educational needs of the recipient, the donor, and their families.

Recommendation II
Policies, procedures, and standards should be developed to ensure effective and safe patient care management. This includes preparative cytoreductive regimens, infection control practices, teaching plans, blood component therapy, drug administration, marrow/stem cell infusion, and complication and symptom management.

Recommendation III
Documentation of the nursing process and evaluation of patient outcomes should occur throughout the transplant process to ensure continuity of care.

Recommendation IV
Quality of life (QOL) should be assessed during the BMT process and QOL efforts should focus on BMT survivors, with consideration of late complications and psychosocial and financial issues.

Recommendation V
Through literature reviews, conferences, in-services, networking, and mentorship, avenues for professional development should be pursued so that nurses can keep up to date in the rapidly changing BMT field.

Recommendation VI
Marrow/stem cell transplant nurses should conduct and participate in medical and nursing research as well as use research findings in nursing practice to promote the evolution of expertise in the arena of BMT nursing.

SOURCE: Ezzone and Camp-Sorrell, 1994.

care of the donor, acute and late complications, education of patient and family, ethical issues, new developments, and nursing research. Table 20.4 illustrates some of the topics included in the manual. A detailed, referenced, outline pro-

vides a comprehensive review of each topic area. Tables and figures throughout the manual provide specific content for nursing management. Appendices for each classification of medication used in transplantation are provided and present the drug, route, action/use, side effects, and special considerations. This manual is the first publication by an internationally recognized oncology organization to provide a foundation for marrow and blood stem cell transplant nursing practice. Currently, a manual for blood stem cell transplantation is being developed through the ONS Clinical Practice Committee and is expected to be available by May 1997.

Another resource developed by the BMT SIG is the directory published by ONS every two years (ONS, 1996). It provides a comprehensive overview of transplant centers in the United States and in Canada and has become a valuable and demanded reference by transplant nurses, other health-care providers, and patients. Demographic information for each center include contact name and phone numbers for nurses, number of beds and transplants per year, adult and/or pediatric facility, type of transplant, type of room, patient acuity, availability of orientation and policy/procedure manual, nursing research conducted, and patient education contact and materials available. The information in the directory is not available through any other resource and allows easy access to contact persons for networking, collaboration, and biannual updates on the standard of care in transplantation.

Nursing Standards in the Community

Transplantation as a treatment modality was traditionally offered at academic and/or research institutions but currently aspects of care are provided through home-care agencies, ambulatory clinics, physicians' offices, and community settings. Each of these settings, new to

TABLE 20.4 Topics in the *Manual for BMT Nursing: Recommendations for Education and Practice*

General Principles

Definition of transplantation	Bone marrow procurement
Sources of stem cells	Marrow treatment options
Patient eligibility criteria	Preparative regimen
Diseases treated	Infusion of stem cells
Donor identification	

Care of the Bone Marrow Donor

Preoperative	Patient education
Postoperative	

Nursing Management of Acute Complications

Acute GVHD	Acute renal failure
Infection	Hemorrhagic cystitis
Bleeding	Nutritional compromise
Veno-occlusive disease	Failed or delayed engraftment
Pulmonary edema	

Nursing Management of Late Complications

Chronic GVHD	Neurologic
Recurrence of disease	Ophthalmic
Secondary malignancy	Musculoskeletal
Sexuality	Endocrine

Patient and Family Education

Pretransplant	Discharge planning
Transplant	Rehabilitation and follow-up

Ethical Issues

Informed consent	Economic issues
Advanced directives	Pediatric issues

New Developments and Research

Cytokines	Gene therapy
Ultraviolet light	Alternative methods of obtaining stem cells

Areas of Nursing Research

Research methodology	Current BMT nursing research

SOURCE: Data from Ezzone and Camp-Sorrell, 1994.

the specialty of transplantation, are struggling to define the standard for providing interdisciplinary care. Many home health care/infusion agencies have recruited transplant nurses as experts in the specialty to provide clinical leadership in developing transplant home-care programs and training staff. Comprehensive re- sources for staff education for care of the transplant patient have been developed by several of the home-care agencies (Lonergan, Kelley, McBride, 1994). These resources are a valuable contribution to developing the standard of care in nontraditional settings in marrow and blood stem cell transplant. Collaboration between the transplant center and the home-care agency should occur to provide continuity of care throughout the transplant continuum.

Patient Education Materials

The challenge of providing education to patients and families undergoing marrow or stem cell transplantation is complicated by the complexity and variation of the treatment modality, as well as the availability of materials. Most transplant programs have developed materials that discuss transplantation specific to the center, but the materials are not widely available. Several patient/family educational resources are available for no cost or for purchase through institutions or the pharmaceutical industry. With permission, some can be adapted to meet the needs of individual transplant centers (see Table 20.5). The development of these and other patient education materials has created a standard for providing patient education materials. One of the most popular materials for patients is a book written by a former transplant patient (Stewart, 1992). In addition, Stewart publishes a bimonthly newsletter on pertinent topics related to bone marrow and blood stem cell transplant; it can be ordered by patients, families, and health-care providers. Each issue of the newsletter provides valuable information on a variety of topics such as types of transplant, treatment of specific diseases, complications of transplant, and resources, as well as articles highlighting individuals' experiences through the transplant process.

In 1990, the Memorial Sloan-Kettering Cancer Center published a manual, available for purchase, that is an excellent resource for the development of standards of care for providing patient education (Ford, Kenny, Slevin, 1990). It includes a detailed outline of topics, educational content and materials, list of educational resources, and a sample documentation tool. Topics across the transplant continuum of care are presented in a manner that assists the nurse or other health-care provider to coordinate the process of educating patients/families.

Several networks provide patient education or information through an international computer network, Internet, such as CompuServe, Prodigy, and America On-Line (AOL). These computer programs offer on-line interactive "chat rooms," which give users access to information from universities, the National Cancer Institute (NCI), and other governmental agencies. The BMT Newsletter described above is available through the Internet, as well as other useful patient education material. Users communicate with others on a variety of topics through typewritten messages and responses, which all users have access to read. A few of the available interactive computer on-line programs include Living with Cancer, BMT Talk, NCI's CancerNET, Cancer-List, Hematology/Oncology List, Breast Cancer List, Ovarian List, and NCI Physicial Data Query (PDQ) (Flatau, 1995; Frankel, 1995). Access to communication through the Internet has provided many transplant recipients the ability to share and receive information about personal experiences.

Medical Standards in Transplantation

Over the past 30 years the specialty of bone marrow transplantation has evolved rapidly and is now considered conventional treatment for leukemia, lymphoma, aplastic anemia, and other diseases. As advances in scientific knowledge and technology have expanded, the use of blood stem cells for transplantation has become a treatment option for many persons who otherwise would be ineligible for transplant. Standards for the use of transplantation as treatment for malignant and nonmalignant disease can be derived from the numerous scientific studies and reports in the medical litera-

TABLE 20.5 Sample of available materials for patient education

Title/Author/Year/Location	Type of material	Content
Bone Marrow Transplants: A Book of Basics for Patients, Stewart (1992)	Book	Detailed description of the fundamentals of transplantation, preparing for transplant, types of transplant, emotional and psychological considerations, GVHD, infection, infertility, liver complications, insurance
BMT Newsletter, Stewart (Ed.)	Newsletter Published bimonthly	Articles discuss various aspects of transplantation including new approaches to treatment, treatment of specific diseases, complications, resources, and individuals' experiences through the transplant process
Bone Marrow Transplants: A Guide for Cancer Patients and Their Families, Shaffer (1994)	Booklet	Detailed descriptions of dealing with the diagnosis of cancer, what is a BMT, making the decision, preparing for transplant, expectations during treatment, outpatient treatment, posttransplant issues
Understanding Your Bone Marrow Transplant: A Patient's Guide, Immunex Corporation (1993), Seattle, WA	Booklet	The basics of BMT, bone marrow donor, preparing for BMT, central venous catheter, preparative regimen, expectations during and after transplant, discharge, life after transplant
"Understanding Your Bone Marrow Transplant: A Videotape for Patients," Immunex Corporation (1993), Seattle, WA	Video	Overview of the transplant process
Myself Resolved: An Artist's Experience with Lymphoma, Lynn (1994)	Book	Paintings reflect the author's experience through cancer treatment and BMT
"Caring for Yourself," Sammons Cancer Center, Baylor University, Dallas, TX	Video	A 25-minute video discusses ways to enable patients undergoing marrow transplant to participate in their care, understand the treatment process and complications
"Central Venous Catheter Care," Davies, Rush Presbyterian-St. Luke's Medical Center, Chicago, IL	Video	Reviews procedure for care of central venous catheter and catheter complications
"A Critical Decision," University of Minnesota, Minneapolis, MN	Video	Overview of BMT; intended to help patients understand the treatment process and make decisions about transplant; conversations with patients throughout
"Gift of Life: Waiting for a Donor," Glaxo-Wellcome Pharmaceuticals, Research Triangle Park, NC	Video	Overview of bone marrow transplant and the need for marrow donors; testimony from patients waiting for donors and volunteer donors; useful tool for educating the public and increasing the donor registry
Dag nul, de Wit and de Wit, Stichting Columbine, Westbroek (1990), Netherlands	Book	Book on bone marrow transplantation written by a patient. Written in Dutch.
Been Nerg Transplantatie, Alewynse and van Dam, Integraal Kankercentrum Limburg, Haastricht (1991), Netherlands	Book	Book on bone marrow transplantation written by a patient. Written in Dutch.

ture. Few documents have been published on the development of standards for medical management of persons undergoing bone marrow or blood stem cell transplantation.

Several publications provide information on the basic and advanced concepts of transplantation, guidelines for the use and practice of transplantation, and scientific investigations. In 1986, the first issue of the journal *Bone Marrow Transplantation* was published through efforts of the EBMT medical group, under the leadership of editor, John Goldman, M.D., London. The journal has become an internationally recognized publication which provides information on all aspects of basic and clinical science of transplantation. In recent years, a very informative newsletter, *Marrow Transplantation Reviews,* has been published by the ASBMT to provide information on numerous topics in the field of transplantation. In the fall of 1995 the ASBMT published the first issue of a new journal titled *Biology of Blood and Marrow Transplantation.* The newsletter and journal will be included in the membership of ASBMT. An IBMTR newsletter distributed to participating centers summarizes the activities of the IBMTR/ABMTR and data on the use and outcomes of transplantation (IBMTR, 1995). Recently published medical textbooks comprehensively discuss the evolution, current approaches, and future directions of transplantation (Atkinson, 1994; Deeg, Klingeman, Gordon, 1992; Forman, Blume, Thomas, 1994). In addition, proceedings of symposia have been published through the BMT journal or independent publications and serve to distribute up-to-date information to transplant centers.

The IBMTR/ABMTR publishes reports on the clinical investigations conducted at transplant centers throughout the world in an effort to determine factors that affect the success and failure of transplantation (Bortin, Horowitz, Rimm, 1992a). Collecting, analyzing, and reporting data from the international registry as-

sists in describing the standard of care and use of transplantation as a therapeutic treatment option. In 1992, Bortin and colleagues through the IBMTR reported survey results that evaluated the use of allogeneic bone marrow transplantation (alloBMT) and determined that the number of alloBMTs and new transplant centers were growing at a rate of 600 patients per year and 25 new centers per year. A recent IBMTR report described changing trends in alloBMT for leukemia, GVHD prophylaxis, and outcomes of transplantation for leukemia and aplastic anemia (Bortin, 1993). From 1980 to 1989 an increase was reported in the use of alloBMT for treatment of CML, transplant for early leukemia, unrelated donors, conditioning regimens without radiation, and use of methotrexate plus cyclosporin for GVHD prophylaxis. The IBMTR conducts periodic assessments through surveys to determine the pattern and frequency of transplantation.

In 1990, ASCO and ASH published in two peer-reviewed journals a special report that described the minimum criteria necessary to provide a safe and successful environment to perform transplantation (ASCO/ASH, 1990a, b). This document was endorsed by the boards of directors of both organizations and is recognized by new transplant centers as the standard for program development. Adherence to these guidelines assist transplant centers with the special preparation and commitment for providing transplant as a treatment modality. Topics in this document include patient volume, facilities, personnel, treatment outcome, and data reporting (see Table 20.6). The ASCO/ASH recommendation of 10 transplants per year as the minimum number is consistent with the IBMTR finding that the number of transplants performed at smaller centers (five or fewer transplants per year) had an increased risk of treatment-related mortality and treatment failure (Bortin et al., 1992b). Similarly, Horowitz and colleagues (1992) found that the 2-year

TABLE 20.6 ASCO/ASH Recommended criteria for centers to perform BMT

Patient Volume
1. A sufficient number of patients must be treated each year.
   a. At least 10–20 patients per year
   b. The unit must never be empty.
2. If both autologous and allogeneic transplants are performed, at least 10 of each type of transplant must be performed annually.
3. For new units, compliance with these goals must be reached within 2 years of operation.

Facilities
1. A designated unit must exist with two or more designated transplant beds.
2. Facilities for handling marrow outside the body must be in place. (i.e., cryopreservation of autologous stem cells, management of ABO-incompatible transplants, certified histocompatibility laboratory).
3. Facilities and policies for isolation and a plan for air handling must be in place.
4. Laboratory, radiology, and transfusion services must have 24-hour availability.
5. Facilities for total body irradiation should be available in most circumstances.

Personnel
1. Physicians should have documented experience with transplantation.
2. Consulting physicians in subspecialties need to be available.
3. A nursing team committed full time to the program with a high ratio of nurses to patients exists.
4. The institution must be committed to have full-time BMT coordinators, social workers and other services.

Treatment Outcome
1. A registry of all transplants performed must be maintained and outcomes compared to other centers.
2. A policy for identifying deficiencies in results, analyzing causes, and implementing changes aimed at improving results must exist.

Data Reporting
1. Data should be reported to the available registries (IBMTR) and observations should be published in the medical literature.

SOURCE: Data from ASCO/ASH, 1990a.

probability for leukemia-free survival was 10% to 15% lower in patients who received an HLA-identical allogeneic BMT at smaller centers when compared to patients who received transplants at larger centers. Rationale for the difference in outcomes consider the volume of procedures; experience of physicians, nurses, and other personnel; complexity of patients' needs; and management of transplant complications such as GVHD. In addition, ASCO published recommendations for the use of hematopoietic colony-stimulating factors (CSFs).

Among other uses, recommendations are given for use of CSFs in patients undergoing high-dose chemotherapy and autologous transplantation and in mobilizing BSCs for transplantation. The routine use of CSFs following allogeneic transplant is not encouraged at this time due to lack of sufficient data to make this recommendation.

The newly formed ASBMT has developed and approved guidelines for clinical centers and training in bone marrow transplantion (Appelbaum et al., 1995; Phillips, 1995). The guidelines discuss requirements to ensure the highest quality of medical practice. Guidelines for clinical centers describe recommendations for program size; type of staff including physicians, consulting physicians, nurses, transplant coordinators, and pharmacy, dietary, social service, physical therapy, and data management staff; data assessment and quality assurance; and inpatient, outpatient, and other facilities (see Table 20.7). Specific guidelines for training of medical staff are recommended and include cognitive and procedural skills; method of training; board certification; and training in the care of transplant patients.

Cooperative oncology groups organized by NCI are conducting clinical trials involving allogeneic and autologous bone marrow and BSC transplantation, allowing large patient samples

TABLE 20.7 Guidelines for clinical centers

Program Size
1. A minimum number of 10 transplants must be performed each year.
2. Programs must perform 10 transplants of each type of transplant performed at the center per year.

Staff
1. A dedicated transplant team must be in place for at least 1 year.
2. Physician staff: The program director should be licensed and board certified in a related specialty as defined by ASBMT and have had at least 1 year of training or 2 years of experience in transplantation.
3. Board-eligible or certified consulting physicians should be available who are capable of assisting in the management of patients requiring intensive medical or pediatric care.
4. Nurses should have formal training in patient care related to hematology/oncology, cytotoxic therapies, infectious complications, administration of blood components, and appropriate intensive medical/pediatric care.
5. Appropriate staff should be available to maintain support services including transplant coordinator, pharmaceutical staff, dietary staff, social services, physical therapy, and data management.

Data, Assessment, and Quality Assurance
1. An institutional review board that meets criteria of the National Institutes of Health should review and approve the program's investigational protocols and consent forms for patients.
2. Each program should keep complete and accurate records that include the data coded in the forms of the IBMTR and/or ABMTR.
3. A written plan for quality assurance/improvement exists and is monitored by the director, and involves all members of the transplant team.

Facilities
1. Inpatient unit should have the following: a designated inpatient unit that minimizes airborne contamination, policies on infection prevention and isolation, a nurse-to-patient ratio that is adequate for the severity of patients' clinical status.
2. Outpatient units should have the following: provisions for prompt 24-hour care, nurses experienced in transplantation, designated outpatient area for infusions of medications or blood components, written policies on outpatient care.
3. Other facilities that must be available include: a processing laboratory that meets established standards, a blood bank providing 24-hour support, and allogeneic centers must have HLA testing laboratory with capability of DNA-based HLA typing and a pathologist experienced in interpretation of GVHD.

SOURCE: Data from Phillips et al., 1995.

TABLE 20.8 ECOG guidelines for management of autologous and allogeneic BMT

GVHD
- Use of recognized diagnosis, grading, and histologic grading and staging of acute and chronic GVHD
- Use of most valid investigational therapies for GVHD

Infection
- *Pneumocysitis carinii:* Bactrim DS one tablet bid, 2–3 times per week, after engraftment, continue for 3–6 months after transplant. (Alternative therapies include dapsone or aerosolized pentamidine.)
- Fungal: continued investigation of fungal prophylaxis. Use either low-dose amphotericin B or fluconazole.
- Cytomegalovirus (CMV)
  Allo BMT seronegative with seronegative donor: should receive CMV negative blood
  Autotransplant seronegative: CMV-negative blood preferred, or use of leukocyte-filtered blood
  Allo seropositive or seropositive donor: IV IG as prophylaxis
  Allo BMT: send blood, urine, throat cultures every week through day +120.
  Allo BMT: culture positive in blood, GI tract, bronchial washing, throat, administer ganciclovir through day +100, or for 2–3 weeks past latest positive culture

Hepatic Veno-Occlusive Disease
- Patients should be entered into controlled clinical trials for prophylaxis and treatment

Hematopoietic Growth Factors
- Encourage use unless disallowed by protocol
- In AML, no definitive recommendation given due to theoretical risk of stimulating leukemic relapse and limited data
- All allo- and auto- patients who do not engraft by day 21 to 28 should receive GM- or G-CSF
- CSFs may have an added role in prevention or treatment of myelosuppression induced by ganciclovir or other agents

Reconstitution of Hematopoiesis after Transplantation
- Autologous BMT: 1×10^8 nucleated cells/kg minimum, prefer 2×10^8 nucleated cells/kg
- Allogeneic BMT: 3×10^8 nucleated cells/kg of recipient's body weight, minimum of 2×10^8

Peripheral Blood Progenitor Cell Transplants
- Autologous: amount of stem cells collected should contain at least $7–8 \times 10^8$ mononuclear cells/kg with a CFU-GM content of 5×10^4/kg
- Allogeneic: no recommendations at this time due to the experimental nature of this area

Cryopreservation of Marrow
- An established method of cryopreservation of stem cells must be developed
- DMSO (dimethylsulfoxide) 10% or hydroxymethyl starch and 5% DMSO for cryopreservation

Immune Reconstitution
- At the end of 1 year, if chronic GVHD is absent, influenza may be given yearly, pneumococcal polysaccharide vaccines and DPT should be considered
- Immunosuppressed patients with chronic GVHD are less likely to develop antibody response after vaccines. Antibody titers should be checked to determine response.
- If 2 years after BMT, without evidence of GVHD, not receiving immunosuppressant drugs, measles-mumps-rubella (MMR) live vaccines can be given.

IV Immunoglobulin
- Administer IV IgG to patients after allo BMT as CMV prophylaxis in seropositve patients and as a antimicrobial prophylaxis in all patients at dose of 500 mg/kg for a minimum of every 2 weeks for the first 3 months after BMT
- Enter patients in clinical trials evaluating this treatment in leukemias, lymphomas, and solid tumors.

Blood Bank Support
- Pretreat blood products with 2500 cGy to 3000 cGy
- Avoid transfusions from family members if possible, prior to transplant, especially from potential donors
- Use leukocyte-depleted blood products whenever possible

SOURCE: Data from Rowe et al., 1994.

to be accrued in short time intervals. The Eastern Cooperative Oncology Group (ECOG) recently published a position paper that recommends guidelines for the management of autologous and allogeneic bone marrow transplantation (Rowe et al., 1994). Because cooperative group clinical trials require uniformity in care and assurance of quality, ECOG developed basic guidelines for the acceptance of centers into the cooperative group trials. A similar set of guidelines has been published by Cancer and Leukemia Group B (CALGB). In addition, the ECOG guidelines may be useful to new transplant centers during program development (see Table 20.8).

The National Marrow Donor Program (NMDP) was established in 1987 to expand the availability of volunteer unrelated HLA-matched marrow donors for transplantation (Welte, 1994). Through the development of this program priniciples were written to describe the standards for evaluation and acceptance of marrow donors, marrow collection, request for donor searches, becoming a donor center, participating NMDP center, histocompatibility, diagnostic criteria, and ethical considerations (see Table 20.9) (Stroncek et al., 1993). In addition, the NMDP has developed detailed standards and minimum guidelines for BMT programs using unrelated donors (see Table 20.10) (NMDP, 1995). The medical director of the participating center is responsible to ensure that the standards, policies, and procedures of the NMDP are strictly adhered to.

The number of transplant centers and the number of transplants done using BSCs is increasing rapidly. In Europe in 1973, only 16 allogeneic transplants were performed and no autologous marrow transplants. More than 20 years later, this number has increased to more than 6000 bone marrow transplants done in 1992 (Gratwohl and Hermans, 1994). At the EBMT conference in Davos, Switzerland, in March 1994, this figure had increased again to

TABLE 20.9 Principles of the National Marrow Donor Program

- Donors will be informed about the marrow donation and will give their consent prior to being listed in the Registry and at each step of the search process.
- Donation of marrow is voluntary.
- Standards for the evaluation of donors and for the collection, preservation, and transportation of marrow have been established.
- Participating donor, marrow collection, and transplant centers must meet minimum performance criteria established by the NMDP.
- Formal search requests are accepted only from physicians at participating transplant centers.
- Marrow is provided for transplants that meet the minimum histocompatibility and diagnostic criteria established by the NMDP.
- Donors undergo examination by a third-party physician prior to a final decision regarding marrow donation.
- The donation process is structured so as to allow the donor to remain as close to home as possible.
- Donor anonymity is maintained.
- The NMDP has an obligation to foster and facilitate research.
- The NMDP has a responsibility to evaluate the outcome of transplants for which donors were provided.
- The NMDP has an obligation to monitor the effects of marrow donation on the donors.

SOURCE: Data from Stroncek et al., 1993.

a total of 8552 autologous and allogeneic blood stem cell transplants. The use of autologous BSC transplant has increased dramatically to more than 5417 in 1994. In 1992, 203 transplant centers in 26 countries submitted data on BSC transplant to the EBMT (Gratwohl and Hermans, 1994).

One of the most controversial and emotional areas of transplantation is the treatment of metastatic breast cancer with high-dose che-

TABLE 20.10 **Summary of standards developed by the National Marrow Donor Program**

- Criteria for participating donor centers
- Criteria for participating donor recruitment groups
- Recruitment of unrelated donors of bone marrow
- Assurance of donor's privacy
- Further tests when a partial HLA match with a recipient has been identified
- Donor information session
- Medical evaluation of the matched prospective donor
- Donor's abnormal findings
- Intent to donate
- Precollection communication
- Criteria for participating collection centers
- Precollection blood samples from donor
- Marrow collection and processing
- Transport of marrow
- Quality control of marrow
- Subsequent donor contracts
- Patient rights
- Criteria for participating marrow transplant centers

SOURCE: National Marrow Donor Program, 1995.

motherapy (HDC) and autologous bone marrow and/or BSC transplant. The effectiveness of HDC with transplant compared to conventional treatment in improving survival rates has been debated by oncologists, hospital administrators, and insurers. Although the lack of data from controlled studies makes it difficult to form conclusions about appropriate treatment for metastatic breast cancer, data are promising that disease-free survival (DFS) can be longer with the use of HDC with transplantation (Eddy, 1992). As this debate continues, it is anticipated that standards for use of HDC with transplantation for the treatment of metastatic breast cancer will be established through the input of health-care providers, administrators, insurers, and patients.

Due to the current focus on reduction of costs in health care it would be remiss not to discuss briefly issues related to costs and benefits of transplantation. Controversies of the medical, social, ethical, and financial consequences of transplantation are debated by hospitals, insurers, governmental agencies, health-care providers, patients, and families. Difficult questions remain regarding the appropriateness of transplantation for the treatment of certain diseases and considerations for end-of-life decisions when complications occur. At times, considerations of cost influence insurers and health-care providers in determining life-and-death decisions. Numerous journal articles in the United States, Europe, and other countries have been published in an attempt to define concretely the cost and benefits of transplantation (Dufoir et al., 1992; Griffiths et al., 1993; Mitchell et al., 1993).

At this point, research findings published about clinical practice are not comparable because great variation exists among centers in techniques of transplantation, preparative regimens, supportive and therapeutic pharmaceutical agents, laboratory, radiology, protective environment, and administrative costs. A survey mailed to pharmacists at 92 United States BMT programs found that inpatient BMT drugs accounted for 12% of the total inpatient drug budget, as well as a significant component of the cost of transplant (King et al., 1994). Transplant centers should consider cost/benefit ratio of medications used in transplantation based on documented scientific and clinical experience. For example, the reduced cost of autologous transplantation with the use of hematopoietic growth factors is reflected in the decreased use of resources such as drug therapy, laboratory testing, transfusion requirements, and hospital days (Petros and Peters, 1993).

Controversy regarding the benefits of autologous transplant for the treatment of metastatic breast cancer raises important questions regarding the use of health-care dollars. There has been wide variation among third-party payers for approval of coverage for transplant so that many women are either being denied treatment or assuming the cost of treatment (Peters and Rogers, 1994; Mahaney, 1994). Although the issues concerning costs are complex and confusing, they will surely influence the continuing development of standards of practice in transplantation.

SUMMARY

Marrow and BSC transplantation continues to be a rapidly growing and changing specialty that requires collaboration and sharing of knowledge and ideas among health-care professionals of multiple disciplines and transplant centers. As trends in this dynamic treatment modality continue to evolve, it will be imperative that health-care professionals develop standards of care for all aspects of transplantation. It has also become essential to facilitate more efficient and timely international networking to expand the knowledge and update the practice of transplantation. Exploration of the Internet may offer new possibilities for international communication through bulletins created for marrow and BSC transplantation. Transplant nurses and members of other disciplines must become familiar with these advanced communication technologies. Ultimately, computer-linked sharing of information could directly affect the care provided to transplant patients.

This chapter has discussed the networks and standards of care in transplantation available at this time. It is evident that research-based standards of care are lacking and need to be developed for many current practices in transplantation. As new approaches to trans-plantation are introduced, it will become mandatory to develop standards to ensure appropriate and cost-effective use of new therapies. Interdisciplinary collaboration among academic research centers, community hospitals, outpatient clinics, home-care agencies, and alternative sites must occur to coordinate care through the treatment process. Nationally recognized oncology organizations must jointly develop recommendations or guidelines for practice to serve as the basis for transplant program development, education of health-care providers caring for transplant patients, and clinical management of transplant recipients and donors.

REFERENCES

Alewynse, L., van Dam, K. 1991. *Been Nerg Transplantatie*. Haastricht, Netherlands: Integraal Kankercentrum Limburg.

American Association of Blood Banks. 1990. *Bone Marrow Transplantation: A Nursing Perspective*. Bethesda, MD: AABB.

Appelbaum, F., Fay, J., Herzig, G., et al. 1995. American society for blood and marrow transplantation guidelines for training. *Bio Blood & Marrow Transplant* 1(1):56.

ASCO. 1994. American Society of Clinical Oncology Recommendations for the use of hematopoietic colony-stimulating factors: evidence-based, clinical practice guidelines. *J Clin Oncol* 12(11):2471-2508.

ASCO/ASH. 1990a. The American Society of Clinical Oncology and American Society of Hematology recommended criteria for the performance of bone marrow transplantation. *J Clin Oncol* 8:563-564.

ASCO/ASH. 1990b. ASCO/ASH recommended criteria for the performance of bone marrow transplantation. *Blood* 75(5):1209.

Atkinson, K. (Ed.) 1994. *Clinical Bone Marrow Transplantation: A Reference Textbook*. New York: Cambridge University Press.

Baylor University. Caring for Yourself. Dallas: Charles A. Sammons Cancer Center. (video)

BMT SIG. 1992. *Bone Marrow Transplant Special Interest Group Strategic Plan*. Pittsburgh: Oncology Nursing Society.

BMT SIG. 1994. *Bone Marrow Transplant Nursing Resource Directory*. Pittsburgh: Oncology Nursing Press.

Bortin, M.M., Horowitz, M.M., Rimm, A.A. 1992a. Increasing utilization of allogeneic bone marrow transplantation. *Ann Intern Med 116*:505-512.

Bortin, M.M., Horowitz, M.M., Rimm, A.A. 1992b. Progress report from the International Bone Marrow Transplant Registry. *BMT 10*:113-122.

Bortin, M.M., Horowitz, M.M, Rowlings, P.A., et al. 1993. Progress report from the International Bone Marrow Transplant Registry. *BMT 12*:97-104.

Buchsel, P.C. 1993. Bone marrow transplantation. In Groenwald, S.L., Frogge, M.H., Goodman, M., Yarbro, C.H. (Eds.) *Cancer Nursing: Principles and Practice*. Boston: Jones & Bartlett, 393-434.

Buchsel, P.C., Ford, R. (Eds.) 1988. Advances in bone marrow transplantation. *Semin Oncol Nurs 4*(1):1-78.

Buchsel, P.C., Kelleher, J. 1989. Bone marrow transplantation. *Nurs Clin North Am 24*(4):907-938.

Buchsel, P.C., Whedon, M.B. (Eds.) 1995. *Bone Marrow Transplantation: Administrative and Clinical Strategies*. Boston: Jones & Bartlett.

Cheson, B.D. 1991. Clinical trials program. *Semin Oncol Nurs 7*(4):235-242.

Coxon, V. 1995. The role of computers. In Buchsel, P.C., Whedon, M.B. (Eds.) *Bone Marrow Transplantation: Administrative and Clinical Strategies*. Boston: Jones & Bartlett, 403-426.

Davies, S. Central Venous Catheter Care. Chicago: Rush Presbyterian-St. Luke's Medical Center. (video)

Davis, B.V. 1991. Injury, potential for, related to graft versus host disease. In McNally, J.C., Somerville, E., Miaskowski, C., Rostad M. (Eds.) *Guidelines for Oncology Nursing Practice*. Philadelphia: Saunders, 223-230.

Deeg, H.J., Klingemann, H.-G., Gordon, P. (Eds.) 1992. *A Guide to Bone Marrow Transplantation*. New York: Springer-Verlag.

de la Montaigne, M., De Mao, J., Nuscher, R., Stutzer, C. 1981. Standards of care for the patient with "graft versus host disease" post bone marrow transplant. *Canc Nurs 4*:191-198.

de Wit, H., de Wit, E.J.L. 1990. *Dag nul*. Westbroek, Netherlands: Stichting Columbine.

Dufoir, T., Saux, M.C., Terraza, et al. 1992. Comparative cost of allogeneic or autologous bone marrow transplantation and chemotherapy in patients with acute myeloid leukaemia in first remission. *BMT 10*:323-329.

Eddy, D.M. 1992. High dose chemotherapy with autologous bone marrow transplantation for the treatment of metastatic breast cancer. *J Clin Oncol 10*(4):657-670.

Eisenberg, S., Maracich, L. 1992. *Bone Marrow Transplant Standards of Nursing Care*. Seattle: Fred Hutchinson Cancer Research Center Nursing Department.

Ezzone, S.A., Camp-Sorrell, D. (Eds.) 1994. *Manual for Bone Marrow Transplant Nursing*. Pittsburgh: Oncology Nursing Press.

Flatau, A. 1995. BMT patients go online: finding information on the Internet. *BMT Newsletter 6*(2):4.

Ford, R., Eisenberg, S. 1990. Bone marrow transplant: recent advances and nursing implications. *Nurs Clin North Am 25*(2):405-422.

Ford, R.N., Kenny, S., Slevin, R. 1990. *Bone Marrow Transplantation Teaching Plan*. New York: Memorial Sloan-Kettering Cancer Center Division of Nursing.

Forman, S.J., Blume, K.G., Thomas, E.D. 1994. *Bone Marrow Transplantation*. Boston: Blackwell Scientific.

Frankel, W. 1995. To tackle their disease: getting support from cyberspace. *BMT Newsletter 6*(2):5.

Glaxo-Wellcome Pharmaceuticals, Gift of Life: Waiting for a Donor. Research Triangle Park, NC. (video)

Gratwohl, A., Hermans, J. 1994. Bone marrow transplantation activity in Europe 1992: report from the European Group for Bone Marrow Transplanation (EBMT). *BMT 13*:5-10.

Griffiths, R.I., Bass, E.B., Powe, N.R., et al. 1993. Factors influencing third party payer costs for allogeneic BMT. *BMT 12*:43-48.

Horowitz, M.M., Przepiorka, D., Champlin, R.E., et al. 1992. Should HLA-identical sibling bone marrow transplants for leukemia be restricted to large centers? *Blood 79*(10):2771-2774.

Hutchinson, M.Mc. (Ed.) 1983. Symposium on bone marrow transplantation. *Nurs Clin North Am 18*(3): 509-610.

Hutchinson, M.Mc., Itoh, K. 1982. Nursing care of the patient undergoing bone marrow transplantation for acute leukemia. *Nurs Clin North Am 17*(4):697-711.

IBMTR. 1995 *IBMTR Newsletter*. Milwaukee: Medical College of Wisconsin Statistical Center.

King, R.S., Wordell, C.J., Haupt, B.A. 1994. Pharmaceutical services and inpatient drug costs in bone marrow transplantation. *Am J Hosp Pharmacists 51*:1339-1344.

Lonergan, J.N., Kelley, C.H., McBride, L.H. 1994. *Homecare Management of the Bone Marrow Transplant Patient*. Northbrook, IL: Caremark.

Lynn, D. 1994. *Myself Resolved: An Artist's Experience with Lymphoma*. Philadelphia: Meniscus.

Mahaney, F.X. 1994. Bone marrow transplants for breast cancer: some insurers pay, some insurers don't. *J Natl Canc Inst 86*(6):420-421.

Mitchell, S.V., Smallwood, R.A., Angus, P.W., Lapsley, H.M. 1993. Can we afford to transplant? *Med J Australia 158*(1):190-194.

National Marrow Donor Program. 1995. *National Marrow Donor Program Standards,* 12th ed. St. Paul, Minnesota: NMDP.

Ohio BMT Consortium. 1992. *Ohio BMT Consortium Mission Statement.*

ONS. 1996. *Bone Marrow Transplant Nursing Resource Directory.* Pittsburgh: Oncology Nursing Press.

Peters, W.P., Rogers, M.C. 1994. Variation in approval by insurance companies of coverage for autologous bone marrow transplantation for breast cancer. *N Engl J Med 330*(7):473-477.

Petros, W.P., Peters, W.P. 1993. Cost implications of haematopoietic growth factors in the BMT setting. *BMT 11*(suppl 2):36-38.

Phillips, G., Armitage, J., Bearman, S., et al. 1995. American Society for Blood and Marrow Transplantation guidelines for clinical centers. *Biol Blood & Marrow Transplant 1*(1):54-55.

Rowe, J.M., Ciobanu, N., Ascensao, J., et al. 1994. Recommended guidelines for the management of autologous and allogeneic bone marrow transplantation: a report from the Eastern Cooperative Oncology Group. *Ann Intern Med 120*:143-158.

Shaffer, M.L. 1994. *Bone Marrow Transplants: A Guide for Cancer Patients and Their Families.* Dallas: Taylor Publishing.

Stewart, S. 1992. *Bone Marrow Transplants: A Book of Basics for Patients.* Highland Park, IL: Author.

Stream, P., Harrington, E., Clark, M. 1980. Bone marrow transplantation: an option for children with leukemia. *Canc Nurs 3*:195-199.

Stroncek, D., Bartsch, G., Perkins, H.A., et al. 1993. The National Marrow Donor Program. *Transfusion 33*(7): 567-577.

Understanding Your Bone Marrow Transplant: A Patient's Guide, 1993. Seattle: Immunex Corporation.

Understanding Your Bone Marrow Transplant: A Videotape for Patients, 1993. Seattle: Immunex Corporation.

University of Minnesota. A Critical Decision. Minneapolis, MN. (video)

Welte, K. 1994. Matched unrelated transplants. *Semin Oncol Nurs 10*(1):20-27.

Whedon, M.B. 1991. *Bone Marrow Transplantation: Priniciples, Practice, and Nursing Insights.* Boston: Jones & Bartlett.

Wikle, T. 1992. Implications of bone marrow transplantation. In Clark, J.C., McGee, R.F. (Eds.) *Oncology Nursing Society Core Curriculum for Oncology Nursing.* Philadelphia: Saunders, 359-370.

Wujcik, D. (Ed.) 1994. Advances in bone marrow transplant. *Semin Oncol Nurs 10*(1).

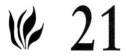

21

Nursing Research in Blood Cell and Marrow Transplantation

Mel R. Haberman

The modern era of blood cell and marrow transplantation (BCMT) nursing research is typified by more sophisticated and clinically relevant studies than any time in history. The steady growth of BCMT nursing research during the past decade can be attributed to several trends. One trend is a new spirit of cooperation among nurse clinicians and nurse scientists. Many practicing clinicians are conducting studies with the assistance of expert research mentors and it is becoming commonplace for nurse investigators to ask clinicians for help in designing studies. Clinicians can evaluate studies for clinical feasibility and potential to fill existing gaps in practice knowledge.

Another trend is the growing tendency of clinical nurses to be critical consumers of research. BCMT nurses are increasingly recognizing the narrow range of outcomes generated by medical transplantation research and, subsequently, are turning to their own discipline for answers. Many of the new generation of nurse scientists entering BCMT research have come directly from clinical practice, resulting in a marked improvement in the clinical relevancy of studies.

Another reason for the emergence of BCMT nursing research as a leading field of oncology nursing research is the current popularity of quality-of-life research. Nurse scien-

tists are leaders in this budding field of inquiry and many investigators have begun programs of research that address the quality of life of BCMT survivors.

Maintaining the momentum of progress will require new research initiatives. Investigators will need to find new mechanisms for conducting large-scale, multi-institutional BCMT nursing research and be creative in securing funding for it. Moreover, a theoretical foundation for BCMT nursing therapies must be conceptualized and tested using intervention and outcome-oriented research designs. If BCMT therapy is to remain a viable treatment option in the future, nursing research must unravel the intricacies of care and link nursing practice and the biopsychosocial outcomes of cancer therapy. We have yet to empirically answer the question, "What nursing therapeutics actually make a difference in the lives of BCMT recipients and their families?"

FOUNDATIONS FOR NURSING RESEARCH

Conceptual Foundations

Nurses researching and practicing BCMT nurses are fortunate to have a diverse and broad-based literature that is conceptually, if not empirically, strong. This body of nursing knowledge provides a beginning theoretical foundation for nursing therapeutics and future research. The literature gives us a snapshot of the developmental history of BCMT nursing. We are indebted to nurses who have taken the time to publish anecdotal, clinically based case histories; guidelines for practice; conceptual overviews; comprehensive reviews of the literature; teaching and documentation tools for nurses and caregivers; and research reports. Moreover, a milestone in the field occurred with the publication of Ezzone and Camp-Sorrell's manual (1994), with the impressive feature of is its attempt to identify and cite the research that supports each practice guideline.

The conceptual foundation that guides BCMT nursing practice is stronger than the existing empirical or research base for practice. Any review of the BCMT nursing literature will show that the number of research studies conducted by nurse investigators remains small when compared to the number of nursing publications in the field (Haberman, 1995a). It is a well-known fact that the current generation of BCMT nursing therapeutics is derived primarily from biomedical research or from other disciplines such as nutrition sciences, psychology, and dentistry (Winters et al., 1994). Our reliance on other disciplines to lend guidance to nursing practice will continue until a sufficient cadre of BCMT nurse investigators is in place to design and test specifically tailored nursing therapies.

Research Foundations

A rudimentary research base for practice is emerging in several areas. Out of a total of 222 BCMT papers published in nursing journals since 1982, 33 papers were empirical, research reports. Table 21.1 lists the topics of these studies, the number of publications by topic, and the investigators.

TABLE 21.1 BCMT nursing research studies organized by topic

Topics	Number of studies	Citations
Quality of life	5	Belec, 1992; Ferrell et al., 1992a; Ferrell et al., 1992b; Haberman et al., 1993; Whedon et al., 1995
Right atrial and central venous catheters	5	Keller, 1994; Kelly et al., 1992; Newman et al., 1984; Shivnan et al., 1991; Ulz et al., 1990
Pediatric issues	3	Mardsen, 1988; Tomlinson et al., 1993; Wood, 1990
Hope	2	Artinian, 1984; Ersek, 1992
Laminar air flow and reverse isolation	2	Collins et al., 1989; Zerbe et al., 1994
Meaning of BMT	2	Haberman, 1995b; Steeves, 1992
Mucositis and oral hygiene	2	Ezzone et al., 1993; McGuire et al., 1993
Cyclosporin regimens	1	Caudell and Adams, 1990
Dimensions of psychosocial nursing	1	Winters et al., 1994
Do-not-resuscitate orders	1	Kern et al., 1992
Graft-versus-host disease	1	Copel and Smith, 1989
Infection prevention measures	1	Poe et al., 1994
Informed consent	1	Carney, 1987
IV Immunoglobulin administration	1	Camp-Sorrell and Wujcik, 1994
Neurological complications	1	Furlong and Gallucci 1994
Nutritional assessment	1	Layton et al., 1981
Pain and psychological distress	1	Gaston-Johannson et al., 1992
Patient acuity	1	Lovett and McMillan, 1993
Symptom perception	1	Larson et al., 1993

As the table shows, quality of life and right atrial/central venous catheters are the most frequently studied topics. Only seven areas of practice have two or more published data-based papers on the same topic. The remaining empirical papers consist of a wide compilation of single studies. No studies were found that represent direct replications of previous research. However, multiple studies on a single topic can be classified as conceptual replication, since the same concept is studied repeatedly from the different vantage points of several studies.

In general, the use of descriptive or correlational designs, small samples, and cross-sectional or single-point-in-time measurement are the hallmarks of the first generation of BCMT nursing research. Only two studies that examined the use of right atrial/central venous catheters used prospective, longitudinal designs; randomized samples; and repeated measurement at several points in time (Shivnan et al., 1991; Ulz et al., 1990). These two studies were the only intervention studies found in the BCMT nursing journals.

In summary, although there is a beginning research base for some areas of practice, the empirical support for all fields of BCMT nursing is either minimal or nonexistent. New investigators should not be unduly worried about selecting a topic for study because every facet of nursing knowledge needs further research and empirical development. Virtually any topic listed in Table 21.1 can serve as a launching point for further investigation.

MECHANISMS FOR CONDUCTING NURSING RESEARCH

Research Conducted by Clinical Nurses

Although several options exist for building a scientific base for BCMT nursing, the present cadre of BCMT nurse researchers is too small to accomplish the research mission of the specialty. More researchers are needed from the ranks of BCMT clinical nurses, new post-master's degree and post-doctorate nurses, as well as senior nurse scientists.

Mechanisms are needed so that more clinical nurses can become involved in research, receive paid release time for research, and obtain research consultation from nurse scientists. At this level of clinical research, staff nurses can either conduct their own independent studies or tag a nursing study onto an existing medical protocol, often referred to as a companion study (Ferrell and Cohen, 1991). Because it is often unrealistic for clinicians to receive paid release time for research, it is advisable to conduct team projects, pool precious resources, and divide the work load. Each member of the team can write a different section of the research protocol or grant and be responsible for assembling the materials for that section (e.g., finding the instruments, preparing the consent form, and so forth). If members of the team are having trouble meeting their writing deadlines, a writing club can be started. Generally, writing clubs require each member to produce a few pages of text either every week or every other week. The members of the club set a realistic timeline for meeting their goals, read and critique each others' work, and keep themselves motivated to finish the project.

Most studies conducted by staff nurses will be small-scale feasibility or pilot studies that may realistically take a couple of years to complete. Most, if not all of these studies, should be designed with the intent of sharing the findings through publication or presentation. Funding for these types of projects may be obtained from many sources: the nursing department, local representatives of the pharmaceutical industry, or local chapters of the Oncology Nursing Society or Sigma Theta Tau International. National funding is available from many nursing specialty organizations. The Oncology Nursing Foundation has an exceptional record of funding small grants and BCMT nursing studies. It is mandatory to begin a new program of BCMT research with some form of feasibility or pilot investigation. Funding agencies like the National Center for Nursing Research, National Cancer Institute, and American Cancer Society will rarely, if ever, fund large grants without first seeing the preliminary data that support a new line of inquiry or that demonstrate a new investigator's track record.

Research Conducted by Undergraduate and Graduate Students

Another mechanism for facilitating BCMT nursing research is to actively recruit bachelor's, master's, and doctoral students and to create an atmosphere of critical inquiry in your setting. Clinically based nurses can go to schools of nursing and invite students to conduct their research in BCMT, suggesting topics for study that have been identified by staff nurses. Clinical nurses can become involved in the development of these student projects and, many times, the projects end up providing staff nurses with the information they need for practice. Students and postdoctorate fellows can be asked to be guest members of the unit's nursing research committee, if such a committee exists.

Many schools of nursing are looking for clinical sites for their baccalaureate nursing students to conduct a feasibility study for their required nursing research course. To fulfill this requirement and to give students the opportunity to be involved in a clinical nursing study, students can be teamed with staff nurses who need additional help with their studies. At the Fred Hutchinson Cancer Research Center, 16 baccalaureate nursing students worked on a half dozen nursing studies over 2 years. They helped staff nurses with literature reviews, locating instruments, data collection, analysis of data, writing up the findings and preparing manuscripts, and preparing research presenta-

tions for local, regional, national, and international conferences. Graduate student research interns also provide an invaluable source of expertise to staff nurses and clinically based nurse investigators. Moreover, research assistance can be obtained from research nurses who are hired specifically to carry out clinical trials for physician investigators.

Research Conducted by Nurse Scientists

External investigators who import their projects to a BCMT unit are generally willing to mentor staff nurses in the research process. Staff nurses can be formally appointed as a clinical mentor to the external researcher and the researcher can act as a research mentor in return. The clinical mentor can smooth the researcher's entry into the institution, teach the clinical realities of BCMT nursing, and critique the clinical feasibility of the researcher's proposed study. In return, staff nurses can negotiate a role in designing and implementing the research project and, many times, external researchers are willing to provide opportunities for staff to help with the preparation of manuscripts and to give presentations at conferences.

Expert Research Consultation

Blood cell and marrow transplantation nursing units should actively seek consultation from advanced nurse scientists by maintaining an ongoing recruitment campaign with local schools of nursing, other comprehensive and community cancer centers, and nursing specialty organizations or honorary societies. Two sources of expertise are the ONS Research Mentorship Program for Chapters and ONS Research Mentorship Program for individual members.

Generally, most nurse investigators provide consultation gratis. However, when extensive work is needed to design a study, pull together a grant application, or provide long-term consultation, it is customary to pay an honorarium or consultation fee. The amount of the honorarium can be negotiated with the nurse investigator. The Oncology Nursing Foundation has two types of special grants for novice researchers and ethnic minority researchers who need consultation and/or a mentor. These mentorship grants provide salary support for the beginning investigator and an honorarium for the research consultant.

Additional sources of expertise are available to BCMT nurses. Many nurse scientists are in private practice and gladly consult with clinical nurses. Many new postdoctorate fellows and mid-career faculty members are looking for clinical sites to start or expand their research program. Nurse scientists working in other agencies are often looking for a comparison sample for their studies. At this level of advanced research preparation, nurses are capable of writing large proposals that include funding for staff nurses to become involved in the research project. The American Cancer Society's Professors of Oncology Nursing are in many localities and are committed to advancing oncology nursing education and research in their communities. Moreover, it is easy to find out which nurse investigators in your community have received federal funding for oncology research by going on-line with the National Cancer Institute or National Center for Nursing Research. Federal funding agencies maintain listings of all publicly funded research on the Internet's World Wide Web. Medical libraries also can obtain this information for investigators who lack on-line access. Also, the Oncology Nursing Society's Research Department maintains a computerized database of research experts in BCMT and can provide these names to members, as well as the names of BCMT nurse investigators both previously and currently funded by the Oncology Nursing Foundation.

Multi-Institutional Research

Research will progress slowly and in a haphazard manner unless a mechanism is developed for multi-institutional oncology nursing research. Many clinical nurses are familiar with the multisite clinical trials conducted by the National Cancer Institute's cooperative research groups such as the Southwest Oncology Group (SWOG) or Eastern Oncology Group (ECOG).

Oncology nursing is ready to instigate its own national, cooperative research group. The Oncology Nursing Society has spent several years developing the infrastructure to facilitate multi-institutional nursing studies. Within a few years, BCMT nurses will be able to submit their research projects to ONS's cooperative group so their studies can be implemented at many BCMT sites across the country. A cooperative BCMT nursing research group will help to focus what is currently a highly fragmented field of research. Clearly, studies conducted in an extensive network of sites can recruit large and diverse samples and obtain data that is generalizable to diverse populations of patients and nursing units.

What is needed immediately is a consensus conference on BCMT nursing. A panel of experts, representing every facet of BCMT nursing, should be convened to identify the current state-of-the-science in BCMT nursing and to reach initial consensus on a national agenda for BCMT nursing research. This agenda would set forward a list of research priorities which, in turn, would guide fund raising for BCMT nursing research and the selection of high priority projects for multi-institutional study.

FUTURE DIRECTIONS FOR RESEARCH

The Role of Oncology Nursing Research

Future research will be precipitated by breakthroughs in transplantation biology, immunology, and genetics. For instance, the advent of new conventional and biological agents, the potential benefits of gene therapy, advances in hematopoietic reconstitution and the mobilization of stem and progenitor cells, and the as yet undiscovered frontiers of BCMT treatment, all hold great promise.

Clinical nursing research focuses on the human experience of wellness and illness and on the clinical therapeutics that are under the control of nurses. Common problems that have faced transplant recipients from the earliest days of bone marrow transplantation will be with us for the foreseeable future and will need ongoing investigation by nurses: acute and chronic graft-versus-host disease, regimen-related toxicities and pancytopenia following intensive chemoradiotherapy, life-threatening infections, and impaired quality of life and long-term survival, to name a few. Table 21.2 lists some additional fruitful lines of inquiry for future research.

TABLE 21.2 Future directions for BCMT nursing research

- Test new strategies to recruit women and ethnic minorities into BCMT clinical trials and to enhance compliance with aggressive therapeutic regimens, including long-term therapy for chronic graft-versus-host disease.
- Design and test new models for research dissemination and utilization.
- Define nursing outcomes both conceptually and empirically at all phases of BCMT therapy and for different types of transplants (e.g., blood cell vs. marrow, autologous vs. allogeneic, single vs. multiple, and unrelated donor).
- Conduct methodological research to obtain reproducible outcome data across multiple research sites (e.g., data on regimen-related toxicities, infection rates, patient safety issues, quality of life, early discharge, length of stay, readmission rates, direct and out-of-pocket costs of care, fatigue and pain intensity).
- Link models of nursing care delivery with clinical outcomes (e.g., models for critical pathways, case management, transition services, continuity of care, ambulatory care, home care, and managed care).
- Test the ability of patient acuity systems to predict nursing outcomes, staff ratios and mix, staff satisfaction and retention, staff psychosocial morbidity, patient safety, cost-containment measures, and quality improvement practices.
- Develop instruments to standardize clinical assessment (e.g., fatigue and pain scales, quality-of-life questionnaires, demands of BCMT transplantation, and multiorgan and multisystems toxicity scales).
- Test models of long-term follow-up and the role of nurses in monitoring chronic symptoms, educating patients and families, and providing specialty referrals.
- Identify caregiver issues (e.g., strategies for psychosocial support, educational needs, methods for monitoring the quality of care given by caregivers, and the long-range aftereffects of the caregiver's role).
- Explore ethical issues, the informed consent process, how information is given in family conferences, nurses' role in genetic counseling, the effect of advanced directives, and how treatment futility and end-of-life issues alter the delivery of care.
- Investigate the nursing therapeutics that support accelerated engraftment, less invasive procedures for progenitor cell collection, and allogeneic stem cell donation.
- Investigate the psychoneuroimmunologic nursing therapeutics that support allogeneic blood cell transplants, immunologically tailored grafts with large infusions of T lymphocytes and natural killer cells, and other new approaches to adoptive immunotherapy (Juttner et al., 1994).
- Examine the nursing therapeutics associated with leukapheresis for blood cell transplants, improved antiemetic therapies, advances in prophylactic antibiotic therapy, the use of cytokines or growth factors and monoclonal antibodies, and protocols of single or multiple courses of high-dose therapy or sequential therapy followed by blood cell transplantation.
- Explore the nursing therapeutics for pediatric and elderly populations of BCMT recipients and for managing the lingering complications of long-range survivorship.
- Conduct research on the psychosocial morbidity of BCMT nursing practice and methods of providing effective support to nurses.

Advances in BCMT nursing science will require investigators to explore the biopsychosocial and spiritual implications of both conventional cancer therapy and BCMT treatment. A greater emphasis will be placed on quantifying nursing outcomes and linking these outcomes to the caring behaviors and interventions of nurses. Although descriptive research is falling out of vogue in favor of intervention trials, there will remain a need to describe and explain the basic human responses to BCMT therapy. Rigorous descriptive research is a prerequisite to the fundamental understanding of concepts that is needed for subsequent intervention trials and outcome-oriented research. Nurse investigators also will be challenged to use multiple and more sophisticated research methodologies to build a solid theoretical foundation for BCMT nursing and our parent specialty, oncology nursing.

Research Collaborations and the Role of Nursing Specialty Organizations

Nursing specialty organizations that fund nursing research will play leading roles in facilitating the work of nurse scientists in the future. This support can be in the form of small grants, research mentorship grants and fellowships, and block grants to build programs of research excellence in cancer care settings. Emphasis will be given to funding BCMT research that involves collaborations between nurse scientists and clinical nurses and that seeks to build nursing knowledge through the conduct of large-scale, multi-institutional projects. The Oncology Nursing Foundation's Fatigue Initiative through Research and Education (FIRE Project™), funded by Ortho Biotech, Inc. (Raritan, NJ), gives all BCMT nurse investigators a model to follow in developing multi-institutional, collaborative projects.

Although there will always be a place for individual investigator-initiated projects, the future of BCMT nursing research must include new collaborative partnerships among nurse investigators. In the current era of federal cuts in funding for research and the emphasis on managed care and cost-containment, nurse researchers must look for novel ways to pool their resources and to maximize the scientific rigor and cost/benefit of their research programs. Existing individual initiated programs of research on a local or statewide level can now be taken to a national arena.

SUMMARY

As we move together into the next millennium and face an unforeseen future, nurses are confronted with the challenge of humanizing the technological breakthroughs that will undoubtedly occur in blood cell and marrow transplantation. Medical science will never provide nursing with the knowledge it needs for nursing therapeutics; it has enough challenges of its own. Our specialty must realize a philosophy of teamwork and a willingness of nurse clinicians, administrators, researchers, and educators to work together to achieve what remains an elusive goal. It is imperative that we anchor our BCMT nursing therapeutics in empirically derived knowledge, and that the best traditions of the art of nursing be embraced and given voice in the emerging science of nursing, while always keeping a clear vision of the ultimate goal—to improve the quality of life of persons with cancer and their families.

Acknowledgments

The author wishes to acknowledge the assistance of Kelli Wisdom in the preparation of this manuscript. Mel Haberman is an employee of the Oncology Nursing Society (ONS). ONS does not assume any responsibility for the content of this publication.

REFERENCES

Artinian, B.M. 1984. Fostering hope in the bone marrow transplant child. *Matern Child Nurs J* 13:57-71.

Belec, K. 1992. Quality of life: perceptions of long-term survivors of bone marrow transplantation. *Oncol Nurs Forum* 19:31-37.

Camp-Sorrell, D., Wujcik, D. 1994. Intravenous immunoglobulin administration: an evaluation of vital sign monitoring. *Oncol Nurs Forum* 21:531-535.

Carney, B. 1987. Bone marrow transplantation: nurses' and physicians' perceptions of informed consent. *Canc Nurs* 10:252-259.

Caudell, K.A., Adams, J. 1990. Cyclosporin administration practices on bone marrow transplant units: a national survey. *Oncol Nurs Forum* 17:563-568.

Collins, C., Upright, C., Aleksich, J. 1989. Reverse isolation: what patients perceive. *Oncol Nurs Forum* 16:675-679.

Copel, L.C., Smith, M. E., 1989. Oncology nurses' knowledge of graft-versus-host disease in bone marrow transplant patients. *Canc Nurs* 12(4):243-249.

Ersek, M. 1992. The process of maintaining hope in adults undergoing bone marrow transplantation for leukemia. *Oncol Nurs Forum* 19(6):883-889.

Ezzone, S., Camp-Sorrell, D. (Eds.) 1994. *Manual for Bone Marrow Transplant Nursing: Recommendations for Practice and Education.* Pittsburgh: Oncology Nursing Society.

Ezzone, S., Kapoor, N., Jolly, D., et al. 1993. Survey of oral hygiene regimes among bone marrow transplant centers. *Oncol Nurs Forum* 20(9):1375-1381.

Ferrell, B.R., Cohen, M.Z. 1991. Companion studies. *Semin Oncol Nurs* 7(4):252-259.

Ferrell, B., Whitehead, C., Grant, M., et al. 1992a. The meaning of the quality of life for bone marrow transplant survivors: improving quality of life for bone marrow transplant survivors. Part 2. *Canc Nurs* 15(4):247-253.

Ferrell, B., Whitehead, C., Grant, M., et al. 1992b. The meaning of the quality of life for bone marrow transplant survivors: improving quality of life for bone marrow transplant survivors. Part 2. *Canc Nurs* 15(3):153-160.

Furlong, T.G., Gallucci, B. B. 1994. Pattern of occurrence and clinical presentation of neurological complications in bone marrow transplant patients. *Canc Nurs* 17(1 Feb):27-36.

Gaston-Johansson, F., Franco, T., Zimmerman, L. 1992. Pain and psychological distress in patients undergoing autologous bone marrow transplant. *Oncol Nurs Forum* 19:41-47.

Haberman M.R. 1995a. Nursing research. In Buchsel, P.C., Whedon, M.B. (Eds.) *Bone Marrow Transplantation: Administrative and Clinical Strategies.* Boston: Jones & Bartlett, 365-402.

Haberman, M.R. 1995b. The meaning of cancer therapy: bone marrow transplantation as an exemplar of therapy. *Semin Oncol Nurs* 11(1):23-31.

Haberman, M., Young, K., Bush, N., et al. 1993. Quality of life of adult long-term survivors of bone marrow transplantation: a qualitative analysis of narrative data. *Oncol Nurs Forum* 10:1545-1553.

Juttner, C.A., Fibbe, W.E., Nemunaitis, J., et al. 1994. Blood cell transplantation: report from an International Consensus Meeting. *BMT* 14:689-693.

Keller, C.A. 1994. Methods of drawing blood samples through central venous catheters in pediatric patients undergoing bone marrow transplant: results of a national survey. *Oncol Nurs Forum* 21(5):879-884.

Kelly, C., McGregor, S.E., Dumenko, L., et al. 1992. A change in flushing protocols of central venous catheters. *Oncol Nurs Forum* 19(4):599-605.

Kern, D., Albrizio, M., Kettner, P. 1992. An exploration of the variables involved when instituting a do-not-resuscitate order for patients undergoing bone marrow transplantation. *Oncol Nurs Forum* 19(4):635-640.

Larson, P.J., Dibble, S.L., Viele, C.S., et al. 1993. Comparison of perceived symptoms of patients undergoing bone marrow transplant and the nurses caring for them (including commentary by Ersek, M.). *Oncol Nurs Forum* 20(1):81-88.

Layton, P.B., Gallucci, B.B., Akar, S.N. 1981. Nutritional assessment of allogeneic bone marrow recipients. *Canc Nurs* 4(2):127-135.

Lovett, R.B., McMillian, S.C. 1993. Validity and reliability of a bone marrow transplant acuity tool. *Oncol Nurs Forum* 20(9):1385-1392.

Marsden, C. 1988. Care giver fidelity in a pediatric bone marrow transplant team. *Heart & Lung* 17:617-625.

McGuire, D.B., Wingard, J.R., Altomonte, V. et al. 1993. Patterns of mucositis and pain in patients receiving chemotherapy and bone marrow transplantation. *Oncol Nurs Forum* 20(10):1493-1502.

Newman K. A., Schnaper, N., Reed, W.P., et al. Effect of Hickman catheters on the self-esteem of patients with leukemia *South Med J* 77:682-685.

Poe, S.S., Larson, E., McGuire, D., et al. 1994. A national survey of infection prevention practices on bone marrow transplant units. *Oncol Nurs Forum* 21(10):1687-1694.

Shivan, J.C., McGuire, D., Freedman, S., et al. 1991. A comparison of transparent adherent and dry sterile gauze dressings for long-term central catheters in patients undergoing bone marrow transplant. *Oncol Nurs Forum* 18:1349-1356.

Steeves, R.H. 1992. Patients who have undergone bone marrow transplantation: their quest for meaning. *Oncol Nurs Forum* 19(6):899-905.

Tomlinson, P.S., Tomczyk, B., Kirshbaum, M., et al. 1993. The relationship of child acuity, maternal responses, nurse attitudes and contextual factors in the bone marrow transplant unit. *Am J Crit Care* 2(3): 246-252.

Ulz, L., Peterson, F.B., Ford, R., et al. 1990. A prospective study of complications in Hickman right-atrial catheters in marrow transplant patiens. *J Parenteral & Enteral Nutr* 14:27-30.

Whedon, M., Sterns, D. and Mills, L.E. 1995. Quality of life of long-term adult survivors of autologous bone marrow transplantation (including commentary by Haberman, M.). *Oncol Nurs Forum* 22(10):1527-1537.

Winters, G., Miller, C., Maracich, L., et al. 1994. Provisional practice: the nature of psychosocial bone marrow transplant nursing. *Oncol Nurs Forum* 21(7) 1147-1154.

Wood, R.M. 1990. Growth patterns in pediatric bone marrow transplant patients. *J Pediatr Nurs* 5:252-258.

Zerbe, M.B., Parkerson, S.G., Spitzer, T. 1994. Laminar air flow versus isolation: nurses' assessments of moods, behaviors, and activity levels in patients receiving bone marrow transplants. *Oncol Nurs Forum* 21(3):565-568.

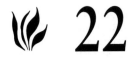

22

Ethical Issues
of Transplantation

Peggy Plunkett

Complex technology leads to ethical dilemmas. The natural lag time between the development of technology and addressing the ethical dilemmas that such technology causes can increase the stress to patients and their families, as well as to the staff involved in managing the technology. Such is the case with bone marrow transplants (BMT). Ethical dilemmas that have been identified include issues around informed consent, marrow donation, resuscitation, advanced directives, futility, allocation of resources, conception for donation, and new therapies.

INFORMED CONSENT

Selection of Patients

The first issue to be considered in the informed consent process is the selection of patients to be offered a BMT. Since this procedure is associated with considerable morbidity and mortality, clinicians debate whether to offer the procedure to patients, realizing that they may not do well. The types of patients who have been offered the choice of BMT is expanding as reduced treatment-related morbidity and mor-

tality have resulted from the use of growth factors and peripheral blood stem cells to restore hematopoiesis following intensive chemotherapy and radiation. Despite such improvement, selection of patients will remain an issue. Franco and Gould (1994) point out that "for those individuals (with acute lymphocytic leukemia) in their first remission, it is not clear whether BMT is the preferred treatment because standard chemotherapeutic regimens offer excellent survival rates." They also state that "controversy surrounds the use of allogeneic BMT in acute myelogenous leukemia patients in first remission" (Franco and Gould, 1994). Marsden (1988) noted this conflict among team members of a pediatric BMT team in a large university hospital. She performed an ethnographic study of team meetings which identified disagreements among the team of physicians and nurses about offering patients a BMT when the chance for a cure was low or when the chance for significant morbidity was high. Potential factors involved in whether a patient is offered a BMT include physician bias about aggressive therapy versus palliation, lack of objective eligibility criteria, and attraction to or identification with the patient and/or his or her family. These factors often contribute to staff discord because they are individualistic in nature, and staff groups often split on either side of the debate. Certainly, if objective and subjective screening eliminates a patient from a BMT, then remaining issues of informed consent are not relevant.

Adequacy of Information

Once the patient is selected to be offered a BMT, one important component of the informed consent includes adequate information. Much debate has occurred over what constitutes adequate information for any informed consent and those for BMTs are no exception. Nurses may not always be fully aware of what the patient has been told, because all nurses are not involved in this process. The consent process is often lengthy, and can occur over several appointments. So, the patient agrees to the procedure, starts the treatment, and then experiences complications or side effects. It is often at this point that they express to the nurse "no one told me it would be like this." Why is this? Was the informed consent faulty? Was the patient not told the information to begin with, did he or she not remember the information, or not appreciate the fact that it "could happen to me"? The nurse is now in the position of having to proceed with the procedure (without returning the hematopoietic stem cells, the patient will die) with a patient whom she or he might believe did not fully understand the dangers of this risky procedure. What are some explanations for how this situation could have developed?

One explanation is that people choose differently when faced with life-or-death decisions. The alternative to the BMT may be death from the disease. The BMT may offer the best chance for survival (or conversely the chance of a quicker death). It can therefore be argued that patients decide solely based on the life-or-death

options. Perhaps for this procedure, the morbidity issues such as those related to side effects are considered less than for procedures in which mortality plays a smaller part.

In a study by Silberfeld and colleagues (1988), 70 volunteers (half were law or medical students, half were lay people) were presented with a hypothetical situation in which they were to choose whether or not to have a BMT. The investigators provided these volunteers with a videotape of actual patients and staff describing the procedure and real patients' experiences. The overwhelming majority (87%) of the volunteers accepted BMT. While there was some exploration of the effect on their choices of the individuals' values about courage and logic as well as negative attributional style, it appeared to the authors that the life-or-death choice was the biggest motivator in the volunteers' decisions (Silberfeld et al., 1988).

Carney (1987) explored the experience of informed consent from the staff's perspective. The striking finding in interviews of BMT nurses (N = 16) and physicians (N = 5) was that the nurses most valued information being told to the patient about potential short- and long-term complications or the process of the procedure, whereas the physicians most valued information about the patient's diagnosis and options, or the outcome of treatment. Carney points out that patients based their decisions on life-or-death (outcome) issues, and suggested that nurses may need to reevaluate their own focus on the process of the treatment and acknowledge that for most patients the outcome of the treatment is most important in making their decisions.

Lesko and colleagues (1989) questioned 39 adult BMT patients, the parents of 61 pediatric BMT patients, and 7 oncologists about their experiences with informed consent. The top three reasons expressed by both adult patients and parents of pediatric patients for choosing the BMT was the "belief that treatment is a cure, fear that the illness will get worse without treatment, and trust in the physician" (Lesko et al., 1989). Most adult patients (95%) and parents (97%) remembered that there was the possibility of complications due to the procedure itself, however, they recalled fewer than half of the complications presented. The complications recalled most often were nausea and graft-versus-host disease/skin reaction. Interestingly, most of the patients and parents thought the content was adequate and not too technical, but the physicians involved thought it contained too much information and was too technical in nature. Although patients and parents thought they had freely expressed their doubts or concerns to the physician, they still withheld some questions. Physicians, on the other hand, thought most of them withheld their doubts and concerns. Almost all of the patients and parents ultimately thought the physicians wanted them to receive the BMT and relied on this advice to make their decisions. The physicians underestimated this reliance on their advice, although they did think that about half of the patients and parents wanted the physician to make the decision.

Lynch (1994) convened focus groups with nurses who worked with BMT patients to learn what they considered their key ethical issues. As in previous studies, nurses in this study struggled with the problems of informed consent for these patients, and were particularly affected when the outcome was bad (the patient suffered complications during the procedure, or died, or the cancer recurred).

Sebban and colleagues (1995) operationalized this debate by constructing a bedside decision-making board for patients who were contemplating BMT for chronic myeloid leukemia during the early phase of the disease. They included information on the procedures, morbidity and mortality at different times throughout the procedure, along with their respective probabilities of occurrence. They pretested the information offered by having 42 healthy volunteers use the board. These volunteers mostly rated the amount of information presented as "about right" (76.2%), but 10 volunteers (23.8%) believed that it was not sufficient. Much emphasis was placed on how decisions were made based on mortality rates. In this study, they adjusted the projected mortality rates to evaluate the point at which the volunteers would choose such a risky procedure. The volunteers shifted their decisions based on whether the BMT option or the chemotherapy option were presented as having the higher mortality rate. Obviously, the debate on the type of information to be presented in an informed consent discussion for BMT continues, but the importance of presenting clear information on mortality rates is gaining emphasis as clinicans appreciate its importance for the patients' decision-making process.

Quality of Life

Quality-of-life studies help to show us what patients experience after the BMT, and give us directions to tailor consent information. Many studies of patients who have had BMT indicate that patients believe their quality of life after the transplant is good (Bush et al., 1995; Hjermstad and Kaasa, 1995). Bush and colleagues (1995) studied 125 adults surviving 6 to 10 years after primarily allogeneic BMTs, although some had syngeneic or autologous BMTs. Eighty-eight percent said that the benefits of the BMT outweighed the side effects. They overwhelmingly (80%) rated their current health status and quality of life as good to excellent, and 74% of these long-term survivors of BMT rated their current quality of life as the same or better than before transplantation (Bush et al., 1995). The persistent complications and demands that they did experience were rated as causing them only a low amount of distress. Hjermstad and Kaasa (1995) reviewed the literature on quality of life for BMT patients, critiquing 48 studies. Although they had concerns about the methods of many of these studies (including the wide range of time since BMT, from 3 months to 5 years), they were impressed by the "consistency (of the) findings that most patients did remarkably well from a physical point of view, the dominating problematic areas being reduced stamina, sexual problems and work-related problems" (Hjermstad and Kaasa, 1995). They also found that, across studies, "many patients seemed to do well after treatment with BMT, . . . (with) up to 25% of the BMT survivors reported moderate to severe problems post-BMT." However, these results were not separated into those who were immediately out from their BMTs and those who were farther out. They speculated that separating this out would help develop appropriate therapeutic interventions (Hjermstad and Kaasa, 1995).

Interestingly, nurses do not necessarily understand the quality of life experienced by these patients. A study by King and colleagues (1995) compared BMT survivors' descriptions and evaluations of their quality of life with 150 BMT nurses' thoughts about this. The results showed that transplant nurses generally perceived patients as having a poorer quality of life than did the patients. With this discrepancy, it is of concern that most of the development of the information presented to prospective BMT patients is prepared by staff who may not rate the quality of life after BMT as actual BMT survivors report. Acknowledging that quality-of-life science is in its infancy, the experiences related by actual survivors should be incorporated into informed consent discussions with patients contemplating BMT.

Related issues that suface during quality-of-life studies concern serious long-term complications. Whedon and Ferrell (1994) reported on multiple problems, from simple, nondistressing ones to development of second cancers. They point out that some prognostic factors predict lesser or greater risk of development of these complications including type of transplant, total body irradiation, the patient's age when the BMT was done, and whether there was immunosuppressive treatment of chronic graft-versus-host disease. Certainly these serious long-term effects must be told to patients considering BMT. However, it would not be surprising if patients ignored much of this information while making their decisions, because the potential development would be far into the future and they might rationalize that their immediate survival and potential of cure from the current life-threatening disease was worth the chance of any long-term complication, even a second cancer.

Do-Not-Resuscitate Orders

Assisting the BMT patient to decide about whether he or she would want resuscitation is fraught with difficulties. Timing of the discussion, the meaning and understanding of the procedure, and the lack of clarity about outcomes of the procedure complicate this informed consent decision. Patients who are candidates for BMT are almost always facing life-threatening illness. If the BMT is not successful, they will die from their diseases. It seems logical that these patients would want to be spared the discomfort, psychological distress, and indignity that performing cardiopulmonary resuscitation (CPR) could cause. After all, it is unlikely that their demises would be due to a sudden life-threatening arrythmia, the situation in which CPR is most effective. This, however, is a strictly logical view, and doesn't take into account the potential reversible causes of cardiopulmonary arrest that might otherwise kill a BMT patient.

The logical viewpoint may be difficult for a patient who is proceeding with aggressive therapy in the hope of cure. Many patients have remarked to me that they "don't want to think about the downside" once they decide to have a BMT, almost as if they believe that thinking about death will magically cause it to happen, as if they could "jinx" the outcome in some way. This belief makes it very difficult for them to participate openly in an informed consent discussion about whether to perform CPR in the event of cardiopulmonary arrest. This same dynamic may affect some staff, who become reluctant to even bring up the subject with a patient, and may become angry with any other staff member who suggests it. This approach contributes to delaying the discussion of CPR until the patient deteriorates, often to the point where he or she cannot participate in the discussion. At this point, staff are left trying to have this difficult discussion with the family.

Another hesitancy of discussing CPR comes from the iatrogenic nature of some complications. Once the patient starts the BMT procedure, he or she is prone to many life-threatening problems. Sepsis and respiratory compromise may, in fact, be reversible, and warrant CPR for the patient until the cause of the deterioration is determined. Staff may feel extra responsibilty to treat aggressively when they believe that these problems are due to their interventions, not to the underlying disease. This is certainly true in the debate about whether patients who have decided against CPR should have that order rescinded during operative procedures. Jacobson (1994) describes that debate and two differing hospital policies and concludes that "decisions regarding do-not-resuscitate orders in the perioperative setting should be made on an individual basis." One could draw some parallels between the situation during surgery, where the procedures themselves could jeopardize the patient's life, and that of BMT, where the treatment can cause a patient to develop life-threatening problems. This issue only complicates the comfort

level of staff in bringing up the issue of CPR with BMT patients. Therefore, it is not surprising that the timing of a discussion of CPR with a BMT patient may be much later than some staff would like.

The difficulty of explaining the procedure of CPR to a patient makes its informed consent even more complicated. Staff often resort to words like "heroics," or "doing everything" when attempting this discussion. These words do not adequately explain to patients what CPR is, nor what it can and cannot do. Often, CPR is lumped in with care in the intensive care unit, including "being kept alive on machines." None of these explanations truly describe the components of CPR to a patient who is facing a life-threatening illness and procedure such as BMT. I have heard patients who believe that CPR will allow them to "live forever," as if you can stimulate a heart and keep someone alive when the rest of the organs are dying. It is not surprising, therefore, that this patient would want CPR, especially if already oriented toward the aggressive therapy of a BMT. However, it is incumbent on staff to attempt to explain the procedure of CPR in such a way that patients and their families understand what it can do and what it cannot do, even while realizing that some patients may still not believe the information.

A central problem with CPR for BMT patients is a lack of outcome data on whether CPR is useful. This is unclear for patients with cancer, let alone for those who are undergoing a BMT. Many authors report poor success with CPR for patients who have "metastatic cancer" (Brown, 1990; Faber-Langendoen, 1991) or "widely metastatic cancer for which the patient is not receiving active therapy" (Alpers and Lo, 1995) or "bedfast metastatic cancer" (Murphy and Finucane, 1993). However, it is unknown whether these authors considered patients for whom their metastatic cancer may be being treated with a BMT. Kern and colleagues

(1992) studied 42 patients who died on a BMT unit, 36 of whom were designated do-not-resuscitate (DNR), and 6 (5 allogeneic BMT, 1 autologous BMT) of whom received CPR. The purposes of this study included identification and comparisons of the variables in patients who had a BMT where DNR was chosen with those in BMT patients where CPR was attempted. "The non-DNR group developed life-threatening complications early in their transplant course as compared to the DNR group" (Kern et al., 1992). Unfortunately, the type and number of organ system(s) failure was not known for the non-DNR group, although "their cause of death identified at autopsy, was primarily infectious (N = 5)" (Kern et al., 1992). This data might have been a start at identifying risk factors for poor outcome in critically ill BMT patients. Kern and colleagues speculated that the non-DNR patients, who died earlier in the course of treatment than the DNR patients, might not have had time to come to terms with their rapid deterioration (and we could speculatively include the staff as well) and therefore did not have time to decide not to have CPR. However, they did not report on patients who might have received CPR and survived, so that we do not have outcome data on that potential group. Without outcome data specific to use of CPR in BMT patients, it is difficult to advise patients on whether this procedure could be beneficial. This problem certainly adversely affects informed consent discussions about CPR with BMT patients.

Transfer to Critical Care Units

A special type of informed consent dilemma is inherent in the decision about whether a BMT patient should go to an intensive care unit (ICU). These patients have a high potential of life-threatening complications during BMT, some of which (e.g., sepsis and respiratory distress) may require ICU care. Usually the devel-

opment of these complications occurs rapidly, and the patient may quickly become incapable of fully participating in the decision about whether to treat in the ICU. One solution would be to discuss this possibility early on with all candidates while describing the BMT procedure. However, this may be difficult, as mentioned before, because patients usually can only pay attention to life-and-death information about the transplant (specifically, whether the BMT has a chance of curing the disease). They might not fully comprehend the seriousness of making a decision about ICU at that time. Clinicians may also despair at having to predict such a dire outcome related to the treatment itself. However, waiting until the patient is developing the complication carries its own problems; the patient with sepsis or respiratory distress may not be cognitively capable of understanding the complexity of information. Also, most patients who have never been to the ICU do not appreciate the discomforts and distressing procedures typical of an ICU stay. They are often simply told euphemistic terms such as *heroics,* and *do you want everything done* when discussing a potential ICU stay. This is not clear enough information upon which to base a decision (Shedd and Whedon, 1991).

Patients need to know that ICU stays for cancer patients, and particularly BMT patients, may not carry good survival outcomes. The term *may* is used because outcomes data are lacking on cancer patients in the ICU (Crawford, 1991; Shedd and Whedon, 1991), let alone BMT patients. Some authors are starting to report APACHE II data for cancer patients. APACHE II (acute physiologic and chronic health evaluation) is a disease classification system that takes data about a variety of basic physiological parameters to predict which patients will survive an ICU stay. Abbott and colleagues (1991) collected retrospective APACHE II data on 451 ICU oncology admissions. These patients represented many types of cancer, with

29.5% having primary lung cancer and 68% with secondary organ involvement. They found that admissions to the ICU were most likely due to respiratory problems, and then second most likely for cardiovascular problems. Almost half of the patients died in the hospital (49.9%). Patients with APACHE II scores of 35 or greater (whether surgical or nonsurgical patients) had very high probabilities of dying (92% and 100%, respectively) (Abbott et al., 1991). It is unlikely that any of these patients were BMT patients since this study was performed in a community hospital. However, their data do support that the use of established prognostic methods, such as the APACHE II system, might help provide outcomes' predictions for some patients with cancer, and possibly BMT patients. However, Honegger (1991) points out that the APACHE system must include an evaluation of the underlying disease, and that a "cancer patient with no evidence of his (former) disease or who is under intensive therapy with intent to cure is entitled to vigorous support for acute medical problems." This would surely apply to BMT patients who are all hoping for cure and may, therefore, be appropriate for intensive care. Shelton (1994) reviewed a number of studies of critical care usage for BMT patients, and states that "poor prognostic variables for survival are older age, active malignancy at the time of BMT, and an HLA mismatched allogeneic transplant." This data does not lend itself to being specific enough to help predict with much certainty which BMT patient will do well in the ICU and which will not.

Therefore, clinicians are still left with less than perfect ability to predict outcomes of ICU stays for BMT patients (Crawford, 1991; Shedd and Whedon, 1991). However, even imperfect information is more than was previously available and should be incorporated into informed consent discussions with patients who are facing ICU stays. Patients may opt out of a grueling and distressing ICU stay if the projected outcome is poor, and instead decide on palliative care with family at their sides in an environment that is less distressing than an ICU. Other patients may decide on ICU stays for the same reasons that they decided on a BMT, namely, they want to live at any cost. Both choices are reasonable, as long as the patient is truly informed to the best of our current knowledge. This knowledge will change, however, as more outcomes information becomes available, and as supportive care for BMT patients continues to improve.

Yet another complication in deciding whether BMT patients should go to the ICU is that many of these patients may have chosen to be DNR due to the life-threatening nature of the illness that led them to the BMT. Some hospitals have had informal or even formal policies restricting DNR patients from ICU care. Although these policies are controversial, the practice continues. In these situations, BMT patients who have bravely confronted the life-threatening nature of their underlying illnesses, have benefited from a good patient-physician relationship so that a difficult subject could be discussed and chosen DNR, may be penalized. The presence of a DNR order does not predict whether the BMT patient is a good candidate for ICU, and therefore should not be considered in a blanket policy related to admission for care.

The American Nurses' Association (1995) states "a DNR order is separate from other aspects of a patient's treatment and there should be no implied or actual abandonment of other types of treatment for patients with DNR orders, which should continue to be evaluated on a burden versus benefits basis." However, this objective stance may be difficult for critical care staff who remember struggling and failing to save a BMT patient who was designated DNR, or the staff who would prefer to see the patient spend his or her last hours or days in a more comfortable and dignified setting than can often be achieved in the ICU.

Pediatric Consent

Informed consent is more complicated with pediatric patients because of their intellectual development. The same issues about the types of information presented to adults apply to children. An additional factor is the child's capacity to comprehend the information. Abramovitz and Senner (1995) point out that information must be explained to children in an "age-appropriate manner." Parents may then need to have a separate meeting to hear more detailed information. Although the parent legally makes the decision, the Academy of Pediatrics believes that "assent (e.g., agreement to participate) must be obtained from children who are intellectually seven years of age or older" (Abramovitz and Senner 1995). This extra "assent" step, however, increases the ethical problems because clinicians may not agree about the type, amount, or delivery of information presented to the parent or to the child. Debate about the information presented to adults is frequent enough without adding the issue of determining the appropriate developmental level of the child. However, it is important that this be attempted, and that the team reach consensus.

Nurses' Concerns

It is understandable that nurses, who grapple with first protecting the patient from the complications and then with promoting the recovery from those complications, would be very concerned with patients' awareness of these problems. Perhaps this is an attempt on the nurses' parts to deal with their own guilt at being part of the process that induces such pain and suffering in these patients. It is logical that one could feel less guilty if the patient were aware of these risks and yet still chose such

risky and uncomfortable treatment. However, the intensity of the life-or-death choice may preclude the ability or interest of a patient to dwell on the process of getting to that end. Carney (1987) therefore poses the challenge that nurses should "work at tailoring the information we disclose to the needs of the patient and not feel that one has failed as a professional because the patient is not completely informed." This advice may assist individual staff to reconcile their frustrations at the informed consent procedure and also decrease interstaff accusations of providing inadequate information, or providing information "too late."

DONOR ISSUES

Donor Autonomy and Confidentiality

Issues of marrow donors addressed include confidentiality, informed consent, and the psychological adjustment of donors, as well as the new issue of conception in order to provide a donor. A case discussed by Caplan and colleagues (1983) explores the dilemma presented when knowledge was acquired by a potential BMT recipient of the existence of a possible matching donor. The dilemma arose because the donor had been tested only because of a family member's need and was not on a public, easily accessible list. The donor was contacted and informed of a general request to donate, and refused to participate. The potential recipient remained unaware of the identity of the donor, but requested that she be contacted again and informed of the specific request, hoping it would persuade her to help him. Obviously, the confidentiality of the donor was at odds with the principle of beneficence, or promoting good, to the potential recipient. The merits, pro or con, of disclosure revolve around the ability of an unrelated transplant to succeed (benefit of the procedure to the recipient versus harm from donating marrow to the donor), coercion of the donor, autonomy of the donor to refuse to donate marrow, as well as the confidentiality of the donor.

These issues are also described in a case study of an 8-year-old sister and donor to a 6-year-old boy with neuroblastoma (Kinrade, 1987). In this case, confidentiality of the donor was not the issue, but coercion and autonomy of the sister to refuse to donate was certainly an issue, complicated by her naive understanding of the procedure and developmental immaturity in understanding the overall ramifications of acceptance or refusal to donate. The same parent's consent was required for both the donor and the recipient, which creates further complications to informed consent. Another case concerning a child donor was described by Fruchtman and colleagues (1993). Similar issues were raised, but in this case, the donor was only 4½ years old and had already donated once to his brother. Younger donors carry more risk than do adults, both for the general anesthesia and because they are unable to donate blood for themselves, so can become profoundly anemic when their bone marrow is harvested. This increased risk further complicates the informed consent process, and choice of a young child for donor. They (Fruchtman et al., 1993) also describe another case in which the adult HLA-identical sibling donor was institutionalized with chronic schizophrenia. They speculated as to whether she would understand what being a marrow donor meant, and furthermore, whether she would be a reliable donor since once the procedure of the BMT occurred, the sick sibling would die without her marrow.

A similar issue was raised by the story of a patient with chronic granulocytic leukemia whose potential donor was a profoundly retarded 28-year-old sister who was "mentally handicapped to the point that she remains like a 6-week-old baby" (Anonymous, 1992). In this case the mother was the sister's legal guardian, and was legally able to consent for the sister to be a bone marrow donor. The hospital's ethics committee became involved and reviewed the case. It was decided that the mother had "every moral and legal right to make the decision for (my) sister." This patient was very impressed with the process and advocates having the ethics committee available whenever there is doubt. These examples are dramatic, but they are not unique and illustrate the dilemma of informed consent for even a relatively simple procedure such as a bone marrow donation.

Effects of Donation

Donating marrow may seem like a small risk relative to the issues facing the recipient of the marrow, but donors should not be ignored. The risky nature of the transplant for the recipient should, in fact, increase our interest and concern for the welfare of the donor. If the donor's experience is negative, it is difficult to promote such a risky procedure as BMT. Risk to the donor has been viewed as mainly psychological; the physical harms are minimal. Most concern has focused on the adverse psychological situation a donor may be in if the recipient experiences serious complications that cause suffering or even death. The ultimate concern is graft-versus-host disease in which the donor's marrow actually rejects the patient and can cause intense discomfort and even death. In a bizarre sense, the donor could actually perceive her "gift of life" to, paradoxically, become the instrument of death (Rappaport, 1988; Wolcott et al., 1986).

Staff become involved if the donor is a member of the patient's family who is present during the patient's hospitalization. Staff may feel a special need to reward and support the donor, whose psychological health may vary according to the patient's physical status. Concern may also be felt about the potential for coercion in the donor's choice, especially if the patient's outcome is poor. Wolcott and colleagues (1986) explored this issue in a questionnaire of 18 donors. They found few reports of ambivalence about donating, and all said they would donate again if asked. There was little emotional distress associated with the donation despite some reported negative consequences if the recipient deteriorated. However, this study looked at donors of marrow to surviving recipients. Therefore, although staff probably do not need to be overly concerned about coercion in this group, the issue of the donor's suffering if the recipient deteriorates is another potential stressor. Supporting family is difficult for the busy, involved BMT staff. It could be even more difficult if the family included the donor who stands by helplessly watching her loved one deteriorate as a result of receiving her marrow.

New Challenges in Donation

Finding an appropriate donor has created the interesting dilemma of parents who choose to conceive a child so that that child's marrow could be donated to another child. In one case, a couple's 17-year-old daughter needed a BMT to cure her otherwise fatal leukemia. No compatible donor had been found, so the couple chose to reverse the husband's vasectomy in order for the wife to become pregnant with the 25% chance that the baby would match. Many people were outraged. How dare this couple conceive simply to bear a child whom they as parents of a minor child, had the legal ability to force to donate its marrow? This case received national publicity and inspired much public and scholarly debate. Some went so far as to speculate that this "could be the newest form of child abuse—and we're by no means ready to

cope with it" (Curtin, 1990). Similar requests prompted Alby (1992) to speculate that the next step would be HLA typing in utero, and he wondered whether it is ethical for the clinician to propose it. The obvious leap from that idea is the request made to physicians from a couple who wanted to have prenatal diagnosis in order to be ensured that the fetus the wife was carrying was HLA identical to their son who suffered from Wiskott-Aldrich syndrome and needed a BMT. They intended to abort fetuses that were not HLA compatible (Clark et al., 1989). These physicians chose not to perform HLA testing, although they would offer prenatal testing for the disorder to allow the parents to know whether a second chid could carry this dread disease.

Another case was illustrated by an example of parents who might choose to conceive to have a child from whom cord blood could provide a stem cell transplant for another child. They point out that they already inform any pregnant mothers of leukemic children that "the cord blood can be easily stored and cryopreserved for a possible graft in case of relapse" (Schaison, 1992).

Many people are horrified by the issues raised by these and similar cases. However, some ethicists argue that what these families are doing is not wrong. Zucker (1992), in analyzing the first case, points out that couples already have many reasons for having children, some of which are clearly selfish, such as parents desiring a child who will fulfill their dream to become a sports star. The desire to have a child in order to save the life of another child may be considered selfish of the parents but could also be considered a parental duty to the other child. Is the danger to the conceived child sufficient to make a determination that the risks outweigh the benefits? Will the risk that the parents might love the second child less be any greater than that risk for any other child conceived for less publicly stated reasons? Zucker also proposes that, in fact, this couple's privacy was wrongly invaded by the ethicists who publicly debated the issue! Downs (1994) believes that "the real issue . . . may not be whether the act can be labeled right or wrong, but how it is viewed by the BMT team," stressing that similar dilemmas will occur as technology continues to expand and options become available to patients for transplantation that we can now hardly imagine. Whether we view these desperate requests as right or wrong, it is incumbent on health-care providers to appreciate the dilemmas that they pose and prepare to understand the full aspects of the related ethical decision making.

ADVANCED DIRECTIVES

Advanced directives, commonly referred to as *living wills* or *durable powers of attorney* (DPOA) for health care, are recognized in almost all states as legally binding. However, the public's knowledge about these documents was sharply increased as a result of the 1990 passage of the Patient Self-Determination Act (Omnibus, 1990), which requires that all health-care institutions receiving Medicaid or Medicare funds inform and educate their patients about these documents and their rights to formulate and use them in their care (ANA, 1995).

One could naively assume that these documents would help deal with some of the issues about CPR and ICU stays mentioned earlier. Many times, that does happen. Certainly, the fact that a staff member does not have to bring up a difficult subject for the first time because the patient already has a living will or DPOA makes the discussion occur much sooner than it might otherwise. However, there remains some concern, even with the presence of advanced directives. The patient may not totally under-

stand what the advanced directive does or does not mean. In a study by Hague and Moody (1993), nearly 60% of their elderly, well-educated sample had "a good deal of confusion regarding living wills," even though 20% of their sample had attended educational offerings about advanced directives. Other, less educated people may understand even less. If the relatively healthy general public does not understand these documents, those under the stress of appraching BMT are even less likely to appreciate their ramifications.

Living wills have some drawbacks to their usefulness in BMT. They usually become effective only when a patient is terminally ill or in a persistent vegetative state, which may not be the case even though a BMT patient is incapable of participating in complex treatment decisions. It may also be difficult to define when the patient's state has changed from a treatable to a terminal situation, especially with acute onset of life-threatening emergencies such as sepsis. Just as staff may be reluctant to talk about DNR orders or ICU stays, they may be reluctant to accept that a BMT patient is in a terminal state and a living will would apply. In that case, the existence of a living will does not ensure its use. The items listed in a living will may also be too limited or too general to help guide staff in making decisions for a BMT patient. Living wills are written by lawmakers and lobbied for language by the public who do not appreciate that terms such as *heroics* or *life-sustaining* do not describe procedures in ways that are precise enough to guide practice. However, when the language is made more specific, it may become too narrow to apply to the actual situation confronted by the BMT patient. All of these issues greatly limit the effectiveness of living wills for BMT patients.

Many people think that a DPOA for health care is more advantageous than a living will because it allows more complex situations to be processed than could possibly be included in a living will. It also becomes effective any time a person is incapable of participating in the decsion-making process, rather than the narrower definition of the living will (e.g., terminal or vegetative state). This would certainly be of use during a BMT, because the patient may rapidly become delirious from sepsis or medications. However, some surrogates admit that they do not know what their loved one would have chosen; the situations that come up during a BMT are not ones that the average layperson may even realize could occur. Even for situations that people expect, it can be difficult to feel confident that the surrogate is knowledgeable about their loved ones' choices.

Libbus and Russell (1995) asked 30 patient-surrogate pairs to respond to vignettes of five treatments (ventilation, CPR, chemotherapy, amputation, tube feeding) and choose which treatments the patient would want. They found agreement between the pairs 60% to 77% of the time. The treatments that created the most disagreement were chemotherapy and amputation, with the surrogate more likely to opt for the care that the patient would refuse. The pairs were also asked to decide which criteria they ranked as most important to the decision making, and they both ranked "likelihood of survival" as the top choice (patients = 67%, surrogates = 57%). However, there was a discrepancy regarding "pain," which was chosen by only 3% of patients as the most important criterion, but by 20% of the surrogates. Although these results could comfort us that surrogates may well know what their loved ones would want, it is of concern that surrogates ranked pain much higher than did patients. How many times have we observed a family member's anguish at the pain that a treatment or disease was causing their loved ones? Would that anguish impair their ability to act as surrogate decision maker during a BMT, when infections and other etiologies can cause great discomfort for patients? Obviously, the concerns continue about the usefulness of advance directives for BMT patients.

FUTILE CARE

The literature concerning futile care, or futility, is increasing rapidly. It is important to be clear about what is meant by the term *futile*. Futile care is not the same as care that is not cost-effective. Determining futility for a patient should not be looked at as helping to allocate scarce resources or forming a basis for cost-control measures. Many authors define *futility* in two ways—by quantitative definitions and by qualitative definitions. Waisel and Truog (1995) summarize these definitions as follows: "Quantitative assessments place a percentage value on the likelihood of something occurring, whereas qualitative assessments define the worth of what may be achieved." For example, Jecker and Schneiderman (1993) propose one method of determining quantitative futility as "a treatment (that) can be shown not to have worked in the last 100 cases." Curtis and colleagues (1995) give an example of qualitative futility as "CPR might be effective in sustaining life, but the quality of life falls well below the threshold considered minimal by general professional judgment."

Many institutions are now forming policies condoning withdrawing or withholding futile care (Waisel and Truog, 1995; Hudson, 1994; Murphy and Barbour, 1994); several states, including New York (Bennett, 1993) and Virginia (Paris, 1993), have directed laws toward this issue. Many professional societies including the American Medical Association, the American Thoracic Society, and the Society for Critical Care Medicine (Jecker and Schneiderman, 1993) are also making statements about guidelines allowing physicians to withhold futile care. How would policies related to futile care affect BMT patients? Issues include the debate about definitions of futile care as well as determining who would make the decision that a treatment would be futile.

Are there problems with instituting policies and laws regarding futile care for BMT patients? One problem occurs with the definitions themselves. Quantitative definitions are not precise, and qualitative definitions require a judgment about values that may or may not fit the patient's values. Van McCrary and colleagues (1994) surveyed 301 physicians, including residents from the second year of residency and higher and attendings, and asked them to determine first the percentage of success that one could expect from a treatment. In other words, if a treatment was successful 15% of the time, the physician would rate it at 15% "success rate." Second, they were asked to define at what percentage of success they would consider a treatment to be futile. Somewhat surprisingly, the range was from 0% to 60% success, and almost 19% defined futility to be at a 20% or higher success rate! That means that some of the physicians would have labeled a treatment as futile even if up to 60% of the time it was successful! It is easy to imagine many BMT-related treatments that would fit that category.

Curtis and colleagues (1995) interviewed internal medicine residents within 1 week after one of their patients had received a DNR order. For the 75 patients whom the residents believed a quantitative futility argument could be applied, they were asked to predict the probability that the patients would survive to discharge, if they had been full-code patients. These residents speculated that between 0 (for 60% of the patients) and 30% (for 1% of the patients) could have survived (e.g., the CPR would not have been futile by a quantitative definition). For 32% of the patients, survival was predicted at 5% or more. These physicians clearly did not understand the concept of quantitative futility. They would determine many BMTs as futile, because the success rate for some BMTs falls

below 20%, and many fall below 60%. Also, the residents studied by Curtis and colleagues (1995) determined qualitative futility to apply for 61 of the patients. However, the residents only discussed quality of life with 65% of the patients who could communicate. How could they have determined a qualitative definition of futility without obtaining input from the patients? How many times have staff been surprised at a BMT patient who chooses to endure treatment that the staff believe significantly impairs his or her quality of life, but is worth it to the patient?

The danger in these definitions is in both the imprecise way they can be used, and the potential for health-care teams to assume they know the patients' views on what is acceptable quality of life (King et al., 1995). The concern about the imprecise way that the definition of futile care can be used is heightened in the field of BMT, where what may be considered futile today is considered standard therapy tomorrow. This rapidly changing field of knowledge is difficult for health-care providers to impose on their quantitative definition of futile care, let alone for laypeople like BMT patients or their surrogates to include in determining their individual qualitative definitions.

There has also been much debate about who should determine whether a treatment is considered futile. One method proposes that the patient and his or her family/surrogate make the decision. This raises several problems for BMT patients. One is related to whether the patient has adequate knowledge of or is involved in the decision. Most policies involve at least informing the patient of the decision, and some that the patient consent to the determination, but some do not (Waisel and, Truog 1995; Hudson, 1994; Murphy and Barbour, 1994). If the patient is not informed of a decision that treatment (such as the BMT itself or a component of supportive care within the BMT such as antibiotics, blood products, or CPR) will be withheld, is that a problem? After all, patients are not informed of other treatments considered futile such as a kidney transplant or emergency heart surgery for a thrombocytopenic and/or neutropenic patient. However, many health-care personnel would be shocked at the thought that patients who are normally so well informed (sometimes verging on overinformed) would not be informed about treatments that are often taken for granted in BMT units. Then, if the patient is informed, what if she disagrees with health-care providers about the definition of futile? Do they have the right to demand treatment, even if health-care providers deem it futile? It seems antithetical to determine that a treatment has no chance of success (quantitative futility) and yet allow the patient to demand it (except that is the current practice with CPR in some instances). Resolution of this dilemma by assisting a patient to switch to a physician or institution that will agree with her choice of futile care begs the question of defining futility. After all, if care is truly futile it does not become acceptable by switching location or provider. In that case, treatment becomes torture, and health-care providers can slip into the ethical trap of maleficence, or doing harm to patients, rather than the ethical principle of beneficence, or promoting good. However, many current and proposed policies on futile care require that a health-care team ensure that the patient's choice will be carried out even if futile.

Others argue that decisions about futile treatments could be determined basically by the health-care team, rather than by the patient or surrogate. One example of such a decision for a BMT patient is that of CPR. If the patient's condition would no longer respond to CPR, then, some argue, physicians could choose not to resuscitate the patient, just as they choose not to give a BMT patient a heart transplant or a liver transplant, if his or her condition does not warrant such treatment. Many people argue that this would allow CPR to be dealt with

more similarly to all other treatments, rather than the current method of assuming all patients should receive CPR unless the patient (rather than the health-care team) chooses not to. Other treatments that require decision making by the BMT patient to discontinue even when the health-care team deems them futile, include antibiotics and blood products. One could envision a futile care policy that allowed the health-care team to make those decisions as well. This could save patients from prolonged suffering and allow staff to provide palliative care earlier, as well as supporting staff who sometimes feel like they are torturing patients with treatments that seem doomed to fail. Also, it might spare surrogates the distressing belief that it was their decision to withhold or withdraw therapy that killed the patient, rather than the inevitable process of the disease state.

Taylor summarizes the debate about who should decide if a treatment is futile in one of three ways. One way is similar to that posed above, with the patient/surrogate deciding all except (she adds) "physiologic futility" (Taylor 1995). However, adding this qualifier itself creates a problem since the definition of futile care (even the quantitative definitions) is so difficult. Another way she describes would be that health-care providers would decide, and a third would be that there be shared decision making, which she calls "mediated compromise" (Taylor, 1995). She points out some of the same pros and cons listed earlier, and concludes that the "mediated compromise" method would work best, instead of "any (one) person or group asserting their primacy of authority" (Taylor, 1995). Although seemingly reasonable, and on first look a great way to resolve the debate, there are certainly circumstances where there can be no compromise between the wishes of the BMT patient/surrogate and those of the health-care providers. When such polarization occurs, there may be no middle ground that is comfortable for both sides, even with the best of mediation. That is always the struggle with any policy— there is often some individual whose wishes are not met by the policy.

One can also envision that futile care policies could create *more* disagreements and stress among health-care personnel, who may not agree with each other's timing or definitions, than does the current lack of clarity. Just as BMT nurses now struggle with situations in which they believe the patient would be better off with a palliative approach, in opposition to the beliefs of other team members, there could be problems with futile care policies that could deny therapies currently provided. However, one could also argue that having a policy or a law would at least sanction and even force needed discussion about such a complex issue.

ALLOCATION OF SCARCE RESOURCES

The ethical dilemma of allocation of scarce resources arises with procedures such as bone marrow transplantation that represent current high-cost technology. Staff are faced with specific issues of resource allocation each time a potential transplant patient is turned away due to lack of funds. Kelleher (1994) reports the bills for the transplant hospitalization as well as "appropriate follow-up out-patient care" to be $70,000 to $135,000 for autologous transplants (both peripheral and bone marrow), $185,000 to $225,000 for allogeneic, and $200,000 to $250,000 for unrelated transplants, although this may change soon as new medications and techniques allow patients to receive a higher proportion of outpatient care. However, Downs (1994) believes that personal costs for patients and their families can add to this up to 60% of the total cost of the BMT. Obviously, few patients can pay for this without insurance. However, prepaid insurances such as health maintenance organizations,

state/federal public insurances such as Medicaid, and some managed care insurances are evaluating the benefits against the financial costs of such procedures and many are denying funding in what Peters and Rogers (1994) describe for breast cancer patients as "arbitrary and capricious." Some states have limited the expenditure of public health funds for BMT (Robinson, 1989).

It is difficult for staff involved with specific potential recipients to accept these decisions about resource allocation. Policy decisions have to be made for a group of people, whereas health-care providers take care of and get to know individual patients. Reconciliation of these two viewpoints is difficult. However, these decisions may become more common as health-care dollars become more scarce. Kelleher (1994) points out that "there is little research to evaluate cost-effectiveness and the cost-benefit ratio." Most transplant staff have experienced the pain of this principle of justice as they watched a leukemia patient well known to them be judged ineligible for transplant because of lack of funds. They now face this issue with patients who could be candidates for the more investigational protocols but are refused by their insurance companies. This happens not only in the United States, but also in countries with national health-care systems (Lie, 1994).

However, at least in the United States, this grief for staff may be much more poignant than the grief of the death of a patient who chooses not to have a transplant for nonfinancial reasons, because it points out the current conflict of whether patients and health-care providers or external authorities choose what treatments are appropriate for an individual. This conflict could leave the health-care providers with some ambivalence or even anger about the ways that the decision was made, and thus create greater grief if the patient dies. It remains important to evaluate the costs of this treatment as well as the outcomes in order to more fully address this issue at the health policy and funding levels. Staff should become involved in policy-making committees at the local, state, and national levels in order to become informed as well as to portray accurately the experience of bone marrow transplantation for these layperson committees. Insurance companies must be lobbied by professionals with information, not just by patients with hopes. Issues of justice will continue to gain in prominence in the ethical decision making as it relates to bone marrow transplantation.

NEW THERAPIES

Improved techniques and medications are reducing the morbidity and mortality associated with BMT, thus allowing it to be used as a treatment for nonmalignant disorders including severe combined immunodeficiency (SCID), aplastic anemia, Wiskott-Aldrich syndrome, thalassemia, severe sickle cell anemia, and some inborn errors of metabolism. Abramovitz and Senner (1995) reviewed these disorders and concluded that "the decision to transplant is clear-cut in some genetic diseases (e.g., SCID) and extremely controversial in others (e.g., sickle cell anemia, inborn errors of metabolism)." Certainly, it is much easier to envision the use of a procedure such as BMT which carries significant morbidity and mortality risks for a disorder or a disease that is always fatal than for a disease that, with proper treatment, allows an individual to live a long life. Kodish and colleagues (1990) describe this tradeoff as the option to "weigh the goal of relieving pain and suffering against the goal of prolonging life." One disorder that illustrates this dilemma is sickle cell anemia. Davies (1993) states that 85% of patients with sickle cell disease (SCD) will live to age 20, and that current and future improvements in clinical care (excluding BMT) may greatly increase that percentage and allow

these patients to live into middle and old age. The hope of a BMT for SCD is that the patient will no longer have circulating sickle cell red blood cells and will therefore suffer no symptoms related to sickle cell disease. It is unknown whether "progression of end organ damage will be halted, or even the optimistic scenario that there may be improvement or resolution of organ damge" (Davies, 1993).

Davies (1993) also speculates "the risk of death or severe morbidity to be in the region of 10% for BMT for sickle cell." This is the reason that the inclusion criteria for BMT are quite limited, and centers in developed countries restrict this procedure to young children who have suffered severe complications of SCD such as stroke or serious retinopathy. Interestingly, centers giving transplants to children from undeveloped countries argue that the risk/benefit ratio differed because they "would have inadequate care for their SCD and would therefore be more likely to die without transplant" (Kodish et al., 1990).

These issues make the process of informed consent for the parents of these children extremely important. First, there is the usual problem of parents consenting for risky treatment for their child, and second, the issue of the risk benefit ratio and whether a parent could truly comprehend its complexities. Kodish and colleagues (1991) studied this problem with parents of children with SCD who were presented with a series of hypothetical percentages of survival and cure rates of SCD with BMT. They found that 37% of the 67 parents sampled were willing to accept at least the 15% short-term mortality risk that this team estimated to be the current figure for BMT, and a 12% were surprisingly willing to accept a short-term mortality rate of 50% or more! This study indicates that parents are willing to consent to risky procedures such as BMT in order to decrease the long-term suffering of their children. One can expect that issues such as this will become commonplace as BMT techniques become more refined and the procedure is contemplated for other nonlethal diseases and disorders.

New therapies such as stem cell transplants may allow cross-species transplants. Altman (1995) reported on the recommendation by the advisory panel to the Food and Drug Administration that a patient with AIDS receive a stem cell transplant from a baboon since baboons are naturally resistant to HIV-1. This would be the second such transplant, the first unsuccessfully done in 1992. However, new technology by Dr. Ildstadt utilizing a facilitating cell supposedly eliminates the risk of graft-versus-host disease in rodents and thus allows such a cross-species or xenotransplant. Ethical concerns include informed consent for the recipient as well as potential risks to health-care workers and even the public. Since this is such new therapy, it is very difficult to speculate about the risks to the recipient, and information for informed consent is therefore sketchy. There is also a concern that a cross-species transplant could introduce a new infectious agent into the human population and thus pose a risk to the health-care workers caring for the patient, as well as to the general public. Also, it is not anticipated that a BMT will cure AIDS, because the patient is expected to always remain infected with HIV. As of December, 1995, the patient had received the transplant, and was "doing well" (Altman, December 1995).

Placental blood transplantation (blood harvested from the umbilical cord immediately after birth) is receiving increasing attention for several reasons: the cells may be used in situations where there is a poor match; they seem to have lower risks of GVHD; and the donors are not exposed to the problems of bone marrow harvesting (Sugarman, Reisner, Kurtzberg, 1995). However, even with all this good news, there are ethical issues involved in these transplants. Sugarman, Reisner, and Kurtzberg

(1995) have performed an initial review that reveals several concerns. They point out that placental tissue in the United States is simply discarded by the hospital or used for experimentation, with the hospital assuming ownership. However, if the blood is used for transplantation, who owns it? Potential owners include the infant, the parents, the hospital, and even private placental blood banks. Informed consent must be considered for the use of this blood for transplantation; simple disposal (or even experimentation) of the placental tissue did not require informed consent. If the blood is used for transplantation, it would need to be tested for infectious diseases. Complex systems would need to be established to inform the parents of the donor infant of any disturbing results of these tests. However, the possibility of contact with the parents raises concerns about privacy and confidentiality, especially because testing of the donated blood would need to be performed multiple times after donation, whenever new mechanisms for testing for infectious or genetic diseases were discovered. Finally, fairness must be practiced to gather, store, and transplant placental blood from and to people of all ethnic and socioeconomic backgrounds.

One can assume that these difficult issues will continue as new therapies expand the horizons and potentials of BMT. After all, it is difficult to speculate about all of the ethical dilemmas inherent in new procedures until they are actually used, and then there is usually no time to deliberate. Once again, expanding technology leads to ethical dilemmas.

REFERENCES

Abbott, R.R., Setter, M., Chan, S., et al. 1991. APACHE II: prediction of outcome of 451 oncology admissions in a community hospital. *Ann Oncol* 2(8):571-574.

Abramovitz, L.Z., Senner, A.M. 1995. Pediatric bone marrow transplantation update. *Oncol Nurs Forum* 22(1): 107-115.

Alby, N. 1992. The child conceived to give life. *BMT 9* (suppl 1):95-96.

Alpers, A., Lo, B. 1995. When is CPR futile? *JAMA 273* (2):156-158.

Altman, L.K. 1995. AIDS test involving baboon is approved. *The New York Times* (July 15):7.

Altman, L.K., 1995. So far, so good for baboon marrow patient. *The New York Times* (Dec. 16):8.

American Nurses' Association. 1995. Position statement on nursing and the patient self-determination act. Washington, DC: Author.

American Nurses' Association. 1995. Position statement on nursing care and do-not-resuscitate decisions. Washington, DC: Author.

Anonymous. 1992. Bedside story: a sister's gift. *Cambr Q Healthcare Ethics* 1(4):409-410.

Bennett, A.J. 1993. When is medical treatment "futile"? *Issues Law & Med* 9(1):35-45.

Brown, C. 1990. Limiting care: is CPR for everyone? *AACN: Clinic Issues Crit Care Nurs* 1(1):161-168.

Bush, N.E., Haberman, M., Donaldson, G., et al. 1995. Quality of life of 125 adults surviving 6–18 years after bone marrow transplantation. *Soc Sci Med* 40(4):479-490.

Caplan, A, Lidz, C.W., Meisel, A., et al. 1983. Mrs. X and the bone marrow transplant, and commentary. *Hastings Ctr Rep* 13(3):17-19.

Carney, B. 1987. Bone marrow transplantation: nurses' and physicians perceptions of informed consent. *Canc Nurs* 10(5):252-259.

Clark, R.D., Fletcher, J., Petersen, G., et al. 1989. Conceiving a fetus for bone marrow donation: an ethical problem in prenatal diagnosis. *Prenatal Diagnosis* 9(5):329-334.

Crawford, S.W. 1991. Decision making in critically ill patients with hematological malignancy. *Western J Med* 155(5):488-493.

Curtin, L.L. 1990 A gift of many parts. *Nurs Manage* 21(6):7-8.

Curtis, J.R., Park, D.R., Krone, M.R., et al. 1995. Use of the medical futility rationale in do-not-attempt-resuscitation orders. *JAMA* 273(2):124-128.

Davies, S.C. 1993. Bone marrow transplant for sickle cell disease—the dilemma. *Blood Rev* 7(1):4-9.

Downs, S. 1994. Ethical issues in bone marrow transplantation. *Semin Oncol Nurs* 10(1):58-63.

Faber-Langendoen, K. 1991. Resuscitation of patients with metastatic cancer: is transient benefit still futile? *Arch Intern Med* 151(2):235-239.

Franco, F., Gould, D.A. 1994. Allogeneic bone marrow transplantation. *Semin Oncol Nurs* 10(1):3-11.

Fruchtman, S.M., Schanzer, H., Schwartz, M.E., et al. 1993. The physician's experience: cases and doubts. *Mount Sinai J Med* 60(1):51-58.

Hague, S.B., Moody, L.E. 1993. A study of the public's knowledge regarding advance directives. *Nurs Econ* 11(5):303-307, 323.

Hjermstad, M.J., Kaasa, S. 1995. Quality of life in adult cancer patients treated with bone marrow transplantation—a review of the literature. *Eur J Canc 31A*(2):163-173.

Honegger, H.P. 1991. Avoiding futility: assessment of cancer patients in intensive care units. *Ann Oncol* 2(8):530-531.

Hudson, T. 1994. Are futile-care policies the answer? *Hosp & Health Networks* (Feb 20):26-32.

Jacobson, B.S. 1994. Ethical dilemmas of do-not-resuscitate orders in surgery. *AORN Journal* 60(3):449-452.

Jecker, N.S., Schneiderman, L J. 1993. Medical futility: the duty not to treat. *Cambr Q Healthcare Ethics* 2(2):151-159.

Kelleher, J. 1994. Issues for designing marrow transplant programs. *Semin Oncol Nurs* 10(1):64-71.

Kern, D., Kettner, P., Albrizio, M. 1992. An exploration of the variables involved when instituting a do-not-resuscitate order for patients undergoing bone marrow transplantation. *Oncol Nurs Forum* 19(4):635-640.

King, C.R., Ferrell, B.R., Grant, M., et al. 1995. Nurses' perceptions of the meaning of quality of life for bone marrow transplant survivors. *Canc Nurs* 18(2):118-129.

Kinrade, L.C. 1987. Preparation of sibling donor for bone marrow transplant harvest procedure. *Canc Nurs* 10(2):77-81.

Kodish, E., Lantos, J., Siegler, M., et al. 1990. Bone marrow transplantation in sickle cell disease: the trade-off between early mortality and quality of life. *Clin Res* 38(4):694-700.

Kodish, E., Lantos, J., Stocking, C., et al. 1991. Bone marrow transplantation for sickle cell disease: a study of parents' decisions. *N Engl J Med* 325(19):1349-1353.

Lesko, L.M, Dermatis, H., Penman, D., et al. 1989. Patients', parents', and oncologists' perceptions of informed consent for bone marrow transplantation. *Med Pediatr Oncol* 17:181-187.

Libbus, M.K., Russell, C. 1995. Congruence of decisions between patients and their potential surrogates about life-sustaining therapies. *Image J Nurs Schol* 27 (2):135-140.

Lie, R.K. 1994. Experimental treatment, values and rationing. *Soc Sci Med* 39(8):1011-1014.

Lynch, A. 1994. Ethical issues in bone marrow transplantation: a nursing perspective. *J Palliative Care* 10(3): 23-26.

Marsden, C. 1988. Care giver fidelity in a pediatric bone marrow transplant team. *Heart & Lung* 17(6, pt. 1): 617-625.

Murphy, D.J., Barbour, E. 1994. GUIDe (guidelines for the use of intensive care in Denver): a community effort to define futile and inappropriate care. *New Horizons* 2(3):326-331.

Murphy, D.J., Finucane, T.E. 1993. New do-not-resuscitate policies: a first step in cost control. *Arch Intern Med* 153:1641-1648.

Omnibus Budget Reconciliation Act of 1990, Public Law 101-508, §4207 and 4751.

Paris, J.J. 1993. Pipes, colanders, and leaky buckets: reflections on the futility debate. *Cambr Q Healthcare Ethics* 2(2):147-149.

Peters, W.P., Rogers, M.C. 1994. Variation in approval by insurance companies of coverage for autologous bone marrow transplantation for breast cancer. *N Engl J Med* 330(7):473-477.

Rappaport, B.S. 1988. Evolution of consultation-liaison services in bone marrow transplantation. *Gen Hosp Psychiatr* 10:346-351.

Robinson, D. 1989. Who should receive medical aid? *Parade Magazine* (May 28):4-5.

Schaison, G.S. 1992. The child conceived to give life: the point of view of the hematologist. *BMT* 9(suppl 1): 93-94.

Sebban, C., Browman, G., Gafni, A., et al. 1995. Design and validation of a bedside decision instrument to elicit a patient's preference concerning allogenic bone marrow transplantation in chronic myeloid leukemia. *Am J Hematol* 48(4):221-227.

Shedd, P., Whedon, M.B. 1991. Oncology patients in critical care: ethical dilemmas. *Dimensions of Crit Care Nurs* 10(2):84-95.

Shelton, B.K. 1994. Cancer critical care: past, present, and future. *Semin Oncol Nurs* 10(3):146-155.

Silberfeld, M., Phoenix, C., Lockwood, G., et al. 1988. Choosing a risky treatment. *Psychiatr J Univ Ottawa* 13(1):9-11.

Sugarman, J., Reisner, E.G., Kurtzberg, J. 1995. Ethical aspects of banking placental blood for transplantation. *JAMA* 274(22):1783-1785.

Taylor, C. 1995. Medical futility and nursing. *Image J Nurs Schol* 27(4):301-306

Van McCrary, S., Swanson, J.W., Younger, S.J., et al. 1994. Physicians' quantitative assessments of medical futility. *J Clin Ethics* 5(2):100-105.

Waisel, D.B., Truog, R.T. 1995. The cardiopulmonary resuscitation-not-indicated order: futility revisited. *Ann Intern Med* 122(4):304-308.

Whedon, M., Ferrell, B.R. 1994. Quality of life in adult bone marrow transplant patients: beyond the first year. *Semin Oncol Nurs* 10(1):42-57.

Wolcott, D.L., Wellisch, D.K., Fawzy, F.I., et al. 1986. Psychological adjustment of adult bone marrow transplant donors whose recipient survives. *Transplantation* 41(4):484-488.

Zucker, A. 1992. Baby marrow: ethics and privacy. *J Med Ethics* 18(3):125-127, 141.

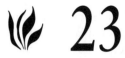

23

Models of Ambulatory Care for Blood Cell and Bone Marrow Transplantation

Patricia Corcoran Buchsel, Pamela M. Kapustay

The modern concept of shifting a large part of care from the hospital to outpatient and home care for blood cell transplantation (BCT) and bone marrow transplantation (BMT) is rooted in recent technological advances, improved clinical support, cost-containment efforts, and new attitudes regarding when and where BCT and BMT transplantation can be performed. Advances in BCT include decreasing numbers of stem cell collections, new and wider applications of hematopoietic growth factors (HGFs), intravenous (IV) antibiotics, and antiemetic medications (Peters et al., 1994). Advances in BMT include enhanced management of graft-versus-host disease (GVHD), improving rates of long-term disease-free survival, increasing availability of donors through the National Marrow Donor Program, and treatment application to a wider scope of diseases (Thomas, 1995). These improvements have led to earlier hospital discharge and creative combinations of the sites of care for transplant recipients (Crump et al., 1992; Klumppit, 1995).

Although recognized for decades as a potential substitute for BMT, BCT has only recently begun to replace autologous BMT. It is estimated that more than 5000 BCTs have been performed to date worldwide (Gale, personal communication, 1995). This growth is expected to be exponential because of the treatment's availability, decreased toxicities, and decreased costs compared to BMT. Some investigators predict that BCT will replace BMT (Bensinger, 1995). It is too early, however, to determine if BCT will provide lasting engraftment and long-term disease-free survival. Only the results of clinical trials collecting long-term data will determine if BCT offers improved treatment efficacy compared to BMT or other conventional oncology treatment protocols.

Outpatient BCT technology is becoming more available in community settings, thereby allowing selected oncologists, other than transplant physicians, to perform this therapy. New models of care for a treatment that was once almost exclusively performed in a hospital is now performed in a number of alternative settings. For many years BMT has been viewed as unique treatment requiring a full complement of highly specialized transplant teams to carry out complex treatment protocols in selected research centers. As the success of BMT has increased and care has become standardized, and more community-based BMT physicians and advanced nurse practitioners emerge, BMT will be performed in more diverse settings.

The goals of an alternative care setting are to offer similar standards of care as hospitals at a lower cost while offering the patient and family an improved quality of life during treatment. Recent studies document that BCT is less costly than BMT, but no published studies exist on economic or psychosocial costs to patients and demands on family caregivers during either treatment (Henon et al., 1992; Peters et al., 1994).

Alternative care models are defined as those designed to provide safe, quality, cost-effective care that reduces or eliminates the need for hospitalization. These designs include combinations of inpatient, outpatient, and home care. The guiding premise in choosing an alternative model of care is that there be no significant differences in mortality, morbidity, costs, and burdens on patients and caregivers between traditional and alternative hospital care.

This chapter is divided into two parts. The first part describes considerations for administrative program design and development. The second part describes clinical concerns in areas that differ from standard inpatient management. These administrative, economic, and clinical issues are explored to assist multidisciplinary transplant teams, oncology nurse administrators, advanced nurse practitioners, nursing researchers, and educators in the process of designing alternative models of care.

HEALTH-CARE ECONOMICS

Alternative models of care for transplant recipients cannot be discussed without understanding the impact of market-driven health-care reform that mandates reductions in the costs of all aspects of health care. BMT is an expensive, investigational therapy often available only to those with financial resources. The role of managed care is to offer quality care with lower costs. This is perhaps the major factor forcing transplant teams to investigate alternative sites of care (Nelson, 1995). Hospital administrators and transplant teams are identifying cost-control measures by integration of similar services, decreasing duplication of services, and eliminating admissions or shortening hospital stays. It is in this milieu that alternative care settings, aimed at reducing costs while offering greater treatment availability, are becoming increasingly important. The changing face of health care in the United States, in both the private and governmental sectors, has made it necessary for institutions to take realistic and immediate stock of health-care utilization. This has led to a change in the overall structure of a primarily physician-driven, fee-for-service model to one of collaboration in which all aspects, both clinical and economic, are evaluated equally to provide the same quality of care in the most cost-effective manner. Consequently, the interest and demand in the development of alternative sites of care to provide safe and cost-effective care is rapidly emerging.

The demand for dedicated outpatient space for transplant recipients often results in the need to adapt existing space, lease or purchase new space. Effective planning calls for the expertise of a visionary multidisciplinary transplant team that works in cooperation with architects familiar with the special considerations of profoundly immunosuppressed outpatients. Although the goal of most alternative models for transplant is to deliver all or most patient care in an ambulatory setting, most recipients will require hospital admissions or readmissions for dose-intensive therapy or for management of acute symptomology such as inetractable pain associated with mucositis, febrile episodes, or the inability of family caregivers to care for multisymptomatic patients.

Numerous reports of "outpatient transplantation" exist. Few, if any, investigators currently report patient management entirely in an outpatient setting. This phenomenon may reflect the lag between treatment and collection and publication of data. Williams and colleagues (1995) recently reported the results of 35 courses of intensive therapy for 20 BCT patients administered partially outside of the hospital. Conditioning chemotherapy for 32 patients was cyclophosphamide based, and for 3 patients was melphalan based. Patients remained hospitalized until they were able to retain food and fluids. The average length of initial hospitalization was 7.7 days (range 3 to 14 days). Blood specimens, prophylactic antibiotics, blood component therapy, and IV fluids were administered at home. Patients were evaluated by home-care nurses five times per week. Patients were evaluated in a clinic twice weekly. Rehospitalization was required during the first 30 days in 17 cases with 64.7% admitted for elevated temperatures. Rehospitalization averaged 7.1 days (range 1 to 16 days) and no death or life-threatening morbidity occurred during therapy. No data was presented determining quality of life or comparing costs to hospitalization (Williams et al., 1995).

Peters and colleagues (1994) reported on intensive outpatient support for autologous BMT in women with breast cancer. Women were hospitalized for dose-intensive chemotherapy, discharged, and assessed daily in a nearby clinic. Readmission rates were reported to be 65% but of short duration. The most common reasons for readmission were culture-negative febrile neutropenia, viral pneumonia, dehydration, persistent nausea, suspected veno-occlusive disease, and thrombocytopenia. In contrast, readmission rates for BMT recipients who have completed the transplant process are noted to be approximately 50% (Buchsel, 1993).

ADMINISTRATIVE PLANNING

The need to establish alternative sites of care depends on the institution's mission to expand oncologic services and the medical staff's desire to offer these options to patients. For example, institutions that have already established BMT programs may expand services to include BCT. Hospitals without previously established BMT programs may choose to enter joint ventures or partnerships with corporate entities or academic institutions offering physician-managed BCT programs. These latter arrangements are emerging with increasing frequency as hospital administrators realize the importance of collaborative care that offers a more cost-effective delivery of care. It is unclear what impact these models will have on quality of care, patient outcomes, costs, and research in clinical trials.

Transplant care is similar to the care of most oncology patients, and can be provided in a variety of settings depending on patients' needs, patient volume, and facility affiliations (Lamkin, 1993). Increasing numbers of private oncology groups are offering this technology outside of standard institutional environments. BCT technology is more available in community settings because it can often be performed in outpatient areas by oncologists other than transplant physicians. Alternative models may arise from already existing oncology or BMT programs. In other cases, BCT programs are instituted as an entirely new product line. Few transplant programs are comprehensive and provide all the critical components such as apheresis, cryopreservation, infusion suites, clinics, and pharmacy. Because of cost-containment issues, similar services may need

TABLE 23.1 Criteria for outpatient care

Recipient must
  Be afebrile (Temp < 38.3°C)
  Have a platelet count >20,000 m³; no active
    bleeding; require no more than 2 transfusions
    per day
  Be able to tolerate physical demands for clinic
    visits for assessments, procedures, and so on
  Be taking adequate oral fluids
  Be taking oral medications
  Have selected IV medications (e.g., antibiotics,
    cyclosporin, ganciclovir)
Caregiver must be able and willing to
  Be responsible for home care
  Transport and accompany patient to and from
    clinic
  Assist with central venous catheter self-care
    management
  Administer IV fluids using ambulatory pumps
  Recognize and report symptoms (e.g., fever,
    shaking chills, uncontrolled nausea and vomiting)
  Monitor patient's compliance with medications
    and self-care
  Maintain written record of medication schedule
  Understand access to emergency care
  Understand and enforce precautions against
    infectious disease
  Acquire medical supplies
  Understand techniques for disposal of hazardous
    materials

to be shared among other departments such as Hematology/Oncology. The need to integrate similar services to reduce costs will continue to prevail.

A key component of alternative models of care is emphasis on supportive care in the outpatient areas with clear patient criteria (see Table 23.1). The ambulatory transplant facility should have easy access to the various departments associated with the transplant (Figure 23.1) and cooperation of many departments necessary for support of transplantation (Table 23.2)

Mission Statement and Strategic Plan

The most dramatic change in planning alternative models for transplantation is aimed at re-engineering or redesigning current systems to meet the cost-reduction goals of the health-care environment. Market-driven managed care demands that traditional care settings change the way they have been or are currently delivering health care. Cancer centers have new attitudes toward the classic strategic plan used to project new growth and directions. Strategic plans now map shifts in patterns of care that sustain, enhance, and prepare their organizations for health care into the next century. For example, physicians' practices offering a broad range of medical services to cancer patients may enter into physician-negotiated contracts to coordinate delivery of BCT in an outpatient setting. These settings may offer quality care that is more cost effective than traditional settings and is increasingly preferred by patients, payers, and physicians. Other approaches may be contracts between home-care companies and transplantation centers to deliver a large portion of care in the home setting rather than the hospital or clinic (Baird, 1995). Whatever model of care administrators choose, a mission statement and a strategic plan are the first steps in moving to innovative directions.

A mission statement should reflect the organization's purpose and values and basic principles that guide the actions of the organization's members (Argenti, 1994, p. 282). A strategic plan is a road map to an organization's future, to define its mission statement, formulate its goals, and develop specific strategies to meet those goals. The basic characteristics of a strategic plan are that decisions are made by all managers, it focuses on short- and long-term goals, and deals with large amounts of resources that directly affect the organization's environment. As oncology groups consider either BCT or BMT as an extension of

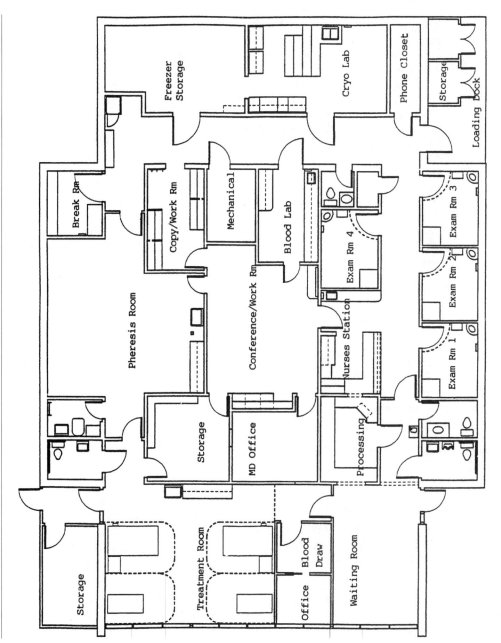

Figure 23.1 A typical floor plan for an ambulatory transplant setting

SOURCE: Reprinted with permission from Duke University Transplant Program, Durham, NC.

TABLE 23.2 Personnel and services necessary for new models of blood cell and marrow transplantation

Administrative	Medical staff or consultants	Nursing staff	Support services	Ancillary services
Chief executive officer	Medical director	Nursing director	Pharmacy	Microbiology, virology, chemistry, pathology genetic assays; cell processing laboratories
Chief financial officer	Attending physicians	Advanced nurse practitioners	Social services	HLA tissue typing
Third-party contract manager	Staff physicians	Insurance coordinator	Volunteer services	Central supply
Fund-raising manager	Psychiatry/Behavioral medicine	Nurse coordinator	Chaplain	Medical records
Legal counsel	Rheumatology	Research nurse	Dietary services	Pulmonary function lab
Human resources manager	Immunology	Licensed practical nurses	Physical therapy	Secretarial services
	Ophthalmology	Certified nursing assistants	Apheresis	Billing office personnel
	Gynecology	Discharge planner		Insurance counselors
	Reproductive medicine	Case managers		Laundry
	Allergist	Home care		Hazardous waste handlers
	Cardiology			Blood bank
	Neurology			
	Radiology			
	Dental			
	Pulmonary medicine			
	Infectious Disease Specialist			
	Oncology			
	Hematology			
	Surgery			
	Stem cell processing			
	Nephrology			
	Urology			

SOURCE: Adapted from Buchsel, P., 1991, p. 298.

their services, important administrative and clinical concerns must be addressed. Program designs and criteria for patient selection are the two major considerations. Other basic questions are:

- Why are we doing this? Is this consistent with our mission statement?
- Do we have the administrative and clinical resources?

- What is the market for skilled practitioners (i.e., medical directors, nurse administrators, advanced practice nurses, etc.)?
- How many transplants need to be done to be clinically and financially feasible?
- What types of transplants will we do?
- What diseases and stages will we treat?
- How long will marrow recipients remain in the area after transplantation?
- What type of family housing is needed?

- What joint partnerships are available?
- Do we want to be a center of excellence or participate in a network?
- What will be the catchment area?
- How will we recruit our patients?
- What technology is changing that will affect the growth or decline of transplantation?
- Can the ambulatory care space be converted for other future uses?
- What therapies will be done in ambulatory care?
- What services will be offered?

Models of Care

Paralleling administrative considerations are clinical guidelines to direct and ensure delivery of optimal care for the transplant recipient. Standards of care should be consistent across care settings. Clinical guidelines are necessary to direct the appropriate care setting for each patient, and depend on the organization's resources. Some models may use focus groups or consensus conferences comprised of oncologists and transplantation experts to determine patients' appropriateness. One national provider network established patients' criteria to define appropriateness for transplant in their diverse clinical setting. A large Texas-based organization uses consensus-based guidelines for care, while another program developed criteria for minimum performance of a transplant program that includes patient selection criteria (Kurowski et al., 1995).

The critical elements for all programs center around patient volume, facility and personnel requirements, treatment outcomes, and data reporting (ASCO/ASH, 1990). Guidelines have been published for the management of autologous and allogenic BMT (Rowe et al., 1994). Scientific consensus conferences are addressing consistency in transplant treatment and terminology (Juttner et al., 1994). Additionally, the World Donor Association issued a special report on recommendations for standardized practice for volunteer donors (Goodman, 1994).

Ideally patients should be treated according to transplant protocols based on critical analyses of data from scientific journals and meetings and/or reported to the International Bone Marrow Transplant Registry and the Autologous Bone Marrow Transplant Registry. These protocols must reflect the team's judgment of the most effective transplant strategy for each disease entity treated. Patients should participate in trials sponsored by The International Cooperative Research Group (ICRG), National Cancer Institute (NCI), Southwest Oncology Group (SWOG), and the other national and international research groups.

Patients who may be candidates for transplantation often visit transplant centers for consultations. Some centers offer a consultation service and physicians are assigned to meet with the patient and family to explore transplantation possibilities. Consultation services may be a shrinking commodity because of health-care reform mandates that direct patients to identified centers of excellence.

The models for transplant in the following chart are currently the most common (courtesy of Marie Bakitas Whedon, 1995).

Traditional BCT	**Outpatient** pretransplant evaluation, central catheter placement, apheresis, mobilization, cryopreservation
	Inpatient admission for dose-intensive chemotherapy/irradiation through supportive care and hematopoietic recovery
	Outpatient care until stabilized engraftment with subsequent return to referring physician
Early-Discharge BCT	**Outpatient** pretransplant evaluation, central catheter placement, apheresis, mobilization, cryopreservation

Early-Discharge BCT (*continued*)

Inpatient dose-intensive chemotherapy/irradiation

Outpatient supportive care during hematopoietic recovery, and stabilized engraftment with subsequent return to referring physician

Inpatient admission per institutional protocol

Outpatient BCT

Outpatient pretransplant evaluation, central catheter placement, apheresis, mobilization, cryopreservation

Outpatient dose-intensive chemotherapy/irradiation, outpatient supportive care during hematopoietic recovery, and stabilized engraftment with subsequent return to referring physician

Inpatient admission per institutional protocol

Traditional BMT

Outpatient evaluation, central catheter placement

Inpatient admission for high-dose chemotherapy and TBI; supportive care until stabilized engraftment and resolution of transplant-related complications; patients discharged on liberal criteria

Early-Discharge BMT

Outpatient evaluation, central catheter placement; supportive care until stabilized engraftment and resolution of transplant-related complication (i.e., infection, mucositis, cystitis); inpatient admission for supportive care as needed

Outpatient BMT

Outpatient evaluation, central catheter placement, selective high-dose conditioning regimens (i.e., busulfan, melphalan, cyclophosphamide, TBI)

Inpatient admission for support care as needed

There are imperative administrative and clinical caveats to the success of any of these models. The ability and clinical condition of the patient and the stamina of a caregiver after a minimal hospitalization in the face of the multiple symptoms and adverse treatment effects are of extreme importance. Included in the program's design are anticipated transitions across sites of care for management of a myriad of transplant-related problems.

The Physical Design

Housing

Patients and family caregivers most often relocate to transplant centers that are some distance from their communities. Availability of safe, affordable, convenient family housing is necessary to attract and maintain steady patient census. Housing needs to be within walking distance of the transplant facility and supported by a 24-hour transportation service. Although a few centers offer their own housing, most transplant centers contract with neighborhood hotel facilities to accommodate patients. In this case, designated spaces should have facilities such as wheelchair ramps, handrails, elevators, and eating areas. Comfortable rooms with television, video camera recorders, and microwave ovens are desirable. Some institutions have created lending closets for household items such as small appliances, cribs, and strollers, as well as lending libraries (Buchsel and Kapustay, 1995; Buchsel, 1995).

Location

Most care for BMT and BCT recipients is given in a location adjacent to the inpatient transplant unit. Dedicated space is often difficult to obtain because of competing requests from other disciplines. Depending on the setting, BCT and BMT outpatients can receive care in a dedicated space or shared space in a hematology or oncology clinic. The BCT and BMT ambulatory care unit is staffed by a knowledgeable multidisciplinary team dedicated to the care of the transplant patients, their donors, and family members. Some clinics have dedicated areas for clinical examinations, but administration of IV therapies such as blood component, antimicrobial, and biological therapies are performed in general or common areas. Likewise, procedures such as peripherally inserted catheters, bone marrow aspirations and biopsies, blood and other specimen collection may be done in another area.

The Clinical Area

Posttransplantation recipients in ambulatory care areas require serious attention to their immunocompromised and fatigued status. Because dose-intensive therapy renders toxicities to every organ system, recipients may present with nausea, vomiting, diarrhea, fever, malaise and fatigue, depression, and anxiety. Clinic waiting areas, examination rooms, infusion areas, and specimen collection areas require considerations of esthetics and space for sick patients and their caregivers. Collaboration with infectious disease physicians is important for minimal cross-contamination of infectious diseases such as airborne parainfluenza, respiratory syncytial virus, and herpes-zoster virus (HZV). Policies must address the occasions when patients or family members bring airborne infectious diseases into waiting areas shared with immunocompromised patients. Acceptable cleaning and maintenance of the setting is a major challenge. Optimally, the cleaning team will be under the direction of the clinic nursing administrator. Careful attention to the ambulatory care environment must include cleaning by a team familiar with the standards of hospital cleaning.

Waiting Areas

Group seating arrangements in waiting areas are ideal to allow a sense of privacy and intimacy. Approximately 15 square feet of space should be allowed per person. Artistic lighting and use of artificial greens can suggest a restful atmosphere without exposing patients to potentially infectious airborne organisms. Centers open after normal business hours will need to maintain this homelike atmosphere with lighting and security measures (Lamkin, 1993). Bathrooms should be equipped with emergency call bells and allow wheelchair access. Waiting rooms can contain refreshment areas with hot water pumps for tea, hot chocolate, or soups. A play area enclosed by plexiglass can contain noise yet allow observation. Toys and play equipment must be made of washable materials and cleaned with bactericidal cleaners daily.

Education Area

Patients and their families require intensive education before and after BCT and BMT, and space must be created to meet this need. Introduction to the transplant process can be performed effectively in a formal didactic classroom environment and supported with audiovisual equipment. Hands-on experiences such as management of central venous catheters, subcutaneous injection of HGFs, and IV pumps can be easily provided. BCT and BMT candidates can be acquainted with the transplant routine of isolation rooms, diet, exercise, staff, and medical rounds. Marrow donors can be taught the process of marrow harvest and have their concerns and expectations explored in this setting.

Clinic Examination Rooms

During and after BCT or BMT recipients require numerous examinations and consultation with the multidisiciplinary care team. Recipients may be seen daily to weekly depending on their needs for assessments and therapies. Clinic examination rooms for physical assessments and procedures must be designed to accommodate an examination table and stool, oxygen and suction, blood pressure monitoring equipment, thermometers, desk, table for supplies, X ray viewing box, computer, and a bathroom with a sink and an emergency call system. The room must allow space for a patient, nurse, physician, and caregiver.

Nurses' Station

Essential to clinical function is a centrally located nurses' station. This area is the hub and houses patients charts, computers, and a medication preparation room. Clerical support areas for charting, patient appointments, and processing of medical records are usually within or in close proximity of the nurses station. A designated admixture area is necessary for mixing medication in emergencies. Reconstitution of chemotherapeutic agents requires appropriate equipment and supplies such as a laminar flow hood, syringes and needles, gowns, masks, goggles, and gloves. Disposal containers should be readily available (Houston and Houston, 1993). Adequate drug storage facilities and disposal arrangements are necessary.

Infusion Areas

Several factors to be considered in the design of infusion areas is length of infusion, patient status, and presence of a family caregiver. Infusions may be administered in minutes to hours. For short-term infusions such as IV "push" medications or subcutaneous injections, an area equipped with reclining clinic chairs is ideal. A second infusion category is infusions that require 1 to 4 hours and may include chemotherapy, hydration, electrolyte replacements, platelet transfusions, biotherapy, or other medications.

Patients receiving these therapies can be seated in reclining chairs unless they are fa-

tigued and require a bed. Other therapies may last longer than 4 hours. Blood component therapy, hydration, and some chemotherapy require that a patient remain in a bed for safety and comfort. Limitations of one family caregiver per patient may be necessary for privacy and efficient delivery of care.

Apheresis Unit

A separate, designated area and/or room should be assigned for blood stem cell collection (Figure 23.1). Space to accommodate several machines, disposable equipment, patient, caregiver, and apheresis personnel requires approximately 40 square feet per patient. Some institutions with limited space and a small amount of procedure space can move machinery between procedures to facilitate alternative uses of the room. Apheresis equipment is easily moved and can be stored until the next procedure. The apheresis procedure generally requires about 3 to 4 hours, so overhead television, videocassette recorders, stereo, and compact disc players are welcomed by patients.

Day Surgery

A day surgery suite can be a profitable service for a transplant setting. All transplant recipients require placement of central venous catheters (CVCs) and some patients require replacement of catheters during the course of treatment. BCT patients, in particular, may require replacement of groin catheters or large-bore catheters after apheresis is completed. Numerous procedures can be performed safely under local or light general anesthesia while providing continuity of care such as placement of CVCs, marrow harvests, endoscopies, biopsies, or blood patches for treatment of spinal headache. Transplant units desiring an independent surgery area need to investigate state and federal requirements for licensure. Third-party payers cannot reimburse for surgical procedures unless these regulations are met (Moskowitz, 1993).

Emergency and After-Hours Care

One of the critical considerations posed during the initial planning of alternative sites is defining the sites for care of patients after clinic hours. The concern in establishing emergency care is clear communication among inpatient, outpatient and emergency room personnel, the patients, and caregivers. Because transplantations are increasingly being performed at community and regional hospitals, after-hours care will differ from the care provided in traditional academic settings. Profoundly immunosuppressed transplant recipients are at considerable risk for life-threatening infections such as gram-negative septicemia with resulting septic shock. Allogeneic recipients are placed on corticosteroid therapy for GVHD management, often masking fever. These patients might present only with chilling, and impending septic shock might not be recognized.

The ability to initiate antibiotic therapy 24 hours a day needs to be coordinated. Patient and caregiver must be aware of communication pathways to receive emergency care. Depending on the institution, patients may be requested to call their physicians, an inpatient unit, 911, or an outpatient nurse on call. Issues of after-hour care need to be incorporated in discharge teaching and reinforced throughout the continuum of care. Institutions should have written materials containing outpatient guidelines and directions for access to emergency care.

Home Care

Home care for the transplant recipient is becoming an increasingly important service to extend IV administration, and assessment and management of a host of transplant-related symptoms (Jassak and Riley, 1994; Schulmeister, 1995; Randolph, 1992). Early discharge from the hospital or exclusive outpatient management of the transplant recipient often depends on sophisticated technology for safely administrating chemotherapy and large volumes of IV fluids. Home care must be approached with caution. Close scrutiny by the hospital team is necessary to determine quality of services and cost-effectiveness if a provider chooses to use a home care service. Mutually beneficial goals are established when inpatient and home-care teams work closely to establish continuity of care, avoidance of duplication of services, and consistent communication with the patient and family. Direct home-care training from the transplant unit's educational staff can ensure that home-care nurses have state-of-the-art transplantation knowledge and that they are familiar with transplant protocols and policies (Schulmeister, 1995).

Outpatient and home care is not always less expensive than inpatient care. In a recent prospective randomized trial of BMT recipients discharged early from the hospital, outpatient and home-care costs were found to be the same as costs for hospitalized recipients (Sullivan et al., 1994). Transplant recipients required assessments for multiorgan toxicities, pain, mucositis, GVHD (allogeneic), failure to thrive, and monitoring of compliance with numerous medications.

Some important administrative concerns surround pharmaceutical revenues lost to corporate home-care providers, because IV therapies such as antimicrobials and immunotherapies are the major revenue source of outpatient care. To ensure consistent pricing, firm contracts that are routinely monitored must be in place. For cancer centers with their own home-care providers, communication and training for the home-care nurses may be necessary. Ethical corporate joint ventures using profit-sharing opportunities may be an option to decrease high cost of inpatient care. With the advent of managed care, health-care providers and patients have few choices of home health-care companies unless patients have the financial resources to select a provider of their choice.

ADMINISTRATIVE ELEMENTS

The elements critical to a successful program rely on collaboration among all disciplines involved in the care of the transplant patient (Buchsel, 1991; Kelleher, 1991).

Nursing Service

The role of the nurse manager in an alternative care model is multidimensional, in constant flux, and varies among institutions. The most common job titles for a nursing administrative role are director, head nurse, vice president, coordinator, or assistant administrator (Martin, 1994). Similar to other nurse administrators, nursing administrators of alternative care are responsible for managing human resources and budgets to create an environment for patients, families, and staff that fosters quality care delivered in a cost-effective manner. The most dramatic changes are increased responsibilities in assuming broader administrative and clinical responsibilities, participation in architectural design of new settings, determining a wider scope of nursing practice, implementing new treatment protocols, and ensuring continuity of care. Because of the dramatic shifts in models of care, nurse managers in these new settings have few role models to direct them through these uncharted areas (Grady-Porter, 1990). Affiliation with professional nursing groups such as the American Organization of Nursing Executives (AONE) and Oncology Nursing Society (ONS) allows networking and sharing of ideas.

Most BCT and BMT treatment sites coexist with other oncology services such as those within a comprehensive cancer treatment center. Current cost-reduction mandates in internal administrative structures are the impetus for new dimensions in nursing responsibilities that are no longer limited to immediate patient care. The nurse manager may supervise not only nursing staff but clerical, housekeeping, operating room, patient services, and other ancillary staff. Changes in health-care policy leading to managed-care contracts have thrust the nurse manger into areas of financial concerns, third-party reimbursement issues, and utilization review (Nelson, 1995). Because alternative care models are an emerging entity, the nurse administrator may also be involved in strategic planning, architectural design, and marketing of these programs.

Changing Practice Environments

In contrast to nursing administrators who manage traditional hospital and clinical areas, the nursing administrator in an alternative care setting works in collaboration with physicians and other clinicians to introduce complex therapies that may not yet be established as nonhospitalized procedures such as dose-intensive chemotherapy for the BCT recipient or total body irradiation for selected BMT recipients. To make the transition from hospital to alternative care, the nurse administrator must gain the support and commitment of the multidisiplinary team to ensure daily 24-hour emergency care.

Rapidly changing technologies and clinical developments in transplantation also pose a challenge to nurse administrators who must be cognizant of new cost-effective treatment modalities that can be integrated into the alternative care setting. For example, patients receiving dose-intensive therapy require copious amounts of hydration. New approaches have allowed selected healthy and capable BCT recipients to forego IV hydration if they can ingest copious amounts of water during therapy. Similarly, selected BMT patients receiving busulfan in conditioning regimens may receive it at home after intensive education. Because of acute nausea and vomiting as a result of this drug, patients and caregivers must be taught to count the number of pills vomited in order to determine ingestion of medication.

Education of Patients and Families

Nursing administrators in transplant settings have had to expand the scope of education for patients and families. The increased responsibility of the patients and families for self-care in an alternative setting demands a comprehensive and organized teaching approach. Transplantation dictates that patients progress through multiple procedures often given by numerous professional caregivers. Effective teaching can alleviate much of the patients' fear and anxiety as they progress through the numerous clinical areas. Patient acuity levels can be equal to or significantly higher than those of traditionally hospitalized patients. Jassak and Porter (1995) divide the marrow transplant education process into six information phases:

1. donor selection,
2. evaluation,
3. preoperative regimens,
4. marrow infusion,
5. treatment complications and engraftment, and
6. discharge planning and ambulatory follow-up.

Similarly, BCT is divided into six phases:

1. evaluation,
2. mobilization,
3. apheresis and cryopreservation,
4. dose-intensive therapy,
5. infusion, and
6. engraftment/recovery (Buchsel and Kapustay, 1995).

Each phase has unique teaching concerns such as orientation to the system, care of CVCs, self-administration of HGFs, symptom identification, and integration into community settings (Walker et al., 1994).

Written materials organized in a comprehensive manner can ease the transition process. Important information consists of documenting the time and place of procedures, clinic and emergency phone numbers, and the names of their various physicians, nurses, and technicians. Patient teaching relative to self-care such as administration of HGFs, CVC care, signs and symptoms of potential problems such as infection, infection control measures, and dietary restrictions are all important aspects of care. Many of these instructions and precautions vary among institutions.

The family caregiver is now recognized as an integral part of the interdisciplinary team who manages the care of the transplant recipient. Common caregiver responsibilities are initiated before the patient arrives at the transplantation center and continues until the patient is reintegrated into his or her community. Clinical and other necessary information for patients and families must be incorporated into a teaching module specifically for the institution's policies and procedures (Table 23.3). Not all patients have willing family caregivers. In these cases, some centers have a pool of approved laypersons capable of assisting patients with some aspects of their outpatient management. Support systems to give caregivers respite can enhance care of the patient while diminishing accumulated caregiver stress.

Critical Pathways

The development, maintenance, and quality of interdisciplinary care is often the responsibility of nurse administrators. This indispensable component of health care is often organized under the umbrella of critical pathways. Critical pathways are designed by interdisciplinary

TABLE 23.3 Education for the patient and family caregiver

PREARRIVAL

Housing Arrangements
  Location
  Rent
  Furnishings
  Lending closets
  Transportation
  Laundry facilities
Community Resources
  Bank
  Post office
  Shopping areas
  Churches

ARRIVAL

General information
Assistance with decision making
Assistance with financial issues
Emotional support
Physical care
Resources
  Social workers
  Psychologists
  Volunteer services
  Chaplain
  Spiritual support groups
  Community support
  Respite service
Support through informed consent procedure
Transportation means and schedules
List of phone numbers
  Hospital
  Clinics
  Emergency care

TRANSPLANTATION PREPARATION

Transplant rationale, process, and expectations
Orientation to health-care team
Written guidelines for all transplant phases
Obtaining emergency and after-hours care
Acquiring and maintaining medical supplies
Management of central catheter
Blood draws from catheter and delivery to
  appropriate locations
Emotional self-care

APHERESIS/MARROW HARVEST

Principles of apheresis or marrow harvest
Donor issues of stem cell or marrow harvest
Risks of general anesthesia
Autostorage of blood
Postoperative complications
Colony-stimulating factors
  Reconstitution
  Administration
  Self-management
Monitoring patient's compliance in self-
  administration of oral and IV medications
Recording medications
Identifying changes in patient's condition
Disposal of hazardous wastes

TRANSPLANTATION/WAITING FOR ENGRAFTMENT

Dietary instruction
Maintaining home environment
Administration of medications via IV pump
Recognition of common symptoms
Symptom management
Handling emergencies
Reporting symptoms
Initial preparation for return home

RECOVERY

Common problems and symptoms
  Fatigue
  Weight loss
  Sexual dysfunction
  Cataracts
  Chronic GVHD
  Herpes-zoster virus
  Depression
  Isolation
Survivorship issues
Reentry into community
Insurance concerns

health-care professionals to treat diseases for specific polulations of patients. These pathways, which differ among institutions, have arisen out of efforts to standardize care to deliver optimal treatment in the most cost-effective manner. Critical elements to this "map" or care plan are time lines for the implementation and expected outcomes of care (Burns et al., 1995). Figures 23.2 and 23.3 are examples of two critical pathways for BCT. Table 23.4 illustrates key questions to be addressed when designing a critical pathway.

New Nursing Roles

Today's nursing leader in an alternative care setting has the challenge of creating new roles and responsibilities for nurses caring for patients who have traditionally been in a hospital setting (Lin and Martin, 1994). One of the greatest challenges is continuity of care as patients obtain their care in multiple departments such as surgery, apheresis, chemotherapy, and follow-up clinics. This multifaceted task demands the ability to communicate with numerous managers. The current nature of transplant is such that a patient may be diagnosed in a physician's office, treated in a medical, surgical, and/or radiology clinic, and referred to a hospital or center for a BCT or BMT. Events can occur rapidly and the nurse administrators are often charged with seamless transition of patients through this system (Kelleher, 1994).

The Transplant Coordinator. Many transplant centers have created a new nursing role called a *transplant coordinator* or *case manager* committed to coordinating care. A coordinator can verify insurance benefits; make clinical appointments for placement of CVCs and stem cell collection procedures, classes for patients, and clinical appointments; and arrange for return to referring physicians. When these nursing positions are not formally established, it often becomes incumbent on the transplant

staff nurse to monitor and ensure the continuity of care.

The Triage Nurse. A triage nurse is an invaluable asset to the daily organization of an alternative care setting. Initial assessment of all patients arriving without appointments or telephoning for emergency care or general information can be initiated without interruption. Emergency situations such as a septic episode or a profusely bleeding patient can be rapidly attended to without impacting regularly scheduled clinic visits. The presence of a triage nurse can also decrease the number of impromptu patient "hall visits" with physicians and nurses.

The Apheresis Nurse. Important administrative decisions about the nursing staff of an apheresis unit need to be made prior to the opening of the unit. Nurses working in the BCT clinical area may be trained in apheresis procedures but the time and costs may not support such cross-training in small BCT units. Lengthy intervals can elapse between stem cell collections and competency may diminish because of underuse of skills. Nurses newly trained in apheresis often lack the skills to interface with problematic equipment or catheters.

Alternative staffing options such as contracted apheresis nursing services can provide a more efficient and cost-effective use of nursing personnel. The use of contracted nurses requires that evaluations be made of their clinical performance and competency to provide special services. Personnel records should be maintained on all contracted nurses and include current RN licensure, cardiopulmonary resuscitation certification, apheresis training certification, continuing education certificates of attendance, competency verification, and ongoing performance evaluations. Each nurse administrator must address the advantages and disadvantages of contracting services for their BCT program (Buchsel and Kapustay, 1995).

TABLE 23.4 Components of a critical pathway for transplant recipients

Disease	Tests and procedures
Hematological	Confirm diagnosis
Solid tumor	Comorbid medical problems
Lymphoma	Allergies
Acquired or congenital	Physiological assessment
Status	Pregnancy
Remission	Sperm or ova storage
Relapse	Tumor staging
Bulky	Electrolyte panel for organ toxicity
Type of transplant	Scans
Blood	Dose-intensity conditioning
Marrow	Chemotherapy
Allogeneic	Total body irradiation
Autologous	BCT mobilization techniques
Syngeneic	Chemotherapy
Clinical consultants	Colony-stimulating factors
Radiologist	Prophylaxis of infection
Anesthesiologist	Management of acute complications
Infectious-disease specialist	Pancytopenia: anemia, thrombocytopenia, neutropenia
Gynecologist	Gastrointestinal toxicities: mucositis, nausea/vomiting. diarrhea
Renal specialist	Acute GVHD
Psychiatrist	Renal insufficiency/hemorrhagic cystitis
Social worker	Central nervous system toxicities: seizures, tremors, change in LOC
Dietitian	Cardiac toxicities: hypertension, hypotension, tachycardia, bradycardia
Blood component therapy	Pulmonary toxcities: shortness of breath, dyspnea, cough, wheezing
RBCs	Veno-occlusive disease
Platelet	Discharge criteria
Typing	Outpatient care
Site of care	Long-term complications, disease-free survival
Inpatient	
Outpatient	
Combination	
Donor status (allogeneic)	
Family of volunteer	
Matched or mismatched	
Blood or marrow	

KEY: BCT = blood cell transplant, GVHD = graft-versus-host disease, LOV = level of consciousness, NVD = nausa/vomiting/diarrhea.

The Advanced Practice Nurse. The presence of an advanced practice nurse (APN) has great potential to provide consistent skilled clinical care for the transplant recipient. *APN,* as recently defined by the Oncology Nursing Society, is an umbrella term for clinical nurse specialists and nurse practitioners who have master's degrees (Hawkins and Holcombe, 1995). Although state limitations relative to prescriptive authority and scope of nursing practice vary, most APNs can offer new roles for care of the transplant patient before, during, and after

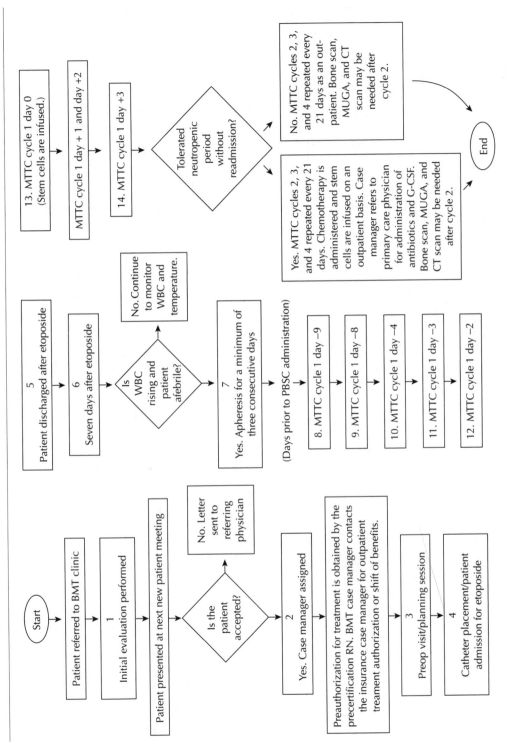

Figure 23.2 The Stanford BMT outpatient critical pathway for sequential high-dose chemotherapy followed by peripheral blood stem cell rescue

SOURCE: Developed by Joanne Burns, Bone Marrow Transplantation Department, Stanford University, Stanford, CA. Used with permission.

Path name: Blood Cell Transplant/NHL

DRG number: _____   **ELOS:** _____ 34

	Adm	Adm phase day –7	Adm phase day –6, –5, –4, –3, –2, –1	BMT day 0	Nadir phase day +1 thru +19	Nadir phase day +20	Recovery/DC phase day +21, +22	Recovery/DC phase day +23, +24, +25
Goals	Initiate consult Blood bank notified Initiate teaching Baseline wt/girth documented Order adm labs/tests IV hydration	Begin condition phase teaching Complete admission teaching Insert foley Complete adm tests/labs Begin antibiotics Begin antifungal Begin antiviral	Foley cath inserted Output balances intake Cytoxan-thiotepa infusion Nausea controlled Day –1: teaching re: BCT complete	Complete bone marrow infusion Nutrition support team consulted Reinfusion supplies to bedside	No active/uncontrolled bleeding Nutritional needs met Fluid/electrolyte imbalances corrected Temp <102.5°F Discomfort controlled No complications DC foley & reduce hydration 48° after cytoxan	ANC >500, platelet transfer <QOD, 1/3 calories and protein p.o.	Team notified of impending discharge Lipids to 10 cc/hr PCXR changed to routine CXR TPN to 40 cc/hr Provisions for output drug therapy	TPN and lipids discontinued Return appt scheduled Pt demonstrates proper med adm Pt demonstrates adequate p.o. intake Pt describes when to call MD Pt knows when to return to MD
Tests & Labs	Admit labs: hemogram/diff chem 6, creat, chem 12 SGPT CXR		Hemogram w/diff chem 6, CR M/Th = chem 12, Mg, PT/PTT, Retic, BCD M/Th port CXR		Temp >100.5°F = blood culture x 2 Urine C&S, portable CXR QM prealbumin 1 hr post plt. ct. QM 24° UUN			→ Thru day 23 M/Th routine CXR
Treatments	VS q shift Wt QD Baseline abd girth	Mouth care BID I&O q 2°	ABD girth QD I&O Insert foley cath Dipstick urine QS		→ Q4° → BID → Q2° → DC foley Pulmonary care QS Accu check BID Neut/throm protocol		→ QD → Q4°	
Diet	Reg diet	NPO before surgery Reg diet after surgery Nutrition assessment			Neutopenic diet TPN		→ Wean calorie counts	Reg diet Verify oral intake

542

Activity							
Consults	Ad lib						
	Pastoral care	Dietician		Nutrition support team			Social services (discharge planning) Pharmacy (DC meds)
Meds/IV	IV hydration			Δ to maintenance rate 48° after cytoxan complete			
			Antiemetics Lasix Mesna		Peridex BID Nystatin QID Pain meds		
			Day-1: acyclovir vanco ofloxicin fluconazole	Start GCSF	Wean antibx day 14–19 Wean GCSF when ANC > 500		
Teaching/DC Plan	Unit introduction	Adm phase: oral hygiene, testing, I&O measurement Condition phase	Continue self-care during BCT incl mouth care & infect control		Neutropenic teaching Thrombocytopenic teaching		Infection/bleeding precautions Activities Meds
Equipment	Omni flow & tubing	Hemocult Foley	Omni flow (meds & hydration)	Reinfusion supplies to bedside			
Chemo	Notify blood bank	VP -16 -7	Cytoxan -6, -5, -4 BCNU -2	Stem cell infusion	2 UPRBC irrad & leukopoor if PCV <25 Pheresis Irrad & leukopoor if plt <20K		

Figure 23.3 **An example of a critical care pathway**

transplantation. For example, a major BMT program in the Pacific Northwest uses the services of gynecological APNs to address women's health issues related to BMT (Schubert et al., 1990). In another case, APNs instituted a quality improvement team to develop skin care regimens for chronic GVHD (DeMeyer, 1995). Typically, APNs are permanently assigned to a transplant unit and can, under the direction of a physician, obtain routine histories; perform physicals, marrow aspirations, biopsies, and intrathecal procedures; prescribe selected medication; or order blood comport therapy. In addition to recipients, APNs can care for blood and marrow donors. As efforts to support the heavily burdened caregiver dramatically increase, some centers may begin to offer family practice care for caregivers. In 1993, the Clinton administration introduced health-care reform that included decreasing costs by using physicians' assistants and nurse practitioners. Many physicians resisted the notion of extended practice for nurses (Hawkins and Holcombe, 1995). However, as the managed-care market continues to demand decreased health-care costs, the role of the APN is becoming increasingly important.

The current status of the above roles are dynamic. Individual transplant nurse administrators are redesigning these roles to offer the most efficient care in the most cost-effective manner. Many responsibilities inherent in these roles will be reassigned to nonclinical staff or to professional nurses without advanced degrees. The use of licensed practice nurses, medical technicians, and other ancillary personnel needs to be evaluated carefully by the nursing administrative staff. Some institutions have successfully used medical technicians to draw blood specimens, assist with procedures, and monitor patients in collaboration with a professional nurse. The economics of health care now demand that nurses demonstrate their value to the institution in terms of economic return (Baird,

1995). In the case of the nurse in the alternative care setting, she or he must demonstrate ability to maintain patients outside of the hospital and decrease rehospitalizations, unnecessary clinic visits, and use of resources. As more budgetary constraints emerge as a result of competition, fewer professional nurses are at the bedside. Nursing administrators of ambulatory BMT settings must carefully and continuously balance optimal patient care with declining nursing personnel budgets.

Recruitment and Retention

Transplantation performed in a nontraditional setting requires recruitment of nurses with unique skills and commitment to patient care. Nurses who are highly skilled, independent clinicians with experience in oncology, critical care, and BCT or BMT may be the ideal candidates, but these nurses may not be available. Graduate nurses, pediatric nurses, or oncology generalists who are trained, educated, and mentored can become experts in this field. A guiding principle in successful recruitment is the nurse manager's sensitivity to the unique skills required for caring for the transplant recipient in a nontraditional setting.

Cross-training must be provided in areas in which the nurse has not had experience. A nurse whose experience has been limited to BCT may not recognize GVHD, whereas those with BMT experience may not have had experience with oncologic diseases. Copel and Smith (1989), in a study to examine BMT nurses' knowledge about the clinical manifestations of GVHD, noted that oncology nurses caring for BMT recipients may need consistent education to assist them in recognizing this common problem in allogeneic recipients. Skills in critical care are desirable in an outpatient setting because the majority of toxic effects experienced by the transplant recipient are generally multisystem. Experience in critical care provides the nurse a sound knowledge base for early recognition of clinical symptomatology and prompt intervention.

Retention of highly skilled nurses is essential to the overall success of a BCT or BMT. Efforts to retain one of the transplant team's most valuable resources is becoming one of the top priorities for nursing administrators. Nursing services typically represent the largest budgetary expenditure in a health provider's budget (Kelleher, 1994). Methods to reduce these costs with the use of the multiskilled workers and targeting nursing budgets to reduce or eliminate professional education, travel, and subscriptions are common (Baird, 1995). Some institutions are creating unique on-site programs conducted by expert transplant nurse consultants with the proceeds targeted to generate financial support for the educational needs of the transplant unit. The Oncology Nursing Society and regional and national transplant centers are offering symposia to help meet educational and networking needs of transplantation nurses in a cost-effective manner.

It has been noted that transplant nursing units are especially stressful due to continuing complex educational needs, managing emergency situations, and the rapid transition between aggressive and terminal care for patients (Ford, 1983; Sarantos, 1988). This may be just as true for the staff of an alternative care site. In efforts to ameliorate stress-related behaviors, stress management programs may be instituted in attempts to reduce absenteeism, optimize job performance, and contribute to the overall well-being of the nurse. Solutions may be on-site support groups, bereavement programs, health club memberships at corporate rates, massage therapy, and legitimate psychological counseling for crisis intervention. Other efforts include participation in the unit's decision making, collaborative relationships with physicians, leadership training, continuing education programs, adequate staffing, and competitive salaries and benefits (Kelleher, 1988; Sarantos, 1988). As

the economics of health care increasingly impinge upon the recruitment and retention of valuable nursing services, nurse administrators will continually need to compete for funding for nursing services. Perhaps one of the most difficult messages that nursing administrators need to relay to their staff is that the onus of job retention now lays with the nurse, who must demonstrate a high level of skill and commitment to patient care with that organization.

Administration

Several levels of administrative responsibilities address clinical and fiscal issues. Typically, a chief executive officer oversees these two areas giving primary responsibilities for day-to-day operations to a nursing administrator and financial manager. Ultimately, the clinical and financial administrators are responsible for profit and loss, revenue generation, managed care, and third-party payer contracts, marketing, risk management, and quality assurance. Some institutions have a nonclinical administrative or operations manager. This role may also be under the responsibility of the nursing director or other clinically oriented managers. As a result of budgetary constraints driven by healthcare reform, middle management is markedly reduced and managerial responsibilities are being consolidated into one role.

Identifying a fee or rate for a transplant is an administrative responsibility. Managed-care contracts dictate global reimbursement rates. Much attention must be given to the determination of the financial feasibility of offering this treatment. An oversimplification of the process is one in which financial officers request that all department managers submit detailed budgets of all transplant-related costs. These costs are subsequently totaled and an estimated aggregate cost per transplant is determined. Some costs are obvious, others are not. For example, who is responsible for the costs of shipping the deceased home if the patient dies during transplant? Adjustments are then made for outliers that represent the lowest to highest cost to perform a transplant.

Medical Staff

Medical Director

The medical director of a transplant program generally oversees all clinical aspects of the program, including writing and implementing research treatment protocols, presenting research findings at scientific symposia, submission of papers to peer review journals, evaluating patients for treatment appropriateness, and documenting medical necessity for insurance clearance. The director is usually the medical oncologist of record, providing direct patient care and supervising the other aspects of the transplant including apheresis, dose-intensive chemotherapy, and stem cell reinfusion. The medical director may also manage the cell processing laboratory where stem cells are processed and cryopreserved.

Physician Staff

Various medical models exist for the physician's role in management of the transplant recipient. Large institutions provide a rotating senior transplant physician who functions as an attending physician and assumes 24-hour responsibility for the patient's care. Depending on the institution, fellows, residents, visiting physicians, and physician extenders such as physician's assistants and advanced nurse practitioners augment patient care. The attending physician and some medical staff often rotate every 30 days. Physician's extenders usually remain as permanent staff or rotate less often. This latter trend is becoming more customary as more emphasis is placed on continuity as patients rapidly move through their care. The advantage of rotating medical staff may be that

it offers a wide diversity and experience in all aspects of marrow transplantation (i.e., infection control, human leukocyte antigen tissue typing, and pediatric, allogeneic or autologous transplant). Disadvantages may be that clinic rotations may distract house staff's writing and research and conflict with administrative responsibilities and ongoing clinical research. Other institutions may hire a permanent full-time outpatient physician to direct daily clinical care under the direction of the medical director. The advantages of a permanently assigned, rather than rotating, staff member are continuity and consistency in patient care. Disadvantages include a budgetary burden of approximately $150,000 to $200,000 per year.

Medical Consultants

Transplant recipients are at high risk for major organ toxicity resulting from pretransplant conditioning regiments, GVHD (allogeneic), and medications used to manage complications (i.e., cyclosporin, corticosteroids). Medical consultants may be required to support patients with neurological, cardiac, renal, or other organ failures.

Medical Dental Services

The oral cavity is a prime target of considerable insult during the transplant process (Lloid, 1995). BCT recipients, however, may not require the medical dental services because of decreased neutropenia compared to marrow recipients. Marrow transplantation recipients have significant morbidity including dental caries, mucositis, and infection. The need for consistent evaluation, early diagnosis, and management for recipients through all stages of the transplant has been well documented (Lloid, 1995; Schubert et al., 1986). Dentists and dental hygienists familiar with the transplant process should be involved in all stages of evaluation and management to identify patients at increased risk for oral complications. It is not unusual for a marrow transplant candidate to be delayed admission for BMT until compromising dental problems are resolved. Dental caries, orthodontic appliances, and peritoneal disease place patients at risk for bacterial, viral, and fungal disease that is exacerbated by parotitis, mucositis, and bleeding problems (Lloid, 1995; Schubert, 1986).

Dental hygienists play an important role in teaching and supporting patients in routine oral care during transplantation and patients are closely followed for ongoing or new oral health problems. Ideally, a dental team is located in the outpatient transplantation setting. Dental chairs, complete with X-ray viewing boxes, sterilizers, medications, oxygen outlets, and emergency equipment are required. A code alarm for emergency situations is necessary because the dental laboratory may be located away from the mainstream clinic traffic.

Ancillary Services

Pharmacy

Transplant recipients may require dose-intensive chemotherapeutic agents, multiple antimicrobials, immunotherapy, hyperalimentation, hydration, lipids, steroids, and symptom management medication. With the rapid emergence of new pharmaceutic agents, the pharmacists have become essential to calculate accurate doses, determine adverse reactions, and understand the synergistic effects of multidosing of medications (Wilkins, 1995). Unstable outpatients, like hospitalized patients, require stat medications that can be more efficiently and safely measured and dispensed by registered pharmacists rather than nursing personnel. Patients require large amounts of self-administered medications. Pharmacists and nurses can collaborate to teach patient and family care-

givers about administration of medications and potential adverse reactions. If the pharmacy is not on-site, various techniques for transporting medications and pharmaceutical supplies are available and include transportation persons and tube systems. Pharmacists with administrative experience in purchasing, dispensing, and controlling expensive medications can ensure efficient management of the on-site pharmacy. The annual costs of a dedicated full-time equivalent can counterbalance otherwise significant losses due to off-site management.

Dietary

Oral intake for transplant recipients can be severely limited during transplantation and patients may be nutritionally depleted as a result of standard chemotherapy and/or radiation administered for their underlying diseases, lengthy hospitalizations, corticosteroid therapy, or psychological stress. Consequently, recipients have unique nutritional requirements and need education to sustain them through periods of neutropenia and subsequent infection, GVHD, and other organ toxicities. Hyperalimentation for nutritional supplements has proved to be a lifesaving measure for transplant recipients. This therapy, however, is not without its particular toxicities and expenses. Expensive medications and therapies are being examined closely to determine the optimal and most cost-effective manner for use in patient care. Decreasing use of TPN is a targeted area. Dieticians are increasingly needed to guide family caregivers in appropriate nutritional needs. In the face of shrinking medical staff, dieticians are responsible for making nutritional recommendations that include hyperalimentation, lipids, hydrations, and possible enteral feedings. Calorie counts and calculating and tracking patients' weights are also the dietician's responsibilities (Stearn and Lenssen, 1995). The dietary area should be close to the nurses' and physicians' areas, and space should accommodate a pediatric and adult stadeometer, regular scales, height charts, and a growth chart for children.

Transplant recipients and family caregivers can spend many hours a day in alternative care settings. Food services must be available to accommodate this population. Small kitchens that have microwave ovens, ice makers, refrigerators, sinks, garbage disposals, disposable dishes, wastepaper disposals, and hot water spigots can support minimal food services. Otherwise, on-site cafeterias or vending machines may be located in halls or near elevators throughout the building.

Behavioral Medicine

Psychosocial support for transplant recipients and their families is essential to address the host of anxiety-producing psychosocial hurdles inherent in the transplant trajectory. Because of the shift from hospitalization to outpatient models of care for recipients, the classic stressors experienced with each phase of transplant may be exacerbated due to the absence of the 24-hour support most often available in the hospital setting. No studies comparing emotional problems of BCT and BMT have been published. It may be expected by some that marrow recipients demand more psychosocial support than BCT recipients secondary to more toxic conditioning regimens, TBI, and GVHD. This judgment, however, may be erroneous. Other factors, such as absence of social support systems, limited economic situations, loss of job security, or preexisting psychological problems, confound the physical demands of transplantation.

Syrjala (1995) notes that each phase of transplant has particular emotional challenges that demand significant energy for coping (Table 23.5). As less hospitalization for BCT and BMT becomes the community standard, more intensive psychological support for family caregivers is needed to assist them in coping with issues of intensive self-care management in an increasingly symptomatic recipient. As healthcare economics continue to be compressed with consequent decrease of dedicated psychosocial support (psychiatrists, psychologists, social workers) for patients and families, oncology nurses will be further pressed to assist with the psychosocial needs of these patients.

Clericals

Clerical staff in transplant settings can be responsible for organization of patients' charts, scheduling patients' appointments and procedures, routing laboratory specimens and results, coordinating billing and reimbursement paperwork, and managing medical supplies. Personnel and space must be allotted for this staff near but not directly in the patient care area. Because of the highly complex nature of transplant technology, nonclinical managers need strong clinical understanding of the transplantation process and sensitivities to the physical and psychological burden of recipients and family caregivers. In some institutions, clerical staff may report to the nursing manager, in others to a nonclinical manager.

Material Supplies

Care and support of transplant recipients require a significant amount of medical and clerical supplies. Adequate space and immediate access to supplies such as IV pumps and tubing, CVC supplies, equipment for various procedures, and specimen collections are critical to efficient and safe patient care. Sufficient space to store supplies for 24 to 48 hours must be available. Daily, clear communication is needed between the nurse and the manager of material supplies. Collection of hazardous waste, disposal of used supplies, and ambulatory home care pumps may be organized under the material supplies department, although some institutions place responsibility of these items with the pharmacy (Buchsel, 1995).

TABLE 23.5 Psychological demands and concerns during transplantation phases

PREARRIVAL FOR TRANSPLANT
Disease status (acceptability for transplant)
Other medical complications or risk factors
Selection
  Finding an appropriate donor or autologous plan
  Selecting a transplant site
  Acceptance by a transplant site
Resources screening
  Insurance, Medicaid, fund raising, or other
    financial support
  Caregiver support
  Family social and assistance supports
Preparing for all possibilities
  Wills, living wills, durable power of attorney
  Job security
  Family needs and home/work maintenance in
    absence
Coping
  Decision making
  Access to and use of information and supports
Psychological responses
  Distress
  Preexisting psychological problems

PRETRANSPLANT
Selection
  Disease status changes
  New medical complications or risk factors identified
Donor
  Retracting consent or pressuring for payment
  Anxieties or phobias
Behavioral medicine
  Heightened sensitivity, decreased pain tolerance
  Phobias to procedures
  Conditioned nausea and vomiting to radiation
    and/or chemotherapy
  Anticipatory anxiety
  Pain from procedures, disease, or prior treatment
Informed consent
  Retaining and comprehending information
  Confronting risks
  Identifying questions or problems
  Maintaining emotional balance with
    preponderance of negative information
  Decision making

Adaptation to new site (if patient traveled for
  transplant)
  Cultural differences
  Daily living difficulties
  Family and home management
  New shopping
  New schools or work
Preexisting psychological and family problems'
  interface with medical system
Ensure safety of family and obtain consent of
  donor
Adjust or discontinue use of psychotropic medi-
  cation
Identify coping style of patient so that staff can
  accomplish necessary care

HOSPITALIZATION PHASE
Survival
Medical complications
Symptom management
  Pain
  Nausea, vomiting
  Oral intake
  Sleep problems
  Anxiety
  Depression
Mental status changes
  Delirium
  Loss of memory and concentration
Neurotoxic effects of medications
  Hallucinations
  Psychosis
Isolation
Medical demands and stress
  Loss of privacy, dignity, control
Behavioral/adherence problems
Family and donor needs
  Food and shelter stresses (if living in a new
    location)
  Multiple roles if caregiver also is parenting or
    working
  Fears, demands related to patient's need for
    blood product from family members
  Grief planning if patient dies
  Discharge safety fears

(Continued)

TABLE 23.5 Psychological demands and concerns during transplantation phases *Continued*

IMMEDIATE POSTTRANSPLANT PHASE	LONG-TERM RECOVERY PHASE
Medical complications	Complications with continued health changes
Symptom management	Physical changes
Strength, stamina	Delayed growth and development
Oral intake	Neurologic sequelae: memory, concentration,
Nausea, vomiting	complex learning and reasoning
Discomfort, uneasiness	Functioning, stamina, strength limitations
Withdrawal	Infertility
Irritation, anger	Changes in sexual functioning
Depression	Psychological adaptation
Anxiety	Changes in sexual functioning
Guilt for thoughts and survival	Medication compliance demands (e.g., steroids
General mental slowing	and cyclosporin)
Memory	Continued isolation requirements
Concentration	Family/caregiver burden and fatigue
Decision making	Posttraumatic stress symptoms
Neurotoxic effects of medications	Uncertainty, waiting
Emotional liability	Medical complications
Seizures	Relapse or secondary cancers
Psychosis	Health and stamina
Continued isolation demands	Role and work limitations
Waiting for something to go wrong	Changes in abilities at job or school
Caregiver burden and fatigue	Family roles and responsibilities
Grief if patient dies	Economic/insurance costs
Safety fears with new responsibilities	Safety fears with return to pre-BMT medical
	providers

SOURCE: Syrjala, K., 1995. Used with permission.

CLINICAL ISSUES DURING THE PHASES OF TRANSPLANTATION

There are six phases of transplantation: (1) evaluation, (2) harvest marrow and/or stem cell harvest and cryopreservation, (3) dose-intensive therapy, (4) reinfusion transplant, (5) engraftment/recovery, and (6) long-term recovery. In new models of care, a large portion of this care is administered in ambulatory care settings which, of course, depends on the philosophies and clinical support of individual institutions.

Evaluation

The first phase of transplantation is the evaluation, which follows pathways that differ among institutions. At this time, the most important questions are (1) does the disease and its present status lend itself to treatment with transplantation? and (2) what is the optimal time for a transplant? These basic questions are imperative due to the growing number of diseases and the growing population now eligible for transplantation. Accordingly, much controversy and considerable debate persist about the optimal time to perform a transplant. For example, the improving physiological status of an aging population now makes it possible to treat older patients with transplants (Ringden et al., 1993). One basic concern in transplant evaluation is the role and timing of standard chemotherapy. The critical question is, does the patient have a significantly improved chance of disease-free survival if traditional chemotherapy is given prior to transplant rather than proceeding directly to transplant?

Some researchers believe that patients without prior extensive exposure to chemotherapeutic agents are at a decreased risk for life-threatening transplant complications. The toxicities of previous chemotherapies may damage marrow, subsequently decreasing stem cell quality and viability. Unfortunately, most managed-care contracts mandate that patients receive conventional chemotherapy rather than "investigational" treatments. Consequently, transplant candidates may arrive at a transplant center having already received chemotherapy and experienced side effects that may compromise the transplant. Conversely, other researchers believe that a positive tumor response to at least one course of adjuvant chemotherapy must be achieved prior to BCT to ensure that harvested stem cells will not suffer tumor cell contamination (Juttner et al., 1994).

Ideally, the potential candidate is evaluated at the initial time of diagnosis using the expertise of the referring oncologist and the transplant physician. If the decision is made to proceed with transplantation, the patient receives treatment dates and plans his or her arrival at the transplantation center. The next priority is to address fertility issues. Because dose-intensive chemotherapy and/or irradiation prior to transplantation usually result in sterility, men should have sperm analysis for possible sperm banking (Sanders, 1988; Corcoran-Buchsel, 1986). Women who want children may require counseling on alternative childbearing methods.

An oncology nurse coordinator who has contacted the patient and family prior to arrival can continue to guide the patients through this process and be a consistent person who directs, reassures, and represents the transplantation center where the patient and caregiver will spend weeks or months.

To spare the patient and family unnecessary expenses and to expedite the transplant, a patient's initial steps prior to transplant are scheduled in rapid succession. The patient's most recent test results, in particular a complete blood count (CBC) and electrolytes, must be sent to the center immediately prior to the patient's arrival to ensure that the patient has no immediate serological indications of complications that may preclude the transplant. If the patient arrives with unforeseen medical problems, transplant may be delayed, which results in increased direct and indirect expenses while exacerbating the patient's and caregiver's anxiety. Health-care providers usually ask that a patient pay cash or demonstrate third-party reimbursement for transplants. Once preauthorization is obtained, all risks and benefits of the transplant are reviewed by a transplant physician with the patient and family. Informed consent is obtained, and the patient is prepared for the specific transplant process.

Clinical Evaluation

The dose-intensive chemotherapy and possible irradiation required to treat the patient's underlying disease can cause major organ dysfunction. A history, physical, and various clinical and laboratory tests are performed prior to or at the time of a patient's arrival at a transplant center. This information indicates that the patient can withstand the dose-intensive therapy. Other factors related to previously administered chemotherapeutic agents must be considered and additional tests performed to validate the candidacy of an individual for transplantation. For example, patients previously treated with doxorubicin require an echocardiogram to determine the present level of cardiac function. The results of the ejection fraction may identify higher risk for the patient but is not the sole determining factor. Abnormal tests should be evaluated in conjunction with other physical and laboratory findings.

Central Venous Catheter Placement

Transplant recipients require a large, surgically placed, multilumen central venous catheter (CVC) for administration of parenteral solutions and collection of blood specimens. BCT recipients require large-bore catheters to collect progenitor cells through apheresis. Placement site depends on the patient's disease status, prior access devices, and the ability of the vessel to support the catheter without perforation of the subclavian wall and/or pneumothorax during placement. BCT recipients presenting with one of these problems or risks may require a catheter placed in the groin, which is usually removed after apheresis because of the risk of contamination and subsequent infection. Such patients will require alternative central and/or peripheral venous access for the administration of dose-intensive chemotherapy, and supportive therapy during BCT recovery is required.

Nursing responsibilities for patients with newly inserted apheresis catheters is based on assessment and management and teaching the patient and caregiver about the time and place of catheter placement, and options for anesthesia (e.g., general or local). CVCs must remain patent with heparin and flushed daily with normal saline to prevent clots. To prevent the risk of heparin-induced hypercoagulation, heparin solutions should not be flushed through the catheter. Daily laboratory studies can be drawn from the catheter after wasting approximately 10 cc of blood. Inadvertent heparinization and/or dilution of the specimen could result in inaccurate laboratory findings. Catheter flush-

ing techniques and care of insertion sites vary slightly among institutions.

Both patients and caregivers should be instructed in and evaluated for signs and symptoms such as pain, swelling, and/or increased temperature of the affected extremity. Significant postoperative bleeding and the subsequent development of a hematoma at the catheter site can occur because of persistent chronic thrombocytopenia related to previous chemotherapy regimens and/or disease process. Patients are placed on restricted activity for the first 24 hours. Sandbags and/or ice packs may be used immediately after surgery to control local bleeding, and the affected extremity should be evaluated frequently for adequate perfusion. Pain may be relieved by 650 mg acetaminophen. Persistent pain should be reported and requires further assessment and intervention for possible pneumothorax (Buchsel and Kapustay, 1995).

Harvest/Apheresis and Cryopreservation

Stem cells for BCT are most often, but not exclusively, harvested after *mobilization*, a technique to increase circulating stem cells and progenitor cells from extravascular sites into the bloodstream. The pheresis procedure occurs exclusively in outpatient areas. The most common agents for mobilization are cyclophosphamide (2–4 g/m^2), granulocyte-macrophage colony-stimulating factor (GM-CSF) or granulocyte colony-stimulating factor (G-CSF). Often the combination of chemotherapy and HGFs result in a more profound mobilization than either agent used alone. Other growth factors that hold promise in clinical trials include erythropoietin, granulocyte-macrophage colony-stimulating factor/interleukin-3 (PIXY 321), and interleukin-3 (Schmidt-Pokorny, 1994).

Approximately 2 days prior to the start of apheresis, daily subcutaneous administration of

HGFs are begun. HGFs have adverse side effects. The predominant symptom is bone pain, which is treated effectively with acetaminophen. Other adverse effects are mild and include nausea, diarrhea, rash, fever, malaise, pleural effusion, increased catheter clotting, vomiting, headache, chills, dyspnea, and edema. Additionally, HGFs can irritate skin at the injection site, and patients must be taught to report this symptom immediately. If left unattended, skin may break down and increase the risk of infection. Patients need to be reassured that symptoms are transient and reversible. Patients and caregivers need to be instructed to store, reconstitute, and administer accurate doses, recognize and manage adverse effects, injection techniques, and appropriate disposal of syringes. Return demonstrations are extremely helpful in evaluating a patient's competency and should be an integral part of any instruction session.

Approximately 9 to 14 liters of blood are processed through a large-bore central-lumen catheter over 2 to 4 hours, and the remaining blood is returned to the patient. The number of aphereses depends on the viability of the collected stem cells and the number of CD34-positive cells collected. In the past, six to eight aphereses were performed over 7 to 10 days. With improved mobilization techniques and cell-separating equipment, adequate cells can be collected in one or two procedures.

The next step is to retrieve stem cells from the blood cell separator and isolate them using a density gradient or another apheresis procedure to reduce the number of contaminating red cells and granulocyte. The average life of stem cells is 3 to 7 days, and cells are usually cryopreserved to prevent damage and ensure cell viability at the time of reinfusion. Recent research in cryopreservation of allogeneic stem cells, however, suggests that for the majority of patients receiving BCT, fresh cells can be administered without major difficulties with stem cell loss. This method decreases expenses by the avoidance of freezing (Bensinger et al., 1995).

Historically, medical care of allogeneic marrow donors, except marrow harvest, takes place almost exclusively in an outpatient setting. Marrow harvest is performed under general or spinal anesthesia in an operating suite in a hospital setting. Patients are usually admitted to day surgery and discharged approximately 24 hours after surgery. Overnight stays have been justified because of rare morbidity associated with the procedure (Buckner et al., 1984; Stronceck et al., 1993). Research data now suggests that it is possible to safely perform marrow harvest as an outpatient procedure for selected donors or autologous patients. Brandwein and colleagues (1989) assessed outpatient marrow harvesting for autologous BMT recipients. During a 13-month period, 39 patients underwent outpatient marrow harvest. Of these patients, 36 were discharged later the same day with oral iron supplements, and no adverse postoperative sequelae. Two patients required hospital admission secondary to postoperative hypotension, and one patient was readmitted due to fever.

Use of allogeneic blood transfusions is diminishing, and administration of rh-Epo to donors to increase production of RBCs may eliminate the need for autostorage of several units of blood, thereby allowing a majority of allogeneic donors to have marrow harvest in outpatient areas. York and colleagues (1992) studied 10 normal marrow donors who received rh-Epo prior to marrow harvest to increase their red blood counts. The mean increase between the initial hematocrit and the postoperative hematocrit was 16%, compared to a decrement of 4% in a control group ($p = 0.001$). As these technologies advance, especially for child donors, alternative sites for transplantation may have on-site outpatient surgeries. BCT allogeneic donors avoid the risk of general anesthesia and postoperative complications because of elimination of marrow harvest.

In efforts to hasten engraftment and decrease morbidity and mortality of BCT recipients, donors are being increasingly treated with HGFs prior to stem cell collection. The role of HGFs in donors is awaiting long-term study that will indicate their effects on long-term engraftment, acute and chronic GVHD, and donor safety (Chatta et al., 1994). Hopes for the future are that with more effective HGF regimens, apheresis will be eliminated and stem cells collected from one or two units of blood (Bensinger, 1995). If these hopes come to fruition, almost all marrow harvesting will be done in outpatient settings in the near future.

Preparative Therapy

Dose-Intensive Chemotherapy

The site of dose-intensive therapy is determined by the type and duration of chemotherapy, after-hour supportive services, and patient and caregiver ability for self-care. Dose-intensive chemotherapeutic protocols for transplantation vary among institutions and among tumor diseases. The overall toxicity of the treatment regimen is a factor in determining its applicability for administration in an outpatient setting, either in its entirety or in part. Patients are generally able to tolerate higher doses of less toxic chemotherapy that do not require administration times longer than 8 to 12 hours. Some dose-intensive regimens that are now administered on an outpatient basis are:

- melpheran
- carmustin/triethylenethiophosphoramide (thiotepa)
- cyclophosphamide/mesna triethylene-thiophosphoramide (thiotepa)
- busulfan

Protocols with longer infusion times can be managed on an outpatient basis by using ambulatory infusion devices at home to administer the remaining hours of the infusion. Some protocols that dictate more toxic levels of chemotherapeutic agents administered over a longer period of time include those containing carmustine, etoposide, cyclophosphamide, and mesna given pre-BCT for some types of lymphoma. Severe adverse effects such as diarrhea, nausea, vomiting, and marrow suppression are immediate and require frequent assessment and immediate intervention to prevent immediate and long-term sequelae. These dose-intensive agents must be evaluated for outpatient safety and efficacy prior to initiation in alternative care settings. This evaluation must include the physical and psychological health of the patient and family caregiver to participate in intensive self-care.

In an alternative model of care, patients may be admitted to an inpatient or to an 18-hour to 24-hour outpatient transplant unit for administration of high-dose chemotherapy that includes pretreatment with aggressive hydration on an average of 1 liter to 4 liters of fluid daily, continuous multiagent antiemetic therapy, and intensive physiologic monitoring. After completion of high-dose chemotherapy and drug elimination, patients are discharged from the hospital, or they return to their temporary housing. Patients must always be accompanied by a competent caregiver because of the high risk of infection, bleeding, and other complications.

Outpatients receiving dose-intensive chemotherapy present unprecedented acuity levels. In spite of aggressive HFG support, life-threatening infections can develop. Mucositis and esophagitis, accompanied by pain, oral infection, nausea, vomiting, diarrhea, and dehydration, are other major concerns; and patients may eventually require IV opioids with monitoring of mental and respiratory status. Attention to oral hygiene is critical and frequent inspection of the oral mucosa is necessary. Fatigue in patients and caregivers is an underreported problem. Certain outpatients need hospital admission for the management of these sequelae.

Educating patients and families is of critical importance and can influence the acuity of symptoms experienced by patients. Instruction should focus on the use of medications to ameliorate adverse effects, the required neutropenic precautions, the value of low-bacterial diets, the need to report symptoms, and the role of emergency care. Consistent assurance is provided to the patient and family with confidence that continuity of care will be maintained as they proceed through the most challenging phase of transplant. Quality of life and burden of care have not been studied in this population and are a rich area of research for oncology nurses.

Total Body Irradiation

Given in high-dose conditioning regimens, TBI for transplant recipients has traditionally been administered in an inpatient setting. Anecdotal reports worldwide are emerging that indicate that selected patients may tolerate outpatient TBI. The most common problems associated with TBI are pain resulting from bilateral parotiditis and generalized fatigue, which can be eased with pain medication, rest, caregiver support, and the patient's desire to remain unhospitalized. As more liberal philosophies emerge as to type of treatments that can be given safely in outpatient settings, more transplant centers may offer TBI as an outpatient procedure.

Reinfusion/Transplant

The process and standard of care for infusion of stem cells or marrow should not change across settings. Expected complications, nursing management, and management of self-care are described elsewhere in this book.

Engraftment/Recovery

Generally speaking, initial hematopoietic recovery after BCT is similar to recovery after autologous BMT. The megakaryocytic cell line is problematic for reasons that remain unclear. It is thought that the phenomenon may be secondary to megakaryocyte fragility caused during cryopreservation, cryoprotectant interaction, or both. New HGFs in clinical trials that hasten megakaryocyte engraftment hold promise for speedier engraftment with subsequent reductions of both cost and risks of multiple platelet transfusions.

For BCT recipients hospitalized for dose-intensive therapy, discharge criteria are similar across care settings, and these criteria are similar to BMT recipients. Particular attention must be given to the family caregiver's ability to care for recipients in an efficacious manner. Parameters of hematopoietic recovery differ slightly among institutions. Minimal criteria are an absolute neutrophil count of greater than $1,000/m^3$, platelet count greater than $20,000/m^3$ with no active bleeding, and a hematocrit of 25% for 1 to 2 weeks.

Patients usually remain near the transplant center for 3 to 4 weeks after treatment for continuous monitoring for febrile episodes, viral pneumonia, dehydration, persistent nausea, suspected veno-occlusive disease, and thrombocytopenia. Prophylactic antibiotics may prevent or decrease episodes of fever, and sequential once-daily antibiotic therapy simplifies care during febrile neutropenia occurrences. The ability to deliver 24-hour care is imperative and a cadre of medical, nursing, pharmacy, and laboratory personnel must be available. Hospital admissions/readmissions peak during this period, and permissions for smooth transition between inpatient, outpatient, and home care are essential. Common reasons for hospital admissions, readmissions, or transitions across sites of care include:

- psychological distress
- IV pain control
- cardiac complications from pretreatment-induced cardiomyopathy
- veno-occlusive disease
- sepsis
- pulmonary complication, CMV
- failure to thrive
- physician's discretion
- financial or third-party payer contract
- undue burden on caregiver

Particular attention must be paid to the family caregiver's ability to administer possible multiple therapies at home or provide transportation to clinical treatment areas.

For the allogenic recipient, similar but more serious complications can exist secondary to more intensive pretransplant conditioning regimens and the presence of GVHD. Initial declarations or exacerbations of acute GVHD usually managed in a hospital setting are being increasingly managed in ambulatory care settings. These symptoms often confound already existing problems of nausea, vomiting, diarrhea, fever, chills, and skin disorders, and require differential diagnosis and management. Nurses, who are usually the first to assess these patients, will require intensive education in the pathophysiology, clinical manifestation, and management of acute GVHD. As allogeneic BMT patients are discharged earlier, nurses will be assessing and managing acute and chronic GVHD.

Long-Term Recovery
Currently, little is known about the long-term recovery of the BCT recipient because of its short existence as a serious treatment option. It is anticipated that long-term sequelae will be similar to but less intense than those associated with BMT (Henon et al., 1995). The classic causes of BMT long-term complications are related to the patient's underlying disease, high-dose conditioning regimens, GVHD, and transplant-related supportive care (i.e., adverse reactions to medications, such as cyclosporin). Because all of these conditions can exist in the BCT recipient, problems such as sterility, immunosuppression, and chronic GVHD (allogenic) may declare themselves before the patient returns home. Consequently, there are insufficient numbers of survivors to determine transplant-related complications and long-term, disease-free survival; but new information will rapidly emerge as researchers publish the results of clinical trials. For example, Bensinger (1995) notes the presence of chronic GVHD in 56% of 23 evaluable allogeneic BCT recipients. In contrast to early fears that GVHD may present serious barriers for allogeneic BCT recipients (Gale, 1995), GVHD was a manageable sequela in this group. More research is needed in this area before it can confidently be documented that GVHD is not a serious complication of BCT. Because allogeneic recipients are returning to their communities sooner, community transplant teams need to evaluate them for chronic GVHD approximately 80 days after BCT.

Compounding this event are barriers preventing complete and consistent long-term follow-up. Patients leave alternative transplant sites only weeks after treatment, and patient follow-up data becomes markedly challenging. Patients are usually followed by their oncologists, rather than their transplant physicians. Obtaining follow-up information is often placed on busy clerical and office staff, making data collection inconsistent.

Retrieval of follow-up information (relapse, death, chronic GVHD) may often depend on the quality of relationships between the oncologist and transplant physician. A transplant coordinator can be of assistance by constantly communicating with primary physicians to collect essential mobidity and mortality data. Establishing this rapport begins at the time of initial referral and continues throughout the transplant process. Patient follow-up can be achieved by direct patient contact, provided this communication is not viewed as intrusive by either the patient or referring physician. In contrast to earlier views of transplant physicians, especially in new models of care and BCT, the transplant is often considered a therapy analogous to the services of an oncologic radiologist or surgeon vis-à-vis the primary care physicians. That is, the referring physician remains the ultimate coordinator of all care required by the patient. Even in case of established long-term, follow-up teams for autologous and allogeneic recipients, long-term, follow-up data is becoming increasingly difficult to gather because of recipients' rapid return to their communities. Five years ago, it was common for marrow recipients to remain at transplant centers up to 100 days after BMT. Current health-care economics mandate earlier return home, further hampering retrieval of vital research data.

Quality of Life
Quality-of-life (QOL) research aimed at patients and caregivers in alternative settings is needed to characterize hurdles incurred during outpatient or combination transplantation. BCT QOL is slowly being recognized. Recently Henon and colleagues (1995) retrospectively compared QOL in 37 patients treated for multiple myeloma. Twelve patients received BCT, 15 received conventional chemotherapy, and 10 patients received polychemotherapy. The investigation noted that BCT recipients demonstrated a quality-of-life score significantly higher than the other study groups ($p = 0.001$).

More studies are under way throughout the world that will illustrate comparative QOL of many patients who receive a variety of toxic treatment options, as the toxicities of transplants decrease due to improvements in current techniques (i.e., decreased apheresis for BCT recipients and supportive care such as GVHD management for allogeneic BMTs). One can expect that QOL in these recipients will surpass that of patients who receive conventional oncologic care. Future research will expand QOL studies to the caregiver as burdens of families increase in direct relationship to decreased or absence of hospital days. As medical costs soar and health-care resources diminish, only treatments that balance successful long-term outcome with the treatment costs will be available. Meaningful nursing research in QOL studies can make an enormous positive contribution to the growing numbers of patients eligible for a lifesaving treatment.

FUTURE TRENDS

The majority of the care of transplant recipients will shift to outpatient or alternative care settings. Advancements with earlier acting cytokines such as IL-3, sequential IL-3 followed by GM-CSF, PIXY 321, stem cell factor (SCF), or G-CSF will enhance engraftment and decrease hospitalizations. Large-scale ex vivo expansion of progenitor cells supplemented with IL-3, GM-CSF, EPO, and SCF may reduce the number of aphereses while facilitating engraftment (Vose and Armitage, 1995). The use of BCT transplantation for a growing number of diseases such as small cell lung, ovarian, and testicular cancer will expand the numbers of eligible candidates. Similar to autologous BMT, stem cells can be stored in healthy persons who are at high risk for certain malignancies (breast cancer) and reinfused, if necessary. Other patients whose cancer is in remission may have their blood stem cells stored in case of relapse (Hooper and Santos, 1993). Preclinical research is investigating opportunities for allogeneic BCT that will further expand this treatment to other patients. Umbilical cord or placenta stem cells obtained at birth may offer less expensive harvesting of stem cells (Issaragrisil et al., 1995). Currently, the procedure is limited to children, and disease-free survival compared to BMT remains unknown (Gale, 1994; Gale et al., 1994). Fetal liver cells, a rich source of hematopoietic stem cells, may hold promise for patients with severe combined immunologic disease. Harvest of fetal liver cells presents serious ethical concerns (Roncarolo et al., 1992; Zanjani et al., 1992).

Future phase III trials will include analysis of the adjusted costs to reduce transplantation expenses. The use of tailor-made monoclonal antibodies in conjunction with BMT to treat patients with large cell lymphoma and leukemia is currently in clinical trials and may hold promise for long-term disease-free survival (McNeil, 1995). As transplant costs diminish, insurance reimbursements will become more available, and the number of candidates will increase exponentially. Patients and families will be asked to participate in a greater portion of their self-management. Nurse-designed computer programs will offer "user-friendly" educational programs (Coxen, 1995). As the results of clinical trials support disease-free survival after BCT or BMT for more diseases, treatment will be more available in the community setting. There will be more patients cared for in the community by advanced nurse practitioners, transplant nurses, and general oncology nurses.

SUMMARY

Historically, the majority of the care of the blood and marrow recipients was given in tra-

ditional hospital settings. Over the past decade, the majority of this care has shifted to new treatment settings that include exclusive outpatient management or combinations of hospital, ambulatory, and home care. Blood and marrow transplant teams who are designing new or renovating existing modes need far-reaching vision to create safe and cost-conscious environments for recipients and their families.

Blood cell and bone marrow transplantation remain dynamic areas of clinical practice and research. Innovations in combining established therapies with novel approaches are occurring rapidly. The primary focus in BCT is aimed at determining appropriateness of current treatment techniques and development of innovative solutions to existing problems. Further investigation through clinical trials is needed to

1. identify optimal dose-intensity regimens,
2. reduce the number of apheresis collections through such innovations as ex vivo expansion,
3. determine the optimal number of stem cells to ensure rapid and enduring engraftment,
4. eliminate tumor contamination, and
5. control allogeneic GVHD.

The ability to perform BCT and BMT in a cost-effective manner is paramount as healthcare reimbursement moves toward an exclusive managed-care environment and payers deem BCT and BMT acceptable, noninvestigational treatments. Challenges for BMT are to

1. increase disease-free survival,
2. improve management of GVHD,
3. decrease infections and toxicities of conditioning regimens, and
4. apply gene therapy to clinical practice.

Furthermore, the emotional and financial burdens on patients, families, and caregivers during transplantation cannot be underestimated. As more of these concerns are addressed, recipients and their families can be managed effectively in alternative care settings. Nurses working in administrative, clinical, educational, and research roles have unique opportunity to collaborate and direct new health-care environments in BCT and BMT.

REFERENCES

Argenti, P. 1994. *The Portable MBA Desk Reference*. New York: Wiley, 368.

ASCO/ASH. 1990. Recommended criteria for performance of bone marrow transplantation. *J Clin Oncol* 8(3):563-564.

Baird, S. 1995. The impact of changing health care delivery on oncology practice. *Oncol Nurs* 2(3):1-12.

Bensinger, W. 1995. Peripheral blood stem cell transplantation. In Buckner, C. (Ed.) *Technical and Biological Components of Marrow Transplantation*. Boston: Kleiver Academic, 68-91.

Bensinger, W., Clift, R., Anasetti, C., et al. 1995. Transplantation of allogeneic peripheral blood stem cells mobilized by recombinant human granaulocyte colony stimuating factor. *Stem Cells* 13:52-66.

Brandwein, J., Callum, J., Rubinger, M., et al. 1989. An evaluation of outpatient bone marrow harvesting. *J Clin Oncol* 7(9):1367-8.

Buchsel, P. 1991. Ambulatory care: before and after BMT. In Whedon, M. (Ed.) *Bone Marrow Transplantation Principles, Practice, and Nursing Insights*. Boston: Jones & Bartlett, 295-313.

Buchsel, P. 1993. Ambulatory care for the bone marrow transplant patient. In Buchsel, P., Yarbro, C. (Eds.) *Oncology Nursing in the Ambulatory Setting: Issues and Models of Care*. Boston: Jones & Bartlett, 185-216.

Buchsel, P. 1995. Administrative issues of an ambulatory care setting. In Buchsel, P., Whedon, M. (Eds.) *Bone Marrow Transplantation: Administrative and Clinical Strategies*. Boston: Jones & Bartlett, 19-38.

Buchsel, P., Kapustay, P. 1995. Peripheral stem cell transplantation. *Oncol Nurs: Patient Treatment and Support* 2(2):1-13.

Buckner, C., Clift, R., Sanders, J., et al. 1984. Marrow harvesting from normal donors. *Blood* 64(3):630-634.

Buckner, C., Petersen, F., Bolonesi, B. 1994. Bone marrow donors. In Foreman, S., Blume, K., Thomas, E. (Eds.) *Bone Marrow Transplantation*. Boston: Blackwell Scientific, 259-270.

Burns, J.M., Tierney, K., Long, G.D., et al. 1995. Critical pathway for administering high-dose chemotherapy followed by peripheral blood stem cell rescue in the outpatient setting. *Oncol Nurs Forum* 22(8):1219-1224.

Chatta, G., Price, T., Allen, R., et al. Effects of in vivo recombinant methionyl human granulocyte colony-stimulating factor on the neutrophil response and peripheral blood colony-forming cells in healthy young and elderly adult volunteers. *Blood* 4(9):2923-2929.

Copel, L., Smith, M. 1989. Oncology nursing knowledge of graft vs host disease in bone marrow transplant patients. *Canc Nurs* 12(4):243-249.

Corcoran-Buchsel P. 1986. Long term complications of allogeneic bone marrow transplant patients. Nursing Implications. *Oncol Nurs Forum* 13(6):61-70.

Coxen, V. 1995. The role of computers. In Buchsel, P., Whedon, M. (Eds.) *Bone Marrow Transplantation: Administrative and Clinical Strategies*. Boston: Jones & Bartlett, 403-426.

Crump, M., Brandwein, J., Smith, A., et al. 1992. A regional autolgous bone marrow transplant network: transfer to designated centers the day after transplant. *BMT* 9(6):445-450.

DeMeyer, E. 1995. Multidisciplinary team contributions in the management of chronic graft versus host disease: a case study. *Oncol Nurs Forum* 22(2):361.

Ford, R. 1983. Reducing nursing staff stress through scheduling orientation, and continuing education. *Nurs Clin North Am* 18(3):597-601.

Gale, R. 1994. Allogeneic peripheral stem cell transplantation. *BMT* 13(3):53-55.

Gale, R. 1995. Cord-blood cell transplantation: a real sleeper? *N Engl J Med* 332(6):392-394.

Gale, R., Juttner, C., Henon, P. 1995. Overview of blood stem cell transplants. In Gale, R., Juttner, C., Henon, P. (Eds.) *Blood Stem Cell Transplants*. New York: New York Press Syndicate of the University of Cambridge, 1.

Gale, R., Reiffers, Juttner, C.A. 1994. What's new in progenitor cell auto transplants? *BMT* 14(3):343-346.

Goodman, J., and the World Donor Association Executive Committee 1994. A special report: bone marrow transplant using volunteer donors—recommendations and requirements for a standardized practice throughout the world. *Blood* 84(9):2833-2839.

Grady-Porter T. 1990. *Reorganization of Nursing Practice: Creating the Corporate Venture*. Rockville, MD: Aspen, 61-88.

Hawkins, R. 1995. Introduction. Proceedings of the State of Knowledge Conference on Advance Practice in Oncology Nursing. *Oncol Nurs Forum* 22(8, suppl 3).

Hawkins, J., Holcombe, J. 1995. Titling for advanced practice nurses. *Oncol Nurs Forum* 22(8):5-9.

Henon, P. Donatini, B., Eisenmann, J., et al. 1995. Comparative survival, quality of life and cost-effectiveness of intensive therapy with autologous blood cell transplantation or conventional chemotherapy in multiple myeloma. *BMT* 16(1):19-25

Henon, P., Liang, H., Beck-Wirth, G., et al. 1992. Comparison of hematopoietic and immune recovery after autologous bone marrow or blood stem cell transplants. *BMT* 9(4):285-291.

Hooper, P., Santos, E. 1993. Peripheral blood stem cell transplantation. *Oncol Nurs Forum* 20(8):1215-1221.

Houston, D., Houston, G. 1993. Administrative issues and concepts in ambulatory care. In Buchsel, P., Yarbro, C. (Eds.) *Oncology Nursing in the Ambulatory Setting: Issues and Models of Care.* Boston: Jones & Bartlett, 3-18.

Issaragrisil, S., Vissuthisakchai, S., Suvatte, V., et al. 1995. Brief report: transplantation of cord-blood stem cells into patient with severe thalassemia. *N Engl J Med* 332(6):367-369.

Jassak, P., Porter, N. 1995. Strategies for education of the BMT patient. In Buchsel, P., Whedon, M. (Eds.) *Bone Marrow Transplantation Administrative and Clinical Strategies.* Boston: Jones & Bartlett, 353-362.

Jassak, P., Riley, M. 1994. Autologous stem cell transplant. *Cancer Practice* 2(2):141-145.

Juttner, C., Fibbie, W., Neumunaitis, J., et al. 1994. Blood cell transplantation: report from an international consensus meeting. *BMT* 14(5):689-693.

Kelleher, J. 1991. Developing a bone marrow transplant program: planning, environmental and personnel challenges, In Whedon, M. (Ed.) *Bone Marrow Transplantation: Principles, Practice, and Nursing Insights.* Boston: Jones & Bartlett, 378-395.

Kelleher, J. 1994. Issues for designing marrow transplant programs. *Semin Oncol Nurs* 10(1):64-71.

Klumpp, T.R., Mangon, K.F., Goldberg, S.L., et al. 1995. Granulocyte colony-stimulating factor accelerates neutrophil engraftment following peripheral-blood stem-cell transplantation: a prospective randomized trial. *J Clin Oncol* 13(6):1323-1327.

Kurowsi, B, Fuller, D., Everson, L. 1995. Oncology managed care/physicians groups. *Oncol Iss* 10(5):27-29.

Lamkin, L. 1993. The new oncology ambulatory clinic. In Buchsel, P., Yarbro, C. (Eds.) *Oncology Nursing in the Ambulatory Setting.* Boston: Jones & Bartlett, 107-131.

Lin, M., Martin, V, 1994. Introduction. *Semin Oncol Nurs* 10(4):227-228.

Lloid, M. 1995. Oral medicine concerns of the BMT patient. In Buchsel, P., Whedon, M. (Eds.) *Bone Marrow Transplantation: Administrative and Clinical Strategies.* Boston: Jones & Bartlett, 257-282.

Martin, V. 1994. Administrative issues in ambulatory oncology care. *Semin Oncol Nurs* 10(4):296-305.

McNeil, C. 1995. A new generation of monoclonal antibodies arrives at the clinic. *J Natl Canc Inst* 22(87): 1658-1660.

Moskowitz, R. 1993. Day surgery for oncology patients. In Buchsel, P., Yarbro, C. (Eds.) *Oncology Nursing in the Ambulatory Setting: Issues and Models of Care.* Boston: Jones & Bartlett, 165-183

Nelson, J. 1995. Centers of excellence for marrow transplantation. In Buchsel, P., Whedon, M. (Eds.) *Bone Marrow Transplantation: Administrative and Clinical Strategies.* Boston: Jones & Bartlett, 443-462.

Peters, W., Rodgers, M. 1994. Variation in approval by insurance companies of coverage for autologous bone marrow transplantation for breast cancer. *N Engl J Med* 33(7):473-477.

Peters, W., Ross, M., Vredenburgh, J., et al. 1994. The use of intensive clinic support to permit outpatient autologous bone marrow transplantation for breast cancer. *Semin Oncol* 21(4 suppl 7):25-31.

Randolph, S.R. 1992. Home care of the bone marrow transplant recipient: high tech, high touch. *Home Healthc Nurse* 11(1):24-28.

Ringden, O., Horowtiz, M., Gale R., et al. 1993. Outcome after allogeneic bone marrow transplantation for leukemia in adults. *JAMA* 270(1):57-60.

Roggerio, M. 1988. The bone marrow donor. *Semin Oncol Nurs* 4(1):9-14.

Roncarolo, M., Bacchetta, R., Touraine, J., et al. 1992. SCID patients reconstituted by fetal liver stem cells; possible role of IL-10 in transplantation tolerance. *J Cellular Biochem Suppl* 16:214.

Rowe, J., Ciobanu, N., Ascensao, J., et al. 1994. Recommended guidelines for the management of autologous and allogeneic bone marrow transplantation: a report from the Eastern Cooperative Oncology Group. *Ann Intern Med* 120(2):143-158.

Sanders, J. 1992. Effects of bone marrow transplantation on reproductive function. In D'Angio, G. (Ed.) *Late Effects of Treatment for Childhood Cancer.* New York: Wiley-Liss, 95-101.

Sarantos, S. 1988. Innovations in psychosocial staff support: a model program for the marrow transplant nurse. *Semin Oncol Nurs* 4(1):69-73.

Schmidt-Pokorny, K. 1994. Nurses must understand the process of mobilization and collection of peripheral blood stem cells. *BMT Newsletter* 5:1-3.

Schubert, M., Sullivan, K., Schubert, M. 1990. Gynecological abnormalities following allogeneic bone marrow transplantation. *BMT* 5:425-430.

Schubert, M., Sullivan, K., Truelove, E. 1986. Oral complication of bone marrow transplantation. In Peterson, D., Sonis, S., Elias, E. (Eds.) *Head and Neck Management of the Cancer Patient.* Boston: Martinus Nijhoff.

Schulmeister, L. 1995. Home care of the BMT recipient. In Buchsel, P., Whedon, M. (Eds.) *Bone Marrow Transplantation: Administrative and Clinical Strategies.* Boston: Jones & Bartlett, 303-322.

Stearn, J., Lenssen, P. 1995. Food and nutritional services for the BMT patient. In Buchsel, P., Whedon, M. (Eds.) *Bone Marrow Transplantation: Administrative and Clinical Strategies.* Boston: Jones & Bartlett, 113-136.

Stroncek, D.F., Holland, P.V., Bartch, G., et al. 1993. Experiences on the first 493 unrelated marrow donors in the National Marrow Donor Program. *Blood* 81(7): 1940-1946.

Sullivan, K., Moinpour, D., Chapko, M., et al. 1994. Reducing the costs of blood and marrow transplantion: a randomized study of early hospital discharge and the results of revised standard practice guidelines. Seattle: American Society of Hematologists.

Syrjala, K. 1995. Meeting the psychological needs of recipients and families. In Buchsel, P., Whedon, M. (Eds.) *Bone Marrow Transplantation: Administrative and Clinical Strategies.* Boston: Jones & Bartlett, 283-299.

Thomas, E. 1995. Foreword. In Buchsel, P., Whedon, M. (Eds.) *Bone Marrow Transplantation: Administrative and Clinical Strategies.* Boston: Jones & Bartlett, xv-xvi.

Vose, J., Armitage, J. 1995. Clinical applications of hematopoietic growth factors. *J Clin Oncol* 33(4): 1023-1035.

Walker, F., Roethke, S., Martin, G. 1994. An overview of the rationale, process, and nursing implications of peripheral blood stem cell transplantation. *Canc Nurs* 17(2):41-148.

Wilkins, V. 1995. Pharmaceutical services for a BMT program. In Buchsel, P., Whedon, M. (Eds.) *Bone Marrow Transplantation: Administrative and Clinical Strategies.* Boston: Jones & Bartlett, 137-151.

Williams, L., Holmes M., Peterson J., et al. 1995. Outpatient management of persons undergoing intensive chemotherapy with or without autologous blood cell support. Fifth International Marrow and Blood Cell Transplantation Conference, Seattle (abstr).

York, A., Clift, R., Sanders, J., et al. 1992. Recombinant human erythropoietin (rh-EPO) administration to normal marrow donors. *BMT* 10(5):415-417.

Zanjani, E., Garrusib, M., Tavassoli, M., et al. 1992. In utero transplantation of fetal hematopoietic stem cells. *J Cellular Biochem Suppl* 16:179.

Index

A

Abdominal distention, VOD and, 315
Academy of Pediatrics, 513
Acanthamoeba, 330-331
Accessibility, 418
Acquired specific host defenses, 34
  cell-mediated immunity, 34-35
  humoral immunity, 35
Acrolein, 89, 102
Acute GVHD, 91-92
  clinical manifestations, 182-184
  pathophysiology, 179-181
  See also Graft-versus-host disease
Acute hemolytic reaction, 304
Acute lymphocytic leukemia (ALL), 429
Acute myelogenous leukemia (AML), 432
Acute nonlymphoblastic leukemia, 18
Acute nonlymphocytic leukemia (ANLL), 9
Acute renal failure (ARF), 88, 298, 301-302
Acute treatment, psychosocial concerns
    during, 361
  psychological factors and occurrence of
    physical symptoms, 361-363
  relationships among psychosocial factors
    and survival outcomes, 363-364
Acute tubular necrosis (ATN), 302-303, 304
Acyclovir, 14, 87
  dosing, administration, and monitoring,
    131
  pharmacology, 129
  therapeutic use, 129-130
  toxicities, 130-131
Addiction, to medications, 368
Adeno-associated virus type 2, 165

Adenosine deaminase deficiency, 167
Adenovirus, 89, 90, 289
  vector, 164-165
  and viral pneumonia, 275
Administrative elements, of alternative care
    models, 536
  ancillary services, 547-548
  clinical and fiscal issues, 545-546
  medical staff, 546-547
  nursing service, 536-545
Administrative planning, of alternative care
    models, 527-528
  mission statement and strategic plan,
    528-531
  models of care, 531-532
  physical design, 532-536
Adria cells, 287
Adriamycin, 287
Adult respiratory distress syndrome (ARDS),
    care of intubated BMT patient with,
    285-286
Advanced directives, 516-517
Advanced practice nurse (APN), 543-544
After-hours care, in alternative care models,
    535
Agglutination, 35
Agranulocytosis, 367
AIDS, 522
Alanine aminotransferase (ALT), 158
Allocation, of scarce resources, 520-521
Allogeneic BCT, source of cells for, 39
Allogeneic BMT, 7, 8, 10, 19, 20, 67-68
  source of bone marrow for, 37-38
Alloimmune versus autoimmune, 210

Alopecia, from total body irradiation, 157
Alternative care models, 525-526, 558-559
  defined, 526
  future trends in, 557-558
  and health-care economics, 526-527
  See also Administrative elements;
    Administrative planning; Phases of
    transplantation
Ambulatory care models, *see* Alternative care
  models
American Association of Sex Educators,
    Counselors and Teachers (AASECT), 391
American Bone Marrow Donor Registry
    (ABMDR), 79
American Cancer Society, 389, 500
  Professors of Oncology Nursing of, 501
American Medical Association, 517
American Nurses' Association, 512
American Organization of Nursing Executives
    (AONE), 536
American Red Cross Blood Services, 11
American Society for Blood and Marrow
    Transplantation (ASBMT), 481, 488,
    489-490
American Society of Clinical Oncologists
    (ASCO), 74, 481, 488, 489
American Society of Hematologists (ASH),
    74, 481, 488
American Society of Histocompatibility and
    Immunogenetics (ASHI), 56
American Thoracic Society, 517
America On-Line (AOL), 486
Amino acids, branched-chain, 258
Amphotericin, 128-129
Amphotericin B, 13, 14, 88
  lipid complex, 129
Amplification, 59
Analgesic agents, neurological effects of, 339
Ancillary services, of alternative care models
  behavioral medicine, 548
  clericals, 548
  dietary, 547-548
  material supplies, 548
  pharmacy, 547

Anemia, 88, 208-209
Anorexia, *see* Emetic response(s)
Anthony Nolan Bone Marrow Trust
    (England), 61
Anthracyclines, cardiac damage from, 287-288
Antibacterials, 125-127
Antibiotics, 87, 88
Antidepressant agents, 367-368
  neurological effects of, 340
Antiemetic agents, neurological effects of,
    338-339
Antifungals, 127-129
Antigen recognition, 180
Antigens, classes I and II, 79-80
Antimicrobial therapy, 12-14
Antipsychotic agents, neurological effects of,
    340
Antithymocyte globulin (ATG), 9, 17
  dosing, administration, and monitoring, 125
  neurological effects, 337
  pharmacology, 124-125
  therapeutic use, 125
  toxicities, 125
Antivirals
  acyclovir, 129-131
  foscarnet, 134-135
  ganciclovir, 131-134
  new, 135
Anxiety
  during pretreatment phase, 357
  psychological symptoms of, during BMT,
    362, 363
  psychopharmacological support for,
    366-367
  visual analogue scales of, 369
Anxiolytic agents, neurological effects of,
    339-340
APACHE (acute physiologic and chronic
    health evaluation) II data, 511-512
Apheresis/harvest and cryopreservation,
    552-554
Apheresis nurse, 542
Apheresis unit, in alternative care models, 534
Aplastic anemia, 9, 18

Area under the curve (AUC), 106
Arousal phase, 381
Ascites, minimizing effects of, in VOD, 319-320
Aspergillosis, invasive pulmonary, 276-277
Aspergillus infections, 13, 14, 88, 90, 128-129, 207
    and cardiac infections, 289
    and fungal infections, 290-291
    and fungal pneumonia, 276-277
    neurological effects of, 329
    secondary hemorrhage from, 283
Australian Bone Marrow Donor Registry, 61
Austria, 476
Austrian Bone Marrow Donor Registry, 61
Autogenic relaxation, 365-366
Autoimmune versus alloimmune, 210
Autologous BCT, source of cells for, 38-39
Autologous Blood and Marrow Transplant Registry–North America (ABMTR), 71, 481, 488, 531
Autologous BMT (ABMT), 7-8, 9, 19, 67
    source of bone marrow for, 38
Autonomy, donor, 513-514
Azathioprine, 17
    neurological effects of, 338

B
Bacterial infections, 87, 206-207, 289-290, 328-329
Bacterial pneumonia, 273-274
Bacterial sepsis, 11
Basophils, 29
Baylor University Medical Center, 418-419, 422
BCNU, *see* Carmustine
Beck Depression Inventory, 357
Behavioral interventions, 365
    biofeedback, 366
    hypnosis, 365
    relaxation training, 365-366
Behavioral medicine, in alternative care models, 548
Benzodiazepines, 339, 367

Benzyl alcohol, 342
Betathalassemia, 9
Biofeedback, 366
Biological response modifiers (BRMs), neurological effects of, 340-342
Biology of Blood and Marrow Transplantation, 488
Biopsy
    open lung (OLB), 271-272
    transbronchial (TBB), 271
Bladder toxicity, 89
Blastomycosis, 276
Bleeding, 213
    ulceration and GI, 234, 241
Bleomycin, 279-280
Blood banking, 10-12
Blood cells (BC), 38, 68
    for allogeneic BCT, source of, 39
    for autologous BCT, source of, 38-39
    precursors, 27-28
    progenitor, 27
    stem cells, 27, 68-69
Blood cell transplantation (BCT), 38, 68-69
    donor issues, 63
    harvest procedures, 80-83
    sources of cells for, 38-39
Blood chemistries, in nursing assessment of renal functions, 305-306
Blood-forming organs
    bone marrow, 25-27
    liver, 27
    spleen, 27
Blood product support, 213-215
Blood stem cells, *see* Blood cells
Blood volume, impaired circulation of, 302
Blue Cross and Blue Shield Association (BCBS), 78
Blue Cross plans, 459
BMT Newsletter, 413, 486
Bone marrow, 25-27
    for allogeneic BMT, source of, 37-38
    for autologous BMT, source of, 38
Bone marrow transplant (BMT), harvest procedures, 83

Bone Marrow Transplantation, 488
"Boost" treatment, 84
Boundary Guidelines, 470
Branched-chain amino acids, 258
Breast cancer, 436, 460, 463, 469
   autologous transplant for, 494
   psychological distress in patients with, 362
   use of HDC with transplantation for,
     492-493
Bronchiolitis obliterans, 282
Bronchiolitis obliterans organizing pneumonia
   (BOOP), 282-283
Bronchoalveolar lavage (BAL), 271
Busulfan, 9
   and cyclophosphamide (BuCy), 9, 101, 105
   dosing, administration, and monitoring, 106
   pharmacology, 105
   pulmonary damage from, 280
   therapeutic use, 105
   toxicities, 105-106
Butyrophenones, 340
Buyers, bargaining power of, 465-468

C
Camphylobacter jejuni, 249-250
Canada
   medical networks in, 482
   nursing networks in, 477
Canadian Association of Nurses in Oncology
   (CANO), 477
Canadian Bone Marrow Transplantation
   medical organization, 482
Canadian Red Cross Society, 61
Cancer, gene therapy for, 166, 167-169
Cancer and Leukemia Group B (CALGB),
   481, 492
Candida albicans, 289, 290
Candida infection, 13, 88, 90, 128-129, 207
   and fungal pneumonia, 276, 277
   neurological effects of, 329
Candidiasis, 239
Capitation, 463
Carbohydrates, and metabolic and nutritional
   alterations, 247

Carboplatin
   dosing, administration, and monitoring, 110
   pharmacology, 109-110
   therapeutic use, 110
   toxicities, 110
Cardiac effects (complications), 266, 287
   bacterial infections, 289-290
   cardiac infections, 289
   cardiac tamponade, 292
   cardiac toxicity, 92-93
   cardiac toxicity associated with infusion of
     cryopreserved cells, 292
   chemotherapy-induced, 287-289
   fungal infections, 290-291
   graft-versus-host disease, 291-292
   long-term, on cardiac function, 292-293
   nursing transplant patient with, 293-294
   radiation-induced, 289
   viral infections, 291
Cardiopulmonary resuscitation (CPR),
   509-511, 516, 518, 519
Caregiver burden, and quality of life, 415-416
Caremaps, 419
Carepaths, 419
"Caring for Yourself," 418-419
Carmustine (BCNU), 93, 280
   dosing, administration, and monitoring, 113
   pharmacology, 113
   therapeutic use, 113
   toxicities, 113
Case management, 462-463
Case manager, 542
Cataracts, and total body irradiation, 158
CD34-positive cells, 36-37, 81
Ceftazidime, 127
Cell-mediated immunity, 34-35
Cell-mediated lympholysis, 183
Cells, identification of, for transplantation, 35
   CD34-positive cells, 36-37
   colony-forming units-spleen (CFU-S), 36
   competitive repopulating unit, 36
   high-proliferative potential cultures, 36
   long-term culture-initiating cells, 36
   number of stem cells, 37

Cells, source of, for transplantation, 37
    blood cells, 38-39
    bone marrow, 37-38
    umbilical cord blood, 39
Cellular HLA typing, 58
Center of excellence, 465
Central nervous system
    infections, neurological effects and, 328-331
    and total body irradiation, 159
Central venous catheter (CVC) placement, 552
Cerebral syndrome, 8
CFU-GM, *see* Colony-forming units-granulocyte and monocyte
Chemoradiotherapy pretransplant conditioning, neurological effects and, 327-328
Chemotaxis, 34
Chemotherapy
    busulfan, 105-106
    carboplatin, 109-110
    carmustine, 113
    cisplatin, 110-111
    cyclophosphamide, 101-105
    cytarabine, 111-112
    dose-intensive, 554-555
    etoposide, 106-108
    gastrointestinal complications from, 91
    high-dose (HDC), for treatment of breast cancer, 492-493
    ifosfamide, 113-115
    -induced cardiac damage, 287-289
    -induced diarrhea, 235
    -induced pulmonary damage, 279-281
    melphalan, 108
    mobilizing stem cells with, 80-81
    preconditioning, 84
    preparative regimens, 84-87, 100-101
    thiotepa, 108-109
Chernobyl nuclear accident, 3-4
Chills, from total body irradiation, 157
Chimera, 3
Chlamydia, 89, 274
Chlorambucil, 280

Choices, giving patients, 419
Chronic GVHD
    clinical manifestations, 184-190
    pathophysiology, 181-182
    See also Graft-versus-host disease
Chronic myelogenous leukemia (CML), 9, 11, 18, 435
Ciprofloxacin, 13, 127
Cisplatin
    dosing, administration, and monitoring, 111
    pharmacology, 110
    therapeutic use, 111
    toxicities, 111
City of Hope Quality-of-Life Conceptual Model, 410
    on physical well-being, 410-412
    on psychological well-being, 412
    on social well-being, 412-413
    on spiritual well-being, 413-414
c-kit ligand, *see* Stem cell factor
Clarithromycin, 127
Clericals, in alternative care models, 548
Clinic examination rooms, in alternative care models, 533-534
Clinical area, in alternative care models, 533
Clinical indications
    bone marrow transplant registries, 71
    malignant diseases, 69-70
    nonmalignant diseases, 70-71
Clinical nurses, research conducted by, 499-500
Clinical nurse specialist (CNS), 74
Clinton, Bill, 460, 544
Clonazepam, 105
Clostridium, 289
    difficile, 235
    perfringens, 250
Cluster of differentiation (CD) antigens, 34
Coagulopathy, treating, in VOD, 320
Coccidioidomycosis, 276
Colony-forming unit blast cell (CFU-blast), 27, 36
Colony-forming units-granulocyte and monocyte (CFU-GM), 81

Colony-forming units-spleen (CFU-S), 36

Colony-stimulating factors, *see* Hematopoietic growth factors

Community, nursing standards in, 484-486

Competitive repopulating unit (CRU), 36

Complement system, 35, 57

Complications, delayed, after transplant, 95-96

Component therapy, 10-11

Computer programs, 486

Conception, for donation, 515-516

Conditioning-induced emetic responses, 225-229

Conditioning regimens, 8-9
  and emetic response, 223

Confidentiality, donor, 513-514

Congestive heart failure, 293

Continuing medical education (CME), 468

Continuous renal replacement therapy (CRRT), 88

Coping strategies, providing, 419

Cord blood, *see* Umbilical cord blood

Corticosteroids
  dosing, administration, and monitoring, 124
  neurological effects, 336-337
  pharmacology, 122-123
  therapeutic use, 123-124
  toxicities, 124

Cotrimoxazole, 127

Coxsackie virus, 289

Critical Care Pathway Guideline, 470

Critical care units, transfer to, 511-513

Critical pathways, in alternative care models, 537-542

Cross-reactive groups (CREGS), 45-46

Cryoprecipitate, and blood product support, 214

Cryopreservation, 83
  harvest/apheresis and, 552-554

Cryopreserved cells, cardiac toxicity associated with infusion of, 292

Cryptococcus, 329
  neoformans, 90, 276

Cryptogenic organizing pneumonia, *see* Bronchiolitis obliterans organizing pneumonia

Cyclophosphamide, 8, 9, 17
  busulfan and (BuCy), 9, 101, 105
  cardiac complications from, 93, 288-289
  dosing, administration, and monitoring, 104-105
  to mobilize stem cells, 81
  pharmacology, 101-102
  pulmonary damage from, 268, 280
  therapeutic use, 102-104
  total body irradiation and (CyTBI), 8-9, 101
  toxicities, 104

Cyclosporin (CyA), 9, 17
  dosing, administration, and monitoring, 118-119
  neurological effects, 333-335
  pharmacology, 115
  therapeutic use, 115-116
  toxicities, 116-118

Cyclosporin-A (CsA), 177, 194-196

Cytarabine
  dosing, administration, and monitoring, 112
  pharmacology, 111
  therapeutic use, 111-112
  toxicities, 112

Cytomegalovirus (CMV), 11, 12, 19, 87, 88, 207-208
  and acyclovir, 129
  and bladder toxicity, 89
  and foscarnet, 134
  and ganciclovir, 131-132
  and intravenous immunoglobulin, 136
  in lungs of BMT patients with IPn, 269
  pneumonia, 14, 274-275
  pneumonitis, 14, 274-275
  and pulmonary toxicity, 89, 90
  viral infections due to, 329, 330

Cytosine arabinoside (Ara-C), 272, 281

D

Dapsone-pyrimethamine, 278

Daunorubicin, 287

Day surgery, in alternative care models, 534-535

Decision making, patients' participation in, 418-419

Delirium, psychopharmacological support for, 367

Dementia Rating Scale, 360

Dental abnormalities, and total body irradiation, 158-159

Dental services, in alternative care models, 546-547

Dependence, on medications, 368

Depression
    during pretreatment phase, 357-358
    psychological symptoms of, during BMT, 362, 363
    psychopharmacological support for, 367-368
    visual analogue scale of, 369

Derogatis Sexual Functioning Inventory, 396

Desire phase, 381

Dexamethasone, 336-337

Diagnosis related groups (DRGs), 462

Diagnostic and Statistical Manual of Mental Disorders, Fourth Edition (DSM-IV), 381-382, 386, 391, 413

Diapedesis, 34

Diarrhea
    chemotherapy-induced, 235
    dismotility-type, 236
    enteritis and, 235-236, 241-242
    exudative, 236
    osmotic, 236
    secretory-type, 235-236
    from total body irradiation, 157

Didanosine (DDI), 134

Dietary services, in alternative care models, 547-548

Diets, *see* Low-microbial diets

Differentiation, 25

Diffuse alveolar hemorrhage (DAH), 283

Difluorodeoxycytidine (dFdC), 359

Dimethylsulfoxide (DMSO), 7, 83

Discharge planning, 93-94

Disease(s)
    malignant and nonmalignant, and clinical indications, 69-71
    status, and patient eligibility, 71-72

Disease-free survival (DFS), 71-72, 493

Dismotility-type diarrhea, 236

Disseminated intravascular coagulation (DIC), 214

Donation
    effects of, 514-515
    new challenges in, 515-516

Donor
    autonomy and confidentiality, 513-514
    availability, 72
    preparation, 80
    registries, unrelated, 60-61
    search, 79
    search, NMDP, 61-63

Do-not-resuscitate (DNR) orders, 509-511, 512, 516, 518

Drug-induced pulmonary damage, 279-281

Drugs, adjusting, in VOD, 320

Duke University, 464

Durable powers of attorney (DPOA), 516-517

Dyspareunia, 385

Dysphagia, esophagitis and, 240-241

E

Eastern Cooperative Oncology Group (ECOG), 481, 492, 501

Economics, health-care, 526-527

Edema
    pulmonary, 89, 272-273, 288, 293
    VOD and, 315

Education
    area, in alternative care models, 533
    reinforcing current, 418
    See also Patient education

Electroencephalographic (EEG) biofeedback, 366

Electrolyte
    balance, maintaining, in VOD, 319
    imbalance, correcting, in renal insufficiency, 309

Electromyographic (EMG) biofeedback, 366

Embolism, pulmonary, 283

Emergency care, in alternative care models, 535

Emetic response(s), 221-222, 362
  causation and character, 222-225
  conditioning-induced, 225-229
  conditioning regimens, 223
  graft-versus-host disease, 224-225
  infection, 224
  other etiologies, 229
  prevention and management, 225-229
  psychoneurologic factors, 225
  supportive pharmaceuticals, 223-224

Emotional support, for total body irradiation, 159-160

Empowering patients, 418-419

Encephalopathy, VOD and, 315

Endocarditis, 289, 291
  vegetations, infective, 290

Energy needs, posttransplant, 247-248

Engraftment and recovery, 93, 555-556
  delayed complications after transplant, 95-96
  discharge planning, 93-94
  follow-up care, 94-95
  posttransplant evaluation, 95
  self-care and home care, 94

Enhancement gene transfer, 163

Enteral nutrition, 253-254
  early, 258-259
  versus TPN, 255
  See also Nutrition for BMT/BCT patient

Enteritis, and diarrhea, 235-236, 241-242

Enterobacter species, 89

Eosinophils, 29

Epoetin (EPO)
  dosing, administration, and monitoring, 138
  pharmacology, 137
  therapeutic use, 137-138
  toxicities, 138

Epstein-Barr virus (EBV), 19, 87, 129, 131, 276

Erythrocytes, 29

Erythropoietin (EPO), 14, 33, 81

Escherichia coli, 87, 138, 139, 236, 250, 328

Esophagitis, 232-234
  treatment of, 240-241

Ethical issues of transplantation, 506
  advanced directives, 516-517
  allocation of scarce resources, 520-521
  donor issues, 513-516
  futile care, 517-520
  informed consent, 506-513
  new therapies, 521-522

Ethics and safety, of gene therapy, 170-171

Etoposide (VP 16), 9
  dosing, administration, and monitoring, 107-108
  pharmacology, 106
  therapeutic use, 106-107
  toxicities, 107

Eugenics gene transfer, 163

European Bone Marrow Transplant (EBMT), 482, 488, 492
  Nurses Group, 476-477

Evaluation
  patient, for transplant process, 75-78
  phase of transplantation, 550-552
  posttransplant, 95

Evolution of BMT, as treatment of human disease, 3-8

Exercise, encouraging, 419

Experimental nutritional therapies, 257
  branched-chain amino acids, 258
  early enteral alimentation, 258-259
  glutamine, 257-258
  growth hormone, 258

Exudative diarrhea, 236

Ex vivo expansion of stem cells, 84

Eyes, and chronic GVHD, 188

F

Famciclovir, 135

Family, 442
  assessment, clinical implications of, 447-449
  framework, 442-447

involvement of, in transplant, 446-447
life cycle, 444
new issues for, in BMT, 454-455
and stress of BMT, 447, 449-454
units in transplant, 444-446
Fatigue, and quality of life, 416-417
Febrile pneumonitis syndrome, 284
Fee for service, 461-462
Fertility, 377
    blood cell and marrow transplantation and
        pregnancy, 379-381
    options, other, 395
    sperm banking for, 394-395
    and total body irradiation, 159
Fever, from total body irradiation, 157
Filgrastim
    dosing, administration, and monitoring,
        139-140
    pharmacology, 138
    therapeutic use, 138-139
    toxicities, 139
Financial issues
    and quality of life, 416
    in transplant process, 78
FK506, see Tacrolimus
Flow centrifugation, 11
Fluconazole, 14, 127-128, 129
Fluid balance
    assessment of, in renal function, 307-308
    maintaining, in VOD, 319
Fluorescence-activated cell sorter (FACS), 37
Fluoxetine, 368
FOCUS/PDSA model, 422
Folinic acid, 119-120, 121
Follow-up care, 94-95
Food
    high-risk, 251
    vehicles of infection, 249-253
Food and Drug Administration (FDA), U.S.,
    32, 129, 134, 135, 139, 170, 414, 522
Foscarnet, 87
    dosing, administration, and monitoring,
        134-135
    pharmacology, 134

therapeutic use, 134
    toxicities, 134
Fractionated radiation therapy, 84, 153, 155
France, 477, 482
Fred Hutchinson Cancer Research Center
    (FHCRC), 299, 475, 483, 500
Fungal infections, 88, 207, 250, 290-291, 329
Fungal pneumonia, 276-277
Futile care, 517-520

G
Ganciclovir, 14
    dosing, administration, and monitoring,
        133-134
    pharmacology, 131
    therapeutic use, 131-132
    toxicities, 132-133
Gastrointestinal bleeding, ulceration and, 234,
    241
Gastrointestinal complications (effects), 91,
    220-221
    of acute GVHD, 182-183
    of chronic GVHD, 188
    emetic response, 221-229
    hepatic response, 243-245
    mucosal response, 230-243
    pathophysiologic responses, 221-245
    salivary gland response, 229-230
    See also Nutrition for BMT/BCT patient
Gastrointestinal syndrome, 8
G-CSF, see Granulocyte colony-stimulating
    factor
Gene therapy, 162
    candidate diseases for, 166
    clinical trials of, in transplant setting,
        167-170
    future directions of, 172-173
    implications of, for nursing, 171-172
    in vitro method of, 163-164
    in vivo method of, 164
    safety and ethics of, 170-171
    types of, 163
    vectors in, 164-166
Genetic code, 162

Genetic diseases, gene therapy for, 166, 167
Germline therapy, 163
Glutamine, 257-258
GM-CSF, *see* Granulocyte-macrophage
  colony-stimulating factor
Gonadal function, cancer treatment and,
  377-378
  blood cell and marrow transplantation,
    378-379
  blood cell and marrow transplantation and
    pregnancy, 379-381
  See also Sexual function(ing)
Graft failure, 210-211
Graft rejection, 68, 210-211
Graft-versus-host disease (GVHD), 10, 13,
  18, 68, 177, 199-200
  acute, 91-92, 179-181, 182-184
  antithymocyte globulin for, 125
  autologous, 20
  and cardiac damage, 291-292
  chronic, 181-182, 184-190
  clinical manifestations of, 182
  corticosteroids for, 123-124
  cyclosporin for, 14, 115-116, 118-119
  developments in control of, 5, 14, 16-17
  diagnosis, grading, and prognosis of,
    190-194
  and emetic response, 224-225
  future considerations of, 19-20, 198-199
  gene therapy and, 167
  and graft-versus-leukemia effect, 181
  incidence of, 177-179
  intravenous immunoglobulin for, 136
  medical management of, 194-197
  methotrexate for, 120
  neurologic complications of, 343-345
  nursing management of, 197-198
  pathophysiology of, 179-182
  prophylaxis of, 194-196
  and pulmonary damage, 282
  transfusions and, 11-12
  treatment of, 196-197
Graft-versus-leukemia (GVL) effect, 17, 19,
  68, 142, 181

Granisetron, 339
Granulocyte colony-stimulating factor
  (G-CSF), 14, 30, 32, 81, 137, 138, 142,
  143
Granulocyte-macrophage colony-stimulating
  factor (GM-CSF), 14, 30, 32-33, 81, 137,
  138, 139, 141-142
Great Britain, 476, 477
Great Depression, 459
Greffe de Moelle (France), 61
Growth, and total body irradiation, 158
Growth hormone, 258
Guillain-Barré syndrome, 344-345

H
Haemophilus influenzae, 208, 274
Haplotypes, 51
Harvest/apheresis and cryopreservation,
  552-554
Harvest procedures, 80
  blood cell transplant, 80-83
  bone marrow transplant, 83
  cryopreservation, 83
  ex vivo expansion of stem cells, 84
  human cord blood, 83
  marrow purging techniques/positive
    selection, 83-84
Health Care Financing Administration
  (HCFA), 78
Health insurance, 78, 460
Health maintenance organization (HMO),
  462
Hematologic disorders
  gene therapy for, 169-170
  psychological distress in patients with, 362
Hematologic effects, 205
  anemia, 208-209
  leukopenia and neutropenia, 205-208
  thrombocytopenia, 209
  See also Immunohematologic
    complications; Myelosuppression
Hematopoiesis, 25
  blood cells, 27-28
  blood-forming organs, 25-27

defined, 25
homeostasis, 30
impact of transplantation on, 35
mature cells, 28-30
patient education related to, 39-40
structure and process, 25-30
Hematopoietic growth factors (HGF), 14-15,
    27, 30
    biologic activity of, 32-33
    classification of, 30-32
    investigational, clinical experience with,
        140-143
    investigational, toxicity of, 143-144
    lineage specific, 30-32
    multilineage, 32
    pharmacology, 137
    side effects of, 553
    for stem cell mobilization, 81
Hematopoietic syndrome, 8
Hemodialysis, 88
Hemolytic uremic syndrome (HUS), 250
Hemorrhagic cystitis (HC)
    etiology of, 309-310
    incidence of, 309
    presentation and clinical course of, 310
    prevention of, 310
    treatment of, 310
Heparin, to prevent VOD, 318
Hepatic blood flow and function,
        consequences of impaired, 313-314
Hepatic disorders, and total body irradiation,
    158
Hepatic response, 243-244
    assessment and management, 245
    causation and character, 244-245
    drug-induced liver injury, 245
    liver infection, 244-245
    veno-occlusive disease, 245
Hepatic toxicity, 88
Hepatic venule occlusion, 312-313
Hepatitis B (HBV) infection, 244
Hepatitis C virus (HCV), 244
Hepatopulmonary syndrome, 284
Heroics, 511, 516

Herpes simplex pneumonitis, 89
Herpes simplex viruses (HSV), 87, 129-130,
    131, 165, 207
    and viral pneumonia, 275, 276
High-dose chemotherapy (HDC), for
    treatment of breast cancer, 492-493
High-efficiency particulate air (HEPA) filters,
    13, 86, 88
High output renal failure, 303
High-proliferative potential cultures (HPPC),
    36
Histocompatibility molecules, 43
Histoplasmosis, 276
HLA complex or region, 49
    See also Human leukocyte antigen
HLA Nomenclature Committee, see World
    Health Organization
Hodgkin's disease, 9
Hodgkin's lymphoma, 18
Home care, 94, 535-536
Homeostasis, 30
"Homing" by cells, 93
Hormonal replacement therapy, 394
Housing, near transplant centers, 532
Human Genome Project, 162, 171
Human herpes virus-6 (HHV-6), 131
Human immunodeficiency virus (HIV), 165,
    166, 167
Human leukocyte antigen (HLA), 11, 43
    complex, structure and function of, 49-51
    nomenclature, 43-49
    role of, in matching for transplantation,
        59-60
    types, inheritance of, 51-52
    types, racial distribution of, 52-53
    See also Human leukocyte antigen (HLA)
        typing
Human-leukocyte-antigen-identical
    (HLA-identical), 60, 67, 79
Human leukocyte antigen (HLA) typing, 43,
    53-56
    cellular methods, 58
    developments in, 9-10, 79-80
    and GVHD, 199

Human leukocyte antigen (HLA) typing
(*continued*)
  molecular methods, 58-59
  serologic methods, 56-58
Humoral immunity, 35
Hybridization, 59
Hydromorphone, 339
4-hydroperoxycyclophosphamide, 19
4-hydroxycyclophosphamide (4-HC), 102
Hydroxyethyl starch (HES), 83
Hydroxymethyl starch, 11, 12
Hypnosis, 365
Hypoactive sexual desire disorder, 382-385
Hypoalbuminemia, VOD and, 315
Hypogammaglobulinemia, 136
Hypomagnesemia, 334
Hyponatremia, VOD and, 315
Hypovolemia, 302

I
ICE (ifosfamide/carboplatin/etoposide), 114
Idiopathic agents, 90
Idiopathic hyperammonemia, 331
Idiopathic pneumonia syndrome, 283, 284
Ifosfamide
  dosing, administration, and monitoring,
    114-115
  pharmacology, 113-114
  therapeutic use, 114
  toxicities, 114
IL-1 (interleukin-1), 141, 142, 143
IL-2, 19, 142-143
  neurological effects of, 340-341
IL-3, 15, 30, 33, 81, 141-142, 143
IL-4, 19
IL-6, 15, 142, 143
IL-11, 15, 142, 144
IL-12, 19
Imipenem, 127
Immune system, and acute GVHD, 183-184
Immunity, 33-34
  acquired specific host defenses, 34-35
  cell-mediated, 34-35

  humoral, 35
  natural nonspecific defenses, 34
Immunoglobulin, 30
Immunohematologic complications, 209-210
  graft failure, 210-211
Immunosuppression, 268
  total body irradiation and, 157
Immunosuppressive agents
  antithymocyte globulin, 124-125, 337
  azathioprine, 338
  corticosteroids, 122-124, 336-337
  cyclosporin, 115-119, 333-335
  methotrexate, 119-121, 335-336
  monoclonal antibody OKT3, 337-338
  neurological effects, 332-338
  tacrolimus, 121-122
  thalidomide, 338
Impaired circulation of blood volume, 302
Infection(s)
  bacterial, 87, 206-207, 289-290, 328-329
  cardiac, 289
  central nervous system, neurological effects
    and, 328-331
  and emetic response, 224
  food vehicles of, 249-253
  fungal, 88, 207, 250, 290-291, 329
  parasitic, 208
  prophylaxis and treatment of, 331
  protozoal, 330-331
  pulmonary, associated with BMT, 273
  treating, in renal insufficiency, 309
  viral, 87, 207-208, 291, 329-330
Infectious pneumonitis, 89
Inflammatory response, 34
Influenza, 276
Information
  adequacy of, 507-508
  providing patients with, 418
Informed consent
  adequacy of information, 507-508
  do-not-resuscitate orders, 509-511
  nurses' concerns, 513
  pediatric consent, 513

quality of life, 508-509
selection of patients, 506-507
transfer to critical care units, 511-513
Informed decision making about BMT, 355-357
Infusion areas, in alternative care models, 534
Inheritance, of HLA types, 51-52
Insertional mutagenesis (IM), 164
Insurance companies, 460
Insurance coverage, 78, 460
Intensive care unit (ICU), 516
transfer to, 511-513
Interferon, 19
neurological effects of, 340-341
Interferon-alpha, 359
Interleukins (ILs), 30
See also IL-1 through IL-12
Intermittent mandatory ventilation with positive airway pressures (IMV/CPAP), 285-286
International Bone Marrow Transplant Registry (IBMTR), 66, 69, 71, 481, 488, 531
International Cooperative Research Group (ICRG), 531
Internet, 486, 501
Interstitial pneumonitis (IPn), 8-9, 90
CMV, 131-132
infectious, 273
nursing assessment and diagnosis of BMT patient with, 285
pulmonary, 267
pulmonary, and pneumonia, diagnosis of, 269
from total body irradiation, 157-158
Intrarenal failure, 301
Intravascular volume, optimizing, in VOD, 319
Intravenous immunoglobulin (IVIg)
dosing, administration, and monitoring, 136-137
pharmacology, 135-136

therapeutic use, 136
toxicities, 136
Invasive pulmonary aspergillosis, 276-277
In vitro fertilization (IVF), 395
In vitro method of gene therapy, 163-164
In vivo method of gene therapy, 164
Isolation techniques, 86, 285
for management of BMT patient with myelosuppression, 211-213
Itraconazole, 14, 128, 129

K
Karnofsky Status, 402
Klebsiella, 87, 89, 236, 274
pneumoniae, 328

L
Laminar air flow (LAF) room, isolation of patient in, 13, 86, 88
Lectin agglutination, 194
Legionella, 89, 272, 274
Leukoagglutinating antibodies, 43
Leukoencephalopathy (LEC), 334, 336
neurological effects of, 342
Leukopenia, and hematologic effects of BMT, 205-208
Leukopheresis, 11
Leukostasis, 11
Lineage specific HGFs, 30-32
Linkage disequilibrium, 52
Lipids, and metabolic and nutritional alterations, 247-248
Listeria monocytogenes, 328-329
Liver, 27
and acute GVHD, 183
infection, 244-245
injury, drug-induced, 245
Living wills, 516-517
Location, of alternative care models, 532-533
Long-term culture-initiating cells (LTC-IC), 36
Long-term marrow culture (LTMC), 36
Lorazepam, 339

Low-microbial diets, 248-249
  food vehicles of infections, 249-253
  high-risk foods, 251
  oral intake, 252-253
  water, 251-252
Lung(s)
  biopsy, open (OLB), 271-272
  and chronic GVHD, 188
  damage, 268-269
Lymphocyte immune globulin, *see*
  Antithymocyte globulin
Lymphocytes, 29-30
Lymphocytic bronchitis, 282
Lymphokine-activated killer (LAK) cells, 19,
  142

M
Macrophage CSF (M-CSF), 33
Macrophages, 29, 34
Major Histocompatibility Complex (MHC),
  49
Malignancies
  second, and total body irradiation, 159
  secondary, and neoplastic recurrence,
    345-346
Malignant diseases, treated with marrow or
  blood stem cell transplantation, 69-70
Malignant infiltration, and pulmonary
  disease, 283
Managed care, 462-463
March of Dimes Birth Defects Foundation,
  171
Margination, 34
Marketplace, BMT and BCT, 459, 471-472
  analyzing external environment, 465-471
  current environment, 463-465
  historical perspectives, 459-461
  preparing for future, 465-471
  reimbursement, 461-463
Marrow purging techniques/positive selection,
  83-84
Marrow Transplantation Reviews, 488
Mast cell growth factor, *see* Stem cell
  factor

Matched unrelated donor (MUD) search,
  79
Material supplies, in alternative care models,
  548
Maturation, 25
Mature cells, 28
  basophils, 29
  eosinophils, 29
  erythrocytes, 29
  lymphocytes, 29-30
  monocytes/macrophages, 29
  neutrophils, 28-29
  thrombocytes, 29
M-CSF, *see* Macrophage CSF; Monocyte CSF
Medicaid, 460, 516, 520
Medical networks
  in Europe and Canada, 482
  in United States, 481-482
Medical staff, of alternative care models
  medical consultants, 546
  medical dental services, 546-547
  medical director, 546
  physician staff, 546
Medical standards, in transplantation,
  486-494
Medicare, 460, 462, 516
Megakaryocyte colony-stimulating activity
  (Meg-CSA), 209
Megakaryocyte growth-promoting activity
  (Meg-GPA), 209
Melphalan, 280-281
  dosing, administration, and monitoring,
    108
  pharmacology, 108
  therapeutic use, 108
  toxicities, 108
Memorial Sloan-Kettering Cancer Center
  (MSKCC), 382, 396, 482, 486
Memory response, 35
Men, gonadal failure in, 379
Menopause, premature, and sexual function,
  386
Mental status assessment, in renal function,
  308-309

Mesna, 89, 310
Metabolic encephalopathy, 331-332
Metabolic and nutritional alterations, 246
  carbohydrates, 247
  lipids, 247-248
  protein, 246-247
Methotrexate (MTX), 17, 177, 194-196
  dosing, administration, and monitoring,
    120-121
  and leukoencephalopathy, 342
  neurological effects of, 335-336
  pharmacology, 119-120
  pulmonary damage from, 268, 280, 281
  therapeutic use, 120
  toxicities, 120
Methylprednisolone, 123-124, 334
  neurological effects of, 336-337
Metoclopramide, 339
MGDF (megakaryocyte growth and
    development factor), 140-141
Microlymphocytotoxicity assay, 10
Mineralizing microangiopathy, 342-343
Mini-Mental State Examination, 347
Minnesota, University of, 286, 476
Minnesota Multiphasic Personality Inventory
    (MMPI), 357
Mission statement, 528-531
Mixed leukocyte culture (MLC), 183-184
Mixed lymphocyte culture, (MLC), 58, 80
Mixed lymphocyte reaction (MLR), 58
Mobilization, 552
Molecular HLA typing, 58-59
Monoamine oxidase inhibitors (MAOIs),
    368
Monoclonal antibody OKT3, 337-338
Monocyte CSF (M-CSF), 30
Monocytes, 29
Mononuclear cells (MNCs), 81
Morphine, PCA versus CI of, 361-362
Mucormycosis, 276
Mucosal response, 230
  assessment and management, 237-243
  causation and character, 230-237
  dysphagia, 240-241

enteritis and diarrhea, 235-236, 241-242
esophagitis, 232-234, 240-241
perirectal abscess, 242-243
perirectal lesions, 236-237
stomatitis, 230-232, 237-240
ulceration and GI bleeding, 234, 241
Mucositis, 87, 91, 105
  from total body irradiation, 157
Multidrug resistance gene (MDR), 169
Multilineage HGFs, 32
Myasthenia gravis, 344
Mycobacteria, 274
Mycoplasma, 274
Mycoplasma pneumonia, 89
Myelodysplastic syndrome (MDS), 430
Myelosuppression, management of BMT
    patient with
  bleeding, 213
  blood product support, 213-215
  neutropenia, 211-213
Myocardial infarction, 291
Myositis, 344

N
National Bone Marrow Transplant Donor
    Registry, 8, 19
National Cancer Act, 460
National Cancer Institute (NCI), 79, 481,
    486, 490-492, 500, 501, 531
National Center for Nursing Research, 500,
    501
National Marrow Donor Program (NMDP),
    53, 60-61, 79, 80, 492, 525
  donor search, 61-63
National Marrow Transplant Nursing
    Consortium, 476
Natural killer (NK) cells, 19
Natural nonspecific defenses, 34
  inflammatory response, 34
Nausea
  during BMT, 362, 363
  from total body irradiation, 155-157
  See also Emetic response(s)
Nebraska, University of, 476

Neoplastic recurrence, and secondary
    malignancy, 345-346
Nephrotoxins, 301
  and acute tubular necrosis, 303
  minimizing, in renal insufficiency, 309
Netherlands, 476, 477, 482
Networks, *see* Medical networks; Nursing
    networks
Neuroendocrine function, and total body
    irradiation, 158-159
Neuroleptic malignant syndrome (NMS),
    367
Neuroleptics, 367
Neurological effects, 90, 326-327, 348
  central nervous system infections,
    328-331
  chemoradiotherapy pretransplant
    conditioning, 327-328
  of graft-versus-host disease, 343-345
  immunosuppressive agents, 332-338
  leukoencephalopathy, 342
  metabolic encephalopathy, 331-332
  neoplastic recurrence and secondary
    malignancy, 345-346
  nursing care for, 346-348
  of other medications, 338-342
  vascular complications, 342-343
Neuromuscular system, and chronic GVHD,
    190
Neuropsychological effects, of previous
    treatment, 359-361
Neutropenia, 11, 12-13, 89
  and hematologic effects of BMT, 205-208
  protective isolation for, 211-213
Neutrophils, 11, 28-29
New therapies, 521-522
Nixon, Richard, 460
Nonbacterial thrombotic endocarditis
    (NBTE), 343
Non-Hodgkin's lymphoma, 9, 18
Nonmalignant diseases, treated with marrow
    or blood stem cell transplantation,
    70-71

Nonviral vectors, in gene therapy, 165-166
Norfloxacin, 13, 127
Nurse coordinators, 74
Nurse practitioner (NP), 74
Nurse scientists, research conducted by,
    500
Nurses' station, in alternative care models,
    534
Nursing
  diagnosis, planning, and intervention, and
    pulmonary complications, 284-286
  implications of gene therapy for, 171-172
  transplant patient with cardiac complica-
    tions, 293-294
Nursing assessment of renal function, 304
  blood chemistries, 305-306
  fluid balance, 307-308
  mental status, 308-309
  pharmacological considerations, 308
  urine assessment, 306-308
Nursing care, 17-18
  of neurological effects, 346-348
Nursing networks
  in Europe and Canada, 476-477
  in United States, 474-476
Nursing research, BCMT, 497, 503
  collaborations and role of nursing specialty
    organizations, 503
  conducted by clinical nurses, 499-500
  conducted by nurse scientists, 500
  conducted by undergraduate and graduate
    students, 500
  consultation, expert, 500
  foundations for, 497-499
  future directions for, 501-503
  multi-institutional, 501
  role of oncology, 501-503
Nursing roles, in alternative care models,
    542-544
Nursing service, in alternative care models,
    536
  changing practice environments, 536-537
  critical pathways, 537-542

education of patients and families, 537
new nursing roles, 542-544
recruitment and retention, 544-545
Nursing specialty organizations, research
    collaborations and role of, 503
Nursing standards
    in community, 484-486
    in transplantation, 482-484
Nursing team, importance of, 74-75
Nutrition for BMT/BCT patient, 15-16, 245
    experimental nutritional therapies,
        257-259
    low-microbial diets, 248-253
    metabolic and nutritional alterations,
        246-248
    nutritional assessment, 248
    parenteral and enteral nutrition, 253-257
Nystatin, oral, 128

O
Occult pulmonary hemorrhage, 283
Ohio Bone Marrow Transplantation
    Consortium (OBMTC), 482
Oligonucleotide probes, 79
Oncology Nursing Foundation, 499-500,
    501
    Fatigue Initiative through Research and
        Education (FIRE Project), 503
Oncology Nursing Society (ONS), 424,
    474-475, 481, 499, 503, 536
    advanced practice nurse defined by, 543
    Bone Marrow Transplant SIG of, 17, 475,
        483, 484
    Clinical Practice Committee of, 483, 484
    Congress and Fall Institute of, 475
    directory of, 484
    manual of, 483-484
    Research Department of, 501
    Research Mentorship Programs of, 500
    symposia offered by, 545
Ondansetron, 106, 339
Oophoropexy, 395
Open lung biopsy (OLB), 271-272

Opioids, 339
Opportunistic microorganisms, 269
Opsonization, 35
Oral Assessment Guide, 237
Oral intake, reintroduction of, 252-253
Orgasm, 381
Orgasmic disorder, 385
Osmotic diarrhea, 236
Outpatient setting, BMT in, 16, 515
    See also Alternative care models
Ovum donation, 395

P
Pain effects during BMT, 361-362, 364
Parainfluenza viruses, 90, 276
Parasitic infections, 208
Parasitic penumonia, 277-279
Parenteral nutrition, see Total parenteral
    nutrition
Parotitis
    bilateral, 229
    from total body irradiation, 157, 229-230
Paroxetine, 368
Path Guidelines, 470
Patient-controlled analgesia (PCA), 361-362
Patient education
    in alternative care models, 537
    materials, 486
    related to hematopoiesis, 39-40
    for total body irradiation, 159-160
    in transplant process, 79
    See also Education
Patient eligibility, 71
    disease status, 71-72
    donor availability, 72
Patient evaluation, for transplant process,
    75-78
Patient selection, 506-507
Patient Self-Determination Act (1990), 516
Pediatric consent, 513
PEG-rHuMGDA, 143
Penicillin, 87, 127
Pentamidine, 278

Pentoxifylline, to prevent VOD, 318

Percutaneous endoscopic gastrostomy (PEG) tube, 254

Pericarditis, 290-291

Peripheral blood stem cell transplant (PBST), 38

See also Blood cell transplantation

Peripheral nerve complications, 345

Perirectal abscess, 242-243

Perirectal lesions, 236-237

Perirectal Skin Assessment Tool (PSAT), 242

Per member per month (PMPM) rate, 463

Pharmaceuticals, supportive, and emetic response, 223-224

Pharmacologic and biologic agents, 100
  antibacterials, 125-127
  antifungals, 127-129
  antivirals, 129-135
  chemotherapy, 100-115
  immunosuppressive agents, 115-125
  miscellaneous, 135-144

Pharmacological considerations, in renal function, 308

Pharmacological treatments, for GVHD, 199

Pharmacotherapy, to improve sexual response, 394

Pharmacy, in alternative care models, 547

Phases of transplantation, clinical issues during, in alternative care models, 550
  engraftment/recovery, 555-556
  evaluation, 550-552
  harvest/apheresis and cryopreservation, 552-554
  long-term recovery, 556-557
  preparative therapy, 554-555
  reinfusion/transplant, 555

Phenothiazenes, 106, 340

Phenotype, 51

Phenytoin, 105, 106

Phosphonoformic acid, *see* Foscarnet

Phosphoramide mustard, 102

Physical design, of alternative care models
  apheresis unit, 534
  clinic examination rooms, 533-534
  clinical area, 533
  day surgery, 534-535
  education area, 533
  emergency and after-hours care, 535
  home care, 535-536
  housing, 532
  infusion areas, 534
  location, 532-533
  nurses' station, 534
  waiting areas, 533

Physical symptoms, psychological factors and occurrence of, 361-363

Physical well-being, City of Hope QOL Conceptual Model on, 410-412

Physician staff, of alternative care models, 546

PIXY 321, 81, 142, 144

Plasma, fresh frozen, and blood product support, 214

Platelets from random/single donor(s), and blood product support, 214

Pleiotropic, 32

PLISSIT model, 389
  intensive treatment (IT), 391
  limited information (LI), 389
  permission (P), 389
  specific suggestions (SS), 389-391

PMNs, *see* Neutrophils

Pneumococcus, 208

Pneumocystis, 272

Pneumocystis carinii (PCP), 88, 90, 208, 245, 269
  and parasitic pneumonia, 277-279
  and protozoal infections, 330

Pneumonia, 14, 273
  bacterial, 273-274
  bronchiolitis obliterans organizing, 282-283
  diagnosis of pulmonary interstitial pneumonitis and, 269
  fungal, 276-277

parastic, 277-279
viral, 274-276
Pneumonitis, 14, 89-90, 274-275
Pneumothorax, 89
Polymerase chain reaction (PCR), 59, 272
Polys, *see* Neutrophils
Positive end-expiratory pressure (PEEP), 285-286
Postprogenitors, *see* Precursors
Postrenal failure, 301
Practice environments, changing, in alternative care models, 536-537
Practice guidelines, 470
Precursors, 27-28
Prednisone, 17, 123, 124
neurological effects of, 336-337
Pregnancy, blood cell and marrow transplantation and, 379-381
Preparative therapy, 554-555
Prerenal failure, 301-302
hypovolemia, 302
impaired circulation of blood volume, 302
renal vascular constriction, 302
syndrome of inappropriate anti-diuretic hormone, 302
Pretreatment phase, psychosocial concerns during, 355
depression and anxiety, 357-358
informed decision making about BMT, 355-357
neuropsychological effects of previous treatment, 359-361
preexisting psychiatric conditions, 358-359
Primary care physicians (PCPs), 462
Primary myelofibrosis, 438
Primers, 59
Private antigens, 44-45
Procarbazine, 281
Prochlorperazine, 339
Prodigy, 486
Products, threat of substitute, 468-469

Progenitor cells, 27
Progressive muscle relaxation, 365
Proliferation, 25
Prospective reimbursement systems, 462
Prostaglandin E_1, to prevent VOD, 318
Protective isolation, 211-213
simple, 212
strict, 212
Protein, and metabolic and nutritional alterations, 246-247
Protozoal infections, 330-331
Pseudomonas, 13, 87, 89, 274, 289
aeruginosa, 127, 236
Psychiatric conditions, preexisting, during pretreatment phase, 358-359
Psychological factors, and occurrence of physical symptoms, 361-363
Psychological interventions, 364
behavioral interventions, 365-366
psychological support, 364-365
psychopharmacological support, 366-368
support groups, 366
Psychological support, 364-365
Psychological well-being, City of Hope QOL Conceptual Model on, 412
Psychoneurologic factors, and emetic response, 225
Psychopharmacological support, 366-368
dependence and addiction, 368
Psychosocial effects (concerns), 355, 370
during acute treatment, 361-364
during pretreatment phase, 355-361
See also Psychological interventions
Psychosocial factors, relationships among survival outcomes and, 363-364
Psychosocial status, measurement of, 368-369
Puberty, and total body irradiation, 159
Public antigens, 44-45
Pulmonary edema, 89, 272-273, 288, 293
Pulmonary effects, 266
adult respiratory distress syndrome, 285-286
bacterial pneumonia, 273-274

Pulmonary effects (*continued*)
  bronchiolitis obliterans organizing
    pneumonia (BOOP), 282-283
  bronchoalveolar lavage and transbronchial
    biopsy, 271
  conventional sputum examination, 270-271
  diagnosis of pulmonary interstitial
    pneumonitis and pneumonia, 269
  diffuse alveolar and pulmonary
    hemorrhage, 283
  drug-induced, 279-281
  fungal pneumonia, 276-277
  graft-versus-host disease, 282
  immunosuppression, 268
  lung damage, 268-269
  malignant infiltration, 283
  miscellaneous, 283-284
  nursing diagnosis, planning, and
    intervention, 284-286
  open lung biopsy (OLB), 271-272
  opportunistic microorganisms, 269
  parasitic pneumonia, 277-279
  pathogenesis, 267
  pulmonary edema, 272-273
  pulmonary infections associated with BMT,
    273
  pulmonary toxicity, 89-90
  radiation-induced, 281-282
  radiological studies, 269-270
  viral pneumonia, 274-276
Pulmonary interstitial pneumonitis (IPn), 267
  and pneumonia, diagnosis of, 269
Purging, *see* Marrow purging techniques/
    positive selection
Pyrimethamine, 278-279

Q
Quality of life (QOL), 400, 425
  in alternative settings, 557
  caregiver burden and, 415-416
  Conceptual Model, City of Hope, 410-414
  cultural considerations, 414
  defining, 401-402
  fatigue and, 416-417
  finances and, 416
  future research on, 424-425
  informed consent and, 508-509
  interventions to improve, 417-419
  as outcome measure, 414-415
  rehabilitation and, 419-424
  research, 403-410
  research, importance of, 400-401
  tools to measure, 402-403

R
Racial distribution, of HLA types, 52-53
Radiation-induced cardiac damage, 289
Radiation-induced pulmonary damage,
    281-282
Radiation nephritis, 303-304
Radiation therapy, 85, 87, 151
  fractionated, 84, 153, 155
  See also Total body irradiation
Radiological studies, 269-270
Recombinant DNA Advisory Committee
    (RAC), 170
Recombinant tPA (r-tPA), 318
Recovery, long-term, 556-557
  See also Engraftment and recovery
Recruitment and retention, in alternative care
    models, 544-545
Red blood cells (RBCs), 27, 88
  and blood product support, 214
Reflex sympathetic dystrophy (RSD), 345
Regional Cooperative Oncology Groups, 481
Registries, bone marrow transplant, 71
  unrelated, 60-61
Rehabilitation, and quality of life, 419-424
Reimbursement, 461
  capitation, 463
  fee for service, 461-462
  managed care, 462-463
  systems, prospective, 462
Reinfusion/transplant, 555
Rejection, 50-51
Relaxation training, 365-366
Renal dysfunction, and total body irradiation,
    158

Renal failure, 298
  high output, 303
  impact of, in transplant, 298-299
Renal function
  basic, 299
  determinants of, 300
  nursing assessment of, 304-309
Renal hemodynamics, altering, in VOD, 319
Renal impairment, 88
Renal insufficiency, 298, 304
  impact of, in transplant, 298-299
  management of, 309
  VOD and, 315-318
Renal physiology, 299-300
Renal toxicity, 88
Renal tubular acidosis (RTA), 305
Renal vascular constriction, 302
Research, *see* Nursing research
Resiliency Model of Family Stress, Adjustment, and Adaptation, 447, 448
Resolution phase, 381
Resources, allocation of, 520-521
Respiratory syncytial virus (RSV), 90, 276
Restriction-fragment length polymorphism (RFLP), 59
Reticulocyte maturation index (RMI), 209
Retroviruses, 164
Reverse isolation, 86
  with special air handling systems, 86
Rifampin, 127

S
Saccaromyces cerevisiae, 138
Safe Drinking Water Act (1974), 251
Safety and ethics, of gene therapy, 170-171
Salivary gland response, 229-230
Salmonella, 249, 250
Sargramostim
  dosing, administration, and monitoring, 139-140
  pharmacology, 138
  therapeutic use, 138-139
  toxicities, 139

Seattle Marrow Transplant Nursing Consortium (SMTNC), 475-476
Second-generation antidepressants, 340
Secretory syndrome (secretory-type diarrhea), 235-236
Segs, *see* Neutrophils
Selection of patients, 506-507
Selective cellular depletion, and GVHD, 199
Selective serotonin reuptake inhibitors (SSRIs), 368
Self-care, 94
Sequence-specific oligonucleotide probe (PCR-SSOP), 59
Sequence-specific primer (PCR-SSP), 59
Serologic HLA typing, 56-58
Serratia, 89
Sertraline, 368
Serum glutamic oxaloacetic transaminase (SGOT), 183
Severe combined immunodeficiency (SCID), 521
Sexual arousal disorder, 385
Sexual counseling and medical treatments, combining, 393-394
  hormone replacement therapy, 394
  other fertility options, 395
  pharmacotherapy, 394
  sperm banking, 394-395
Sexual disorders
  clinical vignettes of, 391-393
  premature menopause and sexual function, 386
  specific, associated with BMT/BCT, 381-386
Sexual function(ing), 377
  assessment of, 386-389
  cancer treatment and gonadal function, 377-381
  interventions to improve, 389-395
  premature menopause and, 386
  recommendations for future research in, 395-396
Sexual pain disorders, 385-386

Sicca syndrome, and chronic GVHD, 188
Sickle cell anemia, gene therapy for, 162,
    169-170
Sickle cell disease (SCD), 521
Sigma Theta Tau International, 499
Silent mutation (silent substitution), 49
Simple protective isolation, 212
Skin conductance level (SCL) biofeedback,
    366
Skin reactions
    to acute GVHD, 182
    to chronic GVHD, 184-188
    to total body irradiation, 157
Social well-being, City of Hope QOL
    Conceptual Model on, 412-413
Society for Critical Care Medicine, 517
Sodium
    imbalance, treating, in VOD, 319
    urine, 307
Somatic cell gene transfer, 163
Soruvidine (BV-ara-U), 135
Southwest Marrow/Stem Cell Transplant
    Nursing Consortium, 476
Southwest Oncology Group (SWOG), 501,
    531
Spanish Bone Marrow Donor Registry
    (REDMO), 61
Special interest groups (SIGs), 17, 475
Sperm banking, 394-395
Spielberger State-Trait Anger Expression
    Inventory, 357
Spielberger State-Trait Anxiety Inventory,
    357
Spiritual well-being, City of Hope QOL
    Conceptual Model on, 413-414
Spleen, 27
Splits, 44
Sputum examination, conventional, 270-271
STAMP V regimen, 109, 110
Standards of care, 474, 482, 494
    medical standards in transplantation,
        486-494
    nursing standards in community, 484-486

nursing standards in transplantation,
    482-484
patient education materials, 486
Staphylococcus, 87
    aureus, 250, 274, 289, 290
    epidermidis, 180, 206
    lactobacillus, 180
    toxoplasmosis, 289
Steel factor, *see* Stem cell factor
Stem cell(s), 27
    blood, 68-69
    cord blood, 69
    ex vivo expansion of, 84
    infusion, 87
    See also Cells, identification of, for
        transplantation; Cells, source of, for
        transplantation
Stem cell factor (SCF), 33, 142
Steroids, 17
    for GVHD, 92
Stomatitis, 230-232
    treatment of, 237-240
Strategic plan, 528-531
Streptococcus, 87, 127, 289
    pneumoniae, 208, 274, 328
    viridans, 127, 289
Streptomyces tsukubaensis, 121, 195
Stress
    family response to, 447
    potential, of BMT for family members,
        449-454
Strict protective isolation, 212
Students, research conducted by
    undergraduate and graduate, 500
Suppliers, bargaining power of, 469-470
Support groups, 366, 418
Supportive care
    acute graft-versus-host disease, 91-92
    anemia and thrombocytopenia, 88
    bladder toxicity, 89
    cardiac toxicity, 92-93
    developments in, 10-16
    gastrointestinal complications, 91

hepatic toxicity, 88
infections, 87-88
neurological complications, 90
pulmonary toxicity, 89-90
renal toxicity, 88
Survival outcomes, relationships among
    psychosocial factors and, 363-364
Survivorship guilt, 413-414
Swedish Medical Center, 475
Swiss Bone Marrow Donor Registry, 61
Switzerland, 476, 482
Sympathomimetic stimulants, 340
Syndrome of inappropriate anti-diuretic
    hormone (SIADH), 104, 105, 302
Syngeneic marrow transplants, 51, 68

T
Tacrolimus
    dosing, administration, and monitoring,
        122
    pharmacology, 121
    therapeutic use, 121
    toxicities, 121-122
T-cell receptor, 50
Team, importance of nursing, 74-75
Temperature biofeedback, 366
TEPA, 108
Thalassemia, 292
    gene therapy for, 162, 165, 169-170
Thalidomide, 17
    neurological effects of, 338
Thiotepa, 9
    dosing, administration, and monitoring,
        109
    pharmacology, 108-109
    therapeutic use, 109
    toxicities, 109
Third-party payers, 460, 461, 465
Thrombocytopenia, 88, 89, 209
Thromboembolism, pulmonary, 284
Thrombopoietin, 15, 33, 140
    See also MGDF
Thyroid, and total body irradiation, 158

Tissue typing, see Human leukocyte antigen
    (HLA) typing
Tolypocladium inflatum Gams, 115
Total abdominal irradiation (TAI), 84
Total body irradiation (TBI), 84, 101, 151,
    160
    acute side effects of, 155-157
    cardiac damage from, 289
    cyclophosphamide and (CyTBI), 8-9, 101
    delayed effects of, 157-159
    neurological effects of, 327-328
    outpatient, 555
    patient education and emotional support
        for, 159-160
    pulmonary damage from, 281-282
    rationale for, 151
    technique of, 152-154
    treatment with, 152
Total lymphoid irradiation (TLI), 9, 84, 289
Total parenteral nutrition (TPN), 15, 16, 253,
    254
    administration, 255-257
    enteral nutrition versus, 255, 258-259
    home, 257
    prophylactic, 254-255
Total protective environment, 212
Toxoplasma gondii, 277, 278-279, 330
Transbronchial biopsy (TBB), 271
Transient hypoxia, 89
Transplantation, marrow and blood cell,
    66-67
    allogeneic, 67-68
    autologous, 67
    blood stem cells, 68-69
    clinical indications for, 69-71
    cord blood stem cells, 69
    defined, 67
    engraftment and recovery, 93-96
    identification of cells from, 35-37
    impact of, on hematopoiesis, 35
    patient eligibility for, 71-72
    role of HLA in matching for, 59-60
    selecting center for, 72-75

Transplantation, marrow and blood cell
(*continued*)
  source of cells for, 37-39
  syngeneic, 68
  See also Supportive care; Transplant
    process
Transplant coordinator, 542
Transplant networks, 474, 494
  history of, 474-482
  international medical networks, 481-482
  international nursing networks, 474-477
Transplant process
  donor preparation, 80
  donor search, 79
  financial issues, 78
  harvest procedures, 80-84
  patient education, 79
  patient evaluation, 75-78
  preconditioning chemotherapy, 84
  preparative regimens, 84-87
  stem cell infusion, 87
  tissue typing, 79-80
  See also Transplantation
Transplant setting, clinical trials of gene
    therapy in, 167-170
Treatment, previous, neuropsychological
    effects of, 359-361
Triage nurse, 542
Tricyclics, 340, 367-368
Trimethoprim-sulfamethoxazole (TMP-SMZ),
    274, 278

U
Ulceration, and GI bleeding, 234, 241
Ultraviolet phototherapy, and GVHD,
    199
Umbilical cord blood
  donor issues, 63-64
  ethical issues, 522
  human, collection of, 83
  as source of cells for transplantation,
    39
  stem cells, 69

Urine assessment, in renal function,
    306-308
Ursodiol, ursodeoxycholic acid, to prevent
    VOD, 318

V
Vagina, and chronic GVHD, 188-190
Vaginismus, 385
Valacyclovir, 135
Vancomycin, 13, 87, 127
Varicella-zoster virus (VZV), 87, 129, 130,
    131, 135, 207, 329
  and viral pneumonia, 275-276
Vascular complications, neurological effects
    and, 342-343
Vascular volume disequilibrium, correcting, in
    renal insufficiency, 309
Vectors, in gene therapy, 164
  nonviral, 165-166
  viral, 164-165
Vegetations, 290
Veno-occlusive disease (VOD), 88, 105-106,
    120, 245, 284, 311
  clinical complications of, 314
  clinical diagnosis of, 314-315
  common additional clinical findings,
    315-318
  consequences of impaired hepatic blood
    flow and function, 313-314
  etiology of, 311-312
  hepatic venule occlusion, 312-313
  incidence and risk factors of, 311
  managing complications of, 318-320
  normal hepatic physiology of, 312
  onset and resolution of, 312
  pathophysiology of, 312
  prevention of, 318
  and total body irradiation, 158
  treatment of, 318
Veteran Affairs, Department of, Medical
    Center, 475
Viral infections, 87, 207-208, 291, 329-330
Viral pneumonia, 274-276

Viral vectors, in gene therapy, 164-165
Virginia Mason Medical Center, 475
Visual analogue scales (VAS), 369
Vomiting, from total body irradiation, 155-157
    See also Emetic response(s)

W
Waiting areas, in alternative care models, 533
Washington, University of, Medical Center, 475
Water, checking, for bacteria, 251-252
Well-being, *see* Physical well-being;
    Psychological well-being; Social
    well-being; Spiritual well-being

White blood count (WBC), 81
Wisconsin, Medical College of, 481
Women, gonadal failure in, 379
World Donor Association, 531
World Health Organization (WHO), HLA
    Nomenclature Committee of, 43, 44, 56
World War II, 459
World Wide Web, 501

XYZ
Xerostomia, partial, 229, 230
Zidovudine (AZT), 134